D0026362

# HCPCS Level II

## Professional Edition

# 2020

**AHIMA**
American Health Information
Management Association®

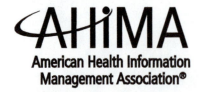

**American Health Information**
**Management Association®**

2020 HCPCS LEVEL II, PROFESSIONAL EDITION

ISBN: 978-1-58426-751-5
Product Code: AC228019

**Copyright © 2020 by Elsevier Inc. All rights reserved.**

No part of this publication may be reproduced or transmitted in any form or by any means, electronic or mechanical, including photocopying, recording, or any information storage and retrieval system, without permission in writing from the publisher. Details on how to seek permission, further information about the Publisher's permissions policies and our arrangements with organizations such as the Copyright Clearance Center and the Copyright Licensing Agency, can be found at our website: www.elsevier.com/permissions.

This book and the individual contributions contained in it are protected under copyright by the Publisher (other than as may be noted herein).

---

**Notice**

Practitioners and researchers must always rely on their own experience and knowledge in evaluating and using any information, methods, compounds or experiments described herein. Because of rapid advances in the medical sciences, in particular, independent verification of diagnoses and drug dosages should be made. To the fullest extent of the law, no responsibility is assumed by Elsevier, authors, editors or contributors for any injury and/or damage to persons or property as a matter of products liability, negligence or otherwise, or from any use or operation of any methods, products, instructions, or ideas contained in the material herein.

---

Previous editions copyrighted 2019, 2018, 2017, 2016, 2015, 2014, 2013, 2012, 2011, 2010, 2009, 2008, 2007, 2006, 2005, 2004, 2003, 2002, 2001, 2000

**International Standard Book Number: 978-1-58426-751-5**

Cover image: draganab/iStockphoto

Printed in the United States of America

Last digit is the print number:   9   8   7   6   5   4   3   2

# DEVELOPMENT OF THIS EDITION

## Lead Technical Collaborator

**Jackie L. Koesterman, CPC**
Coder III/Reimbursement Specialist
Grand Forks, North Dakota

# CONTENTS

Check the Centers for Medicare & Medicaid Services (www.cms.gov/Manuals/IOM/list.asp) website for full IOMs.

# INTRODUCTION

The Centers for Medicare & Medicaid Services (CMS) (formerly Health Care Financing Administration [HCFA]) Healthcare Common Procedure Coding System (HCPCS) is a collection of codes and descriptors that represent procedures, supplies, products, and services that may be provided to Medicare beneficiaries and to individuals enrolled in private health insurance programs. The codes are divided as follows:

**Level I:** Codes and descriptors copyrighted by the American Medical Association's (AMA's) Current Procedural Terminology, ed. 4 (CPT-4). These are five-digit numeric codes representing physician and nonphysician services.

**Level II:** Includes codes and descriptors copyrighted by the American Dental Association's current dental terminology, seventh edition (CDT-7/8). These are five-digit alpha-numeric codes comprising the D series. All other Level II codes and descriptors are alphanumeric and approved and maintained jointly by the editorial panel (consisting of CMS, the Health Insurance Association of America, and the Blue Cross Blue Shield Association). These are five-digit alphanumeric codes representing primarily items and nonphysician services that are not represented in the Level I codes.

**Level III:** The CMS eliminated Level III local codes. See Program Memorandum AB-02-113.

Headings are provided as a means of grouping similar or closely related items. The placement of a code under a heading does not indicate additional means of classification, nor does it relate to any health insurance coverage categories.

HCPCS also contains modifiers, which are two-digit codes and descriptors used to indicate that a service or procedure that has been performed has been altered by some specific circumstance but unchanged in its definition or code. Modifiers are grouped by the levels. Level I modifiers and descriptors are copyrighted by the AMA. Level II modifiers are HCPCS modifiers. Modifiers in the D series are copyrighted by the ADA.

HCPCS is designed to promote uniform reporting and statistical data collection of medical procedures, supplies, products, and services.

## HCPCS Disclaimer

Inclusion or exclusion of a procedure, supply, product, or service does not imply any health insurance coverage or reimbursement policy.

HCPCS makes as much use as possible of generic descriptions, but the inclusion of brand names to describe devices or drugs is intended only for indexing purposes; it is not meant to convey endorsement of any particular product or drug.

## Updating HCPCS

The primary updates are made annually. Quarterly updates are also issued by CMS.

Medical coding has long been a part of the health care profession. Through the years medical coding systems have become more complex and extensive. Today, medical coding is an intricate and immense process that is present in every health care setting. The increased use of electronic submissions for health care services only increases the need for coders who understand the coding process.

*2020 HCPCS Level II* was developed to help meet the needs of today's coder.

All material adheres to the latest government versions available at the time of printing.

## Annotated

Throughout this text, revisions and additions are indicated by the following symbols:

- ▶ **New:** Additions to the previous edition are indicated by the color triangle.

- ↝ **Revised:** Revisions within the line or code from the previous edition are indicated by the color arrow.

- ✔ **Reinstated** indicates a code that was previously deleted and has now been reactivated.

- ✖ ~~Deleted~~ words have been removed from this year's edition.

## HCPCS Symbols

- ✪ **Special coverage instructions** apply to these codes. Usually these special coverage instructions are included in the Internet Only Manuals (IOM). References to the IOM locations are given in the form of Medicare Pub. 100 reference numbers listed below the code.

- ⊘ **Not covered or valid by Medicare** is indicated by the "No" symbol. Usually the reason for the exclusion is included in the Internet Only Manuals (IOM).

- ✳ **Carrier discretion** is an indication that you must contact the individual third-party payers to find out the coverage available for codes identified by this symbol.

- *Other* Drugs approved for Medicare Part B and other FDA-approved drugs are listed as Other.

- A2-Z3 **ASC Payment Indicators** identify the 2019 final payment for the code. A list of Payment Indicators is listed in the front matter of this text.

- A-Y **OPPS Status Indicators** identify the 2019 final status assigned to the code. A list of Status Indicators is listed in the front matter of this text.

- Ⓑ Bill Part B MAC.

- Ⓑ Bill DME MAC.

- *Coding Clinic* Indicates the American Hospital Association *Coding Clinic®* for HCPCS references by year, quarter, and page number.

- ♿ DMEPOS identifies durable medical equipment, prosthetics, orthotics, and supplies that may be eligible for payment from CMS.

- ♀ Indicates a code for female only.

- ♂ Indicates a code for male only.

- Ⓐ Indicates a code with an indication of age.

- 🖐 Indicates a code included in the MIPS Quality Measure Specifications.

- Qp Indicates there is a maximum allowable number of units of service, per day, per patient for physician/provider services.

- Qh Indicates there is a maximum allowable number of units of service, per day, per patient in the outpatient hospital setting.

Red, green, and blue typeface terms within the Table of Drugs and tabular section are terms added by the publisher and do not appear in the official code set. Information supplementing the official HCPCS Index produced by CMS is *italicized*.

# SYMBOLS AND CONVENTIONS

## HCPCS Symbols

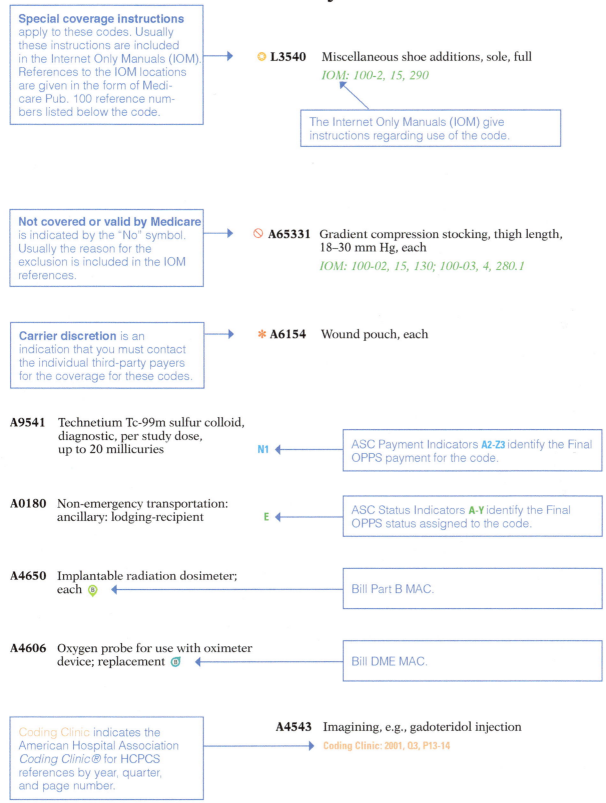

**Special coverage instructions** apply to these codes. Usually these instructions are included in the Internet Only Manuals (IOM). References to the IOM locations are given in the form of Medicare Pub. 100 reference numbers listed below the code.

⊗ **L3540**   Miscellaneous shoe additions, sole, full
*IOM: 100-2, 15, 290*

The Internet Only Manuals (IOM) give instructions regarding use of the code.

**Not covered or valid by Medicare** is indicated by the "No" symbol. Usually the reason for the exclusion is included in the IOM references.

⊘ **A65331**   Gradient compression stocking, thigh length, 18–30 mm Hg, each
*IOM: 100-02, 15, 130; 100-03, 4, 280.1*

**Carrier discretion** is an indication that you must contact the individual third-party payers for the coverage for these codes.

✳ **A6154**   Wound pouch, each

**A9541**   Technetium Tc-99m sulfur colloid, diagnostic, per study dose, up to 20 millicuries

N1

ASC Payment Indicators **A2-Z3** identify the Final OPPS payment for the code.

**A0180**   Non-emergency transportation: ancillary: lodging-recipient

E

ASC Status Indicators **A-Y** identify the Final OPPS status assigned to the code.

**A4650**   Implantable radiation dosimeter; each ⑧

Bill Part B MAC.

**A4606**   Oxygen probe for use with oximeter device; replacement ⑧

Bill DME MAC.

Coding Clinic indicates the American Hospital Association *Coding Clinic®* for HCPCS references by year, quarter, and page number.

**A4543**   Imagining, e.g., gadoteridol injection
**Coding Clinic: 2001, Q3, P13-14**

Codes shown are for illustration purposes only and may not be current codes.

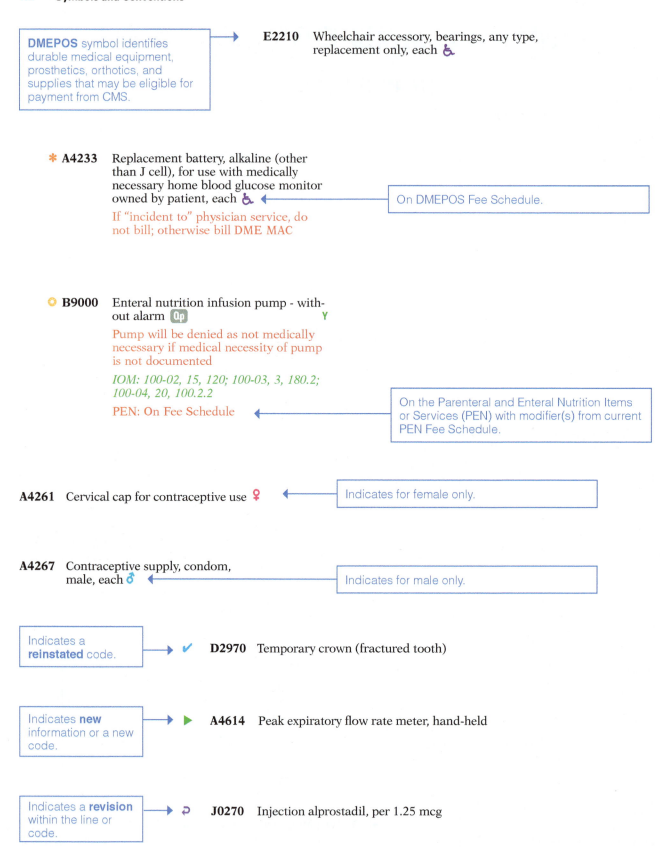

DMEPOS symbol identifies durable medical equipment, prosthetics, orthotics, and supplies that may be eligible for payment from CMS.

E2210    Wheelchair accessory, bearings, any type, replacement only, each ♿

✱ A4233    Replacement battery, alkaline (other than J cell), for use with medically necessary home blood glucose monitor owned by patient, each ♿

If "incident to" physician service, do not bill; otherwise bill DME MAC

On DMEPOS Fee Schedule.

⚙ B9000    Enteral nutrition infusion pump - without alarm Qp    γ

Pump will be denied as not medically necessary if medical necessity of pump is not documented

IOM: 100-02, 15, 120; 100-03, 3, 180.2; 100-04, 20, 100.2.2

PEN: On Fee Schedule

On the Parenteral and Enteral Nutrition Items or Services (PEN) with modifier(s) from current PEN Fee Schedule.

A4261    Cervical cap for contraceptive use ♀

Indicates for female only.

A4267    Contraceptive supply, condom, male, each ♂

Indicates for male only.

Indicates a **reinstated** code.

✔ D2970    Temporary crown (fractured tooth)

Indicates **new** information or a new code.

▶ A4614    Peak expiratory flow rate meter, hand-held

Indicates a **revision** within the line or code.

↻ J0270    Injection alprostadil, per 1.25 mcg

Codes shown are for illustration purposes only and may not be current codes.

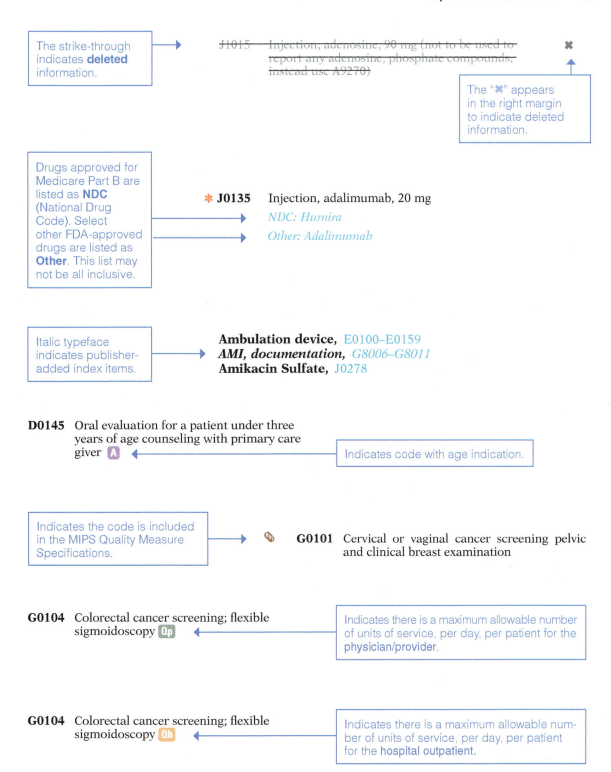

The strike-through indicates **deleted** information.

J1015   Injection, adenosine, 90 mg (not to be used to report any adenosine, phosphate compounds, instead use A9270)

The "✖" appears in the right margin to indicate deleted information.

Drugs approved for Medicare Part B are listed as **NDC** (National Drug Code). Select other FDA-approved drugs are listed as **Other**. This list may not be all inclusive.

✳ **J0135**   Injection, adalimumab, 20 mg
  *NDC: Humira*
  *Other: Adalimumab*

Italic typeface indicates publisher-added index items.

**Ambulation device,** E0100–E0159
**AMI, documentation,** G8006–G8011
**Amikacin Sulfate,** J0278

**D0145**   Oral evaluation for a patient under three years of age counseling with primary care giver **A**

Indicates code with age indication.

Indicates the code is included in the MIPS Quality Measure Specifications.

**G0101**   Cervical or vaginal cancer screening pelvic and clinical breast examination

**G0104**   Colorectal cancer screening; flexible sigmoidoscopy **Qp**

Indicates there is a maximum allowable number of units of service, per day, per patient for the physician/provider.

**G0104**   Colorectal cancer screening; flexible sigmoidoscopy **Qh**

Indicates there is a maximum allowable number of units of service, per day, per patient for the hospital outpatient.

Codes shown are for illustration purposes only and may not be current codes.

## A2-Z3 ASC Payment Indicators

| Final ASC Payment Indicators for CY 2020 | |
|---|---|
| **Payment Indicator** | **Payment Indicator Definition** |
| A2 | Surgical procedure on ASC list in CY 2007; payment based on OPPS relative payment weight. |
| B5 | Alternative code may be available; no payment made. |
| D5 | Deleted/discontinued code; no payment made. |
| F4 | Corneal tissue acquisition, hepatitis B vaccine; paid at reasonable cost. |
| G2 | Non-office-based surgical procedure added in CY 2008 or later; payment based on OPPS relative payment weight. |
| H2 | Brachytherapy source paid separately when provided integral to a surgical procedure on ASC list; payment OPPS rate. |
| J7 | OPPS pass-through device paid separately when provided integral to a surgical procedure on ASC list; payment contractor-priced. |
| J8 | Device-intensive procedure; paid at adjusted rate. |
| K2 | Drugs and biologicals paid separately when provided integral to a surgical procedure on ASC list; payment based on OPPS rate. |
| K7 | Unclassified drugs and biologicals; payment contractor-priced. |
| L1 | Influenza vaccine; pneumococcal vaccine. Packaged item/service; no separate payment made. |
| L6 | New Technology Intraocular Lens (NTIOL); special payment. |
| N1 | Packaged service/item; no separate payment made. |
| P2 | Office-based surgical procedure added to ASC list in CY 2008 or later with MPFS nonfacility PE RVUs; payment based on OPPS relative payment weight. |
| P3 | Office-based surgical procedure added to ASC list in CY 2008 or later with MPFS nonfacility PE RVUs; payment based on MPFS nonfacility PE RVUs. |
| R2 | Office-based surgical procedure added to ASC list in CY 2008 or later without MPFS nonfacility PE RVUs; payment based on OPPS relative payment weight. |
| Z2 | Radiology or diagnostic service paid separately when provided integral to a surgical procedure on ASC list; payment based on OPPS relative payment weight. |
| Z3 | Radiology or diagnostic service paid separately when provided integral to a surgical procedure on ASC list; payment based on MPFS nonfacility PE RVUs. |

CMS-1678-FC, **Final Changes to the ASC Payment System and CY 2020 Payment Rates**, http://www.cms.gov/Medicare/Medicare-Fee-for-Service-Payment/ASCPayment/ASC-Regulations-and-Notices.html.

## A-Y OPPS Status Indicators

| | Final OPPS Payment Status Indicators for CY 2020 | |
|---|---|---|
| **Indicator** | **Item/Code/Service** | **OPPS Payment Status** |
| A | Services furnished to a hospital outpatient that are paid under a fee schedule or payment system other than OPPS,* for example: | Not paid under OPPS. Paid by MACs under a fee schedule or payment system other than OPPS. Services are subject to deductible or coinsurance unless indicated otherwise. |
| | • Ambulance Services | |
| | • Separately Payable Clinical Diagnostic Laboratory Services | Not subject to deductible or coinsurance. |
| | • Separately Payable Non-Implantable Prosthetics and Orthotics | |
| | • Physical, Occupational, and Speech Therapy | |
| | • Diagnostic Mammography | |
| | • Screening Mammography | Not subject to deductible or coinsurance. |
| B | Codes that are not recognized by OPPS when submitted on an outpatient hospital Part B bill type (12x and 13x) | Not paid under OPPS.<br><br>• May be paid by MACs when submitted on a different bill type, for example, 75x (CORF), but not paid under OPPS.<br>• An alternate code that is recognized by OPPS when submitted on an outpatient hospital Part B bill type (12x and 13x) may be available. |
| C | Inpatient Procedures | Not paid under OPPS. Admit patient. Bill as inpatient. |
| D | Discontinued Codes | Not paid under OPPS or any other Medicare payment system. |
| E1 | Items, Codes and Services:<br><br>• Not covered by any Medicare outpatient benefit category<br>• Statutorily excluded by Medicare<br>• Not reasonable and necessary | Not paid by Medicare when submitted on outpatient claims (any outpatient bill type). |
| E2 | Items, Codes and Services:<br>for which pricing information and claims data are not available | Not paid by Medicare when submitted on outpatient claims (any outpatient bill type). |
| F | Corneal Tissue Acquisition; Certain CRNA Services and Hepatitis B Vaccines | Not paid under OPPS. Paid at reasonable cost. |
| G | Pass-Through Drugs and Biologicals | Paid under OPPS; separate APC payment. |
| H | Pass-Through Device Categories | Separate cost-based pass-through payment; not subject to copayment. |
| J1 | Hospital Part B services paid through a comprehensive APC | Paid under OPPS; all covered Part B services on the claim are packaged with the primary "J1" service for the claim, except services with OPPS status indicator of "F," "G," "H," "L," and "U"; ambulance services; diagnostic and screening mammography; all preventive services; and certain Part B inpatient services. |
| J2 | Hospital Part B Services That May Be Paid Through a Comprehensive APC | Paid under OPPS; Addendum B displays APC assignments when services are separately payable.<br><br>(1) Comprehensive APC payment based on OPPS comprehensive-specific payment criteria. Payment for all covered Part B services on the claim is packaged into a single payment for specific combinations of services, except services with OPPS status indicator of "F," "G," "H," "L," and "U"; ambulance services; diagnostic and screening mammography; all preventive services; and certain Part B inpatient services.<br>(2) Packaged APC payment if billed on the same claim as a HCPCS code assigned status indicator "J1."<br>(3) In other circumstances, payment is made through a separate APC payment or packaged into payment for other services. |

## A-Y OPPS Status Indicators—cont'd

| Final OPPS Payment Status Indicators for CY 2020 | | |
|---|---|---|
| **Indicator** | **Item/Code/Service** | **OPPS Payment Status** |
| K | Non-Pass-Through Drugs and Non-Implantable Biologicals, including Therapeutic Radiopharmaceuticals | Paid under OPPS: separate APC payment. |
| L | Influenza Vaccine; Pneumococcal Pneumonia Vaccine | Not paid under OPPS. Paid at reasonable cost; not subject to deductible or coinsurance. |
| M | Items and Services Not Billable to the MAC | Not paid under OPPS. |
| N | Items and Services Packaged into APC Rates | Paid under OPPS; payment is packaged into payment for other services. Therefore, there is no separate APC payment. |
| P | Partial Hospitalization | Paid under OPPS; per diem APC payment. |
| Q1 | STV-Packaged Codes | Paid under OPPS; Addendum B displays APC assignments when services are separately payable.<br>(1) Packaged APC payment if billed on the same claim as a HCPCS code assigned status indicator "S," "T," or "V."<br>(2) Composite APC payment if billed with specific combinations of services based on OPPS composite-specific payment criteria. Payment is packaged into a single payment for specific combinations of services.<br>(3) In other circumstances, payment is made through a separate APC payment. |
| Q2 | T-Packaged Codes | Paid under OPPS; Addendum B displays APC assignments when services are separately payable.<br>(1) Packaged APC payment if billed on the same claim as a HCPCS code assigned status indicator "T."<br>(2) In other circumstances, payment is made through a separate APC payment. |
| Q3 | Codes That May Be Paid Through a Composite APC | Paid under OPPS; Addendum B displays APC assignments when services are separately payable. Addendum M displays composite APC assignments when codes are paid through a composite APC.<br>(1) Composite APC payment based on OPPS composite-specific payment criteria. Payment is packaged into a single payment for specific combinations of service.<br>(2) In other circumstances, payment is made through a separate APC payment or packaged into payment for other services. |
| Q4 | Conditionally packaged laboratory tests | Paid under OPPS or CLFS.<br>(1) Packaged APC payment if billed on the same claim as a HCPCS code assigned published status indicator "J1," "J2," "S," "T," "V," "Q1," "Q2," or "Q3."<br>(2) In other circumstances, laboratory tests should have an SI=A and payment is made under the CLFS. |
| R | Blood and Blood Products | Paid under OPPS; separate APC payment. |
| S | Procedure or Service, Not Discounted when Multiple | Paid under OPPS; separate APC payment. |
| T | Procedure or Service, Multiple Procedure Reduction Applies | Paid under OPPS; separate APC payment. |
| U | Brachytherapy Sources | Paid under OPPS; separate APC payment. |
| V | Clinic or Emergency Department Visit | Paid under OPPS; separate APC payment. |
| Y | Non-Implantable Durable Medical Equipment | Not paid under OPPS. All institutional providers other than home health agencies bill to a DME MAC. |

**\* Note — Payments "under a fee schedule or payment system other than OPPS" may be contractor priced.**

CMS-1678-FC, Final Changes to the ASC Payment System and CY 2020 Payment Rates, http://www.cms.gov/Medicare/Medicare-Fee-for-Service-Payment/HospitalOutpatientPPS/Hospital-Outpatient-Regulations-and-Notices.html.

# 2020 HCPCS New/Revised/Deleted Codes and Modifiers

HCPCS quarterly updates are posted on the companion website (www.codingupdates.com) when available.

## NEW CODES/MODIFIERS

| | | | | | |
|---|---|---|---|---|---|
| MA | G2062 | G2106 | G2149 | J9036 | M1131 |
| MB | G2063 | G2107 | G2150 | J9118 | M1132 |
| MC | G2064 | G2108 | G2151 | J9119 | M1133 |
| MD | G2065 | G2109 | G2152 | J9199 | M1134 |
| ME | G2066 | G2110 | G2153 | J9204 | M1135 |
| MF | G2067 | G2112 | G2154 | J9210 | M1136 |
| MG | G2068 | G2113 | G2155 | J9269 | M1137 |
| MH | G2069 | G2114 | G2156 | J9309 | M1138 |
| A4226 | G2070 | G2115 | G2157 | J9313 | M1139 |
| A9590 | G2071 | G2116 | G2158 | J9356 | M1140 |
| B4187 | G2072 | G2117 | G2159 | K1001 | M1141 |
| C1734 | G2073 | G2118 | G2160 | K1002 | M1142 |
| C1824 | G2074 | G2119 | G2161 | K1003 | M1143 |
| C1839 | G2075 | G2120 | G2162 | K1004 | M1144 |
| C1982 | G2076 | G2121 | G2163 | K1005 | P9099 |
| C2596 | G2077 | G2122 | G2164 | L2006 | Q4205 |
| C9041 | G2078 | G2123 | G2165 | L8033 | Q4206 |
| C9046 | G2079 | G2124 | G2166 | M1106 | Q4208 |
| C9047 | G2080 | G2125 | G2167 | M1107 | Q4209 |
| C9054 | G2081 | G2126 | J0121 | M1108 | Q4210 |
| C9055 | G2082 | G2127 | J0122 | M1109 | Q4211 |
| C9756 | G2083 | G2128 | J0179 | M1110 | Q4212 |
| C9757 | G2086 | G2129 | J0222 | M1111 | Q4213 |
| C9758 | G2087 | G2130 | J0291 | M1112 | Q4214 |
| E0787 | G2088 | G2131 | J0593 | M1113 | Q4215 |
| E2398 | G2089 | G2132 | J0642 | M1114 | Q4216 |
| G1000 | G2090 | G2133 | J1096 | M1115 | Q4217 |
| G1001 | G2091 | G2134 | J1097 | M1116 | Q4218 |
| G1002 | G2092 | G2135 | J1303 | M1117 | Q4219 |
| G1003 | G2093 | G2136 | J1444 | M1118 | Q4220 |
| G1004 | G2094 | G2137 | J1943 | M1119 | Q4221 |
| G1005 | G2095 | G2138 | J1944 | M1120 | Q4222 |
| G1006 | G2096 | G2139 | J2798 | M1121 | Q4226 |
| G1007 | G2097 | G2140 | J3031 | M1122 | Q5112 |
| G1008 | G2098 | G2141 | J3111 | M1123 | Q5113 |
| G1009 | G2099 | G2142 | J7208 | M1124 | Q5114 |
| G1010 | G2100 | G2143 | J7314 | M1125 | Q5115 |
| G1011 | G2101 | G2144 | J7331 | M1126 | Q5116 |
| G2021 | G2102 | G2145 | J7332 | M1127 | Q5117 |
| G2022 | G2103 | G2146 | J7401 | M1128 | Q5118 |
| G2058 | G2104 | G2147 | J7677 | M1129 | |
| G2061 | G2105 | G2148 | J9030 | M1130 | |

## REVISED CODES/MODIFIERS

| | | | | | |
|---|---|---|---|---|---|
| G8650 | G9414 | G9663 | G9798 | J7313 | M1045 |
| G8662 | G9469 | G9727 | G9898 | J9201 | M1046 |
| G8666 | G9510 | G9729 | G9901 | J9355 | M1049 |
| G8670 | G9519 | G9731 | G9910 | L8032 | M1052 |
| G8674 | G9520 | G9733 | G9917 | M1009 | Q4122 |
| G9239 | G9531 | G9735 | G9938 | M1010 | Q4165 |
| G9264 | G9547 | G9737 | G9942 | M1011 | Q4184 |
| G9349 | G9548 | G9739 | G9948 | M1012 | Q5105 |
| G9355 | G9549 | G9772 | G9949 | M1013 | Q5106 |
| G9356 | G9550 | G9781 | J0641 | M1014 | |
| G9359 | G9551 | G9785 | J2794 | M1015 | |
| G9405 | G9595 | G9786 | J7311 | M1043 | |

## DELETED CODES/MODIFIERS

| | | | | | |
|---|---|---|---|---|---|
| GD | C9408 | G8978 | G8996 | G9164 | G9944 |
| C9035 | C9447 | G8979 | G8997 | G9165 | G9947 |
| C9036 | C9746 | G8980 | G8998 | G9166 | J1942 |
| C9037 | D1550 | G8981 | G8999 | G9167 | J9031 |
| C9038 | D1555 | G8982 | G9017 | G9168 | M1000 |
| C9039 | D8691 | G8983 | G9018 | G9169 | M1001 |
| C9040 | D8692 | G8984 | G9019 | G9170 | M1002 |
| C9042 | D8693 | G8985 | G9020 | G9171 | M1030 |
| C9043 | D8694 | G8986 | G9033 | G9172 | M1042 |
| C9044 | G0365 | G8987 | G9034 | G9173 | M1044 |
| C9045 | G0515 | G8988 | G9035 | G9174 | M1047 |
| C9048 | G8649 | G8989 | G9036 | G9175 | M1048 |
| C9049 | G8653 | G8990 | G9158 | G9176 | M1050 |
| C9050 | G8657 | G8991 | G9159 | G9186 | M1053 |
| C9051 | G8665 | G8992 | G9160 | G9472 | S1090 |
| C9052 | G8669 | G8993 | G9161 | G9742 | |
| C9141 | G8673 | G8994 | G9162 | G9743 | |
| C9407 | G8861 | G8995 | G9163 | G9941 | |

## NEW, REVISED, AND DELETED DENTAL CODES

| New | | | Revised | | Deleted |
|---|---|---|---|---|---|
| D0419 | D6084 | D6753 | D5213 | D6067 | D1550 |
| D1551 | D6086 | D6784 | D5214 | D6076 | D1555 |
| D1552 | D6087 | D7922 | D5221 | D6077 | D8691 |
| D1553 | D6088 | D8696 | D5222 | D6094 | D8692 |
| D1556 | D6097 | D8697 | D5223 | D6194 | D8693 |
| D1557 | D6098 | D8698 | D5224 | D6214 | D8694 |
| D1558 | D6099 | D8699 | D6066 | D6794 | |
| D2753 | D6120 | D8701 | | | |
| D5284 | D6121 | D8702 | | | |
| D5286 | D6122 | D8703 | | | |
| D6082 | D6123 | D8704 | | | |
| D6083 | D6195 | D9997 | | | |
| | D6243 | | | | |

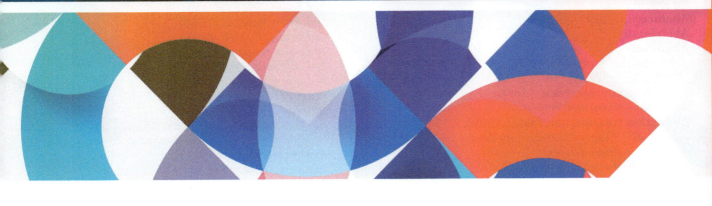

# INDEX

# A

**Abatacept,** J0129
**Abciximab,** J0130
**Abdomen**
  dressing holder/binder, A4462
  pad, low profile, L1270
**Abduction control, each,** L2624
*Abduction restrainer,* A4566
**Abduction rotation bar, foot,** L3140–L3170
  *adjustable shoe style positioning device, L3160*
  *including shoes, L3140*
  *plastic, heel-stabilizer, off-shelf, L3170*
  *without shoes, L3150*
**AbobotulinumtoxintypeA,** J0586
**Absorption dressing,** A6251–A6256
*Access, site, occlusive, device,* G0269
**Access system,** A4301
**Accessories**
  ambulation devices, E0153–E0159
    *crutch attachment, walker, E0157*
    *forearm crutch, platform attachment, E0153*
    *leg extension, walker, E0158*
    *replacement, brake attachment, walker, E0159*
    *seat attachment, walker, E0156*
    *walker, platform attachment, E0154*
    *wheel attachment, walker, per pair, E0155*
  artificial kidney and machine; (see also ESRD),
    E1510–E1699
    *adjustable chair, ESRD patients, E1570*
    *automatic peritoneal dialysis system,*
      *intermittent, E1592*
    *bath conductivity meter, hemodialysis, E1550*
    *blood leak detector, hemodialysis,*
      *replacement, E1560*
    *blood pump, hemodialysis, replacement, E1620*
    *cycler dialysis machine, peritoneal, E1594*
    *deionizer water system, hemodialysis, E1615*
    *delivery/instillation charges, hemodialysis*
      *equipment, E1600*
    *hemodialysis machine, E1590*
    *hemostats, E1637*
    *heparin infusion pump, hemodialysis, E1520*
    *kidney machine, dialysate delivery system, E1510*
    *peritoneal dialysis clamps, E1634*
    *portable travel hemodialyzer, E1635*
    *reciprocating peritoneal dialysis system, E1630*
    *replacement, air bubble detector,*
      *hemodialysis, E1530*
    *replacement, pressure alarm, hemodialysis, E1540*
    *reverse osmosis water system, hemodialysis, E1610*
    *scale, E1639*
    *sorbent cartridges, hemodialysis, E1636*
    *transducer protectors, E1575*
    *unipuncture control system, E1580*
    *water softening system, hemodialysis, E1625*
    *wearable artificial kidney, E1632*

**Accessories** *(Continued)*
  beds, E0271–E0280, E0300–E0326
    *bed board, E0273*
    *bed, board/table, E0315*
    *bed cradle, E0280*
    *bed pan, standard, E0275*
    *bed side rails, E0305–E0310*
    *bed-pan fracture, E0276*
    *hospital bed, extra heavy duty, E0302, E0304*
    *hospital bed, heavy duty, E0301–E0303*
    *hospital bed, pediatric, electric, E0329*
    *hospital bed, safety enclosure frame, E0316*
    *mattress, foam rubber, E0272*
    *mattress, innerspring, E0271*
    *over-bed table, E0274*
    *pediatric crib, E0300*
    *powered pressure-reducing air mattress, E0277*
  wheelchairs, E0950–E1030, E1050–E1298,
    E2300–E2399, K0001–K0109
    *accessory tray, E0950*
    *arm rest, E0994*
    *back upholstery replacement, E0982*
    *calf rest/pad, E0995*
    *commode seat, E0968*
    *detachable armrest, E0973*
    *elevating leg rest, E0990*
    *headrest cushion, E0955*
    *lateral trunk/hip support, E0956*
    *loop-holder, E0951–E0952*
    *manual swingaway, E1028*
    *manual wheelchair, adapter, amputee, E0959*
    *manual wheelchair, anti-rollback device, E0974*
    *manual wheelchair, anti-tipping device, E0971*
    *manual wheelchair, hand rim with*
      *projections, E0967*
    *manual wheelchair, headrest extension, E0966*
    *manual wheelchair, lever-activated, wheel*
      *drive, E0988*
    *manual wheelchair, one-arm drive*
      *attachment, E0958*
    *manual wheelchair, power add-on,*
      *E0983–E0984*
    *manual wheelchair, push activated power*
      *assist, E0986*
    *manual wheelchair, solid seat insert, E0992*
    *medial thigh support, E0957*
    *modification, pediatric size, E1011*
    *narrowing device, E0969*
    *No. 2 footplates, E0970*
    *oxygen related accessories, E1352–E1406*
    *positioning belt/safety belt/pelvic strap, E0978*
    *power-seating system, E1002–E1010*
    *reclining back addition, pediatric size*
      *wheelchair, E1014*
    *residual limb support system, E1020*
    *safety vest, E0980*
    *seat lift mechanism, E0985*
    *seat upholstery replacement, E0981*

◄ New    ↻ Revised    ✔ Reinstated    ~~deleted~~ Deleted

**Accessories** (Continued)
  wheelchairs (Continued)
    shock absorber, E1015–E1018
    shoulder harness strap, E0960
    ventilator tray, E1029–E1030
    wheel lock brake extension, manual, E0961
    wheelchair, amputee, accessories, E1170–E1200
    wheelchair, fully inclining, accessories,
      E1050–E1093
    wheelchair, heavy duty, accessories, E1280–E1298
    wheelchair, lightweight, accessories, E1240–E1270
    wheelchair, semi-reclining, accessories,
      E1100–E1110
    wheelchair, special size, E1220–E1239
    wheelchair, standard, accessories, E1130–E1161
  whirlpool equipment, E1300–E1310
**Ace type, elastic bandage,** A6448–A6450
**Acetaminophen,** J0131
**Acetazolamide sodium,** J1120
**Acetylcysteine**
  inhalation solution, J7604, J7608
  injection, J0132
**Activity, therapy,** G0176
**Acyclovir,** J0133
**Adalimumab,** J0135
**Additions to**
  fracture orthosis, L2180–L2192
    abduction bar, L2300–L2310
    adjustable motion knee joint, L2186
    anterior swing band, L2335
    BK socket, PTB and AFO, L2350
    disk or dial lock, knee flexion, L2425
    dorsiflexion and plantar flexion, L2220
    dorsiflexion assist, L2210
    drop lock, L2405
    drop lock knee joint, L2182
    extended steel shank, L2360
    foot plate, stirrup attachment, L2250
    hip joint, pelvic band, thigh flange, pelvic
      belt, L2192
    integrated release mechanism, L2515
    lacer custom-fabricated, L2320–L2330
    lift loop, drop lock ring, L2492
    limited ankle motion, L2200
    limited motion knee joint, L2184
    long tongue stirrup, L2265
    lower extremity orthrosis, L2200–L2397
    molded inner boot, L2280
    offset knee joint, L2390
    offset knee joint, heavy duty, L2395
    Patten bottom, L2370
    pelvic and thoracic control, L2570–L2680
    plastic shoe insert with ankle joints, L2180
    polycentric knee joint, L2387
    pre-tibial shell, L2340
    quadrilateral, L2188
    ratchet lock knee extension, L2430
    reinforced solid stirrup, L2260

**Additions to** (Continued)
  fracture orthosis (Continued)
    rocker bottom, custom fabricated, L2232
    round caliper/plate attachment, L2240
    split flat caliper stirrups, L2230
    straight knee joint, heavy duty, L2385
    straight knee, or offset knee joints, L2405–L2492
    suspension sleeve, L2397
    thigh/weight bearing, L2500–L2550
    torsion control, ankle joint, L2375
    torsion control, straight knee joint, L2380
    varus/valgus correction, L2270–L2275
    waist belt, L2190
  general additions, orthosis, L2750–L2999
    lower extremity, above knee section, soft
      interface, L2830
    lower extremity, concentric adjustable torsion style
      mechanism, L2861
    lower extremity, drop lock retainer, L2785
    lower extremity, extension, per extension, per
      bar, L2760
    lower extremity, femoral length sock, L2850
    lower extremity, full kneecap, L2795
    lower extremity, high strength, lightweight material,
      hybrid lamination, L2755
    lower extremity, knee control, condylar pad, L2810
    lower extremity, knee control, knee cap, medial or
      lateral, L2800
    lower extremity orthrosis, non-corrosive finish, per
      bar, L2780
    lower extremity orthrosis, NOS, L2999
    lower extremity, plating chrome or nickel, per
      bar, L2750
    lower extremity, soft interface, below knee, L2820
    lower extremity, tibial length sock, L2840
    orthotic side bar, disconnect device, L2768
**Adenosine,** J0151, J0153
**Adhesive,** A4364
  bandage, A6413
  disc or foam pad, A5126
  remover, A4455, A4456
  support, breast prosthesis, A4280
  wound, closure, G0168
**Adjunctive, dental,** D9110–D9999
**Administration, chemotherapy,** Q0083–Q0085
  both infusion and other technique, Q0085
  infusion technique only, Q0084
  other than infusion technique, Q0083
**Administration, Part D**
  vaccine, hepatitis B, G0010
  vaccine, influenza, G0008
  vaccine, pneumococcal, G0009
**Administrative, Miscellaneous and Investigational,**
  A9000–A9999
  alert or alarm device, A9280
  artificial saliva, A9155
  DME delivery set-up, A9901
  exercise equipment, A9300

---

◀ New    ↻ Revised    ✔ Reinstated    ~~deleted~~ **Deleted**

**Administrative, Miscellaneous and Investigational**
  *(Continued)*
  *external ambulatory insulin delivery system, A9274*
  *foot pressure off loading/supportive device, A9283*
  *helmets, A8000–A8004*
  *home glucose disposable monitor, A9275*
  *hot-water bottle, ice cap, heat wrap, A9273*
  *miscellaneous DME, NOS, A9999*
  *miscellaneous DME supply, A9900*
  *monitoring feature/device, stand-alone or
    integrated, A9279*
  *multiple vitamins, oral, per dose, A9153*
  *non-covered item, A9270*
  *non-prescription drugs, A9150*
  *pediculosis treatment, topical, A9180*
  *radiopharmaceuticals, A9500–A9700*
  *reaching grabbing device, A9281*
  *receiver, external, interstitial glucose monitoring
    system, A9278*
  *sensor, invasive, interstitial continuous glucose
    monitoring, A9276*
  *single vitamin/mineral trace element, A9152*
  *spirometer, non-electronic, A9284*
  *transmitter, interstitial continuous glucose
    monitoring system, A9277*
  *wig, any type, A9282*
  *wound suction, disposable, A9272*
**Admission, observation,** G0379
**Ado-trastuzumab,** J9354
**Adrenalin,** J0171
**Advanced life support,** A0390, A0426, A0427, A0433
  *ALS2, A0433*
  *ALS emergency transport, A0427*
  *ALS mileage, A0390*
  *ALS, non-emergency transport, A0426*
**Aerosol**
  compressor, E0571–E0572
  compressor filter, *A7013–A7014,* K0178–K0179
  mask, *A7015,* K0180
**Aflibercept,** J0178
**AFO,** E1815, E1830, L1900–L1990, L4392, L4396
**Afstyla,** J7210
**Agalsidase beta,** J0180
**Aggrastat,** J3245
**A-hydroCort,** J1710
**Aid, hearing,** V5030–V5263
**Aide, home, health,** G0156, S9122, T1021
  *home health aide/certified nurse assistant, in
    home, S9122*
  *home health aide/certified nurse assistant, per
    visit, T1021*
  *home health or hospital setting, G0156*
**Air bubble detector, dialysis,** E1530
**Air fluidized bed,** E0194
**Air pressure pad/mattress,** E0186, E0197
**Air travel and nonemergency transportation,** A0140
**Alarm**
  *not otherwise classified, A9280*
  pressure, dialysis, E1540

**Alatrofloxacin mesylate,** J0200
**Albumin, human,** P9041, P9042
**Albuterol**
  all formulations, inhalation solution, J7620
  all formulations, inhalation solution, concentrated,
    J7610, J7611
  all formulations, inhalation solution, unit dose,
    J7609, J7613
**Alcohol,** A4244
**Alcohol wipes,** A4245
**Alcohol/substance, assessment,** G0396, G0397,
    H0001, H0003, H0049
  *alcohol abuse structured assessment, greater than
    30 min., G0397*
  *alcohol abuse structured assessment,
    15–30 min., G0396*
  *alcohol and/or drug assessment, Medicaid, H0001*
  *alcohol and/or drug screening; laboratory analysis,
    Medicaid, H0003*
  *alcohol and/or drug screening, Medicaid, H0049*
**Aldesleukin (IL2),** J9015
**Alefacept,** J0215
**Alemtuzumab,** J0202
**Alert device,** A9280
**Alginate dressing,** A6196–A6199
  *alginate, pad more than 48 sq. cm, A6198*
  *alginate, pad size 16 sq. cm, A6196*
  *alginate, pad size more than 16 sq. cm, A6197*
  *alginate, wound filler, sterile, A6199*
**Alglucerase,** J0205
**Alglucosidase,** J0220
**Alglucosidase alfa,** J0221
**Allogen,** Q4212 ◄
**Alphanate,** J7186
**Alpha-1–proteinase inhibitor, human,** J0256, J0257
**Alprostadil**
  injection, J0270
  urethral supposity, J0275
**ALS mileage,** A0390
**Alteplase recombinant,** J2997
**Alternating pressure mattress/pad,** A4640, E0180,
    E0181, E0277
  *overlay/pad, alternating, pump, heavy duty, E0181*
  *powered pressure-reducing air mattress, E0277*
  *replacement pad, owned by patient, A4640*
**Alveoloplasty,** D7310–D7321
  *in conjunction with extractions, four or more
    teeth, D7310*
  *in conjunction with extractions, one to three
    teeth, D7311*
  *not in conjunction with extractions, four or more
    teeth, D7320*
  *not in conjunction with extractions, one to three
    teeth, D7321*
**Amalgam dental restoration,** D2140–D2161
  *four or more surfaces, primary or permanent, D2161*
  *one surface, primary or permanent, D2140*
  *three surfaces, primary or permanent, D2160*
  *two surfaces, primary or permanent, D2150*

---

◄ **New**    ⤵ **Revised**    ✔ **Reinstated**    ~~deleted~~ **Deleted**

**Ambulance,** A0021–A0999
air, A0430, A0431, A0435, A0436
  *conventional, transport, one way, fixed wing,* A0430
  *conventional, transport, one way, rotary wing,* A0431
  *fixed wing air mileage,* A0435
  *rotary wing air mileage,* A0436
disposable supplies, A0382–A0398
  *ALS routine disposable supplies,* A0398
  *ALS specialized service disposable supplies,* A0394
  *ALS specialized service, esophageal intubation,* A0396
  *BLS routine disposable,* A0832
  *BLS specialized service disposable supplies, defibrillation,* A0384, A0392
non-emergency transport, fixed wing, S9960
non-emergency transport, rotary wing, S9961
oxygen, A0422

**Ambulation device,** E0100–E0159
*brake attachment, wheeled walker replacement,* E0159
*cane, adjustable or fixed, with tip,* E0100
*cane, quad or three prong, adjustable or fixed, with tip,* E0105
*crutch attachment, walker,* E0157
*crutch forearm, each, with tips and handgrips,* E0111
*crutch substitute, lower leg platform, with or without wheels, each,* E0118
*crutch, underarm, articulating, spring assisted, each,* E0117
*crutches forearm, pair, tips and handgrips,* E0110
*crutches, underarm, other than wood, pair, with pads, tips and handgrips,* E0114
*crutches, underarm, other than wood, with pad, tip, handgrip, with or without shock absorber, each,* E0116
*crutches, underarm, wood, each, with pad, tip and handgrip,* E0113
*leg extensions, walker, set (4),* E0158
*platform attachment, forearm crutch, each,* E0153
*platform attachment, walker,* E0154
*seat attachment, walker,* E0156
*walker, enclosed, four-sided frame, wheeled, posterior seat,* E0144
*walker, folding, adjustable or fixed height,* E0135
*walker, folding, wheeled, adjustable or fixed height,* E0143
*walker, heavy duty, multiple braking system, variable wheel resistance,* E0147
*walker, heavy duty, wheeled, rigid or folding,* E0149
*walker, heavy duty, without wheels, rigid or folding,* E0148
*walker, rigid, adjustable or fixed height,* E0130
*walker, rigid, wheeled, adjustable or fixed height,* E0141
*walker, with trunk support, adjystable or fixed height, any,* E0140
*wheel attachment, rigid, pick up walker, per pair,* E0155
**Amikacin Sulfate,** J0278
**Aminolevulinate,** J7309
~~Aminolevulinic, J7345~~ ✖
**Aminolevulinic acid HCl,** J7308
**Aminophylline,** J0280

**Aminolevulinic**
Ameluz, J7345
**Amiodarone HCl,** J0282
**Amitriptyline HCl,** J1320
**Ammonia N-13,** A9526
**Ammonia test paper,** A4774
**Amnioiwrap2,** Q4221 ◀
**Amnion Bio,** Q4211
**Amniotic membrane,** V2790
**Amobarbital,** J0300
**Amphotericin B,** J0285
Lipid Complex, J0287–J0289
**Ampicillin**
sodium, J0290
sodium/sulbactam sodium, J0295
**Amputee**
adapter, wheelchair, E0959
prosthesis, L5000–L7510, L7520, L7900, L8400–L8465
  *above knee,* L5200–L5230
  *additions to exoskeletal knee-shin systems,* L5710–L5782
  *additions to lower extremity,* L5610–L5617
  *additions to socket insert and suspension,* L5654–L5699
  *additions to socket variations,* L5630–L5653
  *additions to test sockets,* L5618–L5629
  *additions/replacements feet-ankle units,* L5700–L5707
  *ankle,* L5050–L5060
  *below knee,* L5100–L5105
  *component modification,* L5785–L5795
  *endoskeletal,* L5810–L5999
  *endoskeleton, below knee,* L5301–L5312
  *endoskeleton, hip disarticulation,* L5331–L5341
  *fitting endoskeleton, above knee,* L5321
  *fitting procedures,* L5400–L5460
  *hemipelvectomy,* L5280
  *hip disarticulation,* L5250–L5270
  *initial prosthesis,* L5500–L5505
  *knee disarticulation,* L5150–L5160
  *male vacuum erection system,* L7900
  *partial foot,* L5000–L5020
  *preparatory prosthesis,* L5510–L5600
  *prosthetic socks,* L8400–L8485
  *repair, prosthetic device,* L7520
  *tension ring, vacuum erection device,* L7902
  *upper extremity, battery components,* L7360–L7368
  *upper extremity, other/repair,* L7400–L7510
  *upper extremity, preparatory, elbow,* L6584–L6586
  *upper limb, above elbow,* L6250
  *upper limb, additions,* L6600–L6698
  *upper limb, below elbow,* L6100–L6130
  *upper limb, elbow disarticulation,* L6200–L6205
  *upper limb, endoskeletal, above elbow,* L6500
  *upper limb, endoskeletal, below elbow,* L6400
  *upper limb, endoskeletal, elbow disarticulation,* L6450
  *upper limb, endoskeletal, interscapular thoracic,* L6570

---

◀ New   ↻ Revised   ✔ Reinstated   ~~deleted~~ Deleted

**Amputee** (*Continued*)

  prosthesis (*Continued*)

    *upper limb, endoskeletal, shoulder disarticulation,* L6550

    *upper limb, external power, device,* L6920–L6975

    *upper limb, interscapular thoracic,* L6350–L6370

    *upper limb, partial hand,* L6000–L6025

    *upper limb, postsurgical procedures,* L6380–L6388

    *upper limb, preparatory, shoulder, interscapular,* L6588–L6590

    *upper limb, preparatory, wrist,* L6580–L6582

    *upper limb, shoulder disarticulation,* L6300–L6320

    *upper limb, terminal devices,* L6703–L6915, L7007–L7261

    *upper limb, wrist disarticulation,* L6050–L6055

  stump sock, L8470–L8485

    *single ply, fitting above knee,* L8480

    *single ply, fitting, below knee,* L8470

    *single ply, fitting, upper limb,* L8485

  wheelchair, E1170–E1190, E1200, K0100

    *detachable arms, swing away detachable elevating footrests,* E1190

    *detachable arms, swing away detachable footrests,* E1180

    *detachable arms, without footrests or legrest,* E1172

    *detachable elevating legrest, fixed full length arms,* E1170

    *fixed full length arms, swing away detachable footrest,* E1200

    *heavy duty wheelchair, swing away detachable elevating legrests,* E1195

    *without footrests or legrest, fixed full length arms,* E1171

**Amygdalin,** J3570

**Anadulafungin,** J0348

**Analgesia, dental,** D9230

**Analysis**

  *saliva,* D0418

  *semen,* G0027

**Angiography, iliac, artery,** G0278

**Angiography, renal, non-selective,** G0275

  *non-ophthalmic fluorescent vascular,* C9733

  *reconstruction,* G0288

**Anistreplase,** J0350

**Ankle splint, recumbent,** K0126–K0130

**Ankle-foot orthosis (AFO),** L1900–L1990, L2106–L2116, L4361, L4392, L4396

  *ankle gauntlet, custom fabricated,* L1904

  *ankle gauntlet, prefabricated, off-shelf,* L1902

  *double upright free plantar dorsiflexion, olid stirrup, calf-band/cuff, custom,* L1990

  *fracture orthosis, tibial fracture, thermoplastic cast material, custom,* L2106

  *multiligamentus ankle support, prefabricated, off-shelf,* L1906

  *plastic or other material, custom fabricated,* L1940

  *plastic or other material, prefabricated, fitting and adjustment,* L1932, L1951

**Ankle-foot orthosis** (*Continued*)

  *plastic or other material, with ankle joint, prefabricated, fitting and adjustment,* L1971

  *plastic, rigid anterior tibial section, custom fabricated,* L1945

  *plastic, with ankle joint, custom,* L1970

  *posterior, single bar, clasp attachment to shoe,* L1910

  *posterior, solid ankle, plastic, custom,* L1960

  *replacement, soft interface material, static AFO,* L4392

  *single upright free plantar dorsiflection, solid stirrup, calf-band/cuff, custom,* L1980

  *single upright with static or adjustable stop, custom,* L1920

  *spiral, plastic, custom fabricated,* L1950

  *spring wire, dorsiflexion assist calf band,* L1900

  *static or dynamic AFO, adjustable for fit, minimal ambulation,* L4396

  *supramalleolar with straps, custom fabricated,* L1907

  *tibial fracture cast orthrosis, custom,* L2108

  *tibial fracture orthrosis, rigid, prefabricated, fitting and adjustment,* L2116

  *tibial fracture orthrosis, semi-rigid, prefabricated, fitting and adjustment,* L2114

  *tibial fracture orthrosis, soft prefabricated, fitting and adjustment,* L2112

  *walking boot, prefabricated, off-the-shelf,* L4361

**Anterior-posterior-lateral orthosis,** L0700, L0710

**Antibiotic,** G8708–G8712

  *antibiotic not prescribed or dispensed,* G8712

  *patient not prescribed or dispensed antibiotic,* G8708

  *patient prescribed antibiotic, documented condition,* G8709

  *patient prescribed or dispensed antibiotic,* G8710

  *prescribed or dispensed antibiotic,* G8711

**Antidepressant, documentation,** G8126–G8128

**Anti-emetic, oral,** J8498, J8597, Q0163–Q0181

  *antiemetic drug, oral NOS,* J8597

  *antiemetic drug, rectal suppository, NOS,* J8498

  *diphenhydramine hydrochloride, 50 mg, oral,* Q0163

  *dolasetron mesylate, 100 mg, oral,* Q0180

  *dronabinol, 2.5 mg,* Q0167

  *granisetron hydrochloride, 1 mg, oral,* Q0166

  *hydroxyzine pomoate, 25 mg, oral,* Q0177

  *perphenazine, 4 mg, oral,* Q0175

  *prochlorperazine maleate, 5 mg, oral,* Q0164

  *promethazine hydrochloride, 12.5 mg, oral,* Q0169

  *thiethylperazine maleate, 10 mg, oral,* Q0174

  *trimethobenzamide hydrochloride, 250 mg, oral,* Q0173

  *unspecified oral dose,* Q0181

**Anti-hemophilic factor (Factor VIII),** J7190–J7192

**Anti-inhibitors, per I.U.,** J7198

**Antimicrobial, prophylaxis, documentation,** D4281, G8201

**Anti-neoplastic drug, NOC,** J9999

**Antithrombin III,** J7197

**Antithrombin recombinant,** J7196

---

◀ **New** ↻ **Revised** ✔ **Reinstated** ~~deleted~~ **Deleted**

*Antral fistula closure, oral,* D7260
*Apexification, dental,* D3351–D3353
*Apicoectomy,* D3410–D3426
  *anterior, periradicular surgery,* D3410
  *biscuspid (first root),* D3421
  *(each additional root),* D3426
  *molar (first root),* D3425
**Apomorphine,** J0364
**Appliance**
  cleaner, A5131
  pneumatic, E0655–E0673
    *non-segmental pneumatic appliance,* E0655,
      E0660, E0665, E0666
    *segmental gradient pressure, pneumatic appliance,*
      E0671–E0673
    *segmental pneumatic appliance,* E0656–E0657,
      E0667–E0670
*Application, heat, cold,* E0200–E0239
  *electric heat pad, moist,* E0215
  *electric heat pad, standard,* E0210
  *heat lamp with stand,* E0205
  *heat lamp without stand,* E0200
  *hydrocollator unit, pads,* E0225
  *hydrocollator unit, portable,* E0239
  *infrared heating pad system,* E0221
  *non-contact wound warming device,* E0231
  *paraffin bath unit,* E0235
  *phototherapy (bilirubin),* E0202
  *pump for water circulating pad,* E0236
  *therapeutic lightbox,* E0203
  *warming card,* E0232
  *water circulating cold pad with pump,* E0218
  *water circulating heat pad with pump,* E0217
**Aprotinin,** J0365
**Aqueous**
  shunt, L8612
  sterile, J7051
*ARB/ACE therapy,* G8473–G8475
**Arbutamine HCl,** J0395
**Arch support,** L3040–L3100
  *hallus-valgus night dynamic splint, off-shelf,* L3100
  intralesional, J3302
  *non-removable, attached to shoe, longitudinal,* L3070
  *non-removable, attached to shoe, longitudinal/*
    *metatarsal, each,* L3090
  *non-removable, attached to shoe, metatarsal,* L3080
  *removable, premolded, longitudinal,* L3040
  *removable, premolded, longitudinal/metatarsal,*
    *each,* L3060
  *removable, premolded, metatarsal,* L3050
**Arformoterol,** J7605
**Argatroban,** J0883–J0884
**Aripiprazole,** J0400, J0401 ↻
**Aripiprazol lauroxil, (aristada),** J1944 ◄
  aristada initio, H1943 ◄
**Arm, wheelchair,** E0973
**Arsenic trioxide,** J9017
**Artacent cord,** Q4216 ◄

*Arthrography, injection, sacroiliac, joint,*
  G0259, G0260
*Arthroscopy, knee, surgical,* G0289, S2112
  *chondroplasty, different compartment,*
    *knee,* G0289
  *harvesting of cartilage, knee,* S2112
**Artificial**
  cornea, L8609
  heart system, miscellaneous component, supply or
    accessory, L8698
  kidney machines and accessories (see also Dialysis),
    E1510–E1699
  larynx, L8500
  saliva, A9155
**Ascent,** Q4213 ◄
**Asparaginase,** J9019–J9020
*Aspirator, VABRA,* A4480
**Assessment**
  *alcohol/substance (see also Alcohol/substance,*
    *assessment),* G0396, G0397, H0001,
    H0003, H0049
  *assessment for hearing aid,* V5010
  audiologic, V5008–V5020
  *cardiac output,* M0302
  *conformity evaluation,* V5020
  *fitting/orientation, hearing aid,* V5014
  *hearing screening,* V5008
  *repair/modification hearing aid,* V5014
  speech, V5362–V5364
**Assistive listening devices and accessories,**
  V5281–V5290
  *FMlDM system, monaural,* V5281
**Astramorph,** J2275
**Atezolizumab,** J9022
*Atherectomy, PTCA,* C9602, C9603
**Atropine**
  inhalation solution, concentrated, J7635
  inhalation solution, unit dose, J7636
**Atropine sulfate,** J0461
*Attachment, walker,* E0154–E0159
  *brake attachment, wheeled walker,*
    *replacement,* E0159
  *crutch attachment, walker,* E0157
  *leg extension, walker,* E0158
  *platform attachment, walker,* E0154
  *seat attachment, walker,* E0156
  *wheel attachment, rigid pick up walker,* E0155
**Audiologic assessment,** V5008–V5020
**Auditory osseointegrated device,** L8690–L8694
*Auricular prosthesis,* D5914, D5927
**Aurothioglucose,** J2910
**Avelumab,** J9023
**Axobiomembrane,** Q4211 ◄
**Axolotl ambient or axolotl cryo,** Q4215 ◄
**Axolotl graft or axoloti dualgraft,** Q4210 ◄
**Azacitidine,** J9025
**Azathioprine,** J7500, J7501
**Azithromycin injection,** J0456

◄ New   ↻ Revised   ✔ Reinstated   ~~deleted~~ Deleted

# B

**Back supports,** L0621–L0861, L0960
*lumbar orthrosis,* L0625–L0627
*lumbar orthrosis, sagittal control,* L0641–L0648
*lumbar-sacral orthrosis,* L0628–L0640
*lumbar-sacral orthrosis, sagittal-coronal control,* L0640, L0649–L0651
*sacroiliac orthrosis,* L0621–L0624
**Baclofen,** J0475, J0476
**Bacterial sensitivity study,** P7001
**Bag**
drainage, A4357
*enema, A4458*
irrigation supply, A4398
*urinary, A4358, A5112*
***Bandage, conforming***
*elastic, >5", A6450*
*elastic, >3", <5", A6449*
*elastic, load resistance 1.25 to 1.34 foot pounds, >3", <5", A6451*
*elastic, load resistance <1.35 foot pounds, >3", <5", A6452*
*elastic, <3", A6448*
*non-elastic, non-sterile, >5", A6444*
*non-elastic, non-sterile, width greater than or equal to 3", <5", A6443*
*non-elastic, non-sterile, width <3", A6442*
*non-elastic, sterile, >5", A6447*
*non-elastic, sterile, >3" and <5", A6446*
**Basiliximab,** J0480
***Bath, aid,*** E0160–E0162, E0235, E0240–E0249
*bath tub rail, floor base, E0242*
*bath tub wall rail, E0241*
*bath/shower chair, with/without wheels, E0240*
*pad for water circulating heat unit, replacement, E0249*
*paraffin bath unit, portable, E0235*
*raised toilet seat, E0244*
*sitz bath chair, E0162*
*sitz type bath, portable, with faucet attachment, E0161*
*sitz type bath, portable, with/without commode, E0160*
*toilet rail, E0243*
*transfer bench, tub or toilet, E0248*
*transfer tub rail attachment, E0246*
*tub stool or bench, E0245*
**Bathtub**
chair, E0240
stool or bench, E0245, E0247–E0248
transfer rail, E0246
wall rail, E0241–E0242
**Battery,** L7360, L7364–L7368
charger, E1066, L7362, L7366
replacement for blood glucose monitor, A4233–A4236

**Battery** *(Continued)*
replacement for cochlear implant device, L8618, L8623–L8625
replacement for TENS, A4630
ventilator, A4611–A4613
~~BCG live, intravesical, J9031~~
**Beclomethasone inhalation solution,** J7622
**Bed**
*accessories,* E0271–E0280, E0300–E0326
*bed board, E0273*
*bed cradle, E0280*
*bed pan, fracture, metal, E0276*
*bed pan, standard, metal, E0275*
*mattress, foam rubber, E0272*
*mattress innerspring, E0271*
*over-bed table, E0274*
*power pressure-reducing air mattress, E0277*
air fluidized, E0194
cradle, any type, E0280
drainage bag, bottle, A4357, A5102
hospital, E0250–E0270, E0300–E0329
pan, E0275, E0276
rail, E0305, E0310
safety enclosure frame/canopy, E0316
***Behavioral, health, treatment services (Medicaid),*** H0002–H2037
*activity therapy, H2032*
*alcohol/drug services, H0001, H0003, H0005–H0016, H0020–H0022, H0026–H0029, H0049–H0050, H2034–H2036*
*assertive community treatment, H0040*
*community based wrap-around services, H2021–H2022*
*comprehensive community support, H2015–H2016*
*comprehensive medication services, H2010*
*comprehensive multidisciplinary evaluation, H2000*
*crisis intervention, H2011*
*day treatment, per diem, H2013*
*day treatment, per hour, H2012*
*developmental delay prevention activities, dependent child of client, H2037*
*family assessment, H1011*
*foster care, child, H0041–H0042*
*health screening, H0002*
*hotline service, H0030*
*medication training, H0034*
*mental health clubhouse services, H2030–H2031*
*multisystemic therapy, juveniles, H2033*
*non-medical family planning, H1010*
*outreach service, H0023*
*partial hospitalization, H0035*
*plan development, non-physician, H0033*
*prenatal care, at risk, H1000–H1005*
*prevention, H0024–H0025*
*psychiatric supportive treatment, community, H0036–H0037*
*psychoeducational service, H2027*
*psychoscial rehabilitation, H2017–H2018*

◀ **New**  ↻ **Revised**  ✔ **Reinstated**  ~~deleted~~ **Deleted**

*Behavioral, health, treatment services (Medicaid)*
   *(Continued)*
  *rehabilitation program, H2010*
  *residential treatment program, H0017–H0019*
  *respite care, not home, H0045*
  *self-help/peer services, H0039*
  *sexual offender treatment, H2028–H2029*
  *skill training, H2014*
  *supported employment, H2024–H2026*
  *supported housing, H0043–H0044*
  *therapeutic behavioral services, H2019–H2020*
*Behavioral therapy, cardiovascular disease, G0446*
**Belatacept,** J0485
**Belimumab,** J0490
**Bellacell,** Q4220 ◄
**Belt**
  belt, strap, sleeve, garment, or covering, any
    type, A4467
  extremity, E0945
  ostomy, A4367
  pelvic, E0944
  safety, K0031
  wheelchair, E0978, E0979
**Bench, bathtub; (see also Bathtub),** E0245
**Bendamustine HCl**
  Bendeka, 1 mg, J9034
  Treanda, 1 mg, J9033
**Bendamustine HCI (Belrapzo/bendamustine),**
  J9036 ◄
**Benesch boot,** L3212–L3214
**Benztropine,** J0515
*Beta-blocker therapy, G9188–G9192*
**Betadine,** A4246, A4247
**Betameth,** J0704
**Betamethasone**
  acetate and betamethasone sodium
    phosphate, J0702
  inhalation solution, J7624
**Bethanechol chloride,** J0520
**Bevacizumab,** J9035, Q2024
  bvzr (Zirabez), Q5118 ◄
**Bezlotoxuman,** J0565
*Bicuspid (excluding final restoration), D3320*
  *retreatment, by report, D3347*
  *surgery, first root, D3421*
**Bifocal, glass or plastic,** V2200–V2299
  *aniseikonic, bifocal, V2218*
  *bifocal add-over 3.25 d, V2220*
  *bifocal seg width over 28 mm, V2219*
  *lenticular, bifocal, myodisc, V2215*
  *lenticular lens, V2221*
  *specialty bifocal, by report, V2200*
  *sphere, bifocal, V2200–V2202*
  *spherocylinder, bifocal, V2203–V2214*
**Bilirubin (phototherapy) light,** E0202
**Binder,** A4465
**Biofeedback device,** E0746
**Bioimpedance, electrical, cardiac output,** M0302

**Biosimilar (infliximab),** Q5102–Q5110
**BioWound,** Q4217 ◄
**Biperiden lactate,** J0190
*Bitewing, D0270–D0277*
  *four radiographic images, D0274*
  *single radiographic image, D0270*
  *three radiographic images, D0273*
  *two radiographic images, D0272*
  *vertical bitewings, 7–8 radiographic images, D0277*
**Bitolterol mesylate, inhalation solution**
  concentrated, J7628
  unit dose, J7629
**Bivalirudin,** J0583
*Bivigam, 500 mg, J1556*
**Bladder calculi irrigation solution,** Q2004
**Bleomycin sulfate,** J9040
**Blood**
  *count, G0306, G0307, S3630*
    *complete CBC, automated, without platelet*
      *count, G0307*
    *complete CBC, automated without platelet count,*
      *automated WBC differential, G0306*
    *eosinophil count, blood, direct, S3630*
  component/product not otherwise classified,
    P9099 ◄
  fresh frozen plasma, P9017
  glucose monitor, E0607, E2100, E2101, *S1030,*
    *S1031, S1034*
    *blood glucose monitor, integrated voice*
      *synthesizer, E2100*
    *blood glucose monitor with integrated lancing/*
      *blood sample, E2101*
    *continuous noninvasive device, purchase, S1030*
    *continuous noninvasive device, rental, S1031*
    *home blood glucose monitor, E0607*
  glucose test, A4253
  *glucose, test strips, dialysis, A4772*
  granulocytes, pheresis, P9050
  ketone test, A4252
  leak detector, dialysis, E1560
  leukocyte poor, P9016
  mucoprotein, P2038
  platelets, P9019
  platelets, irradiated, P9032
  platelets, leukocytes reduced, P9031
  platelets, leukocytes reduced, irradiated, P9033
  platelets, pheresis, P9034, P9072, P9073, P9100
  platelets, pheresis, irradiated, P9036
  platelets, pheresis, leukocytes reduced, P9035
  platelets, pheresis, leukocytes reduced,
    irradiated, P9037
  pressure monitor, A4660, A4663, A4670
  pump, dialysis, E1620
  red blood cells, deglycerolized, P9039
  red blood cells, irradiated, P9038
  red blood cells, leukocytes reduced, P9016
  red blood cells, leukocytes reduced,
    irradiated, P9040

◄ **New**   ⊋ **Revised**   ✔ **Reinstated**   ~~deleted~~ **Deleted**

**Blood** (*Continued*)
  red blood cells, washed, P9022
  strips, A4253
  supply, P9010–P9022
  testing supplies, A4770
  tubing, A4750, A4755
**Blood collection devices accessory,** A4257, E0620
***BMI,*** *G8417–G8422*
**Body jacket**
  scoliosis, L1300, L1310
***Body mass index,*** *G8417–G8422*
**Body sock,** L0984
**Bond or cement, ostomy skin,** A4364
***Bone***
  *density, study, G0130*
**Boot**
  pelvic, E0944
  surgical, ambulatory, L3260
**Bortezomib,** J9041
**Brachytherapy radioelements,** Q3001
  *brachytherapy, LDR, prostate, G0458*
  *brachytherapy planar source, C2645*
  *brachytherapy, source, hospital outpatient,*
    *C1716–C1717, C1719*
**Breast prosthesis,** L8000–L8035, **L8600**
  adhesive skin support, A4280
  *custom breast prosthesis, post mastectomy, L8035*
  *garment with mastectomy form, post*
    *mastectomy, L8015*
  *implantable, silicone or equal, L8600*
  *mastectomy bra, with integrated breast prosthesis*
    *form, unilateral, L8001*
  *mastectomy bra, with prosthesis form,*
    *bilateral, L8002*
  *mastectomy bra, without integrated breast prosthesis*
    *form, L8000*
  *mastectomy form, L8020*
  *mastectomy sleeve, L8010*
  *nipple prosthesis, L8032*
  *silicone or equal, with integral adhesive, L8031*
  *silicone or equal, without integral adhesive, L8030*
**Breast pump**
  accessories, A4281–A4286
    *adapter, replacement, A4282*
    *cap, breast pump bottle, replacement, A4283*
    *locking ring, replacement, A4286*
    *polycarbonate bottle, replacement, A4285*
    *shield and splash protector, replacement, A4284*
    *tubing, replacement, A4281*
  electric, any type, E0603
  heavy duty, hospital grade, E0604
  manual, any type, E0602
**Breathing circuit,** A4618
**Brentuximab Vedotin,** J9042
***Bridge***
  *repair, by report, D6980*
  *replacement, D6930*
**Brolucizumab-dbll,** J0179 ◀

**Brompheniramine maleate,** J0945
**Budesonide inhalation solution,** J7626, J7627,
  J7633, J7634
**Bulking agent,** L8604, L8607
**Buprenorphine hydrochlorides,** J0592
**Buprenorphine/Naloxone,** J0571–J0575
***Burn, compression garment,*** *A6501–A6513*
  *bodysuit, head-foot, A6501*
  *burn mask, face and/or neck, A6513*
  *chin strap, A6502*
  *facial hood, A6503*
  *foot to knee length, A6507*
  *foot to thigh length, A6508*
  *glove to axilla, A6506*
  *glove to elbow, A6505*
  *glove to wrist, A6504*
  *lower trunk, including leg openings, A6511*
  *trunk, including arms, down to leg openings, A6510*
  *upper trunk to waist, including arm openings, A6509*
**Bus, nonemergency transportation,** A0110
**Busulfan,** J0594, J8510
**Butorphanol tartrate,** J0595
***Bypass, graft, coronary, artery***
  *surgery, S2205–S2209*

## C

**C-1 Esterase Inhibitor,** J0596–J0598
**Cabazitaxel,** J9043
**Cabergoline, oral,** J8515
***Cabinet/System, ultraviolet,*** *E0691–E0694*
  *multidirectional light system, 6 ft. cabinet, E0694*
  *timer and eye protection, 4 foot, E0692*
  *timer and eye protection, 6 foot, E0693*
  *ultraviolet light therapy system, treatment area*
    *2 sq ft., E0691*
**Caffeine citrate,** J0706
**Calaspargase pegol injection-mknl,** J9118 ◀
**Calcitonin-salmon,** J0630
**Calcitriol,** J0636, *S0169*
**Calcium**
  disodium edetate, J0600
  gluconate, J0610
  glycerophosphate and calcium lactate, J0620
  lactate and calcium glycerophosphate, J0620
  leucovorin, J0640
**Calibrator solution,** A4256
**Canakinumab,** J0638
***Cancer, screening***
  *cervical or vaginal, G0101*
  *colorectal, G0104–G0106, G0120–G0122, G0328*
    *alternative to screening colonoscopy, barium*
      *enema, G0120*
    *alternative to screening sigmoidoscopy, barium*
      *enema, G0106*
    *barium enema, G0122*
    *colonoscopy, high risk, G0105*

◀ New   ↻ Revised   ✔ Reinstated   ~~deleted~~ Deleted

*Cancer, screening* (Continued)
   *colorectal* (Continued)
     *colonoscopy, not at high-risk, G0121*
     *fecal occult blood test-1–3 simultaneous, G0328*
     *flexible sigmoidoscopy, G0104*
   *prostate, G0102, G0103*
**Cane,** E0100, E0105
   accessory, A4636, A4637
**Canister**
   disposable, used with suction pump, A7000
   non-disposable, used with suction pump, A7001
**Cannula, nasal,** A4615
**Capecitabine, oral,** J8520, J8521
**Capsaicin patch,** J7336
**Carbidopa 5 mg/levodopa 20 mg enteral suspension,** J7340
**Carbon filter,** A4680
**Carboplatin,** J9045
**Cardia Event, recorder, implantable,** E0616
**Cardiokymography,** Q0035
**Cardiovascular services,** M0300–M0301
   *Fabric wrapping abdominal aneurysm, M0301*
   *IV chelation therapy, M0300*
***Cardioverter-defibrillator,*** *G0448*
***Care, coordinated,*** *G9001–G9011*, *H1002*
   *coordinated care fee, home monitoring, G9006*
   *coordinated care fee, initial rate, G9001*
   *coordinated care fee, maintenance rate, G9002*
   *coordinated care fee, physician coordinated care oversight, G9008*
   *coordinated care fee, risk adjusted high, initial, G9003*
   *coordinated care fee, risk adjusted low, initial, G9004*
   *coordinated care fee, risk adjusted maintenance, G9005*
   *coordinated care fee, risk adjusted maintenance, level 3, G9009*
   *coordinated care fee, risk adjusted maintenance, level 4, G9010*
   *coordinated care fee, risk adjusted maintenance, level 5, G9011*
   *coordinated care fee, scheduled team conference, G9007*
   *prenatal care, at-risk, enhanced service, care coordination, H1002*
***Care plan,*** *G0162*
**Carfilzomib,** J9047
***Caries susceptibility test,*** *D0425*
**Carmustine,** J9050
**Case management,** T1016, T1017
   *dental, D9991–D9994*
**Caspofungin acetate,** J0637
**Cast**
   *diagnostic, dental, D0470*
   hand restoration, L6900–L6915
   materials, special, A4590
   supplies, A4580, A4590, Q4001–Q4051
     *body cast, adult, Q4001–Q4002*
     *cast supplies (e.g., plaster), A4580*

**Cast** (Continued)
   supplies (Continued)
     *cast supplies, unlisted types, Q4050*
     *finger splint, static, Q4049*
     *gauntlet cast, adult, Q4013–Q4014*
     *gauntlet cast, pediatric, Q4015–Q4016*
     *hip spica, adult, Q4025–Q4026*
     *hip spica, pediatric, Q4027–Q4028*
     *long arm cast, adult, Q4005–Q4006*
     *long arm cast, pediatric, Q4007–Q4008*
     *long arm splint, adult, Q4017–Q4018*
     *long arm splint, pediatric, Q4019–Q4020*
     *long leg cast, adult, Q4029–Q4030*
     *long leg cast, pediatric, Q4031–Q4032*
     *long leg cylinder cast, adult, Q4033–Q4034*
     *long leg cylinder cast, pediatric, Q4035–Q4036*
     *long leg splint, adult, Q4041–Q4042*
     *long leg splint, pediatric, Q4043–Q4044*
     *short arm cast, adult, Q4009–Q4010*
     *short arm cast, pediatric, Q4011–Q4012*
     *short arm splint, adult, Q4021–Q4022*
     *short arm splint, pediatric, Q4023–Q4024*
     *short leg cast, adult, Q4037–Q4038*
     *short leg cast, pediatric, Q4039–Q4040*
     *short leg splint, adult, Q4045–Q4046*
     *short leg splint, pediatric, Q4047–Q4048*
     *shoulder cast, adult, Q4003–Q4004*
     *special casting material (fiberglass), A4590*
     *splint supplies, miscellaneous, Q4051*
   thermoplastic, L2106, L2126
**Caster**
   front, for power wheelchair, K0099
   wheelchair, E0997, E0998
**Catheter,** A4300–A4355
   anchoring device, A4333, A4334, A5200
   cap, disposable (dialysis), A4860
   external collection device, A4327–A4330, A4347–A7048
   *female external, A4327–A4328*
   indwelling, A4338–A4346
   insertion tray, A4354
   insulin infusion catheter, A4224
   intermittent with insertion supplies, A4353
   irrigation supplies, A4355
   male external, A4324, A4325, A4326, A4348
   oropharyngeal suction, A4628
   starter set, A4329
   trachea (suction), A4609, A4610, A4624
   *transluminal angioplasty, C2623*
   transtracheal oxygen, A4608
   *vascular, A4300–A4301*
**Catheterization, specimen collection,** P9612, P9615
***CBC,*** *G0306, G0307*
**Cefazolin sodium,** J0690
**Cefepime HCl,** J0692
**Cefotaxime sodium,** J0698
**Ceftaroline fosamil,** J0712
**Ceftazidime,** J0713, J0714

◄ New    ↻ Revised    ✔ Reinstated    ~~deleted~~ Deleted

**Ceftizoxime sodium,** J0715
**Ceftolozane 50 mg and tazobactam 25 mg,** J0695
**Ceftriaxone sodium,** J0696
**Cefuroxime sodium,** J0697
**CellCept,** K0412
**Cellesta cord,** Q4214 ◀
**Cellesta or cellesta duo,** Q4184 ◀
**Cellular therapy,** M0075
**Cement, ostomy,** A4364
**Cemiplimab injection-rwlc,** J9119 ◀
**Centrifuge,** A4650
**Centruroides Immune F(ab),** J0716
**Cephalin Floculation, blood,** P2028
**Cephalothin sodium,** J1890
**Cephapirin sodium,** J0710
*Certification, physician, home, health (per calendar month),* G0179–G0182
　*Physician certification, home health,* G0180
　*Physician recertification, home health,* G0179
　*Physician supervision, home health, complex care, 30 min or more,* G0181
　*Physician supervision, hospice 30 min or more,* G0182
**Certolizumab pegol,** J0717
*Cerumen, removal,* G0268
**Cervical**
　*cancer, screening,* G0101
　*cytopathology,* G0123, G0124, G0141–G0148
　　*screening, automated thin layer, manual rescreening, physician supervision,* G0145
　　*screening, automated thin layer preparation, cytotechnologist, physician interpretation,* G0143
　　*screening, automated thin layer preparation, physician supervision,* G0144
　　*screening, by cytotechnologist, physician supervision,* G0123
　　*screening, cytopathology smears, automated system, physician interpretation,* G0141
　　*screening, interpretation by physician,* G0124
　　*screening smears, automated system, manual rescreening,* G0148
　　*screening smears, automated system, physician supervision,* G0147
　halo, L0810–L0830
　head harness/halter, E0942
　orthosis, L0100–L0200
　　*cervical collar molded to patient,* L0170
　　*cervical, flexible collar,* L0120–L0130
　　*cervical, multiple post collar, supports,* L0180–L0200
　　*cervical, semi-rigid collar,* L0150–L0160, L0172, L0174
　　*cranial cervical,* L0112–L0113
　traction, E0855, E0856
**Cervical cap contraceptive,** A4261
**Cervical-thoracic-lumbar-sacral orthosis (CTLSO),** L0700, L0710
**Cetuximab,** J9055

**Chair**
　adjustable, dialysis, E1570
　lift, E0627
　rollabout, E1031
　sitz bath, E0160–E0162
　*transport,* E1035–E1039
　　*chair, adult size, heavy duty, greater than 300 pounds,* E1039
　　*chair, adult size, up to 300 pounds,* E1038
　　*chair, pediatric,* E1037
　　*multi-positional patient transfer system, extra-wide, greater than 300 pounds,* E1036
　　*multi-positional patient transfer system, up to 300 pounds,* E1035
**Chelation therapy,** M0300
**Chemical endarterectomy,** M0300
**Chemistry and toxicology tests,** P2028–P3001
**Chemotherapy**
　administration (hospital reporting only), Q0083–Q0085
　drug, oral, not otherwise classified, J8999
　drugs; (see also drug by name), J9000–J9999
**Chest shell (cuirass),** E0457
**Chest Wall Oscillation System,** E0483
　hose, replacement, A7026
　vest, replacement, A7025
**Chest wrap,** E0459
**Chin cup, cervical,** L0150
**Chloramphenicol sodium succinate,** J0720
**Chlordiazepoxide HCl,** J1990
**Chloromycetin sodium succinate,** J0720
**Chloroprocaine HCl,** J2400
**Chloroquine HCl,** J0390
**Chlorothiazide sodium,** J1205
**Chlorpromazine HCl,** J3230
　*Chlorpromazine HCL, 5 mg, oral,* Q0161
**Chorionic gonadotropin,** J0725
*Choroid, lesion, destruction,* G0186
**Chromic phosphate P32 suspension,** A9564
**Chromium CR-51 sodium chromate,** A9553
**Cidofovir,** J0740
**Cilastatin sodium, imipenem,** J0743
**Cinacalcet,** J0604
**Ciprofloxacin**
　for intravenous infusion, J0744
　octic suspension, J7342
**Cisplatin,** J9060
**Cladribine,** J9065
**Clamp**
　dialysis, A4918
　external urethral, A4356
**Cleanser, wound,** A6260
**Cleansing agent, dialysis equipment,** A4790
**Clofarabine,** J9027
**Clonidine,** J0735
*Closure, wound, adhesive, tissue,* G0168
**Clotting time tube,** A4771
**Clubfoot wedge,** L3380

---

◀ New　　↩ Revised　　✔ Reinstated　　deleted Deleted

◄ New   ↻ Revised   ✔ Reinstated   ~~deleted~~ Deleted

**Contracts, maintenance, ESRD,** A4890
*Contrast,* Q9951–Q9969
   *HOCM,* Q9958–Q9964
   *injection, iron based magnetic resonance, per ml,* Q9953
   *injection, non-radioactive, non-contrast, visualization adjunct,* Q9968
   *injection, octafluoropropane microspheres, per ml,* Q9956
   *injection, perflexane lipid microspheres, per ml,* Q9955
   *injection, perflutren lipid microspheres, per ml,* Q9957
   *LOCM,* Q9965–Q9967
   *LOCM, 400 or greater mg/ml iodine, per ml,* Q9951
   *oral magnetic resonance contrast,* Q9954
   *Tc-99m per study dose,* Q9969
**Contrast material**
   injection during MRI, A4643
   low osmolar, A4644–A4646
*Coordinated, care,* G9001–G9011
   *CORF, registered nurse- face-face,* G0128
**Corneal tissue processing,** V2785
**Corset, spinal orthosis,** L0970–L0976
   *LSO, corset front,* L0972
   *LSO, full corset,* L0976
   *TLSO, corset front,* L0970
   *TLSO, full corset,* L0974
**Corticorelin ovine triflutate,** J0795
**Corticotropin,** J0800
**Corvert (see Ibutilide fumarate)**
**Cosyntropin,** J0833, J0834
**Cough stimulating device,** A7020, E0482
*Counseling*
   *alcohol misuse,* G0443
   *cardiovascular disease,* G0448
   *control of dental disease,* D1310, D1320
   *obesity,* G0447
   *sexually transmitted infection,* G0445
*Count, blood,* G0306, G0307
*Counterpulsation, external,* G0166
**Cover, wound**
   alginate dressing, A6196–A6198
   foam dressing, A6209–A6214
   hydrogel dressing, A6242–A6248
   non-contact wound warming cover, and accessory, A6000, E0231, E0232
   specialty absorptive dressing, A6251–A6256
**CPAP (continuous positive airway pressure) device,** E0601
   headgear, K0185
   humidifier, A7046
   intermittent assist, E0452
**Cradle, bed,** E0280
**Cranial electrotherapy stimulation (CES),** K1002 ◀
**Crib,** E0300
**Cromolyn sodium, inhalation solution, unit dose,** J7631, J7632
**Crotalidae polyvalent immune fab,** J0840

*Crowns,* D2710–D2983, D4249, D6720–D6794
   *clinical crown lengthening-hard tissue,* D4249
   *fixed partial denture retainers, crowns,* D6710–D6794
   *single restoration,* D2710–D2983
**Crutches,** E0110–E0118
   accessories, A4635–A4637, K0102
   *crutch substitute, lower leg,* E0118
   *forearm,* E0110–E0111
   *underarm,* E0112–E0117
**Cryoprecipitate, each unit,** P9012
**CTLSO,** L0700, L0710, L1000–L1120
   *addition, axilla sling,* L1010
   *addition, cover for upright, each,* L1120
   *addition, kyphosis pad,* L1020
   *addition, kyphosis pad, floating,* L1025
   *addition, lumbar bolster pad,* L1030
   *addition, lumbar rib pad,* L1040
   *addition, lumbar sling,* L1090
   *addition, outrigger,* L1080
   *addition, outrigger bilateral, vertical extensions,* L1085
   *addition, ring flange,* L1100
   *addition, ring flange, molded to patient model,* L1110
   *addition, sternal pad,* L1050
   *addition, thoracic pad,* L1060
   *addition, trapezius sling,* L1070
   *anterior-posterior-lateral control, molded to patient model (CTLSO),* L0710
   *cervical, thoracic, lumbar, sacral orthrosis (CTLSO),* L0700
   *furnishing initial orthrosis,* L1000
   *immobilizer, infant size,* L1001
   *tension based scoliosis orthosis, fitting,* L1005
**Cuirass,** E0457
**Culture sensitivity study,** P7001
**Cushion, wheelchair,** E0977
**Cyanocobalamin Cobalt C057,** A9559
**Cycler dialysis machine,** E1594
**Cyclophosphamide,** J9070
   oral, J8530
**Cyclosporine,** J7502, J7515, J7516
**Cytarabine,** J9100
   liposome, J9098
**Cytomegalovirus immune globulin (human),** J0850
*Cytopathology, cervical or vaginal,* G0123, G0124, G0141–G0148

# D

**Dacarbazine,** J9130
**Daclizumab,** J7513
**Dactinomycin,** J9120
**Dalalone,** J1100
**Dalbavancin, 5mg,** J0875
**Dalteparin sodium,** J1645
**Daptomycin,** J0878
**Daratumumab,** J9145

---

◀ New   ↪ Revised   ✔ Reinstated   ~~deleted~~ Deleted

**Darbepoetin Alfa,** *J0881–J0882*

**Daunorubicin**
Citrate, *J9151*
HCl, *J9150*

**DaunoXome (see Daunorubicin citrate)**

**Decitabine,** *J0894*

**Decubitus care equipment,** *E0180–E0199*
*air fluidized bed, E0194*
*air pressure mattress, E0186*
*air pressure pad, standard mattress, E0197*
*dry pressure mattress, E0184*
*dry pressure pad, standard mattress, E0199*
*gel or gel-like pressure pad mattress, standard, E0185*
*gel pressure mattress, E0196*
*heel or elbow protector, E0191*
*positioning cushion, E0190*
*power pressure reducing mattress overlay, with pump, E0181*
*powered air flotation bed, E0193*
*pump, alternating pressure pad, replacement, E0182*
*synthetic sheepskin pad, E0189*
*water pressure mattress, E0187*
*water pressure pad, standard mattress, E0198*

**Deferoxamine mesylate,** *J0895*

**Defibrillator, external,** *E0617, K0606*
battery, *K0607*
electrode, *K0609*
garment, *K0608*

**Degarelix,** *J9155*

**Deionizer, water purification system,** *E1615*

**Delivery/set-up/dispensing,** *A9901*

**Denileukin diftitox,** *J9160*

**Denosumab,** *J0897*

**Density, bone, study,** *G0130*

**Dental procedures**
*adjunctive general services, D9110–D9999*
*alveoloplasty, D7310–D7321*
*analgesia, D9230*
*diagnostic, D0120–D0999*
*endodontics, D3000–D3999*
*evaluations, D0120–D0180*
*implant services, D6000–D6199*
*implants, D3460, D5925, D6010–D6067, D6075–D6199*
*laboratory, D0415–D0999*
*maxillofacial, D5900–D5999*
*orthodontics, D8000–D8999*
*periodontics, D4000–D4999*
*preventive, D1000–D1999*
*prosthetics, D5911–D5960, D5999*
*prosthodontics, fixed, D6200–D6999*
*prosthodontics, removable, D5000–D5999*
*restorative, D2000–D2999*
*scaling, D4341–D4346, D6081*

**Dentures,** *D5110–D5899*

**Depo-estradiol cypionate,** *J1000*

**Dermacell, dermacell awn or dermacell awn porous,** *Q4122* ◀

*Dermal filler injection, G0429*

**Desmopressin acetate,** *J2597*

*Destruction, lesion, choroid, G0186*

**Detector, blood leak, dialysis,** *E1560*

*Developmental testing, G0451*

*Devices, other orthopedic, E1800–E1841*
*assistive listening device, V5267–V5290*

**Dexamethasone**
acetate, *J1094*
inhalation solution, concentrated, *J7637*
inhalation solution, unit dose, *J7638*
intravitreal implant, *J7312*
lacrimal ophthalmic insert, *J1096* ◀
oral, *J8540*
sodium phosphate, *J1100*

**Dextran,** *J7100*

**Dextrose**
saline (normal), *J7042*
water, *J7060, J7070*

**Dextrose, 5% in lactated ringers infusion,** *J7121*

**Dextrostick,** *A4772*

*Diabetes*
*evaluation, G0245, G0246*
*shoes (fitting/modifications), A5500–A5508*
*deluxe feature, depth-inlay shoe, A5508*
*depth inlay shoe, A5500*
*molded from cast patient's foot, A5501*
*shoe with metatarsal bar, A5505*
*shoe with off-set heel(s), A5506*
*shoe with rocker or rigid-bottom rocker, A5503*
*shoe with wedge(s), A5504*
*specified modification NOS, depth-inlay shoe, A5507*
*training, outpatient, G0108, G0109*

**Diagnostic**
*dental services, D0100–D0999*
florbetaben, *Q9983*
flutemetamol F18, *Q9982*
*mammography, digital image, G9899, G9900*
radiology services, *R0070–R0076*

**Dialysate**
concentrate additives, *A4765*
solution, *A4720–A4728*
testing solution, *A4760*

**Dialysis**
air bubble detector, *E1530*
bath conductivity, meter, *E1550*
chemicals/antiseptics solution, *A4674*
disposable cycler set, *A4671*
*emergency, G0257*
equipment, *E1510–E1702*
extension line, *A4672–A4673*
filter, *A4680*
fluid barrier, *E1575*
*home, S9335, S9339*
kit, *A4820*
pressure alarm, *E1540*

---

◀ New    ↻ Revised    ✔ Reinstated    ~~deleted~~ Deleted

**15**

**Dialysis** *(Continued)*
    shunt, A4740
    supplies, A4650–A4927
    tourniquet, A4929
    unipuncture control system, E1580
    *unscheduled,* G0257
    venous pressure clamp, A4918
**Dialyzer,** A4690
**Diaper,** T1500, T4521–T4540, **T4543, T4544**
    adult incontinence garment, A4520, A4553
    incontinence supply, rectal insert, any type,
        each, A4337
    disposable penile wrap, T4545
**Diathermy low frequency ultrasonic treatment**
    **device for home use,** K1004 ◀
**Diazepam,** J3360
**Diazoxide,** J1730
**Diclofenac,** J1130
**Dicyclomine HCl,** J0500
**Diethylstilbestrol diphosphate,** J9165
**Digoxin,** J1160
**Digoxin immune fab (ovine),** J1162
**Dihydroergotamine mesylate,** J1110
**Dimenhydrinate,** J1240
**Dimercaprol,** J0470
**Dimethyl sulfoxide (DMSO),** J1212
**Diphenhydramine HCl,** J1200
**Dipyridamole,** J1245
**Disarticulation**
    lower extremities, prosthesis, L5000–L5999
      *above knee, L5200–L5230*
      *additions exoskeletal-knee-shin system,*
        *L5710–L5782*
      *additions to lower extremities, L5610–L5617*
      *additions to socket insert, L5654–L5699*
      *additions to socket variations, L5630–L5653*
      *additions to test sockets, L5618–L5629*
      *additions/replacements, feet-ankle units,*
        *L5700–L5707*
      *ankle, L5050–L5060*
      *below knee, L5100–L5105*
      *component modification, L5785–L5795*
      *endoskeletal, L5810–L5999*
      *endoskeletal, above knee, L5321*
      *endoskeletal, hip disarticulation, L5331–L5341*
      *endoskeleton, below knee, L5301–L5312*
      *hemipelvectomy, L5280*
      *hip disarticulation, L5250–L5270*
      *immediate postsurgical fitting, L5400–L5460*
      *initial prosthesis, L5500–L5505*
      *knee disarticulation, L5150–L5160*
      *partial foot, L5000–L5020*
      *preparatory prosthesis, L5510–L5600*
    upper extremities, prosthesis, L6000–L6692
      *above elbow, L6250*
      *additions to upper limb, L6600–L6698*
      *below elbow, L6100–L6130*
      *elbow disarticulation, L6200–L6205*

**Disarticulation** *(Continued)*
    upper extremities, prosthesis *(Continued)*
      *endoskeletal, below elbow, L6400*
      *endoskeletal, interscapular thoracic, L6570–L6590*
      *endoskeletal, shoulder disarticulation, L6550*
      *immediate postsurgical procedures, L6380–L6388*
      *interscapular/thoracic, L6350–L6370*
      *partial hand, L6000–L6026*
      *shoulder disarticulation, L6300–L6320*
      *wrist disarticulation, L6050–L6055*
***Disease***
    *status, oncology, G9063–G9139*
***Dispensing, fee, pharmacy,*** *G0333,*
    *Q0510–Q0514,* **S9430**
    *dispensing fee inhalation drug(s), 30 days, Q0513*
    *dispensing fee inhalation drug(s), 90 days, Q0514*
    *inhalation drugs, 30 days, as a beneficiary, G0333*
    *initial immunosuppressive drug(s), post*
      *transplanr, G0510*
    *oral anti-cancer, oral anti-emetic,*
      *immunosuppressive, first prescription, Q0511*
    *oral anti-cancer, oral anti-emetic,*
      *immunosuppressive, subsequent*
      *preparation, Q0512*
**Disposable collection and storage bag for breast**
    **milk,** K1005 ◀
**Disposable supplies, ambulance,** A0382, A0384,
    A0392–A0398
***DME***
    *miscellaneous, A9900–A9999*
      *DME delivery, set up, A9901*
      *DME supple, NOS, A9999*
      *DME supplies, A9900*
**DMSO,** J1212
**Dobutamine HCl,** J1250
**Docetaxel,** J9171
***Documentation***
    *antidepressant, G8126–G8128*
    *blood pressure, G8476–G8478*
    *bypass, graft, coronary, artery, documentation,*
      *G8160–G8163*
    *CABG, G8160–G8163*
    *dysphagia, G8232*
    *dysphagia, screening, G8232, V5364*
    *ECG, 12–lead, G8705, G8706*
    *eye, functions, G8315–G8333*
    *influenza, immunization, G8482–G8484*
    *pharmacologic therapy for osteoporosis, G8635*
    *physician for DME, G0454*
    *prophylactic antibiotic, G8702, G8703*
    *prophylactic parenteral antibiotic, G8629–G8632*
    *prophylaxis, DVT, G8218*
    *prophylaxis, thrombosis, deep, vein, G8218*
    *urinary, incontinence, G8063, G8267*
**Dolasetron mesylate,** J1260
**Dome and mouthpiece (for nebulizer),** A7016
**Dopamine HCl,** J1265
**Doripenem,** J1267

**Dornase alpha, inhalation solution, unit dose form,** J7639

**Doxercalciferol,** J1270

**Doxil,** J9001

**Doxorubicin HCl,** J9000, J9002

**Drainage**

    bag, A4357, A4358

    board, postural, E0606

    bottle, A5102

**Dressing; (see also Bandage),** A6020–A6406

    alginate, A6196–A6199

    collagen, A6020–A6024

    composite, A6200–A6205

    contact layer, A6206–A6208

    foam, A6209–A6215

    gauze, A6216–A6230, A6402–A6406

    holder/binder, A4462

    hydrocolloid, A6234–A6241

    hydrogel, A6242–A6248

    specialty absorptive, A6251–A6256

    transparent film, A6257–A6259

    tubular, A6457

    *wound, K0744–K0746*

**Droperidol,** J1790

    and fentanyl citrate, J1810

**Dropper,** A4649

**Drugs; (see also Table of Drugs)**

    administered through a metered dose inhaler, J3535

    *antiemetic, J8498, J8597, Q0163–Q0181*

    chemotherapy, J8500–J9999

    disposable delivery system, 50 ml or greater per hour, A4305

    disposable delivery system, 5 ml or less per hour, A4306

    immunosuppressive, J7500–J7599

    infusion supplies, A4221, A4222, A4230–A4232

    inhalation solutions, J7608–J7699

    *non-prescription, A9150*

    not otherwise classified, J3490, J7599, J7699, J7799, J7999, J8499, J8999, J9999

    *oral, NOS, J8499*

    prescription, oral, J8499, J8999

**Dry pressure pad/mattress,** E0179, E0184, E0199

**Durable medical equipment (DME),** E0100–E1830, K Codes

    *additional oxygen related equipment, E1352–E1406*

    *arm support, wheelchair, E2626–E2633*

    *artificial kidney machines/accessories, E1500–E1699*

    *attachments, E0156–E0159*

    *bath and toilet aides, E0240–E0249*

    *canes, E0100–E0105*

    *commodes, E0160–E0175*

    *crutches, E0110–E0118*

    *decubitus care equipment, E0181–E0199*

    *DME, respiratory, inexpensive, purchased, A7000–A7509*

    *gait trainer, E8000–E8002*

    *heat/cold application, E0200–E0239*

**Durable medical equipment** *(Continued)*

    *hospital beds and accessories, E0250–E0373*

    *humidifiers/nebulizers/compressors, oxygen IPPB, E0550–E0585*

    *infusion supplies, E0776–E0791*

    *IPPB machines, E0500*

    *jaw motion rehabilitation system, E1700–E1702*

    *miscellaneous, E1902–E2120*

    *monitoring equipment, home glucose, E0607*

    *negative pressure, E2402*

    *other orthopedic devices, E1800–E1841*

    *oxygen/respiratory equipment, E0424–E0487*

    *pacemaker monitor, E0610–E0620*

    *patient lifts, E0621–E0642*

    *pneumatic compressor, E0650–E0676*

    *rollout chair/transfer system, E1031–E1039*

    *safety equipment, E0700–E0705*

    *speech device, E2500–E2599*

    *suction pump/room vaporizers, E0600–E0606*

    *temporary DME codes, regional carriers, K0000–K9999*

    *TENS/stimulation device(s), E0720–E0770*

    *traction equipment, E0830–E0900*

    *trapeze equipment, fracture frame, E0910–E0948*

    *walkers, E0130–E0155*

    *wheelchair accessories, E2201–E2397*

    *wheelchair, accessories, E0950–E1030*

    *wheelchair, amputee, E1170–E1200*

    *wheelchair cusion/protection, E2601–E2621*

    *wheelchair, fully reclining, E1050–E1093*

    *wheelchair, heavy duty, E1280–E1298*

    *wheelchair, lightweight, E1240–E1270*

    *wheelchair, semi-reclining, E1100–E1110*

    *wheelchair, skin protection, E2622–E2625*

    *wheelchair, special size, E1220–E1239*

    *wheelchair, standard, E1130–E1161*

    *whirlpool equipment, E1300–E1310*

**Duraclon, (see Clonidine)**

**Dyphylline,** J1180

***Dysphagia, screening, documentation,*** G8232, V5364

***Dystrophic, nails, trimming,*** G0127

## E

**Ear mold,** V5264, V5265

**Ecallantide,** J1290

**Echocardiography injectable contrast material,** A9700

    *ECG, 12–lead, G8704*

**Eculizumab,** J1300

***ED, visit,*** G0380–G0384

**Edetate**

    calcium disodium, J0600

    disodium, J3520

***Educational Services***

    *chronic kidney disease, G0420, G0421*

**Eggcrate dry pressure pad/mattress,** E0184, E0199

---

◄ New    ↻ Revised    ✔ Reinstated    ~~deleted~~ Deleted

**EKG,** *G0403–G0405*
**Elbow**
  disarticulation, endoskeletal, *L6450*
  orthosis (EO), *E1800, L3700–L3740, L3760, L3671*
    *dynamic adjustable elbow flexion device, E1800*
    *elbow arthrosis, L3702–L3766*
  protector, *E0191*
*Electric hand, L7007–L7008*
*Electric, nerve, stimulator, transcutaneous, A4595, E0720–E0749*
  *conductive garment, E0731*
  *electric joint stimulation device, E0762*
  *electrical stimulator supplies, A4595*
  *electromagnetic wound treatment device, E0769*
  *electronic salivary reflex stimulator, E0755*
  *EMG, biofeedback device, E0746*
  *functional electrical stimulator, nerve and/or muscle groups, E0770*
  *functional stimulator sequential muscle groups, E0764*
  *incontinence treatment system, E0740*
  *nerve stimulator (FDA), treatment nausea and vomiting, E0765*
  *osteogenesis stimulator, electrical, surgically implanted, E0749*
  *osteogenesis stimulator, low-intensity ultrasound, E0760*
  *osteogenesis stimulator, non-invasive, not spinal, E0747*
  *osteogenesis stimulator, non-invasive, spinal, E0748*
  *radiowaves, non-thermal, high frequency, E0761*
  *stimulator, electrical shock unit, E0745*
  *stimulator for scoliosis, E0744*
  *TENS, four or more leads, E0730*
  *TENS, two lead, E0720*
**Electrical stimulation device used for cancer treatment,** *E0766*
**Electrical work, dialysis equipment,** *A4870*
**Electrodes, per pair,** *A4555, A4556*
*Electromagnetic, therapy, G0295, G0329*
*Electronic medication compliance, T1505*
**Electronic positional obstructive sleep apnea treatment,** K1001 ◄
**Elevating leg rest,** *K0195*
**Elliotts b solution,** *J9175*
**Elotuzumab,** *J9176*
*Emapalumab injection-lzsg, J9210* ◄
*Emergency department, visit, G0380–G0384*
**EMG,** *E0746*
**Eminase,** *J0350*
**Endarterectomy, chemical,** *M0300*
*Endodontic procedures, D3000–D3999*
  *periapical services, D3410–D3470*
  *pulp capping, D3110, D3120*
  *root canal therapy, D3310–D3353*
  *therapy, D3310–D3330*
*Endodontics, dental, D3000–D3999*
**Endoscope sheath,** *A4270*

**Endoskeletal system, addition,** *L5848, L5856–L5857, L5925, L5961, L5969*
*Enema, bag, A4458*
**Enfuvirtide,** *J1324*
**Enoxaparin sodium,** *J1650*
**Enteral**
  feeding supply kit (syringe) (pump) (gravity), *B4034–B4036*
  formulae, *B4149–B4156, B4157–B4162*
  nutrition infusion pump (with alarm) (without), *B9000,* **B9002**
  *therapy, supplies, B4000–B9999*
    *enteral and parenteral pumps, B9002–B9999*
    *enteral formula/medical supplies, B0434–B4162*
    *parenteral solutions/supplies, B4164–B5200*
**Epinephrine,** *J0171*
**Epirubicin HCl,** *J9178*
**Epoetin alpha,** *J0885, Q4081*
**Epoetin alpha-epbx, (Retacrit) (for ESRD on dialysis),** Q5105 ◄
**Epoetin alpha-epbx, (Retacrit) (non ESRD use),** Q5106 ◄
**Epoetin beta,** *J0887–J0888*
**Epoprostenol,** *J1325*
*Equipment*
  *decubitus, E0181–E0199*
  *exercise, A9300, E0935, E0936*
  *orthopedic, E0910–E0948, E1800–E8002*
  *oxygen, E0424–E0486, E1353–E1406*
  *pump, E0781, E0784, E0791*
  *respiratory, E0424–E0601*
  *safety, E0700, E0705*
  *traction, E0830–E0900*
  *transfer, E0705*
  *trapeze, E0910–E0912, E0940*
  *whirlpool, E1300, E1310*
**Eravacycline injection,** J0122 ◄
*Erection device, tension ring, L7902*
**Ergonovine maleate,** *J1330*
**Eribulin mesylate,** *J9179*
**Ertapenem sodium,** *J1335*
**Erythromycin lactobionate,** *J1364*
**ESRD (End-Stage Renal Disease); (see also Dialysis)**
  machines and accessories, *E1500–E1699*
    *adjustable chair, ESRD, E1570*
    *centrifuge, dialysis, E1500*
    *dialysis equipment, NOS, E1699*
    *hemodialysis, air bubble detector, replacement, E1530*
    *hemodialysis, bath conductivity meter, E1550*
    *hemodialysis, blood leak detector, replacement, E1560*
    *hemodialysis, blood pump, replacement, E1620*
    *hemodialysis equipment, delivery/instillation charges, E1600*
    *hemodialysis, heparin infusion pump, E1520*
    *hemodialysis machine, E1590*

◄ New    ⮌ Revised    ✔ Reinstated    ~~deleted~~ Deleted

**ESRD** *(Continued)*
  machines and accessories *(Continued)*
    *hemodialysis, portable travel hemodialyzer*
      *system, E1635*
    *hemodialysis, pressure alarm, E1540*
    *hemodialysis, reverse osmosis water system, E1615*
    *hemodialysis, sorbent cartridges, E1636*
    *hemodialysis, transducer protectors, E1575*
    *hemodialysis, unipuncture control system, E1580*
    *hemodialysis, water softening system, E1625*
    *hemostats, E1637*
    *peritoneal dialysis, automatic intermittent*
      *system, E1592*
    *peritoneal dialysis clamps, E1634*
    *peritoneal dialysis, cycler dialysis machine, E1594*
    *peritoneal dialysis, reciprocating system, E1630*
    *scale, E1639*
    *wearable artificial kidney, E1632*
  plumbing, A4870
  supplies, A4651–A4929
    *acetate concentrate solution, hemodialysis, A4708*
    *acid concentrate solution, hemodialysis, A4709*
    *activated carbon filters, hemodialysis, A4680*
    *ammonia test strip, dialysis, A4774*
    *automatic blood pressure monitor, A4670*
    *bicarbonate concentrate, powder,*
      *hemodialysis, A4707*
    *bicarbonate concentrate, solution, A4706*
    *blood collection tube, vaccum, dialysis, A4770*
    *blood glucose test strip, dialysis, A4772*
    *blood pressure cuff only, A4663*
    *blood tubing, arterial and venous,*
      *hemodialysis, A4755*
    *blood tubing, arterial or venous, hemodialysis, A4750*
    *chemicals/antiseptics solution, clean dialysis*
      *equipment, A4674*
    *dialysate solution, non-dextrose, A4728*
    *dialysate solution, peritoneal dialysis,*
      *A4720–A4726, A4760–A4766*
    *dialyzers, hemodialysis, A4690*
    *disposable catheter tips, peritoneal dialysis, A4860*
    *disposable cycler set, dialysis machine, A4671*
    *drainage extension line, dialysis, sterile, A4672*
    *extension line easy lock connectors, dialysis, A4673*
    *fistula cannulation set, hemodialysis, A4730*
    *injectable anesthetic, dialysis, A4737*
    *occult blood test strips, dialysis, A4773*
    *peritoneal dialysis, catheter anchoring device, A4653*
    *protamine sulfate, hemodialysis, A4802*
    *serum clotting timetube, dialysis, A4771*
    *shunt accessory, hemodialysis, A4740*
    *sphygmomanometer, cuff and stethoscope, A4660*
    *syringes, A4657*
    *topical anesthetic, dialysis, A4736*
    *treated water, peritoneal dialysis, A4714*
    *"Y set" tubing, peritoneal dialysis, A4719*
**Estrogen conjugated,** J1410
**Estrone (5, Aqueous),** J1435

**Etelcalcetide,** J0606
**Eteplirsen,** J1428
**Ethanolamine oleate,** J1430
**Etidronate disodium,** J1436
**Etonogestrel implant system,** J7307
**Etoposide,** J9181
  oral, J8560
**Euflexxa,** J7323
*Evaluation*
  *conformity, V5020*
  *contact lens, S0592*
  *dental, D0120–D0180*
  *diabetic, G0245, G0246*
  *footwear, G8410–G8416*
  *hearing, S0618, V5008, V5010*
  *hospice, G0337*
  *multidisciplinary, H2000*
  *nursing, T1001*
  *ocularist, S9150*
  *performance measurement, S3005*
  *resident, T2011*
  *speech, S9152*
  *team, T1024*
**Everolimus,** J7527
*Examination*
  *gynecological, S0610–S0613*
  *ophthalmological, S0620, S0621*
  *oral, D0120–D0160*
  *pinworm, Q0113*
**Exercise**
  *class, S9451*
  equipment, A9300
**External**
  ambulatory infusion pump, E0781, E0784
  ambulatory infusion pump continuous glucose
    sensing, E0787 ◄
  ambulatory insulin delivery system, A9274
  power, battery components, L7360–L7368
  power, elbow, L7160–L7191
  urinary supplies, A4356–A4359
*Extractions; (see also Dental procedures),*
  *D7111–D7140, D7251*
**Extremity**
  belt/harness, E0945
  *traction, E0870–E0880*
**Eye**
  case, V2756
  *functions, documentation, G8315–G8333*
  lens (contact) (spectacle), V2100–V2615
  *pad, patch, A6410–A6412*
  prosthetic, V2623, V2629
  service (miscellaneous), V2700–V2799

## F

**Face tent, oxygen,** A4619
**Faceplate, ostomy,** A4361

---

◄ New    ↻ Revised    ✔ Reinstated    ~~deleted~~ Deleted

**Factor IX,** J7193, J7194, J7195, J7200–J7202
**Factor VIIA coagulation factor, recombinant,** J7189, J7205
**Factor VIII, anti-hemophilic factor,** J7182, J7185, J7190–J7192, J7207–J7209 ↻
**Factor X,** J7175
**Factor XIII, anti-hemophilic factor,** J7180, J7188
**Factor XIII, A-subunit,** J7181
**Family Planning Education,** H1010
*Fee*
   *coordinated care, G9001–G9011*
   *dispensing, pharmacy, G0333, Q0510–Q0514, S9430*
**Fentanyl citrate,** J3010
   and droperidol, J1810
**Fern test,** Q0114
**Ferric pyrophosphate citrate powder,** J1444 ◄
**Ferumoxytol,** Q0138, Q0139
**Filgrastim (G-CSF & TBO),** J1442, J1447, Q5101
**Filler, wound**
   alginate dressing, A6199
   foam dressing, A6215
   hydrocolloid dressing, A6240, A6241
   hydrogel dressing, A6248
   not elsewhere classified, A6261, A6262
**Film, transparent (for dressing),** A6257–A6259
**Filter**
   aerosol compressor, A7014
   dialysis carbon, A4680
   ostomy, A4368
   tracheostoma, A4481
   ultrasonic generator, A7014
**Fistula cannulation set,** A4730
**Flebogamma,** J1572
**Florbetapir F18,** A9586
**Flowmeter,** E0440, E0555, E0580
**Floxuridine,** J9200
**Fluconazole, injection,** J1450
**Fludarabine phosphate,** J8562, J9185
**Fluid barrier, dialysis,** E1575
**Fluid flow,** Q4206 ◄
**Flunisolide inhalation solution,** J7641
**Fluocinolone,** J7311, J7313
   (Yutiq), J7314 ◄
*Fluoride treatment, D1201–D1205*
**Fluorodeoxyglucose F-18 FDG,** A9552
**Fluorouracil,** J9190
*Fluphenazine decanoate, J2680*
**Foam**
   dressing, A6209–A6215
   pad adhesive, A5126
**Folding walker,** E0135, E0143
**Foley catheter,** A4312–A4316, A4338–A4346
   *indwelling catheter, specialty type, A4340*
   *indwelling catheter, three-way, continuous*
     *irrigation, A4346*
   *indwelling catheter, two-way, all silicone, A4344*
   *indwelling catheter, two-way latex, A4338*
   *insertion tray with drainage bag, A4312*

**Foley catheter** *(Continued)*
   *insertion tray with drainage bag, three-way,*
     *continuous irrigation, A4316*
   *insertion tray with drainage bag, two-way*
     *latex, A4314*
   *insertion tray with drainage bag, two-way,*
     *silicone, A4315*
   *insertion tray without drainage bag, A4313*
**Fomepizole,** J1451
**Fomivirsen sodium intraocular,** J1452
**Fondaparinux sodium,** J1652
*Foot care, G0247*
**Footdrop splint,** L4398
**Footplate,** E0175, E0970, L3031
**Footwear, orthopedic,** L3201–L3265
   *additional charge for split size, L3257*
   *Benesch boot, pair, child, L3213*
   *Benesch boot, pair, infant, L3212*
   *Benesch boot, pair, junior, L3214*
   *custom molded shoe, prosthetic shoe, L3250*
   *custom shoe, depth inlay, L3230*
   *ladies shoe, hightop, L3217*
   *ladies shoe, oxford, L3216*
   *ladies shoe, oxford/brace, L3224*
   *mens shoe, depth inlay, L3221*
   *mens shoe, hightop, L3222*
   *mens shoe, oxford, L3219*
   *mens shoe, oxford/brace, L3225*
   *molded shoe, custom fitted, Plastazote, L3253*
   *non-standard size or length, L3255*
   *non-standard size or width, L3254*
   *Plastazote sandal, L3265*
   *shoe, hightop, child, L3206*
   *shoe, hightop, infant, L3204*
   *shoe, hightop, junior, L3207*
   *shoe molded/patient model, Plastazote, L3252*
   *shoe, molded/patient model, silicone, L3251*
   *shoe, oxford, child, L3202*
   *shoe, oxford, infant, L3201*
   *shoe, oxford, junior, L3203*
   *surgical boot, child, L3209*
   *surgical boot, infant, L3208*
   *surgical boot, junior, L3211*
   *surgical boot/shoe, L3260*
**Forearm crutches,** E0110, E0111
**Formoterol,** J7640
   fumarate, J7606
**Fosaprepitant,** J1453
**Foscarnet sodium,** J1455
**Fosphenytoin,** Q2009
**Fracture**
   bedpan, E0276
   frame, E0920, E0930, E0946–E0948
     *attached to bed/weights, E0920*
     *attachments for complex cervical traction, E0948*
     *attachments for complex pelvic traction, E0947*
     *dual, cross bars, attached to bed, E0946*
     *free standing/weights, E0930*

---

◄ New    ↻ Revised    ✔ Reinstated    ~~deleted~~ Deleted

**Fracture** *(Continued)*
  orthosis, L2106–L2136, L3980–L3984
    *ankle/foot orthosis, fracture, L2106–L2128*
    *KAFO, fracture orthosis, L2132–L2136*
    *upper extremity, fracture orthosis, L3980–L3984*
  orthotic additions, L2180–L2192, L3995
    *addition to upper extremity orthosis, sock,*
      *fracture, L3995*
    *additions lower extremity fracture, L2180–L2192*
**Fragmin, (see Dalteparin sodium),** *J1645*
**Frames (spectacles),** V2020, V2025
  *deluxe frame, V2025*
  *purchases, V2020*
**Fremanezumab-vfrm,** J3031 ◄
**Fulvestrant,** J9395
**Furosemide,** J1940

# G

**Gadobutrol,** A9585
**Gadofosveset trisodium,** A9583
**Gadoxetate disodium,** A9581
**Gait trainer,** E8000–E8002
**Gallium Ga67,** A9556
**Gallium nitrate,** J1457
**Galsulfase,** J1458
**Gamma globulin,** J1460, J1560
  *injection, gamma globulin (IM), 1cc, J1460*
  *injection, gamma globulin (IM), over 10cc, J1560*
**Gammagard liquid,** J1569
**Gammaplex,** J1557
**Gamunex,** J1561
**Ganciclovir**
  implant, J7310
  sodium, J1570
**Garamycin,** J1580
**Gas system**
  compressed, E0424, E0425
  gaseous, E0430, E0431, E0441, E0443
  liquid, E0434–E0440, E0442, E0444
*Gastric freezing, hypothermia, M0100*
**Gatifloxacin,** J1590
**Gauze; (see also Bandage)**
  impregnated, A6222–A6233, A6266
  non-impregnated, A6402–A6404
**Gefitinib,** J8565
**Gel**
  conductive, A4558
  pressure pad, E0185, E0196
**Gemcitabine HCl, not otherwise specified,**
  J9201 ↻
  Infugem, J9199 ◄
**Gemtuzumab ozogamicin,** J9203
**Generator**
  *neurostimulator (implantable), high frequency, C1822*
  ultrasonic with nebulizer, E0574–E0575
**Gentamicin (Sulfate),** J1580

*Gingival procedures, D4210–D4240*
  *gingival flap procedure, D4240–D4241*
  *gingivectomy or gingivoplasty, D4210–D4212*
**Glasses**
  air conduction, V5070
  binaural, V5120–V5150
    *behind the ear, V5140*
    *body, V5120*
    *glasses, V5150*
    *in the ear, V5130*
  bone conduction, V5080
  frames, V2020, V2025
  hearing aid, V5230
*Glaucoma*
  *screening, G0117, G0118*
**Gloves,** A4927
**Glucagon HCl,** J1610
**Glucose**
  monitor includes all supplies, K0553
  monitor with integrated lancing/blood sample
    collection, E2101
  monitor with integrated voice synthesizer, E2100
  receiver (monitor) dedicated, K0554
  test strips, A4253, A4772
**Gluteal pad,** L2650
**Glycopyrrolate, inhalation solution,**
  **concentrated,** J7642
**Glycopyrrolate, inhalation solution, unit dose,** J7643
**Gold**
  *foil dental restoration, D2410–D2430*
    *gold foil, one surface, D2410*
    *gold foil, two surfaces, D2420*
    *gold foli, three surfaces, D2430*
  sodium thiomalate, J1600
**Golimumab,** J1602
**Gomco drain bottle,** A4912
**Gonadorelin HCl,** J1620
**Goserelin acetate implant; (see also Implant),** J9202
**Grab bar, trapeze,** E0910, E0940
**Grade-aid, wheelchair,** E0974
*Gradient, compression stockings, A6530–A6549*
  *below knee, 18–30 mmHg, A6530*
  *below knee, 30–40 mmHg, A6531*
  *below knee, thigh length, 18–30 mmHg, A6533*
  *full length/chap style, 18–30 mmHg, A6536*
  *full length/chap style, 30–40 mmHg, A6537*
  *full length/chap style, 40–50 mmHg, A6538*
  *garter belt, A6544*
  *non-elastic below knee, 30–50 mmhg, A6545*
  *sleeve, NOS, A6549*
  *thigh length, 30–40 mmHg, A6534*
  *thigh length, 40–50 mmHg, A6535*
  *waist length, 18–30 mmHg, A6539*
  *waist length, 30–40 mmHg, A6540*
  *waist length, 40–50 mmHg, A6541*
**Granisetron HCl,** J1626
  XR, J1627
**Gravity traction device,** E0941

◄ **New**   ↻ **Revised**   ✔ **Reinstated**   ~~deleted~~ **Deleted**

**Gravlee jet washer,** A4470
*Guidelines, practice, oncology,* G9056–G9062

## H

**Hair analysis (excluding arsenic),** P2031
*Halaven, Injection, eribulin mesylate, 0.1 mg,* J9179
**Hallus-Valgus dynamic splint,** L3100
**Hallux prosthetic implant,** L8642
**Halo procedures,** L0810–L0860
  *addition HALO procedure, MRI compatible*
    *systems,* L0859
  *addition HALO procedure, replacement liner,* L0861
  *cervical halo/jacket vest,* L0810
  *cervical halo/Milwaukee type orthosis,* L0830
  *cervical halo/plaster body jacket,* L0820
**Haloperidol,** J1630
  *decanoate,* J1631
**Halter, cervical head,** E0942
**Hand finger orthosis, prefabricated,** L3923
**Hand restoration,** L6900–L6915
  orthosis (WHFO), E1805, E1825, L3800–L3805,
    L3900–L3954
  partial prosthesis, L6000–L6020
    *partial hand, little and/or ring finger*
      *remaining,* L6010
    *partial hand, no finger,* L6020
    *partial hand, thumb remaining,* L6000
    *transcarpal/metacarpal or partial hand*
      *disarticulation prosthesis,* L6025
  rims, wheelchair, E0967
**Handgrip (cane, crutch, walker),** A4636
**Harness,** E0942, E0944, **E0945**
**Headgear (for positive airway pressure device),** K0185
**Hearing**
  *aid,* V5030–V5267, V5298
    *aid-body worn,* V5100
    *assistive listening device,* V5268–V5274,
      V5281–V5290
    *battery, use in hearing device,* V5266
    *contralateral routing,* V5171–V5172, V5181,
      V5211–V5115, V5221
    *dispensing fee, binaural,* V5160
    *dispensing fee, monaural hearing aid, any*
      *type,* V5241
    *dispensing fee, unspecified hearing aid,* V5090
    *ear impression, each,* V5275
    *ear mold/insert, disposable, any type,* V5265
    *ear mold/insert, not disposable,* V5264
    *glasses, air conduction,* V5070
    *glasses, bone conduction,* V5080
    *hearing aid, analog, binaural, CIC,* V5248
    *hearing aid, analog, binaural, ITC,* V5249
    *hearing aid, analog, monaural, CIC,* V5242
    *hearing aid, analog, monaural, ITC,* V5243
    *hearing aid, BICROS,* V5210–V5240
    *hearing aid, binaural,* V5120–V5150

**Hearing** *(Continued)*
  *aid (Continued)*
    *hearing aid, CROS,* V5170–V5200
    *hearing aid, digital,* V5254–V5261
    *hearing aid, digitally programmable,* V5244–V5247,
      V5250–V5253
    *hearing aid, disposable, any type, binaural,* V5263
    *hearing aid, disposable, any type, monaural,* V5262
    *hearing aid, monaural,* V5030–V5060
    *hearing aid, NOC,* V5298
    *hearing aid or assistive listening device/supplies/*
      *accessories, NOS,* V5267
    *hearing service, miscellaneous,* V5299
    *semi-implantable, middle ear,* V5095
  *assessment,* S0618, V5008, V5010
  *devices,* L8614, V5000–V5169, V5171–V5179,
    V5181–V5209, V5211–V5219, V5221–V5299 ↻
  *services,* V5000–V5999
**Heat**
  application, E0200–E0239
  infrared heating pad system, A4639, E0221
  lamp, E0200, E0205
  pad, A9273, E0210, E0215, E0237, E0249
**Heater (nebulizer),** E1372
***Heavy duty, wheelchair,*** E1280–E1298, K0006,
  K0007, K0801–K0886
  *detachable arms, elevating legrests,* E1280
  *detachable arms, swing away detachable*
    *footrest,* E1290
  *extra heavy duty wheelchair,* K0007
  *fixed full length arms, elevating legrest,* E1295
  *fixed full length arms, swing away detachable*
    *footrest,* E1285
  *heavy duty wheelchair,* K0006
  *power mobility device, not coded by DME PDAC or*
    *no criteria,* K0900
  *power operated vehicle, group 2,* K0806–K0808
  *power operated vehicle, NOC,* K0812
  *power wheelchair, group 1,* K0813–K0816
  *power wheelchair, group 2,* K0820–K0843
  *power wheelchair, group 3,* K0848–K0864
  *power wheelchair, group 4,* K0868–K0886
  *power wheelchair, group 5, pediatric,* K0890–K0891
  *power wheelchair, NOC,* K0898
  *power-operated vehicle, group 1,* K0800–K0802
  *special wheelchair seat depth and/or width, by*
    *construction,* E1298
  *special wheelchair seat depth, by upholstery,* E1297
  *special wheelchair seat height from floor,* E1296
**Heel**
  elevator, air, E0370
  protector, E0191
  shoe, L3430–L3485
  stabilizer, L3170
**Helicopter, ambulance; (see also Ambulance)**
**Helmet**
  cervical, L0100, L0110
  head, A8000–A8004

---

◀ New    ↻ Revised    ✔ Reinstated    ~~deleted~~ Deleted

**Hemin,** J1640

**Hemipelvectomy prosthesis,** L5280

**Hemi-wheelchair,** E1083–E1086

**Hemodialysis machine,** E1590

~~*Hemodialysis, vessel mapping, G0365*~~ ✖

**Hemodialyzer, portable,** E1635

**Hemofil M,** J7190

**Hemophilia clotting factor,** J7190–J7198

   *anti-inhibitor, per IU,* J7198

   *anti-thrombin III, human, per IU,* J7197

   *Factor IX, complex, per IU,* J7194

   *Factor IX, purified, non-recombinant, per IU,* J7193

   *Factor IX, recombinant,* J7195

   *Factor VIII, human, per IU,* J7190

   *Factor VIII, porcine, per IU,* J7191

   *Factor VIII, recombinant, per IU, NOS,* J7192

   *injection, antithrombin recombinant, 50 i.u.,* J7196

   NOC, J7199

**Hemostats,** A4850, E1637

**Hemostix,** A4773

**Hepagam B**

   IM, J1571

   IV, J1573

**Heparin**

   infusion pump, dialysis, E1520

   lock flush, J1642

   sodium, J1644

*Hepatitis B, vaccine, administration,* G0010

**Hep-Lock (U/P),** J1642

**Hexalite,** A4590

**High osmolar contrast material,** Q9958–Q9964

   *HOCM, 400 or greater mg/ml iodine,* Q9964

   *HOCM, 150–199 mg/ml iodine,* Q9959

   *HOCM, 200–249 mg/ml iodine,* Q9960

   *HOCM, 250–299 mg/ml iodine,* Q9961

   *HOCM, 300–349 mg/ml iodine,* Q9962

   *HOCM, 350–399 mg/ml iodine,* Q9963

   *HOCM, up to 149 mg/ml iodine,* Q9958

**Hip**

   disarticulation prosthesis, L5250, L5270

   orthosis (HO), L1600–L1690

**Hip-knee-ankle-foot orthosis (HKAFO),** L2040–L2090

**Histrelin**

   acetate, J1675

   implant, J9225

**HKAFO,** L2040–L2090

*Home*

   *certification, home health,* G0180

   *glucose, monitor,* E0607, E2100, E2101, S1030, S1031

   *health, aide,* G0156, S9122, T1021

   *health, aide, in home, per hour,* S9122

   *health, aide, per visit,* T1021

   *health, clinical, social worker,* G0155

   *health, hospice, each 15 min,* G0156

   *health, occupational, therapist,* G0152

*Home (Continued)*

   *health, physical therapist,* G0151

   *health, physician, certification,* G0179–G0182

   *health, respiratory therapy,* S5180, S5181

   *recerticication, home health,* G0179

   *supervision, home health,* G0181

   *supervision, hospice,* G0182

   *therapist, speech,* S9128

**Home Health Agency Services,** T0221, T1022

   *care improvement home visit assessment,* G9187

*Home sleep study test,* G0398–G0400

*HOPPS,* C1000–C9999

*Hospice care*

   *assisted living facility,* Q5002

   *hospice facility,* Q5010

   *inpatient hospice facility,* Q5006

   *inpatient hospital,* Q5005

   *inpatient psychiatric facility,* Q5008

   *long term care facility,* Q5007

   *nursing long-term facility,* Q5003

   *patient's home,* Q5001

   *skilled nursing facility,* Q5004

*Hospice, evaluation, pre-election,* G0337

*Hospice physician supervision,* G0182

*Hospital*

   *bed,* E0250–E0304, E0328, E0329

   *observation,* G0378, G0379

   *outpatient clinic visit, assessment,* G0463

*Hospital Outpatient Payment System,* C1000–C9999

**Hot water bottle,** A9273

**Human fibrinogen concentrate,** J7178

**Humidifier,** A7046, E0550–E0563

   *durable, diring IPPB treatment,* E0560

   *durable, extensive, IPPB,* E0550

   *durable glass bottle type, for regulator,* E0555

   *heated, used with positive airway pressure device,* E0562

   *non-heated, used with positive airway pressure,* E0561

   *water chamber, humidifier, replacement, positive airway device,* A7046

**Hyalgan,** J7321

*Hyalomatrix,* Q4117

**Hyaluronan,** J7326, J7327

   derivative, J7332 ◀

   durolane, J7318

   gel-Syn, J7328

   genvisc, J7320

   hymovis, J7322

   trivisc, J7329 ◀

**Hyaluronate, sodium,** J7317

**Hyaluronidase,** J3470

   ovine, J3471–J3473

**Hydralazine HCl,** J0360

**Hydraulic patient lift,** E0630

**Hydrocollator,** E0225, E0239

**Hydrocolloid dressing,** A6234–A6241

---

◀ **New**    ↻ **Revised**    ✔ **Reinstated**    ~~deleted~~ **Deleted**

**Hydrocortisone**
  acetate, J1700
  sodium phosphate, J1710
  sodium succinate, J1720
**Hydrogel dressing,** A6231–A6233, A6242–A6248
**Hydromorphone,** J1170
**Hydroxyprogesterone caproate,** J1725–J1726, J1729
**Hydroxyzine HCl,** J3410
**Hygienic item or device, disposable or non-disposable, any type, each,** A9286
**Hylan G-F 20,** J7322
**Hyoscyamine Sulfate,** J1980
**Hyperbaric oxygen chamber, topical,** A4575
**Hypertonic saline solution,** J7130, *J7131*

# I

**Ibandronate sodium,** J1740
**Ibuprofen,** J1741
**Ibutilide Fumarate,** J1742
**Icatibant,** J1744
**Ice**
  cap, E0230
  collar, E0230
**Idarubicin HCl,** J9211
**Idursulfase,** J1743
**Ifosfamide,** J9208
*Iliac, artery, angiography,* G0278
**Iloprost,** Q4074
*Imaging, PET,* G0219, G0235
  *any site, NOS,* G0235
  *whole body, melanoma, non-covered indications,* G0219
**Imiglucerase,** J1786
**Immune globulin,** J1575
  Bivigam, 500 mg, J1556
  Cuvitru, J1555
  Flebogamma, J1572
  Gammagard liquid, J1569
  Gammaplex, J1557
  Gamunex, J1561
  HepaGam B, J1571
  Hizentra, J1559
  Intravenous services, supplies and accessories, Q2052
  NOS, J1566
  Octagam, J1568
  Privigen, J1459
  Rho(D), J2788, J2790, *J2791*
  Rhophylac, J2791
  Subcutaneous, J1562
**Immunosuppressive drug, not otherwise classified,** J7599
**Implant**
  access system, A4301
  aqueous shunt, L8612
  breast, L8600
  buprenorphine implant, J0570
  cochlear, L8614, L8619

**Implant** *(Continued)*
  collagen, urinary tract, L8603
  *dental,* D3460, D5925, D6010–D6067, D6075–D6199
    *crown, provisional,* D6085
    *endodontic endosseous implant,* D3460
    *facial augmentation implant prosthesis,* D5925
    *implant supported prosthetics,* D6055–D6067, D6075–D6077
    *other implant services,* D6080–D6199
    *surgical placement,* D6010–D6051
  dextranomer/hyaluronic acid copolymer, L8604
  ganciclovir, J7310
  hallux, L8642
  infusion pump, programmable, E0783, E0786
    *implantable, programmable,* E0783
    *implantable, programmable, replacement,* E0786
  joint, L8630, L8641, L8658
    *interphalangeal joint spacer, silicone or equal,* L8658
    *metacarpophalangeal joint implant,* L8630
    *metatarsal joint implant,* L8641
  lacrimal duct, A4262, A4263
  *maintenance procedures,* D6080
  *maxillofacial,* D5913–D5937
    *auricular prosthesis,* D5914
    *auricular prosthesis, replacement,* D5927
    *cranial prosthesis,* D5924
    *facial augmentation implant prosthesis,* D5925
    *facial prosthesis,* D5919
    *facial prosthesis, replacement,* D5929
    *mandibular resection prosthesis, with guide flange,* D5934
    *mandibular resection prosthesis, without guide flange,* D5935
    *nasal prosthesis,* D5913
    *nasal prosthesis, replacement,* D5926
    *nasal septal prosthesis,* D5922
    *obturator prosthesis, definitive,* D5932
    *obturator prosthesis, modification,* D5933
    *obturator prosthesis, surgical,* D5931
    *obturator/prosthesis, interim,* D5936
    *ocular prosthesis,* D5916
    *ocular prosthesis, interim,* D5923
    *orbital prosthesis,* D5915
    *orbital prosthesis, replacement,* D5928
    *trismus appliance, not for TM treatment,* D5937
  metacarpophalangeal joint, L8630
  metatarsal joint, L8641
  neurostimulator pulse generator, L8679, L8681–L8688
  not otherwise specified, L8699
  ocular, L8610
  ossicular, L8613
  osteogenesis stimulator, E0749
  percutaneous access system, A4301
  *removal, dental,* D6100
  *repair, dental,* D6090
  replacement implantable intraspinal catheter, E0785
  synthetic, urinary, L8606
  urinary tract, L8603, L8606
  vascular graft, L8670

◀ New    ⤵ Revised    ✔ Reinstated    ~~deleted~~ Deleted

**Implantable radiation dosimeter,** A4650
**Impregnated gauze dressing,** A6222–A6230, *A6231–A6233*
**Incobotulinumtoxin a,** J0588
**Incontinence**
  appliances and supplies, A4310, A4331, A4332, A4360, A5071–A5075, *A5081–A5093,* A5102–A5114
  *garment, A4520, T4521–T4543*
    *adult sized disposable incontinence product, T4522–T4528*
    *any type, e.g. brief, diaper, A4520*
    *pediatric sized disposable incontinence product, T4529–T4532*
    *youth sized disposable incontinence product, T4533–T4534*
  *supply, A4335, A4356–A4360*
    *bedside drainage bag, A4357*
    *disposable external urethral clamp/compression device, A4360*
    *external urethral clamp or compression device, A4356*
    *incontinence supply, miscellaneous, A4335*
    *urinary drainage bag, leg or abdomen, A4358*
  treatment system, E0740
**Indium IN-111**
  carpromab pendetide, A9507
  ibritumomab tiuxetan, A9542
  labeled autologous platelets, A9571
  labeled autologous white blood cells, A9570
  oxyquinoline, A9547
  pentetate, A9548
  pentetreotide, A9572
  satumomab, A4642
**Infliximab injection,** J1745
***Influenza***
  *afluria, Q2035*
  *agriflu, Q2034*
  *flulaval, Q2036*
  *fluvirin, Q2037*
  *fluzone, Q2038*
  *immunization, documentation, G8482–G8484*
  *not otherwise specified, Q2039*
  *vaccine, administration, G0008*
  *virus vaccine, Q2034–Q2039*
**Infusion**
  pump, ambulatory, with administrative equipment, E0781
  pump, continuous glucose sensing supplies for maintenance, A4226 ◀
  pump, heparin, dialysis, E1520
  pump, implantable, E0782, E0783
  pump, implantable, refill kit, A4220
  pump, insulin, E0784
  pump, mechanical, reusable, E0779, E0780
  pump, uninterrupted infusion of Epiprostenol, K0455
  replacement battery, A4602
  *saline, J7030–J7060*
  supplies, A4219, A4221, A4222, A4225, A4230–A4232, E0776–E0791
  therapy, other than chemotherapeutic drugs, Q0081

**Inhalation solution; (see also drug name),** J7608–J7699, Q4074
***Injection device, needle-free, A4210***
**Injections; (see also drug name),** J0120–J2504, J2794, J2798, J1303, J1943–J1944, J2506, J3031, J7311, J7313, J7314, J7320, J7332, J7208, J9032, J9036, J9039, J9044, J9057, J9153, J9118, J9173, J9199, J9201, J9210, J9229, J9269, J9271, J9299, J9308, J9309, J9313, J9355, J9356, Q5112–Q5118, Q9950, Q9991, Q9992 ↻
  *ado-trastuzumab emtansine, 1 mg, J9354*
  *aripiprazole, extended release, J0401*
  *arthrography, sacroiliac, joint, G0259, G0260*
  *carfilzomib, 1 mg, J9047*
  *certolizumab pegol, J0717*
  *dental service, D9610, D9630*
    *other drugs/medicaments, by report, D9630*
    *therapeutic parenteral drug, single administration, D9610*
    *therapeutic parenteral drugs, two or more administrations, different medications, D9612*
  *dermal filler (LDS), G0429*
  *filgrastim, J1442*
  *interferon beta-1a, IM, Q3027*
  *interferon beta-1a, SC, Q3028*
  *omacetaxtine mepesuccinate, 0.01 mg, J9262*
  *pertuzumb, 1 mg, J9306*
  *sculptra, 0.5 mg, Q2028*
  *supplies for self-administered, A4211*
  *vincristine, 1 mg, J9371*
  *ziv-aflibercept, 1 mg, J9400*
***Inlay/onlay dental restoration,*** *D2510–D2664*
***INR, monitoring,*** *G0248–G0250*
  *demonstration prior to initiation, home INR, G0248*
  *physician review and interpretation, home INR, G0250*
  *provision of test materials, home INR, G0249*
**Insertion tray,** A4310–A4316
**Instillation, hexaminolevulinate hydrochloride,** A9589
**Insulin,** J1815, J1817, S5550–S5571
  *ambulatory, external, system, A9274*
  *treatment, outpatient, G9147*
***Integra flowable wound matrix,*** *Q4114*
**Interferon**
  Alpha, J9212–J9215
  Beta-1a, J1826, Q3027, Q3028
  Beta-1b, J1830
  Gamma, J9216
**Intermittent**
  assist device with continuous positive airway pressure device, E0470–E0472
  limb compression device, E0676
  peritoneal dialysis system, E1592
  positive pressure breathing machine (IPPB), E0500
**Interphalangeal joint, prosthetic implant,** L8658, L8659

---

◀ New   ↻ Revised   ✔ Reinstated   ~~deleted~~ Deleted

**Interscapular thoracic prosthesis**
  endoskeletal, L6570
  upper limb, L6350–L6370
*Intervention, alcohol/substance (not tobacco),*
  *G0396–G0397*
*Intervention, tobacco, G9016*
**Intraconazole,** J1835
**Intraocular**
  lenses, V2630–V2632
*Intraoral radiographs, dental, D0210–D0240*
  *intraoral-complete series, D0210*
  *intraoral-occlusal image, D0420*
  *intraoral-periapical-each additional*
    *image, D0230*
  *intraoral-periapical-first radiographic*
    *image, D0220*
**Intrapulmonary percussive ventilation**
  **system,** E0481
**Intrauterine copper contraceptive,** J7300
**Inversion/eversion correction device,** A9285
**Iodine I-123**
  iobenguane, A9582
  ioflupane, A9584
  sodium iodide, A9509, A9516
**Iodine I-125**
  serum albumin, A9532
  sodium iodide, A9527
  sodium iothalamate, A9554
**Iodine I-131**
  iodinated serum albumin, A9524
  sodium iodide capsule, A9517, A9528
  sodium iodide solution, A9529–A9531
**Iodine Iobenguane sulfate I-131,** A9508
**Iodine swabs/wipes,** A4247
**IPD**
  system, E1592
**Ipilimumab,** J9228
**IPPB machine,** E0500
**Ipratropium bromide, inhalation solution, unit**
  **dose,** J7644, J7645
**Irinotecan,** J9205, J9206
**Iron**
  Dextran, J1750
  sucrose, J1756
**Irrigation solution for bladder calculi,** Q2004
**Irrigation supplies,** A4320–A4322, A4355,
  A4397–A4400
  *irrigation supply, sleeve, each, A4397*
  *irrigation syringe, bulb, or piston, each, A4320*
  *irrigation tubing set, bladder irrigation, A4355*
  *ostomy irrigation set, A4400*
  *ostomy irrigation supply, bag, A4398*
  *ostomy irrigation supply, cone/catheter, A4399*
**Irrigation/evacuation system, bowel**
  control unit, E0350
  disposable supplies for, E0352
  manual pump enema, A4459
**Isavuconazonium,** J1833

*Islet, transplant, G0341–G0343, S2102*
**Isoetharine HCl, inhalation solution**
  concentrated, J7647, J7648
  unit dose, J7649, J7650
**Isolates,** B4150, B4152
**Isoproterenol HCl, inhalation solution**
  concentrated, J7657, J7658
  unit dose, J7659, J7660
**Isosulfan blue,** Q9968
*Item, non-covered, A9270*
*IUD, J7300, S4989*
**IV pole, each,** E0776, K0105
**Ixabepilone,** J9207

## J

**Jacket**
  scoliosis, L1300, L1310
*Jaw, motion, rehabilitation system, E1700–E1702*
**Jenamicin,** J1580
*Jetria, (ocriplasmin), J7316*

## K

*Kadcyla, ado-trastuzumab emtansine,*
  *1 mg, J9354*
**Kanamycin sulfate,** J1840, J1850
**Kartop patient lift, toilet or bathroom; (see also**
  **Lift),** E0625
**Keramatrix or kerasorb,** J4165 ◄
**Ketorolac thomethamine,** J1885
**Kidney**
  ESRD supply, A4650–A4927
  *machine, E1500–E1699*
  *machine, accessories, E1500–E1699*
  system, E1510
  wearable artificial, E1632
**Kits**
  enteral feeding supply (syringe) (pump) (gravity),
    B4034–B4036
  fistula cannulation (set), A4730
  parenteral nutrition, B4220–B4224
    *administration kit, per day, B4224*
    *supply kit, home mix, per day, B4222*
    *supply kit, premix, per day, B4220*
  surgical dressing (tray), A4550
  tracheostomy, A4625
**Knee**
  *arthroscopy, surgical, G0289, S2112, S2300*
    *knee, surgical, harvesting cartilage, S2112*
    *knee, surgical, removal loose body, chondroplasty,*
      *different compartment, G0289*
    *shoulder, surgical, thermally-induced,*
      *capsulorraphy, S2300*
  disarticulation, prosthesis, L5150, L5160
  joint, miniature, L5826

**Knee** *(Continued)*
orthosis (KO), E1810, L1800–L1885
*dynamic adjustable elbow extension/flexion device, E1800*
*dynamic adjustable knee extension/flexion device, E1810*
*static-progressive devices, E1801, E1806, E1811, E1816–E1818, E1831, E1841*
**Knee-ankle-foot device with microprocessor control, L2006**
**Knee-ankle-foot orthosis (KAFO), L2000–L2039, L2126–L2136**
addition, high strength, lightweight material, L2755
*base procedure, used with any knee joint, double upright, double bar, L2020*
*base procedure, used with any knee joint, full plastic double upright, L2036*
*base procedure, used with any knee joint, single upright, single bar, L2000*
*foot orthrosis, double upright, double bar, without knee joint, L2030*
*foot orthrosis, single upright, single bar, without knee joint, L2010*
**Kovaltry,** J7211
**Kyphosis pad,** L1020, L1025

# L

*Laboratory*
*dental, D0415–D0999*
*adjunctive pre-diagnostic tests, mucosal abnormalities, D0431*
*analysis saliva sample, D0418*
*caries risk assessment, low, D0601*
*caries risk assessment, moderate, D0602*
*caries susceptibility tests, D0425*
*collection and preparation, saliva sample, D0417*
*collection of microorganisms for culture and sensitivity, D0415*
*diagnostic casts, D0470*
*oral pathology laboratory, D0472–D0502*
*processing, D0414*
*pulp vitality tests, D0460*
*services, P0000–P9999*
*viral culture, D0416*
**Laboratory tests**
chemistry, P2028–P2038
*cephalin flocculation, blood, P2028*
*congo red, blood, P2029*
*hair analysis, excluding arsenic, P2031*
*mucoprotein, blood, P2038*
*thymol turbidity, blood, P2033*
microbiology, P7001
miscellaneous, P9010–P9615, Q0111–Q0115
*blood, split unit, P9011*
*blood, whole, transfusion, unit, P9010*

**Laboratory tests** *(Continued)*
miscellaneous *(Continued)*
*catheterization, collection specimen, multiple patients, P9615*
*catheterization, collection specimen, single patient, P9612*
*cryoprecipitate, each unit, P9012*
*fern test, Q0114*
*fresh frozen plasma, donor retested, each unit, P9060*
*fresh frozen plasma (single donor), frozen within 8 hours, P9017*
*fresh frozen plasma, within 8–24 hours of collection, each unit, P9059*
*granulocytes, pheresis, each unit, P9050*
*infusion, albumin (human), 25%, 20 ml, P9046*
*infusion, albumin (human), 25%, 50 ml, P9047*
*infusion, albumin (human), 5%, 250 ml, P9045*
*infusion, albumin (human), 5%, 50 ml, P9041*
*infusion, plasma protein fraction, human, 5%, 250 ml, P9048*
*infusion, plasma protein fraction, human, 5%, 50 ml, P9043*
*KOH preparation, Q0112*
*pinworm examinations, Q0113*
*plasma, cryoprecipitate reduced, each unit, P9044*
*plasma, pooled, multiple donor, frozen, P9023*
*platelet rich plasma, each unit, P9020*
*platelets, each unit, P9019*
*platelets, HLA-matched leukocytes reduced, apheresis/pheresis, each unit, P9052*
*platelets, irradiated, each unit, P9032*
*platelets, leukocytes reduced, CMV-neg, aphresis/pheresis, each unit, P9055*
*platelets, leukocytes reduced, each unit, P9031*
*platelets, leukocytes reduced, irradiated, each unit, P9033*
*platelets, pheresis, each unit, P9034*
*platelets, pheresis, irradiated, each unit, P9036*
*platelets, pheresis, leukocytes reduced, CMV-neg, irradiated, each unit, P9053*
*platelets, pheresis, leukocytes reduced, each unit, P9035*
*platelets, pheresis, leukocytes reduced, irradiated, each unit, P9037*
*post-coital, direct qualitative, vaginal or cervical mucous, Q0115*
*red blood cells, deglycerolized, each unit, P9039*
*red blood cells, each unit, P9021*
*red blood cells, frozen/deglycerolized/washed, leukocytes reduced, irradiated, each unit, P9057*
*red blood cells, irradiated, each unit, P9038*
*red blood cells, leukocytes reduced, CMV-neg, irradiated, each unit, P9058*
*red blood cells, leukocytes reduced, each unit, P9016*

---

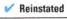 ◀ New   ⏎ Revised   ✔ Reinstated   ~~deleted~~ **Deleted**

**Laboratory tests** *(Continued)*
 miscellaneous *(Continued)*
  *red blood cells, leukocytes reduced, irradiated, each unit, P9040*
  *red blood cells, washed, each unit, P9022*
  *travel allowance, one way, specimen collection, home/nursing home, P9603, P9604*
  *wet mounts, vaginal, cervical, or skin, Q0111*
  *whole blood, leukocytes reduced, irradiated, each unit, P9056*
  *whole blood or red blood cells, leukocytes reduced, CMV-neg, each unit, P9051*
  *whole blood or red blood cells, leukocytes reduced, frozen, deglycerol, washed, each unit, P9054*
 toxicology, P3000–P3001, Q0091
**Lacrimal duct, implant**
 permanent, A4263
 temporary, A4262
**Lactated Ringer's infusion,** J7120
**Laetrile,** J3570
**Lanadelumab-flyo,** J0593 ◄
**Lancet,** A4258, A4259
*Language, screening, V5363*
**Lanreotide,** J1930
**Laronidase,** J1931
**Larynx, artificial,** L8500
**Laser blood collection device and accessory,** A4257, E0620
*LASIK, S0800*
**Lead investigation,** T1029
**Lead wires, per pair,** A4557
**Leg**
 bag, A4358, A5105, A5112
  *leg or abdomen, vinyl, with/without tubes, straps, each, A4358*
  *urinary drainage bag, leg bag, leg/abdomen, latex, with/without tube, straps, A5112*
  *urinary suspensory, leg bag, with/without tube, each, A5105*
 extensions for walker, E0158
 rest, elevating, K0195
 rest, wheelchair, E0990
 strap, replacement, A5113–A5114
**Legg Perthes orthosis,** L1700–L1755
 *Newington type, L1710*
 *Patten bottom type, L1755*
 *Scottish Rite type, L1730*
 *Tachdjian type, L1720*
 *Toronto type, L1700*
**Lens**
 aniseikonic, V2118, V2318
 contact, V2500–V2599
  *gas permeable, V2510–V2513*
  *hydrophilic, V2520–V2523*
  *other type, V2599*
  *PMMA, V2500–V2503*
  *scleral, gas, V2530–V2531*

**Lens** *(Continued)*
 eye, V2100–V2615, V2700–V2799
  *bifocal, glass or plastic, V2200–V2299*
  *contact lenses, V2500–V2599*
  *low vision aids, V2600–V2615*
  *miscellaneous, V2700–V2799*
  *single vision, glass or plastic, V2100–V2199*
  *trifocal, glass or plastic, V2300–V2399*
  *variable asphericity, V2410–V2499*
 intraocular, V2630–V2632
  *anterior chamber, V2630*
  *iris supported, V2631*
  *new technology, category 4, IOL, Q1004*
  *new technology, category 5, IOL, Q1005*
  *posterior chamber, V2632*
  *telescopic lens, C1840*
 low vision, V2600–V2615
  *hand held vision aids, V2600*
  *single lens spectacle mounted, V2610*
  *telescopic and other compound lens system, V2615*
 progressive, V2781
**Lepirudin,** J1945
*Lesion, destruction, choroid, G0186*
**Leucovorin calcium,** J0640
**Leukocyte poor blood, each unit,** P9016
**Leuprolide acetate,** J1950, J9217, J9218, J9219
 *for depot suspension, 7.5 mg, J9217*
 *implant, 65 mg, J9219*
 *injection, for depot suspension, per 3.75 mg, J1950*
 *per 1 mg, J9218*
**Levalbuterol, all formulations, inhalation solution**
 concentrated, J7607, J7612
 unit dose, J7614, J7615
**Levetiracetam,** J1953
**Levocarnitine,** J1955
**Levofloxacin,** J1956
**Levoleucovorin injection,** J0641 ⮌
**Levoleucovorin injection (khapzory),** J0642 ◄
**Levonorgestrel, (contraceptive), implants and supplies,** J7306
**Levorphanol tartrate,** J1960
**Lexidronam,** A9604
**Lidocaine HCl,** J2001
**Lift**
 patient (includes seat lift), E0621–E0635
  *bathroom or toilet, E0625*
  *mechanism incorporated into a combination lift-chair, E0627*
  *patient lift, electric, E0635*
  *patient lift, hydraulic or mechanical, E0630*
  *separate seat lift mechanism, patient owned furniture, non-electric, E0629*
  *sling or seat, canvas or nylon, E0621*
 shoe, L3300–L3334
  *lift, elevation, heel, L3334*
  *lift, elevation, heel and sole, cork, L3320*
  *lift, elevation, heel and sole, Neoprene, L3310*

---

◄ **New**  ⮌ **Revised**  ✔ **Reinstated**  ~~deleted~~ **Deleted**

**Lift** *(Continued)*
  shoe *(Continued)*
    *lift, elevation, heel, tapered to metatarsals, L3300*
    *lift, elevation, inside shoe, L3332*
    *lift, elevation, metal extension, L3330*
*Lightweight, wheelchair, E1087–E1090, E1240–E1270*
  *detachable arms, swing away detachable, elevating leg rests, E1240*
  *detachable arms, swing away detachable footrest, E1260*
  *fixed full length arms, swing away detachable elevating legrests, E1270*
  *fixed full length arms, swing away detachable footrest, E1250*
  *high strength, detachable arms desk, E1088*
  *high strength, detachable arms desk or full length, E1090*
  *high strength, fixed full length arms, E1087*
  *high strength, fixed length arms swing away footrest, E1089*
**Lincomycin HCl,** J2010
**Linezolid,** J2020
**Liquid barrier, ostomy,** A4363
*Listening devices, assistive, V5281–V5290*
  *personal blue tooth FM/DM, V5286*
  *personal FM/DM adapter/boot coupling device for receiver, V5289*
  *personal FM/DM binaural, 2 receivers, V5282*
  *personal FM/DM, direct audio input, V5285*
  *personal FM/DM, ear level receiver, V5284*
  *personal FM/DM monaural, 1 receiver, V5281*
  *personal FM/DM neck, loop induction receiver, V5283*
  *personal FM/DM transmitter assistive listening device, V5288*
  *transmitter microphone, V5290*
**Lodging, recipient, escort nonemergency transport,** A0180, A0200
*LOPS, G0245–G0247*
  *follow-up evaluation and management, G0246*
  *initial evaluation and management, G0245*
  *routine foot care, G0247*
**Lorazepam,** J2060
*Loss of protective sensation, G0245–G0247*
**Low osmolar contrast material,** Q9965–Q9967
**Loxapine, for inhalation,** J2062
**LSO,** L0621–L0640
**Lubricant,** A4332, A4402
**Lumbar flexion,** L0540
**Lumbar-sacral orthosis (LSO),** L0621–L0640
*LVRS, services, G0302–G0305*
**Lymphocyte immune globulin,** J7504, J7511

# M

*Machine*
  *IPPB, E0500*
  *kidney, E1500–E1699*

**Magnesium sulphate,** J3475
**Maintenance contract, ESRD,** A4890
*Mammography, screening, G9899, G9900*
**Mannitol,** J2150, J7665
~~Mapping, vessel, for hemodialysis access, G0365~~ ✖
*Marker, tissue, A4648*
**Mask**
  aerosol, K0180
  oxygen, A4620
**Mastectomy**
  bra, L8000
  form, L8020
  prosthesis, L8030, L8600
  sleeve, L8010
*Matristem, Q4118*
  *micromatrix, 1 mg, Q4118*
**Mattress**
  air pressure, E0186
  alternating pressure, E0277
  dry pressure, E0184
  gel pressure, E0196
  hospital bed, E0271, E0272
  non-powered, pressure reducing, E0373
  overlay, E0371–E0372
  powered, pressure reducing, E0277
  water pressure, E0187
*Measurement period*
  *left ventricular function testing, G8682*
**Mecasermin,** J2170
**Mechlorethamine HCl,** J9230
*Medicaid, codes, T1000–T9999*
**Medical and surgical supplies,** A4206–A8999
*Medical nutritional therapy, G0270, G0271*
*Medical services, other, M0000–M9999*
**Medroxyprogesterone acetate,** J1050
**Melphalan**
  HCl, J9245
  oral, J8600
**Membrane graft/wrap,** Q4205 ◄
*Mental, health, training services, G0177*
**Meperidine,** J2175
  and promethazine, J2180
**Mepivacaine HCl,** J0670
**Mepolizumab,** J2182
**Meropenem,** J2185
**Mesna,** J9209
**Metacarpophalangeal joint, prosthetic implant,** L8630, L8631
**Metaproterenol sulfate, inhalation solution**
  concentrated, J7667, J7668
  unit dose, J7669, J7670
**Metaraminol bitartrate,** J0380
**Metatarsal joint, prosthetic implant,** L8641
**Meter, bath conductivity, dialysis,** E1550
**Methacholine chloride,** J7674
**Methadone HCl,** J1230
*Methergine, J2210*
**Methocarbamol,** J2800

---

◄ New    ⟳ Revised    ✔ Reinstated    ~~deleted~~ Deleted

**Methotrexate**
  oral, J8610
  sodium, J9250, J9260
**Methyldopate HCl,** J0210
**Methylene blue,** Q9968
**Methylnaltrexone,** J2212
**Methylprednisolone**
  acetate, J1020–J1040
    *injection, 20 mg, J1020*
    *injection, 40 mg, J1030*
    *injection, 80 mg, J1040*
  oral, J7509
  sodium succinate, J2920, J2930
**Metoclopramide HCl,** J2765
**Micafungin sodium,** J2248
**Microbiology test,** P7001
**Midazolam HCl,** J2250
**Mileage**
  *ALS, A0390*
  ambulance, A0380, A0390
**Milrinone lactate,** J2260
**Mini-bus, nonemergency transportation,** A0120
**Minocycline hydrochloride,** J2265
*Miscellaneous and investigational, A9000–A9999*
**Mitomycin,** J7315, J9280
**Mitoxantrone HCl,** J9293
*MNT, G0270, G0271*
*Mobility device, physician, service, G0372*
**Modalities, with office visit,** M0005–M0008
**Mogamulizumab injection-kpkc,** J9201 ◄
**Moisture exchanger for use with invasive mechanical ventilation,** A4483
**Moisturizer, skin,** A6250
*Molecular pathology procedure, G0452*
**Mometasone furoate sinus implant,** J7401 ◄
**Monitor**
  blood glucose, home, E0607
  blood pressure, A4670
  pacemaker, E0610, E0615
**Monitoring feature/device,** A9279
*Monitoring, INR, G0248–G0250*
  *demonstration prior to initiation, G0248*
  *physician review and interpretation, G0250*
  *provision of test materials, G0249*
**Monoclonal antibodies,** J7505
**Morphine sulfate,** J2270
  epidural or intrathecal use, J2274
*Motion, jaw, rehabilitation system, E1700–E1702*
  *motion rehabilitation system, E1700*
  *replacement cushions, E1701*
  *replacement measuring scales, E1702*
**Mouthpiece (for respiratory equipment),** A4617
**Moxetumomab pasudotox-tdfx,** J9313 ◄
**Moxifloxacin,** J2280
**Mucoprotein, blood,** P2038
**Multiaxial ankle,** L5986
**Multidisciplinary services,** H2000–H2001, T1023–T1028

**Multiple post collar, cervical,** L0180–L0200
  *occipital/mandibular supports, adjustable, L0180*
  *occipital/mandibular supports, adjustable cervical bars, L0200*
  *SQMI, Guilford, Taylor types, L0190*
**Multi-Podus type AFO,** L4396
**Muromonab-CD3,** J7505
**Mycophenolate mofetil,** J7517
**Mycophenolic acid,** J7518
**MyOwn skin,** Q4226 ◄

# N

**Nabilone,** J8650
*Nails, trimming, dystrophic, G0127*
**Nalbuphine HCl,** J2300
**Naloxone HCl,** J2310
**Naltrexone,** J2315
**Nandrolone**
  decanoate, J2320
**Narrowing device, wheelchair,** E0969
**Nasal**
  application device, K0183
  pillows/seals (for nasal application device), K0184
  vaccine inhalation, J3530
**Nasogastric tubing,** B4081, B4082
**Natalizumab,** J2323
**Nebulizer,** E0570–E0585
  aerosol compressor, E0571, *E0572*
  aerosol mask, A7015
  corrugated tubing, disposable, A7010
  filter, disposable, A7013
  filter, non-disposable, A7014
  heater, E1372
  large volume, disposable, prefilled, A7008
  large volume, disposable, unfilled, A7007
  not used with oxygen, durable, glass, A7017
  pneumatic, administration set, A7003, A7005, A7006
  pneumatic, nonfiltered, A7004
  portable, E0570
  small volume, A7003–A7005
  ultrasonic, E0575
  ultrasonic, dome and mouthpiece, A7016
  ultrasonic, reservoir bottle, non-disposable, A7009
  water collection device, large volume nebulizer, A7012
**Necitumumab,** J9295
**Needle,** A4215
  *bone marrow biopsy, C1830*
  non-coring, A4212
  with syringe, A4206–A4209
**Negative pressure wound therapy pump,** E2402
  accessories, A6550
**Nelarabine,** J9261
**Neonatal transport, ambulance, base rate,** A0225
**Neostigmine methylsulfate,** J2710

---

◄ **New**    ⮌ **Revised**    ✔ **Reinstated**    ~~deleted~~ **Deleted**

*Nerve, conduction, sensory, test,* G0255
**Nerve stimulator with batteries,** E0765
**Nesiritide injection,** J2324, *J2325*
*Neupogen, injection, filgrastim, 1 mcg,* J1442
**Neuromuscular stimulator,** E0745
*Neurophysiology, intraoperative, monitoring,* G0453
**Neurostimulator**
  battery recharging system, L8695
  external antenna, L8696
  *implantable pulse generator,* L8679
  pulse generator, L8681–L8688
    *dual array, non-rechargeable, with extension,* L8688
    *dual array, rechargeable, with extension,* L8687
    *patient programmer (external), replacement only,* L8681
    *radiofrequency receiver,* L8682
    *radiofrequency transmitter (external), sacral root receiver, bowel and bladder management,* L8684
    *radiofrequency transmitter (external), with implantable receiver,* L8683
    *single array, rechargeable, with extension,* L8686
**Nipple prosthesis, custom fabricated, reusable,** L8033 ◄
**Nipple prosthesis, prefabricated, reusable,** L8032 ◄
**Nitrogen N-13 ammonia,** A9526
*NMES,* E0720–E0749
**Nonchemotherapy drug, oral, NOS,** J8499
**Noncovered services,** A9270
**Nonemergency transportation,** A0080–A0210
**Nonimpregnated gauze dressing,** A6216–A6221, A6402–A6404
**Nonprescription drug,** A9150
**Not otherwise classified drug,** J3490, J7599, J7699, J7799, J8499, J8999, J9999, Q0181
**Novafix,** Q4208 ◄
*NPH,* J1820
*NPWT, pump,* E2402
**NTIOL category 3,** Q1003
**NTIOL category 4,** Q1004
**NTIOL category 5,** Q1005
**Nursing care,** T1030–T1031
*Nursing service, direct, skilled, outpatient,* G0128
**Nusinersen,** J2326
**Nutrition**
  *counseling, dental,* D1310, *D1320*
  enteral infusion pump, B9002
  parenteral infusion pump, B9004, B9006
  parenteral solution, B4164–B5200
  *therapy, medical,* G0270, G0271

## O

**O & P supply/accessory/service,** L9900
*Observation*
  *admission,* G0379
  *hospital,* G0378

*Obturator prosthesis*
  *definitive,* D5932
  *interim,* D5936
  *surgical,* D5931
**Occipital/mandibular support, cervical,** L0160
*Occlusive device, placement,* G0269
*Occupational, therapy,* G0129, S9129
**Ocrelizumab,** J2350
**Ocriplasmin,** J7316
**Octafluoropropane,** Q9956
**Octagam,** J1568
**Octreotide acetate,** J2353, J2354
**Ocular prosthetic implant,** L8610
**Ofatumumab,** J9302
**Olanzapine,** J2358
**Olaratumab,** J9285
**Omacetaxine Mepesuccinate,** J9262
**Omadacycline,** J0121 ◄
**Omalizumab,** J2357
**Omegaven,** B4187 ◄
**OnabotulinumtoxinA,** J0585
*Oncology*
  *disease status,* G9063–G9139
  *practice guidelines,* G9056–G9062
  *visit,* G9050–G9055
**Ondansetron HCl,** J2405
**Ondansetron oral,** Q0162
**One arm, drive attachment,** K0101
*Ophthalmological examination, refraction,* S0621
**Oprelvekin,** J2355
*Oral and maxillofacial surgery,* D7111–D7999
  *alveoloplasty,* D7310–D7321
  *complicated suturing,* D7911–D7912
  *excision of bone tissue,* D7471–D7490
  *extractions, local,* D7111–D7140
  *other repair procedures,* D7920–D7999
  *other surgical procedures,* D7260–D7295
  *reduction of dislocation/TMJ dysfunction,* D7810–D7899
  *repair of traumatic wounds,* D7910
  *surgical excision, intra-osseous lesions,* D7440–D7465
  *surgical excision, soft tissue lesions,* D7410–D7415
  *surgical extractions,* D7210–D7251
  *surgical incision,* D7510–D7560
  *treatment of fractures, compound,* D7710–D7780
  *treatment of fractures, simple,* D7610–D7680
  *vestibuloplasty,* D7340–D7350
**Oral device/appliance,** E0485–E0486
**Oral interface,** A7047
*Oral, NOS, drug,* J8499
**Oral/nasal mask,** A7027
  nasal pillows, A7029
  oral cushion, A7028
**Oritavancin,** J2407
**Oropharyngeal suction catheter,** A4628
**Orphenadrine,** J2360
*Orthodontics,* D8000–D8999

---

◄ New    ↻ Revised    ✔ Reinstated    ~~deleted~~ Deleted

**Orthopedic shoes**
  arch support, L3040–L3100
  footwear, *L3000–L3649*, L3201–L3265
  insert, L3000–L3030
  lift, L3300–L3334
  miscellaneous additions, L3500–L3595
  positioning device, L3140–L3170
  transfer, L3600–L3649
  wedge, L3340–L3420
**Orthotic additions**
  carbon graphite lamination, L2755
  fracture, L2180–L2192, L3995
  halo, L0860
  lower extremity, L2200–L2999, L4320
  ratchet lock, L2430
  scoliosis, L1010–L1120, L1210–L1290
  shoe, L3300–L3595, L3649
  spinal, L0970–L0984
  upper limb, L3810–L3890, *L3900, L3901,*
    L3970–L3974, *L3975–L3978,* L3995
**Orthotic devices**
  ankle-foot (AFO); (see also Orthopedic shoes),
    E1815, E1816, E1830, L1900–L1990,
    L2102–L2116, L3160, L4361, *L4397*
  anterior-posterior-lateral, L0700, L0710
  cervical, L0100–L0200
  cervical-thoracic-lumbar-sacral (CTLSO),
    L0700, L0710
  elbow (EO), E1800, E1801, L3700–L3740,
    L3760–L3761, *L3762*
  fracture, L2102–L2136, L3980–L3986
  halo, L0810–L0830
  hand, (WHFO), E1805, E1825, L3807,
    L3900–L3954, *L3956*
  hand, finger, prefabricated, L3923
  hip (HO), L1600–L1690
  hip-knee-ankle-foot (HKAFO), L2040–L2090
  interface material, E1820
  knee (KO), E1810, E1811, L1800–L1885
  knee-ankle-foot (KAFO); (see also Orthopedic
    shoes), L2000–L2038, L2126–L2136
  Legg Perthes, L1700–L1755
  *lumbar, L0625–L0651*
  multiple post collar, L0180–L0200
  not otherwise specified, L0999, L1499, L2999,
    L3999, L5999, L7499, L8039, L8239
  pneumatic splint, L4350–L4380
  pronation/supination, E1818
  repair or replacement, L4000–L4210
  replace soft interface material, L4390–L4394
  sacroiliac, L0600–L0620, *L0621–L0624*
  scoliosis, L1000–L1499
  shoe, (see Orthopedic shoes)
  shoulder (SO), L1840, L3650, L3674, *L3678*
  shoulder-elbow-wrist-hand (SEWHO),
    L3960–L3978
  side bar disconnect, L2768
  spinal, cervical, L0100–L0200

**Orthotic devices** *(Continued)*
  spinal, DME, K0112–K0116
  thoracic, L0210, *L0220*
  thoracic-hip-knee-ankle (THKO), L1500–L1520
  toe, E1830
  wrist-hand-finger (WHFO), E1805, E1806, E1825,
    *L3806–L3809,* L3900–L3954, *L3956*
**Orthovisc,** J7324
**Ossicula prosthetic implant,** L8613
**Osteogenesis stimulator,** E0747–E0749, E0760
***Osteotomy, segmented or subapical,*** *D7944*
**Ostomy**
  accessories, A5093
  belt, A4396
  pouches, A4416–A4435, *A5056, A5057*
  skin barrier, A4401–A4449, *A4462*
  supplies, A4361–A4421, A5051–A5149, *A5200*
***Otto Bock, prosthesis,*** *L7007*
***Outpatient payment system, hospital,***
    *C1000–C9999*
***Overdoor, traction,*** *E0860*
**Oxacillin sodium,** J2700
**Oxaliplatin,** J9263
**Oxygen**
  ambulance, A0422
  battery charger, E1357
  battery pack/cartridge, E1356
  catheter, transtracheal, A7018
  chamber, hyperbaric, topical, A4575
  concentrator, E1390–E1391
  DC power adapter, E1358
  delivery system (topical), E0446
  *equipment, E0424–E0486, E1353–E1406*
  Liquid oxygen system, E0433
  mask, A4620
  medication supplies, A4611–A4627
  rack/stand, E1355
  regulator, E1352, E1353
  respiratory equipment/supplies, E0424–E0480,
    A4611–A4627, *E0481*
  supplies and equipment, E0425–E0444, E0455
  tent, E0455
  tubing, A4616
  water vapor enriching system, E1405, E1406
  wheeled cart, E1354
**Oxymorphone HCl,** J2410
**Oxytetracycline HCl,** J2460
**Oxytocin,** J2590

## P

**Pacemaker monitor,** E0610, E0615
**Paclitaxel,** J9267
**Paclitaxel protein-bound particles,** J9264
**Pad**
  *correction, CTLSO, L1020–L1060*
  gel pressure, E0185, E0196

◀ New    ↻ Revised    ✔ Reinstated    ~~deleted~~ Deleted

**Pad** *(Continued)*
   heat, *A9273*, E0210, E0215, E0217, E0238, E0249
     *electric heat pad, moist, E0215*
     *electric heat pad, standard, E0210*
     *hot water bottle, ice cap or collar, heat and/or cold*
       *wrap, A9273*
     *pad for water circulating heat unit, replacement*
       *only, E0249*
     *water circulating heat pad with pump, E0217*
   orthotic device interface, E1820
   sheepskin, E0188, E0189
   water circulating cold with pump, E0218
   water circulating heat unit, E0249
   water circulating heat with pump, E0217
**Pail, for use with commode chair,** E0167
***Pain assessment,*** *G8730–G8732*
**Palate, prosthetic implant,** L8618
**Palifermin,** J2425
**Paliperidone palmitate,** J2426
**Palonosetron,** J2469, J8655
**Pamidronate disodium,** J2430
**Pan, for use with commode chair,** E0167
**Panitumumab,** J9303
**Papanicolaou screening smear (Pap),** P3000,
   P3001, Q0091
   *cervical or vaginal, up to 3 smears, by*
     *technician, P3000*
   *cervical or vaginal, up to 3 smears, physician*
     *interpretation, P3001*
   *obtaining, preparing and conveyance, Q0091*
**Papaverine HCl,** J2440
**Paraffin,** A4265
   bath unit, E0235
**Parenteral nutrition**
   administration kit, B4224
   not otherwise specified, B4185 ◄
   pump, B9004, B9006
   solution, B4164, B4184, B4186 ↺
     *compounded amino acid and carbohydrates, with*
       *electrolytes, B4189–B4199, B5000–B5200*
     *nutrition additives, homemix, B4216*
     *nutrition administration kit, B4224*
     *nutrition solution, amino acid, B4168–B4178*
     *nutrition solution, carbohydrates, B4164, B4180*
     *nutrition solution, per 10 grams, liquid, B4185*
     *nutrition supply kit, homemix, B4222*
   supply kit, B4220, B4222
**Paricalcitol,** J2501
**Parking fee, nonemergency transport,** A0170
***Partial Hospitalization, OT,*** *G0129*
**Pasireotide long acting,** J2502
**Paste, conductive,** A4558
**Pathology and laboratory tests, miscellaneous,**
   P9010–P9615
***Pathology, surgical,*** *G0416*
**Patient support system,** E0636
**Patient transfer system,** E1035–E1036
**Patisiran injection,** J0222 ◄

***Pediculosis (lice) treatment,*** *A9180*
**PEFR, peak expiratory flow rate meter,** A4614
**Pegademase bovine,** J2504
**Pegaptanib,** J2503
**Pegaspargase,** J9266
**Pegfilgrastim,** J2505
**Peginesatide,** J0890
**Pegloticase,** J2507
**Pelvic**
   belt/harness/boot, E0944
   *traction, E0890, E0900, E0947*
**Pemetrexed,** J9305
**Penicillin**
   G benzathine/G benzathine and penicillin G
     procaine, J0558, J0561
   G potassium, J2540
   G procaine, aqueous, J2510
**Pentamidine isethionate,** J2545, J7676
**Pentastarch, 10% solution,** J2513
**Pentazocine HCl,** J3070
**Pentobarbital sodium,** J2515
**Pentostatin,** J9268
**Peramivir,** J2547
**Percussor,** E0480
**Percutaneous access system,** A4301
**Perflexane lipid microspheres,** Q9955
**Perflutren lipid microspheres,** Q9957
***Periapical service,*** *D3410–D3470*
   *apicoectomy, bicuspid, first root, D3421*
   *apicoectomy, each additional root, D3426*
   *apicoectomy, molar, first root, D3425*
   *apicoectomy/periradicular surgery-anterior, D3410*
   *biological materials, aid soft and osseous tissue*
     *regeneration/periradicular surgery, D3431*
   *bone graft, per tooth, periradicular surgery, D3429*
   *endodonic endosseous implant, D3460*
   *guided tissue regeneration/periradicular surgery, D3432*
   *intentional replantation, D3470*
   *periradicular surgery without apicoectomy, D3427*
   *retrograde filling, per root, D3430*
   *root amputation, D3450*
***Periodontal procedures,*** *D4000–D4999*
***Periodontics, dental,*** *D4000–D4999*
**Peroneal strap,** L0980
**Peroxide,** A4244
**Perphenazine,** J3310
**Personal care services,** T1019–T1021
   *home health aide or CAN, per visit, T1021*
   *per diem, T1020*
   *provided by home health aide or CAN, per*
     *15 minutes, T1019*
**Pertuzumab,** J9306
**Pessary,** A4561, A4562
***PET,*** *G0219, G0235, G0252*
***Pharmacologic therapy,*** *G8633*
***Pharmacy, fee,*** *G0333*
**Phenobarbital sodium,** J2560
**Phentolamine mesylate,** J2760

---

◄ New   ↺ Revised   ✔ Reinstated   ~~deleted~~ Deleted

Phenylephrine HCl, J2370
Phenylephrine/ketorolac ophthalmic solution, J1097 ◄
Phenytoin sodium, J1165
Phisohex solution, A4246
Photofrin, (see Porfimer sodium)
*Photorefraction keratectomy, (PRK), S0810*
*Phototherapeutic keratectomy, (PTK), S0812*
Phototherapy light, E0202
Phytonadione, J3430
Pillow, cervical, E0943
*Pin retention (per tooth), D2951*
Pinworm examination, Q0113
Plasma
    multiple donor, pooled, frozen, P9023, P9070
    single donor, fresh frozen, P9017, P9071
Plastazote, L3002, L3252, L3253, L3265, L5654–L5658
    *addition to lower extremity socket insert, L5654*
    *addition to lower extremity socket insert, above knee, L5658*
    *addition to lower extremity socket insert, below knee, L5655*
    *addition to lower extremity socket insert, knee disarticulation, L5656*
    *foot insert, removable, plastazote, L3002*
    *foot, molded shoe, custom fitted, plastazote, L3253*
    *foot, shoe molded to patient model, plastazote, L3252*
    *plastazote sandal, L3265*
Platelet, P9073, P9100
    concentrate, each unit, P9019
    rich plasma, each unit, P9020
*Platelets, P9031–P9037, P9052–P9053, P9055*
Platform attachment
    forearm crutch, E0153
    walker, E0154
Plazomicin injection, J0291 ◄
Plerixafor, J2562
Plicamycin, J9270
Plumbing, for home ESRD equipment, A4870
Pneumatic
    appliance, E0655–E0673, L4350–L4380
    compressor, E0650–E0652
    splint, L4350–L4380
    ventricular assist device, Q0477, Q0480–Q0505
Pneumatic nebulizer
    administration set, small volume, filtered, A7006
    administration set, small volume, nonfiltered, A7003
    administration set, small volume, nonfiltered, nondisposable, A7005
    small volume, disposable, A7004
*Pneumococcal*
    *vaccine, administration, G0009*
Polatuzumab vedotin-piiq, J9309 ◄
*Pontics, D6210–D6252*
Porfimer, J9600

Portable
    equipment transfer, R0070–R0076
    gaseous oxygen, K0741, K0742
    hemodialyzer system, E1635
    liquid oxygen system, E0433
    x-ray equipment, Q0092
Positioning seat, T5001
Positive airway pressure device, accessories, A7030–A7039, E0561–E0562
Positive expiratory pressure device, E0484
Post-coital examination, Q0115
Postural drainage board, E0606
Potassium
    chloride, J3480
    hydroxide preparation(KOH), Q0112
Pouch
    fecal collection, A4330
    ostomy, A4375–A4378, A5051–A5054, A5061–A5065
    urinary, A4379–A4383, A5071–A5075
*Practice, guidelines, oncology, G9056–G9062*
Pralatrexate, J9307
Pralidoxime chloride, J2730
Prednisolone
    acetate, J2650
    oral, J7510
Prednisone, J7512
*Prefabricated crown, D2930–D2933*
Preparation kits, dialysis, A4914
Preparatory prosthesis, L5510–L5595
    chemotherapy, J8999
    nonchemotherapy, J8499
Pressure
    alarm, dialysis, E1540
    pad, A4640, E0180–E0199
*Preventive dental procedures, D1000–D1999*
Privigen, J1459
Procainamide HCl, J2690
*Procedure*
    *HALO, L0810–L0861*
    *noncovered, G0293, G0294*
    *scoliosis, L1000–L1499*
Prochlorperazine, J0780
Progenamatrix, Q4222 ◄
Prolotherapy, M0076
Promazine HCl, J2950
Promethazine
    and meperdine, J2180
    HCl, J2550
Propranolol HCl, J1800
*Prostate, cancer, screening, G0102, G0103*
Prosthesis
    artificial larynx battery/accessory, L8505
    *auricular, D5914*
    breast, L8000–L8035, L8600
    *dental, D5911–D5960, D5999*
    eye, L8610, L8611, V2623–V2629
    fitting, L5400–L5460, L6380–L6388
    foot/ankle one piece system, L5979

◄ New    ↻ Revised    ✔ Reinstated    ~~deleted~~ Deleted

**Prosthesis** *(Continued)*
   hand, L6000–L6020, L6026
   implants, L8600–L8690
   larynx, L8500
   lower extremity, L5700–L5999, L8640–L8642
   mandible, L8617
   maxilla, L8616
   maxillofacial, provided by a non-physician, L8040–L8048
   miscellaneous service, L8499
   *obturator, D5931–D5933, D5936*
   ocular, V2623–V2629
   repair of, L7520, L8049
   socks (shrinker, sheath, stump sock), L8400–L8485
   taxes, orthotic/prosthetic/other, L9999
   tracheo-esophageal, L8507–L8509
   upper extremity, L6000–L6999
   vacuum erection system, L7900
**Prosthetic additions**
   lower extremity, L5610–L5999
   Powered Upper extremity range of motion assist device, L8701–L8702 ↻
   upper extremity, L6600–L7405
**Prosthetic, eye,** *V2623*
**Prosthodontic procedure**
   *fixed, D6200–D6999*
   *removable, D5000–D5899*
**Prosthodontics, removable,** *D5110–D5899*
**Protamine sulfate,** J2720
**Protectant, skin,** A6250
**Protector, heel or elbow,** E0191
**Protein C Concentrate,** J2724
**Protirelin,** J2725
**Psychotherapy, group, partial hospitalization,** *G0410–G0411*
**Pulp capping,** *D3110, D3120*
**Pulpotomy,** *D3220*
   *partial, D3222*
   *vitality test, D0460*
**Pulse generator,** E2120
**Pump**
   alternating pressure pad, E0182
   ambulatory infusion, E0781
   ambulatory insulin, E0784
   blood, dialysis, E1620
   breast, E0602–E0604
   enteral infusion, B9000, B9002
   external infusion, E0779
   heparin infusion, E1520
   implantable infusion, E0782, E0783
   implantable infusion, refill kit, A4220
   infusion, supplies, A4230, A4232
   negative pressure wound therapy, E2402
   parenteral infusion, B9004, B9006
   suction, portable, E0600
   water circulating pad, E0236
   *wound, negative, pressure, E2402*
**Purification system,** E1610, E1615
**Pyridoxine HCl,** J3415

# Q

**Quad cane,** E0105
**Quinupristin/dalfopristin,** J2770

# R

**Rack/stand, oxygen,** E1355
**Radiesse,** Q2026
**Radioelements for brachytherapy,** Q3001
**Radiograph, dental,** *D0210–D0340*
**Radiological, supplies,** *A4641, A4642*
**Radiology service,** R0070–R0076
**Radiopharmaceutical diagnostic and therapeutic imaging agent,** A4641, A4642, A9500–A9699
**Radiosurgery, robotic,** *G0339–G0340*
**Radiosurgery, stereotactic,** *G0339, G0340*
**Rail**
   bathtub, E0241, E0242, E0246
   bed, E0305, E0310
   toilet, E0243
**Ranibizumab,** J2778
**Rasburicase,** J2783
**Ravulizumab injection-cwvz,** J1303 ◄
**Reaching/grabbing device,** A9281
**Reagent strip,** A4252
*Re-cement*
   *crown, D2920*
   *inlay, D2910*
**Reciprocating peritoneal dialysis system,** E1630
**Reclast,** *J3488, J3489*
**Reclining, wheelchair,** *E1014, E1050–E1070, E1100–E1110*
**Reconstruction, angiography,** *G0288*
**Rectal Control System for Vaginal insertion,** A4563 ↻
**Red blood cells,** P9021, P9022
**Regadenoson,** J2785
**Regular insulin,** *J1815, J1820*
**Regulator, oxygen,** E1353
*Rehabilitation*
   *cardiac, S9472*
   *program, H2001*
   *psychosocial, H2017, H2018*
   *pulmonary, S9473*
   *system, jaw, motion, E1700–E1702*
   *vestibular, S9476*
**Removal, cerumen,** *G0268*
**Repair**
   contract, ESRD, A4890
   durable medical equipment, E1340
   maxillofacial prosthesis, L8049
   orthosis, L4000–L4130
   prosthetic, L7500, L7510

---

◄ New    ↻ Revised   ✔ Reinstated   ~~deleted~~ Deleted

**Replacement**
    battery, A4630
    pad (alternating pressure), A4640
    tanks, dialysis, A4880
    tip for cane, crutches, walker, A4637
    underarm pad for crutches, A4635
***Resin dental restoration**, D2330–D2394*
**Reslizumab**, J2786
**RespiGam, (see Respiratory syncytial virus immune globulin)**
***Respiratory***
    *DME, A7000–A7527*
    *equipment, E0424–E0601*
    *function, therapeutic, procedure, G0237–G0239, S5180–S5181*
    *supplies, A4604–A4629*
***Restorative nerve dental procedure**, D2000–D2999*
**Restraint, any type**, E0710
**Reteplase**, J2993
***Revascularization**, C9603–C9608*
**Revefenacin inhalation solution**, J7677 ◄
**Rho(D) immune globulin, human**, J2788, J2790, J2791, J2792
**Rib belt, thoracic**, A4572, L0220
**Rilanocept**, J2793
**RimabotulinumtoxinB**, J0587
**Ring, ostomy**, A4404
**Ringers lactate infusion**, J7120
***Risk-adjusted functional status***
    *elbow, wrist or hand, G8667–G8670*
    *hip, G8651–G8654*
    *lower leg, foot or ankle, G8655–G8658*
    *lumbar spine, G8659–G8662*
    *neck, cranium, mandible, thoracic spine, ribs, or other, G8671–G8674*
    *shoulder, G8663–G8666*
**Risperidone (risperdal consta)**, J2794 ↻
    **(perseris)**, J2798 ◄
**Rituximab**, J9310
    abbs (Truxina), Q5115 ◄
**Robin-Aids**, L6000, L6010, L6020, L6855, L6860
**Rocking bed**, E0462
**Rolapitant**, J8670
**Rollabout chair**, E1031
**Romidepsin**, J9315
**Romiplostim**, J2796
**Romosozumab injection-aqqg**, J3111 ◄
***Root canal therapy**, D3310–D3353*
**Ropivacaine HCl**, J2795
**Rubidium Rb-82**, A9555

## S

**Sacral nerve stimulation test lead**, A4290
**Safety equipment**, E0700
    vest, wheelchair, E0980

**Saline**
    hypertonic, J7130, *J7131*
    *infusion, J7030–J7060*
    solution, A4216–A4218, J7030–J7050
***Saliva***
    *artificial, A9155*
    *collection and preparation, D0417*
**Samarium SM 153 Lexidronamm**, A9605
**Sargramostim (GM-CSF)**, J2820
**Scale**, E1639
**Scoliosis**, L1000–L1499
    additions, L1010–L1120, L1210–L1290
***Screening***
    *alcohol misuse, G0442*
    *cancer, cervical or vaginal, G0101*
    *colorectal, cancer, G0104–G0106, G0120–G0122, G0328*
    *cytopathology cervical or vaginal, G0123, G0124, G0141–G0148*
    *depression, G0444*
    *dysphagia, documentation, V5364*
    *enzyme immunoassay, G0432*
    *glaucoma, G0117, G0118*
    *infectious agent antibody detection, G0433, G0435*
    *language, V5363*
    *mammography, digital image, G9899, G9900*
    *prostate, cancer, G0102, G0103*
    *speech, V5362*
**Sculptra**, Q2028
**Sealant**
    skin, A6250
    *tooth, D1351*
**Seat**
    attachment, walker, E0156
    insert, wheelchair, E0992
    lift (patient), E0621, E0627–E0629
    upholstery, wheelchair, E0975, *E0981*
**Sebelipase alfa ,** J2840
**Secretin**, J2850
**Semen analysis**, G0027
***Semi-reclining, wheelchair**, E1100, E1110*
**Sensitivity study**, P7001
***Sensory nerve conduction test**, G0255*
**Sermorelin acetate**, Q0515
**Serum clotting time tube**, A4771
***Service***
    *Allied Health, home health, hospice, G0151–G0161*
    *behavioral health and/or substance abuse, H0001–H9999*
    *hearing, V5000–V5999*
    *laboratory, P0000–P9999*
    *mental, health, training, G0177*
    *non-covered, A9270*
    *physician, for mobility device, G0372*
    *pulmonary, for LVRS, G0302–G0305*
    *skilled, RN/LPN, home health, hospice, G0162*
    *social, psychological, G0409–G0411*
    *speech-language, V5336–V5364*
    *vision, V2020–V2799*

◄ New     ↻ Revised     ✔ Reinstated     ~~deleted~~ Deleted

**SEWHO,** L3960–L3974, *L3975–L3978*
*SEXA, G0130*
**Sheepskin pad,** E0188, E0189
**Shoes**
   arch support, L3040–L3100
   for diabetics, A5500–A5514
   insert, L3000–L3030, *L3031*
   lift, L3300–L3334
   miscellaneous additions, L3500–L3595
   orthopedic, L3201–L3265
   positioning device, L3140–L3170
   transfer, L3600–L3649
   wedge, L3340–L3485
**Shoulder**
   disarticulation, prosthetic, L6300–L6320, L6550
   orthosis (SO), L3650–L3674
   spinal, cervical, L0100–L0200
**Shoulder sling,** A4566
**Shoulder-elbow-wrist-hand orthosis (SEWHO),** L3960–L3969, *L3971–L3978*
**Shunt accessory for dialysis,** A4740
   aqueous, L8612
**Sigmoidoscopy, cancer screening,** G0104, G0106
**Siltuximab,** J2860
**Sincalide,** J2805
**Sipuleucel-T,** Q2043
**Sirolimus,** J7520
**Sitz bath,** E0160–E0162
**Skin**
   barrier, ostomy, A4362, A4363, A4369–A4373, A4385, A5120
   bond or cement, ostomy, A4364
   sealant, protectant, moisturizer, A6250
   substitute, Q4100–Q4222 ↵
*Skyla, 13.5 mg, J7301*
**Sling,** A4565
   patient lift, E0621, E0630, E0635
*Smear, Papanicolaou, screening, P3000, P3001, Q0091*
*SNCT, G0255*
*Social worker, clinical, home, health, G0155*
*Social worker, nonemergency transport, A0160*
*Social work/psychological services, CORF, G0409*
**Sock**
   body sock, L0984
   prosthetic sock, *L8417,* L8420–L8435, L8470, L8480, L8485
   stump sock, L8470–L8485
**Sodium**
   chloride injection, J2912
   ferric gluconate complex in sucrose, J2916
   fluoride F-18, A9580
   hyaluronate
     Euflexxa, J7323
     GELSYN-3, J7328
     Hyalgan, J7321
     Orthovisc, J7324
     Supartz, J7321

**Sodium** *(Continued)*
   hyaluronate *(Continued)*
     Synvisc and Synvisc-One, J7325
     Visco-3, J7321
   phosphate P32, A9563
   pyrophosphate, J1443
   succinate, J1720
**Solution**
   calibrator, A4256
   dialysate, A4760
   elliotts b, J9175
   enteral formulae, B4149–B4156, *B4157–B4162*
   parenteral nutrition, B4164–B5200
*Solvent, adhesive remover, A4455*
**Somatrem,** J2940
**Somatropin,** J2941
**Sorbent cartridge, ESRD,** E1636
*Special size, wheelchair, E1220–E1239*
**Specialty absorptive dressing,** A6251–A6256
*Spectacle lenses, V2100–V2199*
**Spectinomycin HCl,** J3320
**Speech assessment,** V5362–V5364
**Speech generating device,** E2500–E2599
*Speech, pathologist, G0153*
*Speech-Language pathology, services, V5336–V5364*
*Spherocylinder, single vision, V2100–V2114*
   *bifocal, V2203–V2214*
   *trifocal, V2303–V2314*
**Spinal orthosis**
   cervical, L0100–L0200
   cervical-thoracic-lumbar-sacral (CTLSO), L0700, L0710
   DME, K0112–K0116
   halo, L0810–L0830
   multiple post collar, L0180–L0200
   scoliosis, L1000–L1499
   torso supports, L0960
**Splint,** A4570, L3100, L4350–L4380
   ankle, L4390–L4398
   dynamic, E1800, E1805, E1810, E1815, E1825, E1830, E1840
   footdrop, L4398
   *supplies, miscellaneous, Q4051*
*Standard, wheelchair, E1130, K0001*
**Static progressive stretch,** E1801, E1806, E1811, E1816, E1818, E1821
*Status*
   *disease, oncology, G9063–G9139*
*STELARA, ustekinumab, 1 mg, J3357*
*Stent, transcatheter, placement, C9600, C9601*
*Stereotactic, radiosurgery, G0339, G0340*
**Sterile cefuroxime sodium,** J0697
**Sterile water,** A4216–A4217
*Stimulation, electrical, non-attended, G0281–G0283*
**Stimulators**
   neuromuscular, E0744, E0745
   osteogenesis, electrical, E0747–E0749
   salivary reflex, E0755

**Stimulators** (Continued)
  stoma absorptive cover, A5083
  *transcutaneous, electric, nerve,* A4595, E0720–E0749
  ultrasound, E0760
**Stockings**
  *gradient, compression,* A6530–A6549
  *surgical,* A4490–A4510
**Stoma, plug or seal,** A5081
**Stomach tube,** B4083
**Streptokinase,** J2995
**Streptomycin,** J3000
**Streptozocin,** J9320
**Strip, blood glucose test,** A4253–A4772
  urine reagent, A4250
**Strontium-89 chloride, supply of,** A9600
**Study, bone density,** G0130
**Stump sock,** L8470–L8485
**Stylet,** A4212
**Substance/Alcohol, assessment,** G0396, G0397,
  H0001, H0003, H0049
**Succinylcholine chloride,** J0330
**Suction pump**
  gastric, home model, E2000
  portable, E0600
  respiratory, home model, E0600
**Sumatriptan succinate,** J3030
**Supartz,** J7321
**Supplies**
  *battery,* A4233–A4236, A4601, A4611–A4613, A4638
  *cast,* A4580, A4590, Q4001–Q4051
  *catheters,* A4300–A4306
  *contraceptive,* A4267–A4269
  *diabetic shoes,* A5500–A5513
  *dialysis,* A4653–A4928
  *DME, other,* A4630–A4640
  *dressings,* A6000–A6513
  *enteral, therapy,* B4000–B9999
  *incontinence,* A4310–A4355, A5102–A5200
  *infusion,* A4221, A4222, A4230–A4232,
    E0776–E0791
  *needle,* A4212, A4215
  *needle-free device,* A4210
  *ostomy,* A4361–A4434, A5051–A5093, A5120–A5200
  *parenteral, therapy,* B4000–B9999
  *radiological,* A4641, A4642
  *refill kit, infusion pump,* A4220
  *respiratory,* A4604–A4629
  *self-administered injections,* A4211
  *splint,* Q4051
  *sterile water/saline and/or dextrose,* A4216–A4218
  *surgical, miscellaneous,* A4649
  *syringe,* A4206–A4209, A4213, A4232
  *syringe with needle,* A4206–A4209
  *urinary, external,* A4356–A4360
**Supply/accessory/service,** A9900
**Support**
  arch, L3040–L3090
  cervical, L0100–L0200

**Support** (Continued)
  spinal, L0960
  stockings, L8100–L8239
**Surederm,** Q4220 ◀
**Surgery, oral,** D7000–D7999
**Surgical**
  *arthroscopy, knee,* G0289, S2112
  boot, L3208–L3211
  dressing, A6196–A6406
  *procedure, noncovered,* G0293, G0294
  stocking, A4490–A4510
  supplies, A4649
  tray, A4550
**Surgicord,** Q4218–Q4219 ◀
**Surgraft,** Q4209 ◀
**Swabs, betadine or iodine,** A4247
**Synojoynt,** J7331 ◀
**Synvisc and Synvisc-One,** J7325
**Syringe,** A4213
  with needle, A4206–A4209
**System**
  *external, ambulatory insulin,* A9274
  *rehabilitation, jaw, motion,* E1700–E1702
  *transport,* E1035–E1039

# T

**Tables, bed,** E0274, E0315
**Tacrolimus**
  oral, J7503, J7507, J7508
  parenteral, J7525
**Tagraxofusp injections-erzs,** J9269 ◀
**Taliglucerase,** J3060
**Talimogene laheroareovec,** J9325
**Tape,** A4450–A4452
**Taxi, non-emergency transportation,** A0100
**Team, conference,** G0175, G9007, S0220,
  S0221
**Technetium TC 99M**
  Arcitumomab, A9568
  Bicisate, A9557
  Depreotide, A9536
  Disofenin, A9510
  Exametazine, A9521
  Exametazine labeled autologous white blood
    cells, A9569
  Fanolesomab, A9566
  Glucepatate, A9550
  Labeled red blood cells, A9560
  Macroaggregated albumin, A9540
  Mebrofenin, A9537
  Mertiatide, A9562
  Oxidronate, A9561
  Pentetate, A9539, A9567
  Pertechnetate, A9512
  Pyrophosphate, A9538
  Sestamibi, A9500

◀ **New**   ↻ **Revised**   ✔ **Reinstated**   ~~deleted~~ **Deleted**

**Technetium TC 99M** *(Continued)*
  Succimer, A9551
  Sulfur colloid, A9541
  Teboroxime, A9501
  Tetrofosmin, A9502
  Tilmanocept, A9520
**Tedizolid phosphate,** J3090
**TEEV,** J0900
**Telavancin,** J3095
**Telehealth,** Q3014
**Telehealth transmission,** T1014
**Temozolomide**
  injection, J9328
  oral, J8700
*Temporary codes,* *Q0000–Q9999, S0009–S9999*
*Temporomandibular joint,* *D0320, D0321*
**Temsirolimus,** J9330
**Tenecteplase,** J3101
**Teniposide,** Q2017
**TENS,** A4595, E0720–E0749
**Tent, oxygen,** E0455
**Terbutaline sulfate,** J3105
  inhalation solution, concentrated, J7680
  inhalation solution, unit dose, J7681
**Teriparatide,** J3110
**Terminal devices,** L6700–L6895
*Test*
  *sensory, nerve, conduction,* *G0255*
**Testosterone**
  cypionate and estradiol cypionate, J1071
  enanthate, J3121
  undecanoate, J3145
**Tetanus immune globulin, human,** J1670
**Tetracycline,** J0120
**Thallous Chloride TL 201,** A9505
**Theophylline,** J2810
**Therapeutic lightbox,** A4634, E0203
**Therapy**
  *activity,* *G0176*
  *electromagnetic,* *G0295, G0329*
  *endodontic,* *D3222–D3330*
  *enteral, supplies,* *B4000–B9999*
  *medical, nutritional,* *G0270, G0271*
  occupational, *G0129, H5300, S9129*
  *occupational, health,* *G0152*
  *parenteral, supplies,* *B4000–B9999*
  *respiratory, function, procedure,* *G0237–S0239,*
    *S5180, S5181*
  *speech, home,* *G0153, S9128*
  *wound, negative, pressure, pump,* *E2402*
*Theraskin,* *Q4121*
**Thermometer,** A4931–A4932
  dialysis, A4910
**Thiamine HCl,** J3411
**Thiethylperazine maleate,** J3280
**Thiotepa,** J9340
**Thoracic orthosis,** L0210
**Thoracic-hip-knee-ankle (THKAO),** L1500–L1520

**Thoracic-lumbar-sacral orthosis (TLSO)**
  scoliosis, L1200–L1290
  spinal, L0450–L0492
**Thymol turbidity, blood,** P2033
**Thyrotropin Alfa,** J3240
**Tigecycline,** J3243
**Tinzarparin sodium,** J1655
**Tip (cane, crutch, walker) replacement,** A4637
*Tire, wheelchair,* *E2211–E2225, E2381–E2395*
**Tirofiban,** J3246
**Tisagenlecleucel,** Q2040
**Tissue marker,** A4648
**TLSO,** L0450–L0492, L1200–L1290
*Tobacco*
  *intervention,* *G9016*
**Tobramycin**
  inhalation solution, unit dose, J7682, J7685
  sulfate, J3260
**Tocilizumab,** J2362
*Toe device,* *E1831*
**Toilet accessories,** E0167–E0179, E0243, E0244, E0625
**Tolazoline HCl,** J2670
**Toll, non emergency transport,** A0170
*Tomographic radiograph, dental,* *D0322*
**Topical hyperbaric oxygen chamber,** A4575
**Topotecan,** J8705, J9351
**Torsemide,** J3265
**Trabectedin,** J9352
**Tracheostoma heat moisture exchange system,**
  A7501–A7509
**Tracheostomy**
  care kit, A4629
  filter, A4481
  speaking valve, L8501
  supplies, A4623, A4629, A7523–A7524
  tube, A7520–A7522
**Tracheotomy mask or collar,** A7525–A7526
**Traction**
  *cervical,* *E0855, E0856*
  device, ambulatory, E0830
  equipment, E0840–E0948
  *extremity,* *E0870–E0880*
  *pelvic,* *E0890, E0900, E0947*
*Training*
  *diabetes, outpatient,* *G0108, G0109*
  *home health or hospice,* *G0162*
  *services, mental, health,* *G0177*
**Transcutaneous electrical nerve stimulator**
  **(TENS),** E0720–E0770
**Transducer protector, dialysis,** E1575
**Transfer (shoe orthosis),** L3600–L3640
**Transfer system with seat,** E1035
**Transparent film (for dressing),** A6257–A6259
*Transplant*
  *islet,* *G0341–G0343, S2102*
*Transport*
  *chair,* *E1035–E1039*
  *system,* *E1035–E1039*
  *x-ray,* *R0070–R0076*

---

◄ New    ↵ Revised    ✔ Reinstated    ~~deleted~~ Deleted

**Transportation**
- ambulance, A0021–A0999, Q3019, Q3020
- corneal tissue, V2785
- EKG (portable), R0076
- handicapped, A0130
- non-emergency, A0080–A0210, T2001–T2005
- service, including ambulance, A0021, A0999, T2006
- taxi, non-emergency, A0100
- toll, non-emergency, A0170
- volunteer, non-emergency, A0080, A0090
- x-ray (portable), R0070, R0075, *R0076*

*Transportation services*
- *air services, A0430, A0431, A0435, A0436*
- *ALS disposable supplies, A0398*
- *ALS mileage, A0390*
- *ALS specialized service, A0392, A0394, A0396*
- *ambulance, ALS, A0426, A0427, A0433*
- *ambulance, outside state, Medicaid, A0021*
- *ambulance oxygen, A0422*
- *ambulance, waiting time, A0420*
- *ancillary, lodging, escort, A0200*
- *ancillary, lodging, recipient, A0180*
- *ancillary, meals, escort, A0210*
- *ancillary, meals, recipient, A0190*
- *ancillary, parking fees, tolls, A0170*
- *BLS disposable supplies, A0382*
- *BLS mileage, A0380*
- *BLS specialized service, A0384*
- *emergency, neonatal, one-way, A0225*
- *extra ambulance attendant, A0424*
- *ground mileage, A0425*
- *non-emergency, air travel, A0140*
- *non-emergency, bus, A0110*
- *non-emergency, case worker, A0160*
- *non-emergency, mini-bus, A0120*
- *non-emergency, no vested interest, A0080*
- *non-emergency, taxi, A0100*
- *non-emergency, wheelchair van, A0130*
- *non-emergency, with vested interest, A0090*
- *paramedic intercept, A0432*
- *response and treat, no transport, A0998*
- *specialty transport, A0434*

**Transtracheal oxygen catheter,** A7018
**Trapeze bar,** E0910–E0912, E0940
*Trauma, response, team, G0390*
**Tray**
- insertion, A4310–A4316
- irrigation, A4320
- surgical; (see also kits), A4550
- wheelchair, E0950

**Trastuzumab injection excludes biosimilar,** J9355 ◄
- anns (kanjinti), Q5117 ◄
- dkst (Ogivri), Q5114 ◄
- dttb (Ontruzant), Q5112 ◄
- pkrb (Herzuma), Q5113 ◄
- qyyp (trazimera), Q5116 ◄

**Trastuzumab and Hyaluronidase-oysk,** J9356 ◄

*Treatment*
- *bone, G0412–G0415*
- *pediculosis (lice), A9180*
- *services, behavioral health, H0002–H2037*

**Treprostinil,** J3285
**Triamcinolone,** J3301–J3303
- acetonide, J3300, J3301
- diacetate, J3302
- hexacetonide, J3303
- inhalation solution, concentrated, J7683
- inhalation solution, unit dose, J7684

**Triflupromazine HCl,** J3400
**Trifocal, glass or plastic,** V2300–V2399
- *aniseikonic, V2318*
- *lenticular, V2315, V2321*
- *specialty trifocal, by report, V2399*
- *sphere, plus or minus, V2300–V2302*
- *spherocylinder, V2303–V2314*
- *trifocal add-over 3.25d, V2320*
- *trifocal, seg width over 28 mm, V2319*

*Trigeminal division block anesthesia, D9212*
**Triluron intraarticular injection,** J7332 ◄
**Trimethobenzamide HCl,** J3250
**Trimetrexate glucuoronate,** J3305
*Trimming, nails, dystrophic, G0127*
**Triptorelin pamoate,** J3315
*Trismus appliance, D5937*
**Truss,** L8300–L8330
- *addition to standard pad, scrotal pad, L8330*
- *addition to standard pad, water pad, L8320*
- *double, standard pads, L8310*
- *single, standard pad, L8300*

**Tube/Tubing**
- anchoring device, A5200
- blood, A4750, A4755
- corrugated tubing, non-disposable, used with large volume nebulizer,10 feet, A4337
- drainage extension, A4331
- gastrostomy, B4087, B4088
- irrigation, A4355
- larynectomy, A4622
- nasogastric, B4081, B4082
- oxygen, A4616
- serum clotting time, A4771
- stomach, B4083
- suction pump, each, A7002
- tire, K0091, K0093, K0095, K0097
- tracheostomy, A4622
- urinary drainage, K0280

## U

**Ultrasonic nebulizer,** E0575
*Ultrasound, S8055, S9024*
- *paranasal sinus ultrasound, S9024*
- *ultrasound guidance, multifetal pregnancy reduction, technical component, S8055*

---

◄ New ↻ Revised ✔ Reinstated ~~deleted~~ Deleted

*Ultraviolet, cabinet/system,* E0691, E0694
**Ultraviolet light therapy system,** A4633, E0691–E0694
*light therapy system in 6 foot cabinet,* E0694
*replacement bulb/lamp,* A4633
*therapy system panel, 4 foot,* E0692
*therapy system panel, 6 foot,* E0693
*treatment area 2 sq feet or less,* E0691
**Unclassified drug,** J3490
*Underpads, disposable,* A4554
**Unipuncture control system, dialysis,** E1580
**Upper extremity addition, locking elbow,** L6693
**Upper extremity fracture orthosis,** L3980–L3999
**Upper limb prosthesis,** L6000–L7499
**Urea,** J3350
**Ureterostomy supplies,** A4454–A4590
**Urethral suppository, Alprostadil,** J0275
**Urinal,** E0325, E0326
**Urinary**
  catheter, A4338–A4346, A4351–A4353
    *indwelling catheter,* A4338–A4346
    *intermittent urinary catheter,* A4351–A4353
    *male external catheter,* A4349
  collection and retention (supplies), A4310–A4360
    *bedside drainage bag,* A4357
    *disposable external urethral clamp,* A4360
    *external urethral clamp,* A4356
    *female external urinary collection device,* A4328
    *insertion trays,* A4310–A4316, A4354–A4355
    *irrigation syringe,* A4322
    *irrigation tray,* A4320
    *male external catheter/integral collection chamber,* A4326
    *perianal fecal collection pouch,* A4330
    *therapeutic agent urinary catheter irrigation,* A4321
    *urinary drainage bag, leg/abdomen,* A4358
  supplies, external, A4335, A4356–A4358
    *bedside drainage bag,* A4357
    *external urethral clamp/compression device,* A4356
    *incontinence supply,* A4335
    *urinary drainage bag, leg or abdomen,* A4358
  tract implant, collagen, L8603
  tract implant, synthetic, L8606
**Urine**
  sensitivity study, P7001
  tests, A4250
**Urofollitropin,** J3355
**Urokinase,** J3364, J3365
**Ustekinumab,** J3357, J3758
**U-V lens,** V2755

## V

**Vabra aspirator,** A4480
**Vaccination, administration**
  flublok, Q2033
  hepatitis B, G0010

**Vaccination, administration** *(Continued)*
  influenza virus, G0008
  pneumococcal, G0009
*Vaccine*
  *administration, influenza,* G0008
  *administration, pneumococcal,* G0009
  *hepatitis B, administration,* G0010
*Vaginal*
  *cancer, screening,* G0101
  *cytopathologist,* G0123
  *cytopathology,* G0123, G0124, G0141–G0148
  *screening, cervical/vaginal, thin-layer, cytopathologist,* G0123
  *screening, cervical/vaginal, thin-layer, physician interpretation,* G0124
  *screening cytopathology smears, automated,* G0141–G0148
**Vancomycin HCl,** J3370
**Vaporizer,** E0605
**Vascular**
  catheter (appliances and supplies), A4300–A4306
    *disposable drug delivery system, >50 ml/hr,* A4305
    *disposable drug delivery system, <50 ml/hr,* A4306
    *implantable access catheter, external,* A4300
    *implantable access total, catheter,* A4301
  graft material, synthetic, L8670
**Vasoxyl,** J3390
**Vedolizumab,** J3380
*Vehicle, power-operated,* K0800–K0899
**Velaglucerase alfa,** J3385
**Venous pressure clamp, dialysis,** A4918
**Ventilator**
  battery, A4611–A4613
  home ventilator, any type, E0465, E0466
    used with invasive interface (e.g., tracheostomy tube), E0465
    used with non-invasive interface (e.g., mask, chest shell), E0466
  moisture exchanger, disposable, A4483
**Ventricular assist device,** Q0478–Q0504, Q0506–Q0509
  *battery clips, electric or electric/pneumatic, replacement,* Q0497
  *battery, lithium-ion, electric or electric/pneumatic, replacement,* Q0506
  *battery, other than lithium-ion, electric or electric/ pneumatic, replacement,* Q0496
  *battery, pneumatic, replacement,* Q0503
  *battery/power-pack charger, electric or electric/ pneumatic, replacement,* Q0495
  *belt/vest/bag, carry external components, replacement,* Q0499
  *driver, replacement,* Q0480
  *emergency hand pump, electric or electric/pneumatic, replacement,* Q0494
  *emergency power source, electric, replacement,* Q0490
  *emergency power source, electric/pneumatic, replacement,* Q0491

◄ New   ↻ Revised   ✔ Reinstated   ~~deleted~~ Deleted

**Ventricular assist device** *(Continued)*
  *emergency power supply cable, electric, replacement,* Q0492
  *emergency power supply cable, electric/pneumatic, replacement,* Q0493
  *filters, electric or electric/pneumatic, replacement,* Q0500
  *holster, electric or electric/pneumatic, replacement,* Q0498
  *leads (pneumatic/electrical), replacement,* Q0487
  *microprocessor control unit, electric/pneumatic combination, replacement,* Q0482
  *microprocessor control unit, pneumatic, replacement,* Q0481
  *miscellaneous supply, external VAD,* Q0507
  *miscellaneous supply, implanted device,* Q0508
  *miscellaneous supply, implanted device, payment not made under Medicare Part A,* Q0509
  *mobility cart, replacement,* Q0502
  *monitor control cable, electric, replacement,* Q0485
  *monitor control cable, electric/pneumatic,* Q0486
  *monitor/display module, electric, replacement,* Q0483
  *monitor/display module, electric/electric pneumatic, replacement,* Q0484
  *power adapter, pneumatic, replacement, vehicle type,* Q0504
  *power adapter, vehicle type,* Q0478
  *power module, replacement,* Q0479
  *power-pack base, electric, replacement,* Q0488
  *power-pack base, electric/pneumatic, replacement,* Q0489
  *shower cover, electric or electric/pneumatic, replacement,* Q0501
**Verteporfin,** J3396
**Vest, safety, wheelchair,** E0980
**Vinblastine sulfate,** J9360
**Vincristine sulfate,** J9370, J9371
**Vinorelbine tartrate,** J9390
**Vision service,** V2020–V2799
  *bifocal, glass or plastic,* V2200–V2299
  *contact lenses,* V2500–V2599
  *frames,* V2020–V2025
  *intraocular lenses,* V2630–V2632
  *low-vision aids,* V2600–V2615
  *miscellaneous,* V2700–V2799
  *prosthetic eye,* V2623–V2629
  *spectacle lenses,* V2100–V2199
  *trifocal, glass or plastic,* V2300–V2399
  *variable asphericity,* V2410–V2499
***Visit, emergency department,*** G0380–G0384
***Visual, function, postoperative cataract surgery,*** G0915–G0918
**Vitamin B-12 cyanocobalamin,** J3420
**Vitamin K,** J3430
**Voice**
  amplifier, L8510
  prosthesis, L8511–L8514

**Von Willebrand Factor Complex, human,** J7179, J7183, J7187
**Voriconazole,** J3465

# W

**Waiver,** T2012–T2050
  *assessment/plan of care development,* T2024
  *case management, per month,* T2022
  *day habilitation, per 15 minutes,* T2021
  *day habilitation, per diem,* T2020
  *habilitation, educational, per diem,* T2012
  *habilitation, educational, per hour,* T2013
  *habilitation, prevocational, per diem,* T2014
  *habilitation, prevocational, per hour,* T2015
  *habilitation, residential, 15 minutes,* T2017
  *habilitation, residential, per diem,* T2016
  *habilitation, supported employment, 15 minutes,* T2019
  *habilitation, supported employment, per diem,* T2018
  *targeted case management, per month,* T2023
  *waiver services NOS,* T2025
**Walker,** E0130–E0149
  accessories, A4636, A4637
  attachments, E0153–E0159
  *enclosed, four-sided frame,* E0144
  *folding (pickup),* E0135
  *folding, wheeled,* E0143
  *heavy duty, multiple braking system,* E0147
  *heavy duty, wheeled, rigid or folding,* E0149
  *heavy duty, without wheels,* E0148
  *rigid (pickup),* E0130
  *rigid, wheeled,* E0141
  *with trunk support,* E0140
**Walking splint,** L4386
***Washer, Gravlee jet,*** A4470
**Water**
  *dextrose,* J7042, J7060, J7070
  distilled (for nebulizer), A7018
  pressure pad/mattress, E0187, E0198
  purification system (ESRD), E1610, E1615
  softening system (ESRD), E1625
  sterile, A4714
***WBC/CBC,*** G0306
**Wedges, shoe,** L3340–L3420
***Wellness visit; annual,*** G0438, G0439
**Wet mount,** Q0111
**Wheel attachment, rigid pickup walker,** E0155
**Wheelchair,** E0950–E1298, K0001–K0108, K0801–K0899
  accessories, E0192, E0950–E1030, E1065–E1069, E2211–E2230, E2300–E2399, E2626–E2633
  amputee, E1170–E1200
  back, fully reclining, manual, E1226
  component or accessory, not otherwise specified, K0108
  cushions, E2601–E2625

---

◄ **New**    ↻ **Revised**    ✔ **Reinstated**    ~~deleted~~ **Deleted**

**Wheelchair** (*Continued*)

  *custom manual wheelchair base, K0008*

  *custom motorized/power base, K0013*

  dynamic positioning hardware for back, E2398 ◄

  foot box, E0954

  *heavy duty, E1280–E1298, K0006, K0007, K0801–K0886*

  lateral thigh or knee support, E0953

  *lightweight, E1087–E1090, E1240–E1270*

  narrowing device, E0969

  power add-on, E0983–E0984

  *reclining, fully, E1014, E1050–E1070, E1100–E1110*

  *semi-reclining, E1100–E1110*

  shock absorber, E1015–E1018

  specially sized, E1220, E1230

  *standard, E1130, K0001*

  stump support system, K0551

  tire, E0999

  transfer board or device, E0705

  tray, K0107

  van, non-emergency, A0130

  youth, E1091

**WHFO with inflatable air chamber,** L3807

**Whirlpool equipment,** E1300–E1310

**Whirlpool tub, walk-in, portable,** K1003 ◄

**WHO, wrist extension,** L3914

**Wig,** A9282

**Wipes,** A4245, A4247

**Wound**

  cleanser, A6260

  *closure, adhesive, G0168*

  cover

    alginate dressing, A6196–A6198

    collagen dressing, A6020–A6024

    foam dressing, A6209–A6214

    hydrocolloid dressing, A6234–A6239

    hydrogel dressing, A6242–A6247

    non-contact wound warming cover, and accessory, E0231–E0232

    specialty absorptive dressing, A6251–A6256

**Wound** (*Continued*)

  filler

    alginate dressing, A6199

    collagen based, A6010

    foam dressing, A6215

    hydrocolloid dressing, A6240–A6241

    hydrogel dressing, A6248

    not elsewhere classified, A6261–A6262

**Woundfix, Woundfix Plus,** Q4217 ◄

  *matrix, Q4114*

  pouch, A6154

  *therapy, negative, pressure, pump, E2402*

  *wound suction, A9272, K0743*

**Wrapping, fabric, abdominal aneurysm,** *M0301*

**Wrist**

  disarticulation prosthesis, L6050, L6055

  electronic wrist rotator, L7259

  hand/finger orthosis (WHFO), E1805, E1825, L3800–L3954

# X

**Xenon Xe 133,** A9558

**X-ray**

  equipment, portable, Q0092, R0070, R0075

  *single, energy, absorptiometry (SEXA), G0130*

  *transport, R0070–R0076*

**Xylocaine HCl,** J2000

# Y

**Yttrium Y-90 ibritumomab,** A9543

# Z

**Ziconotide,** J2278

**Zidovudine,** J3485

**Ziprasidone mesylate,** J3486

**Zoledronic acid,** J3489

# TABLE OF DRUGS

| IA | Intra-arterial administration |
|---|---|
| IU | International unit |
| IV | Intravenous administration |
| IM | Intramuscular administration |
| IT | Intrathecal |
| SC | Subcutaneous administration |
| INH | Administration by inhaled solution |
| VAR | Various routes of administration |
| OTH | Other routes of administration |
| ORAL | Administered orally |

Intravenous administration includes all methods, such as gravity infusion, injections, and timed pushes. The "VAR" posting denotes various routes of administration and is used for drugs that are commonly administered into joints, cavities, tissues, or topical applications, in addition to other parenteral administrations. Listings posted with "OTH" indicate other administration methods, such as suppositories or catheter injections.

**Blue typeface terms are added by publisher.**

| DRUG NAME | DOSAGE | METHOD OF ADMINISTRATION | HCPCS CODE |
|---|---|---|---|
| **A** | | | |
| Abatacept | 10 mg | IV | **J0129** |
| Abbokinase | 5,000 IU vial | IV | J3364 |
| | 250,000 IU vial | IV | J3365 |
| Abbokinase, Open Cath | 5,000 IU vial | IV | J3364 |
| Abciximab | 10 mg | IV | **J0130** |
| Abelcet | 10 mg | IV | J0287-J0289 |
| Abilify Maintena | 1 mg | | J0401 |
| ABLC | 50 mg | IV | J0285 |
| AbobotulinumtoxintypeA | 5 units | IM | **J0586** |
| Abraxane | 1 mg | | J9264 |
| Accuneb | 1 mg | | J7613 |
| Acetadote | 100 mg | | J0132 |
| Acetaminophen | 10 mg | IV | **J0131** |
| Acetazolamide sodium | up to 500 mg | IM, IV | **J1120** |
| Acetylcysteine | | | |
| injection | 100 mg | IV | **J0132** |
| unit dose form | per gram | INH | **J7604, J7608** |
| Achromycin | up to 250 mg | IM, IV | J0120 |
| Actemra | 1 mg | | J3262 |
| ACTH | up to 40 units | IV, IM, SC | J0800 |
| Acthar | up to 40 units | IV, IM, SC | J0800 |
| Acthib | | | J3490 |
| Acthrel | 1 mcg | | J0795 |
| Actimmune | 3 million units | SC | J9216 |
| Activase | 1 mg | IV | J2997 |

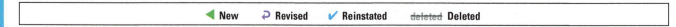

◀ New    ↻ Revised    ✔ Reinstated    ~~deleted~~ Deleted

| DRUG NAME | DOSAGE | METHOD OF ADMINISTRATION | HCPCS CODE |
|---|---|---|---|
| Acyclovir | 5 mg | | J0133 |
| | | | J8499 |
| Adagen | 25 IU | | J2504 |
| Adalimumab | 20 mg | SC | J0135 |
| Adcetris | 1 mg | IV | J9042 |
| Adenocard | 1 mg | IV | J0153 |
| Adenoscan | 1 mg | IV | J0153 |
| Adenosine | 1 mg | IV | J0153 |
| Ado-trastuzumab Emtansine | 1 mg | IV | J9354 |
| Adrenalin Chloride | up to 1 ml ampule | SC, IM | J0171 |
| Adrenalin, epinephrine | 0.1 mg | SC, IM | J0171 |
| Adriamycin, PFS, RDF | 10 mg | IV | J9000 |
| Adrucil | 500 mg | IV | J9190 |
| Advate | per IU | | J7192 |
| Aflibercept | 1 mg | OTH | J0178 |
| Agalsidase beta | 1 mg | IV | J0180 |
| Aggrastat | 0.25 mg | IM, IV | J3246 |
| A-hydrocort | up to 50 mg | IV, IM, SC | J1710 |
| | up to 100 mg | | J1720 |
| Akineton | per 5 mg | IM, IV | J0190 |
| Akynzeo | 300 mg and 0.5 mg | | J8655 |
| Alatrofloxacin mesylate, injection | 100 mg | IV | J0200 |
| Albumin | | | P9041, P9045, P9046, P9047 |
| Albuterol | 0.5 mg | INH | J7620 |
|    concentrated form | 1 mg | INH | J7610, J7611 |
|    unit dose form | 1 mg | INH | J7609, J7613 |
| Aldesleukin | per single use vial | IM, IV | J9015 |
| Aldomet | up to 250 mg | IV | J0210 |
| Aldurazyme | 0.1 mg | | J1931 |
| Alefacept | 0.5 mg | IM, IV | J0215 |
| Alemtuzumab | 1 mg | | J0202 |
| Alferon N | 250,000 IU | IM | J9215 |
| Alglucerase | per 10 units | IV | J0205 |
| Alglucosidase alfa | 10 mg | IV | J0220, J0221 |
| Alimta | 10 mg | | J9305 |
| Alkaban-AQ | 1 mg | IV | J9360 |
| Alkeran | 2 mg | ORAL | J8600 |
| | 50 mg | IV | J9245 |
| AlloDerm | per square centimeter | | Q4116 |

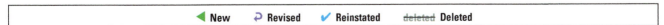

◄ New    ⟲ Revised    ✔ Reinstated    ~~deleted~~ Deleted

| DRUG NAME | DOSAGE | METHOD OF ADMINISTRATION | HCPCS CODE |
|---|---|---|---|
| AlloSkin | per square centimeter | | Q4115 |
| Aloxi | 25 mcg | | J2469 |
| Alpha 1-proteinase inhibitor, human | 10 mg | IV | J0256, J0257 |
| Alphanate | | | J7186 |
| AlphaNine SD | per IU | | J7193 |
| Alprolix | per IU | | J7201 |
| Alprostadil | | | |
|   injection | 1.25 mcg | OTH | J0270 |
|   urethral suppository | each | OTH | J0275 |
| Alteplase recombinant | 1 mg | IV | J2997 |
| Alupent | per 10 mg | INH | J7667, J7668 |
|   noncompounded, unit dose | 10 mg | INH | J7669 |
|   unit does | 10 mg | INH | J7670 |
| AmBisome | 10 mg | IV | J0289 |
| Amcort | per 5 mg | IM | J3302 |
| A-methaPred | up to 40 mg | IM, IV | J2920 |
| | up to 125 mg | IM, IV | J2930 |
| Amgen | 1 mcg | SC | J9212 |
| Amifostine | 500 mg | IV | J0207 |
| Amikacin sulfate | 100 mg | IM, IV | J0278 |
| Aminocaproic Acid | | | J3490 |
| Aminolevalinic acid HCl | unit dose (354 mg) | OTH | J7308 |
| Aminolevulinic acid HCl 10% Gel | 10 mg | OTH | J7345 |
| Aminolevulinate | 1 g | OTH | J7309 |
| Aminophylline/Aminophyllin | up to 250 mg | IV | J0280 |
| Amiodarone HCl | 30 mg | IV | J0282 |
| Amitriptyline HCl | up to 20 mg | IM | J1320 |
| Amobarbital | up to 125 mg | IM, IV | J0300 |
| Amphadase | 1 ml | | J3470 |
| Amphocin | 50 mg | IV | J0285 |
| Amphotericin B | 50 mg | IV | J0285 |
| Amphotericin B, lipid complex | 10 mg | IV | J0287-J0289 |
| Ampicillin | | | |
|   sodium | up to 500 mg | IM, IV | J0290 |
|   sodium/sulbactam sodium | per 1.5 g | IM, IV | J0295 |
| Amygdalin | | | J3570 |
| Amytal | up to 125 mg | IM, IV | J0300 |
| Anabolin LA 100 | up to 50 mg | IM | J2320 |
| Anadulafungin | 1 mg | IV | J0348 |
| Anascorp | up to 120 mg | IV | J0716 |

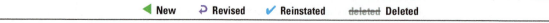

◀ New    ↺ Revised    ✔ Reinstated    ~~deleted~~ Deleted

| DRUG NAME | DOSAGE | METHOD OF ADMINISTRATION | HCPCS CODE |
|---|---|---|---|
| Anastrozole | 1 mg | | J8999 |
| Ancef | 500 mg | IV, IM | J0690 |
| Andrest 90-4 | 1 mg | IM | J3121 |
| Andro-Cyp | 1 mg | | J1071 |
| Andro-Cyp 200 | 1 mg | | J1071 |
| Andro L.A. 200 | 1 mg | IM | J3121 |
| Andro-Estro 90-4 | 1 mg | IM | J3121 |
| Andro/Fem | 1 mg | | J1071 |
| Androgyn L.A. | 1 mg | IM | J3121 |
| Androlone-50 | up to 50 mg | | J2320 |
| Androlone-D 100 | up to 50 mg | IM | J2320 |
| Andronaq-50 | up to 50 mg | IM | J3140 |
| Andronaq-LA | 1 mg | | J1071 |
| Andronate-100 | 1 mg | | J1071 |
| Andronate-200 | 1 mg | | J1071 |
| Andropository 100 | 1 mg | IM | J3121 |
| Andryl 200 | 1 mg | IM | J3121 |
| Anectine | up to 20 mg | IM, IV | J0330 |
| Anergan 25 | up to 50 mg | IM, IV | J2550 |
| | 12.5 mg | ORAL | Q0169 |
| Anergan 50 | up to 50 mg | IM, IV | J2550 |
| | 12.5 mg | ORAL | Q0169 |
| Angiomax | 1 mg | | J0583 |
| Anidulafungin | 1 mg | IV | J0348 |
| Anistreplase | 30 units | IV | J0350 |
| Antiflex | up to 60 mg | IM, IV | J2360 |
| Anti-Inhibitor | per IU | IV | J7198 |
| Antispas | up to 20 mg | IM | J0500 |
| Antithrombin III (human) | per IU | IV | J7197 |
| Antithrombin recombinant | 50 IU | IV | J7196 |
| Anzemet | 10 mg | IV | J1260 |
| | 50 mg | ORAL | S0174 |
| | 100 mg | ORAL | Q0180 |
| Apidra Solostar | per 50 units | | J1817 |
| A.P.L. | per 1,000 USP units | IM | J0725 |
| Apligraf | per square centimeter | | Q4101 |
| Apomorphine Hydrochloride | 1 mg | SC | J0364 |
| Aprepitant | 1 mg | IV | J0185 |
| Aprepitant | 5 mg | ORAL | J8501 |
| Apresoline | up to 20 mg | IV, IM | J0360 |

◀ New   ↪ Revised   ✔ Reinstated   ~~deleted~~ Deleted

| DRUG NAME | DOSAGE | METHOD OF ADMINISTRATION | HCPCS CODE |
|---|---|---|---|
| Aprotinin | 10,000 kiu | | **J0365** |
| AquaMEPHYTON | per 1 mg | IM, SC, IV | J3430 |
| Aralast | 10 mg | IV | J0256 |
| Aralen | up to 250 mg | IM | J0390 |
| Aramine | per 10 mg | IV, IM, SC | J0380 |
| Aranesp | | | |
| ESRD use | 1 mcg | | J0882 |
| Non-ESRD use | 1 mcg | | J0881 |
| Arbutamine | 1 mg | IV | **J0395** |
| Arcalyst | 1 mg | | J2793 |
| Aredia | per 30 mg | IV | J2430 |
| Arfonad, *see* Trimethaphan camsylate | | | |
| Arformoterol tartrate | 15 mcg | INH | **J7605** |
| Argatroban | | | |
| (for ESRD use) | 1 mg | IV | **J0884** |
| (for non-ESRD use) | 1 mg | IV | **J0883** |
| Aridol | 25% in 50 ml | IV | J2150 |
| | 5 mg | INH | J7665 |
| Arimidex | | | J8999 |
| Aripiprazole | 0.25 mg | IM | **J0400** |
| Aripiprazole, extended release | 1 mg | IV | **J0401** |
| Aripiprazole lauroxil (aristada) | 1 mg | IV | **J1944** ◄ |
| Aripiprazole lauroxil (aristada initio) | 1 mg | IV | **J1943** ◄ |
| ~~Aripiprazole lauroxil~~ | ~~1 mg~~ | ~~IV~~ | ~~J1942~~ ✖ |
| ~~Aristada~~ | ~~3.9 ml~~ | | ~~J1942~~ ✖ |
| Aristocort Forte | per 5 mg | IM | J3302 |
| Aristocort Intralesional | per 5 mg | IM | J3302 |
| Aristospan Intra-Articular | per 5 mg | VAR | J3303 |
| Aristospan Intralesional | per 5 mg | VAR | J3303 |
| Arixtra | per 0.5 m | | J1652 |
| Aromasin | | | J8999 |
| Arranon | 50 mg | | J9261 |
| Arrestin | up to 200 mg | IM | J3250 |
| | 250 mg | ORAL | Q0173 |
| Arsenic trioxide | 1 mg | IV | **J9017** |
| Arzerra | 10 mg | | J9302 |
| Asparaginase | 1,000 units | IV, IM | **J9019** |
| | 10,000 units | IV, IM | **J9020** |
| Astagraf XL | 0.1 mg | | J7508 |
| Astramorph PF | up to 10 mg | IM, IV, SC | J2270 |

◄ New    ↻ Revised    ✔ Reinstated    ~~deleted~~ Deleted

| DRUG NAME | DOSAGE | METHOD OF ADMINISTRATION | HCPCS CODE |
|---|---|---|---|
| Atezolizumab | 10 mg | IV | J9022 |
| Atgam | 250 mg | IV | J7504 |
| Ativan | 2 mg | IM, IV | J2060 |
| Atropine | | | |
| concentrated form | per mg | INH | J7635 |
| unit dose form | per mg | INH | J7636 |
| sulfate | 0.01 mg | IV, IM, SC | J0461, J7636 |
| Atrovent | per mg | INH | J7644, J7645 |
| ATryn | 50 IU | IV | J7196 |
| Aurothioglucose | up to 50 mg | IM | J2910 |
| Autologous cultured chondrocytes implant | | OTH | J7330 |
| Autoplex T | per IU | IV | J7198, J7199 |
| AUVI-Q | 0.15 mg | | J0171 |
| Avastin | 10 mg | | J9035 |
| Avelox | 100 mg | | J2280 |
| Avelumab | 10 mg | IV | J9023 |
| Avonex | 30 mcg | IM | J1826 |
| | 1 mcg | IM | Q3027 |
| | 1 mcg | SC | Q3028 |
| Azacitidine | 1 mg | SC | J9025 |
| Azasan | 50 mg | | J7500 |
| Azathioprine | 50 mg | ORAL | J7500 |
| Azathioprine, parenteral | 100 mg | IV | J7501 |
| Azithromycin, dihydrate | 1 gram | ORAL | Q0144 |
| Azithromycin, injection | 500 mg | IV | J0456 |
| **B** | | | |
| Baciim | | | J3490 |
| Bacitracin | | | J3490 |
| Baclofen | 10 mg | IT | J0475 |
| Baclofen for intrathecal trial | 50 mcg | OTH | J0476 |
| Bactocill | up to 250 mg | IM, IV | J2700 |
| BAL in oil | per 100 mg | IM | J0470 |
| Banflex | up to 60 mg | IV, IM | J2360 |
| Basiliximab | 20 mg | IV | J0480 |
| ~~BCG (Bacillus Calmette and Guerin), live~~ | ~~per vial~~ | ~~IV~~ | ~~J9031~~ ✖ |
| BCG live intravesical instillation | 1 mg | OTH | J9030 ◀ |
| Bebulin | per IU | | J7194 |
| Beclomethasone inhalation solution, unit dose form | per mg | INH | J7622 |
| Belatacept | 1 mg | IV | J0485 |
| Beleodaq | 10 mg | | J9032 |

◀ New    ↻ Revised    ✔ Reinstated    ~~deleted~~ Deleted

| DRUG NAME | DOSAGE | METHOD OF ADMINISTRATION | HCPCS CODE |
|---|---|---|---|
| Belimumab | 10 mg | IV | J0490 |
| Belinostat | 10 mg | IV | J9032 |
| Bena-D 10 | up to 50 mg | IV, IM | J1200 |
| Bena-D 50 | up to 50 mg | IV, IM | J1200 |
| Benadryl | up to 50 mg | IV, IM | J1200 |
| Benahist 10 | up to 50 mg | IV, IM | J1200 |
| Benahist 50 | up to 50 mg | IV, IM | J1200 |
| Ben-Allergin-50 | up to 50 mg | IV, IM | J1200 |
|  | 50 mg | ORAL | Q0163 |
| Bendamustine HCl |  |  |  |
|    Bendeka | 1 mg | IV | J9034 |
|    Treanda | 1 mg | IV | J9033 |
| Bendamustine HCl (Belrapzo/bendamustine) | 1 mg | IV | J9036 ◄ |
| Benefix | per IU | IV | J7195 |
| Benlysta | 10 mg |  | J0490 |
| Benoject-10 | up to 50 mg | IV, IM | J1200 |
| Benoject-50 | up to 50 mg | IV, IM | J1200 |
| Benralizumab | 1 mg | IV | J0517 |
| Bentyl | up to 20 mg | IM | J0500 |
| Benzocaine |  |  | J3490 |
| Benztropine mesylate | per 1 mg | IM, IV | J0515 |
| Berinert | 10 units |  | J0597 |
| Berubigen | up to 1,000 mcg | IM, SC | J3420 |
| Beta amyloid | per study dose | OTH | A9599 |
| Betalin 12 | up to 1,000 mcg | IM, SC | J3420 |
| Betameth | per 3 mg | IM, IV | J0702 |
| Betamethasone Acetate |  |  | J3490 |
| Betamethasone Acetate & Betamethasone Sodium Phosphate | per 3 mg | IM | J0702 |
| Betamethasone inhalation solution, unit dose form | per mg | INH | J7624 |
| Betaseron | 0.25 mg | SC | J1830 |
| Bethanechol chloride | up to 5 mg | SC | J0520 |
| Bethkis | 300 mg |  | J7682 |
| Bevacizumab | 10 mg | IV | J9035 |
| Bevacizumab-awwb | 10 mg | IV | Q5107 |
| Bevacizumab-bvzr (Zirabev) | 10 mg | IV | Q5118 ◄ |
| Bezlotoxumab | 10 mg | IV | J0565 |
| Bicillin C-R | 100,000 units |  | J0558 |
| Bicillin C-R 900/300 | 100,000 units | IM | J0558, J0561 |
| Bicillin L-A | 100,000 units | IM | J0561 |
| BiCNU | 100 mg | IV | J9050 |

◄ New    ↻ Revised    ✔ Reinstated    ~~deleted~~ Deleted

| DRUG NAME | DOSAGE | METHOD OF ADMINISTRATION | HCPCS CODE |
|---|---|---|---|
| Biperiden lactate | per 5 mg | IM, IV | J0190 |
| Bitolterol mesylate | | | |
|    concentrated form | per mg | INH | J7628 |
|    unit dose form | per mg | INH | J7629 |
| Bivalirudin | 1 mg | IV | J0583 |
| Blenoxane | 15 units | IM, IV, SC | J9040 |
| Bleomycin sulfate | 15 units | IM, IV, SC | J9040 |
| Blinatumomab | 1 microgram | IV | J9039 |
| Blincyto | 1 mcg | | J9039 |
| Boniva | 1 mg | | J1740 |
| Bortezomib | 0.1 mg | IV | J9041 |
| Bortezomib, not otherwise specified | 0.1 mg | | J9044 |
| Botox | 1 unit | | J0585 |
| Bravelle | 75 IU | | J3355 |
| Brentuximab Vedotin | 1 mg | IV | J9042 |
| Brethine | | | |
|    concentrated form | per 1 mg | INH | J7680 |
|    unit dose | per 1 mg | INH | J7681 |
| | up to 1 mg | SC, IV | J3105 |
| Bricanyl Subcutaneous | up to 1 mg | SC, IV | J3105 |
| Brompheniramine maleate | per 10 mg | IM, SC, IV | J0945 |
| Bronkephrine, *see* Ethylnorepinephrine HCl | | | |
| Bronkosol | | | |
|    concentrated form | per mg | INH | J7647, J7648 |
|    unit dose form | per mg | INH | J7649, J7650 |
| Brovana | | | J7605 |
| Budesonide inhalation solution | | | |
|    concentrated form | 0.25 mg | INH | J7633, J7634 |
|    unit dose form | 0.5 mg | INH | J7626, J7627 |
| Bumetanide | | | J3490 |
| Bupivacaine | | | J3490 |
| Buprenex | 0.3 mg | | J0592 |
| Buprenorphine Hydrochloride | 0.1 mg | IM | J0592 |
| Buprenorphine/Naloxone | 1 mg | ORAL | J0571 |
| | < = 3 mg | ORAL | J0572 |
| | > 3 mg but < = 6 mg | ORAL | J0573 |
| | > 6 mg but < = 10 mg | ORAL | J0574 |
| | > 10 mg | ORAL | J0575 |
| Buprenorphine extended release | < = 100 mg | ORAL | Q9991 |
| | > 100 mg | ORAL | Q9992 |

◀ New    ↻ Revised    ✔ Reinstated    ~~deleted~~ Deleted

| DRUG NAME | DOSAGE | METHOD OF ADMINISTRATION | HCPCS CODE |
|---|---|---|---|
| Burosumab-twza | 1 mg | IV | J05894 |
| Busulfan | 1 mg | IV | J0594 |
| | 2 mg | ORAL | J8510 |
| Butorphanol tartrate | 1 mg | | J0595 |
| **C** | | | |
| C1 Esterase Inhibitor | 10 units | IV | J0596-J0599 |
| Cabazitaxel | 1 mg | IV | J9043 |
| Cabergoline | 0.25 mg | ORAL | J8515 |
| Cafcit | 5 mg | IV | J0706 |
| Caffeine citrate | 5 mg | IV | J0706 |
| Caine-1 | 10 mg | IV | J2001 |
| Caine-2 | 10 mg | IV | J2001 |
| Calaspargase pegol-mknl | 10 units | IV | J9118 |
| Calcijex | 0.1 mcg | IM | J0636 |
| Calcimar | up to 400 units | SC, IM | J0630 |
| Calcitonin-salmon | up to 400 units | SC, IM | J0630 |
| Calcitriol | 0.1 mcg | IM | J0636 |
| Calcitrol | | | J8499 |
| Calcium Disodium Versenate | up to 1,000 mg | IV, SC, IM | J0600 |
| Calcium gluconate | per 10 ml | IV | J0610 |
| Calcium glycerophosphate and calcium lactate | per 10 ml | IM, SC | J0620 |
| Caldolor | 100 mg | IV | J1741 |
| Calphosan | per 10 ml | IM, SC | J0620 |
| Camptosar | 20 mg | IV | J9206 |
| Canakinumab | 1 mg | SC | J0638 |
| Cancidas | 5 mg | | J0637 |
| Capecitabine | 150 mg | ORAL | J8520 |
| | 500 mg | ORAL | J8521 |
| Capsaicin patch | per sq cm | OTH | J7336 |
| Carbidopa 5 mg/levodopa 20 mg enteral suspension | | IV | J7340 |
| Carbocaine | per 10 ml | VAR | J0670 |
| Carbocaine with Neo-Cobefrin | per 10 ml | VAR | J0670 |
| Carboplatin | 50 mg | IV | J9045 |
| Carfilzomib | 1 mg | IV | J9047 |
| Carimune | 500 mg | | J1566 |
| Carmustine | 100 mg | IV | J9050 |
| Carnitor | per 1 g | IV | J1955 |
| Carticel | | | J7330 |
| Caspofungin acetate | 5 mg | IV | J0637 |
| Cathflo Activase | 1 mg | | J2997 |

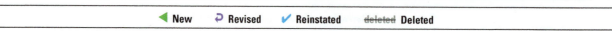

◀ New    ↻ Revised    ✔ Reinstated    ~~deleted~~ Deleted

| DRUG NAME | DOSAGE | METHOD OF ADMINISTRATION | HCPCS CODE |
|---|---|---|---|
| Caverject | per 1.25 mcg | | J0270 |
| Cayston | 500 mg | | S0073 |
| Cefadyl | up to 1 g | IV, IM | J0710 |
| Cefazolin sodium | 500 mg | IV, IM | J0690 |
| Cefepime hydrochloride | 500 mg | IV | J0692 |
| Cefizox | per 500 mg | IM, IV | J0715 |
| Cefotaxime sodium | per 1 g | IV, IM | J0698 |
| Cefotetan | | | J3490 |
| Cefoxitin sodium | 1 g | IV, IM | J0694 |
| Ceftaroline fosamil | 1 mg | | J0712 |
| Ceftazidime | per 500 mg | IM, IV | J0713 |
| Ceftazidime and avibactam | 0.5 g/0.125 g | IV | J0714 |
| Ceftizoxime sodium | per 500 mg | IV, IM | J0715 |
| Ceftolozane 50 mg and Tazobactam 25 mg | | IV | J0695 |
| Ceftriaxone sodium | per 250 mg | IV, IM | J0696 |
| Cefuroxime sodium, sterile | per 750 mg | IM, IV | J0697 |
| Celestone Soluspan | per 3 mg | IM | J0702 |
| CellCept | 250 mg | ORAL | J7517 |
| Cel-U-Jec | per 4 mg | IM, IV | Q0511 |
| Cenacort A-40 | 1 mg | | J3300 |
| | per 10 mg | IM | J3301 |
| Cenacort Forte | per 5 mg | IM | J3302 |
| Centruroides Immune F(ab) | up to 120 mg | IV | J0716 |
| Cephalothin sodium | up to 1 g | IM, IV | J1890 |
| Cephapirin sodium | up to 1 g | IV, IM | J0710 |
| Ceprotin | 10 IU | | J2724 |
| Ceredase | per 10 units | IV | J0205 |
| Cerezyme | 10 units | | J1786 |
| Cerliponase alfa | 1 mg | IV | J0567 |
| Certolizumab pegol | 1 mg | SC | J0717 |
| Cerubidine | 10 mg | IV | J9150 |
| Cetuximab | 10 mg | IV | J9055 |
| Chealamide | per 150 mg | IV | J3520 |
| Chirhostim | 1 mcg | IV | J2850 |
| Chloramphenicol Sodium Succinate | up to 1 g | IV | J0720 |
| Chlordiazepoxide HCl | up to 100 mg | IM, IV | J1990 |
| Chloromycetin Sodium Succinate | up to 1 g | IV | J0720 |
| Chloroprocaine HCl | per 30 ml | VAR | J2400 |
| Chloroquine HCl | up to 250 mg | IM | J0390 |
| Chlorothiazide sodium | per 500 mg | IV | J1205 |

◀ New    ↩ Revised    ✔ Reinstated    ~~deleted~~ Deleted

| DRUG NAME | DOSAGE | METHOD OF ADMINISTRATION | HCPCS CODE |
|---|---|---|---|
| Chlorpromazine | 5 mg | ORAL | Q0161 |
| Chlorpromazine HCl | up to 50 mg | IM, IV | J3230 |
| Cholografin Meglumine | per ml | | Q9961 |
| Chorex-5 | per 1,000 USP units | IM | J0725 |
| Chorex-10 | per 1,000 USP units | IM | J0725 |
| Chorignon | per 1,000 USP units | IM | J0725 |
| Chorionic Gonadotropin | per 1,000 USP units | IM | J0725 |
| Choron 10 | per 1,000 USP units | IM | J0725 |
| Cidofovir | 375 mg | IV | J0740 |
| Cilastatin sodium, imipenem | per 250 mg | IV, IM | J0743 |
| Cimzia | 1 mg | SC | J0717 |
| Cinacalcet | | ORAL | J0604 |
| Cinryze | 10 units | | J0598 |
| Cipro IV | 200 mg | IV | J0706 |
| Ciprofloxacin | 200 mg | IV | J0706 |
| octic suspension | 6 mg | OTH | J7342 |
| | | | J3490 |
| Cisplatin, powder or solution | per 10 mg | IV | J9060 |
| Cladribine | per mg | IV | J9065 |
| Claforan | per 1 gm | IM, IV | J0698 |
| Cleocin Phosphate | | | J3490 |
| Clindamycin | | | J3490 |
| Clofarabine | 1 mg | IV | J9027 |
| Clolar | 1 mg | | J9027 |
| Clonidine Hydrochloride | 1 mg | Epidural | J0735 |
| Cobex | up to 1,000 mcg | IM, SC | J3420 |
| Codeine phosphate | per 30 mg | IM, IV, SC | J0745 |
| Codimal-A | per 10 mg | IM, SC, IV | J0945 |
| Cogentin | per 1 mg | IM, IV | J0515 |
| Colistimethate sodium | up to 150 mg | IM, IV | J0770 |
| Collagenase, Clostridium Histolyticum | 0.01 mg | OTH | J0775 |
| Coly-Mycin M | up to 150 mg | IM, IV | J0770 |
| Compa-Z | up to 10 mg | IM, IV | J0780 |
| Copanlisib | 1 mg | IV | J9057 |
| Compazine | up to 10 mg | IM, IV | J0780 |
| | 5 mg | ORAL | Q0164 |
| | | | J8498 |
| Compounded drug, not otherwise classified | | | J7999 |
| Compro | | | J8498 |
| Conray | per ml | | Q9961 |

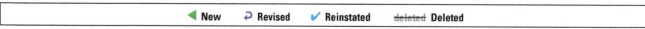

◄ New   ↩ Revised   ✔ Reinstated   ~~deleted~~ Deleted

| DRUG NAME | DOSAGE | METHOD OF ADMINISTRATION | HCPCS CODE |
|---|---|---|---|
| Conray 30 | per ml | | Q9958 |
| Conray 43 | per ml | | Q9960 |
| Copaxone | 20 mg | | J1595 |
| Cophene-B | per 10 mg | IM, SC, IV | J0945 |
| Copper contraceptive, intrauterine | | OTH | J7300 |
| Cordarone | 30 mg | IV | J0282 |
| Corgonject-5 | per 1,000 USP units | IM | J0725 |
| Corifact | 1 IU | | J7180 |
| Corticorelin ovine triflutate | 1 mcg | | J0795 |
| Corticotropin | up to 40 units | IV, IM, SC | J0800 |
| Cortisone Acetate Micronized | | | J3490 |
| Cortrosyn | per 0.25 mg | IM, IV | J0835 |
| Corvert | 1 mg | | J1742 |
| Cosmegen | 0.5 mg | IV | J9120 |
| Cosyntropin | per 0.25 mg | IM, IV | J0833, J0834 |
| Cotranzine | up to 10 mg | IM, IV | J0780 |
| Crofab | up to 1 gram | | J0840 |
| Cromolyn Sodium | | | J8499 |
| Cromolyn sodium, unit dose form | per 10 mg | INH | J7631, J7632 |
| Crotalidae immune f(ab')2 (equine) | 120 mg | IV | J0841 |
| Crotalidae Polyvalent Immune Fab | up to 1 gram | IV | J0840 |
| Crysticillin 600 A.S. | up to 600,000 units | IM, IV | J2510 |
| Cubicin | 1 mg | | J0878 |
| Cuvitru | | | J7799 |
| Cyclophosphamide | 100 mg | IV | J9070 |
| oral | 25 mg | ORAL | J8530 |
| Cyclosporine | 25 mg | ORAL | J7515 |
| | 100 mg | ORAL | J7502 |
| parenteral | 250 mg | IV | J7516 |
| Cymetra | 1 cc | | Q4112 |
| Cyramza | 5 mg | | J9308 |
| Cysto-Cornray II | per ml | | Q9958 |
| Cystografin | per ml | | Q9958 |
| Cytarabine | 100 mg | SC, IV | J9100 |
| Cytarabine liposome | 10 mg | IT | J9098 |
| CytoGam | per vial | | J0850 |
| Cytomegalovirus immune globulin intravenous (human) | per vial | IV | J0850 |
| Cytosar-U | 100 mg | SC, IV | J9100 |
| Cytovene | 500 mg | IV | J1570 |
| Cytoxan | 100 mg | IV | J8530, J9070 |

◀ New   ↻ Revised   ✔ Reinstated   ~~deleted~~ Deleted

| DRUG NAME | DOSAGE | METHOD OF ADMINISTRATION | HCPCS CODE |
|---|---|---|---|
| **D** | | | |
| D-5-W, infusion | 1000 cc | IV | **J7070** |
| Dacarbazine | 100 mg | IV | **J9130** |
| Daclizumab | 25 mg | IV | **J7513** |
| Dacogen | 1 mg | | J0894 |
| Dactinomycin | 0.5 mg | IV | **J9120** |
| Dalalone | 1 mg | IM, IV, OTH | J1100 |
| Dalalone L.A. | 1 mg | IM | J1094 |
| Dalbavancin | 5 mg | IV | **J0875** |
| Dalteparin sodium | per 2500 IU | SC | **J1645** |
| Daptomycin | 1 mg | IV | **J0878** |
| Daratumumab | 10 mg | IV | **J9145** |
| Darbepoetin Alfa | 1 mcg | IV, SC | **J0881, J0882** |
| Darzalex | 10 mg | | J9145 |
| Daunorubicin citrate, liposomal formulation | 10 mg | IV | **J9151** |
| Daunorubicin HCl | 10 mg | IV | **J9150** |
| Daunoxome | 10 mg | IV | J9151 |
| DDAVP | 1 mcg | IV, SC | J2597 |
| Decadron | 1 mg | IM, IV, OTH | J1100 |
| | 0.25 mg | | J8540 |
| Decadron Phosphate | 1 mg | IM, IV, OTH | J1100 |
| Decadron-LA | 1 mg | IM | J1094 |
| Deca-Durabolin | up to 50 mg | IM | J2320 |
| Decaject | 1 mg | IM, IV, OTH | J1100 |
| Decaject-L.A. | 1 mg | IM | J1094 |
| Decitabine | 1 mg | IV | **J0894** |
| Decolone-50 | up to 50 mg | IM | J2320 |
| Decolone-100 | up to 50 mg | IM | J2320 |
| De-Comberol | 1 mg | | J1071 |
| Deferoxamine mesylate | 500 mg | IM, SC, IV | **J0895** |
| Definity | per ml | | J3490, Q9957 |
| Degarelix | 1 mg | SC | **J9155** |
| Dehist | per 10 mg | IM, SC, IV | J0945 |
| Deladumone | 1 mg | IM | J3121 |
| Deladumone OB | 1 mg | IM | J3121 |
| Delatest | 1 mg | IM | J3121 |
| Delatestadiol | 1 mg | IM | J3121 |
| Delatestryl | 1 mg | IM | J3121 |
| Delestrogen | up to 10 mg | IM | J1380 |
| Delta-Cortef | 5 mg | ORAL | J7510 |

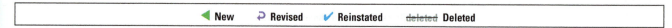

◄ New      ↻ Revised      ✔ Reinstated      ~~deleted~~ Deleted

| DRUG NAME | DOSAGE | METHOD OF ADMINISTRATION | HCPCS CODE |
|---|---|---|---|
| Demadex | 10 mg/ml | IV | J3265 |
| Demerol HCl | per 100 mg | IM, IV, SC | J2175 |
| Denileukin diftitox | 300 mcg | IV | **J9160** |
| Denosumab | 1 mg | SC | **J0897** |
| DepAndro 100 | 1 mg | | J1071 |
| DepAndro 200 | 1 mg | | J1071 |
| DepAndrogyn | 1 mg | | J1071 |
| DepGynogen | up to 5 mg | IM | J1000 |
| DepMedalone 40 | 20 mg | IM | J1020 |
| | 40 mg | IM | J1030 |
| | 80 mg | IM | J1040 |
| DepMedalone 80 | 20 mg | IM | J1020 |
| | 40 mg | IM | J1030 |
| | 80 mg | IM | J1040 |
| DepoCyt | 10 mg | | J9098 |
| Depo-estradiol cypionate | up to 5 mg | IM | **J1000** |
| Depogen | up to 5 mg | IM | J1000 |
| Depoject | 20 mg | IM | J1020 |
| | 40 mg | IM | J1030 |
| | 80 mg | IM | J1040 |
| Depo-Medrol | 20 mg | IM | J1020 |
| | 40 mg | IM | J1030 |
| | 80 mg | IM | J1040 |
| Depopred-40 | 20 mg | IM | J1020 |
| | 40 mg | IM | J1030 |
| | 80 mg | IM | J1040 |
| Depopred-80 | 20 mg | IM | J1020 |
| | 40 mg | IM | J1030 |
| | 80 mg | IM | J1040 |
| Depo-Provera Contraceptive | 1 mg | | J1050 |
| Depotest | 1 mg | | J1071 |
| Depo-Testadiol | 1 mg | | J1071 |
| Depo-Testosterone | 1 mg | | J1071 |
| Depotestrogen | 1 mg | | J1071 |
| Dermagraft | per square centimeter | | Q4106 |
| Desferal Mesylate | 500 mg | IM, SC, IV | J0895 |
| Desmopressin acetate | 1 mcg | IV, SC | **J2597** |
| Dexacen-4 | 1 mg | IM, IV, OTH | J1100 |
| Dexacen LA-8 | 1 mg | IM | J1094 |

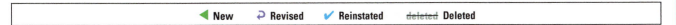

◀ New    ↻ Revised    ✔ Reinstated    ~~deleted~~ Deleted

| DRUG NAME | DOSAGE | METHOD OF ADMINISTRATION | HCPCS CODE |
|---|---|---|---|
| Dexamethasone | | | |
|    concentrated form | per mg | INH | J7637 |
|    intravitreal implant | 0.1 mg | OTH | J7312 |
|    lacrimal ophthalmic insert | 0.1 mg | OTH | J1096 |
|    unit form | per mg | INH | J7638 |
|    oral | 0.25 mg | ORAL | J8540 |
|    acetate | 1 mg | IM | J1094 |
|    sodium phosphate | 1 mg | IM, IV, OTH | J1100 |
| Dexasone | 1 mg | IM, IV, OTH | J1100 |
| Dexasone L.A. | 1 mg | IM | J1094 |
| Dexferrum | 50 mg | | J1750 |
| Dexone | 0.25 mg | ORAL | J8540 |
| | 1 mg | IM, IV, OTH | J1100 |
| Dexone LA | 1 mg | IM | J1094 |
| Dexpak | 0.25 mg | ORAL | J8540 |
| Dexrazoxane hydrochloride | 250 mg | IV | J1190 |
| Dextran 40 | 500 ml | IV | J7100 |
| Dextran 75 | 500 ml | IV | J7110 |
| Dextrose 5%/normal saline solution | 500 ml = 1 unit | IV | J7042 |
| Dextrose/water (5%) | 500 ml = 1 unit | IV | J7060 |
| D.H.E. 45 | per 1 mg | | J1110 |
| Diamox | up to 500 mg | IM, IV | J1120 |
| Diazepam | up to 5 mg | IM, IV | J3360 |
| Diazoxide | up to 300 mg | IV | J1730 |
| Dibent | up to 20 mg | IM | J0500 |
| Diclofenac sodium | 37.5 | IV | J1130 |
| Dicyclomine HCl | up to 20 mg | IM | J0500 |
| Didronel | per 300 mg | IV | J1436 |
| Diethylstilbestrol diphosphate | 250 mg | IV | J9165 |
| Diflucan | 200 mg | IV | J1450 |
| DigiFab | per vial | | J1162 |
| Digoxin | up to 0.5 mg | IM, IV | J1160 |
| Digoxin immune fab (ovine) | per vial | | J1162 |
| Dihydrex | up to 50 mg | IV, IM | J1200 |
| | 50 mg | ORAL | Q0163 |
| Dihydroergotamine mesylate | per 1 mg | IM, IV | J1110 |
| Dilantin | per 50 mg | IM, IV | J1165 |
| Dilaudid | up to 4 mg | SC, IM, IV | J1170 |
| | 250 mg | OTH | S0092 |
| Dilocaine | 10 mg | IV | J2001 |

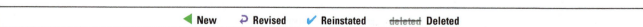

◄ New    ↻ Revised    ✔ Reinstated    ~~deleted~~ Deleted

| DRUG NAME | DOSAGE | METHOD OF ADMINISTRATION | HCPCS CODE |
|---|---|---|---|
| Dilomine | up to 20 mg | IM | J0500 |
| Dilor | up to 500 mg | IM | J1180 |
| Dimenhydrinate | up to 50 mg | IM, IV | J1240 |
| Dimercaprol | per 100 mg | IM | J0470 |
| Dimethyl sulfoxide | 50%, 50 ml | OTH | J1212 |
| Dinate | up to 50 mg | IM, IV | J1240 |
| Dioval | up to 10 mg | IM | J1380 |
| Dioval 40 | up to 10 mg | IM | J1380 |
| Dioval XX | up to 10 mg | IM | J1380 |
| Diphenacen-50 | up to 50 mg | IV, IM | J1200 |
|  | 50 mg | ORAL | Q0163 |
| Diphenhydramine HCl |  |  |  |
| injection | up to 50 mg | IV, IM | J1200 |
| oral | 50 mg | ORAL | Q0163 |
| Diprivan | 10 mg |  | J2704 |
|  |  |  | J3490 |
| Dipyridamole | per 10 mg | IV | J1245 |
| Disotate | per 150 mg | IV | J3520 |
| Di-Spaz | up to 20 mg | IM | J0500 |
| Ditate-DS | 1 mg | IM | J3121 |
| Diuril Sodium | per 500 mg | IV | J1205 |
| D-Med 80 | 20 mg | IM | J1020 |
|  | 40 mg | IM | J1030 |
|  | 80 mg | IM | J1040 |
| DMSO, Dimethyl sulfoxide 50% | 50 ml | OTH | J1212 |
| Dobutamine HCl | per 250 mg | IV | J1250 |
| Dobutrex | per 250 mg | IV | J1250 |
| Docefrez | 1 mg |  | J9171 |
| Docetaxel | 20 mg | IV | J9170 |
| Dolasetron mesylate |  |  |  |
| injection | 10 mg | IV | J1260 |
| tablets | 100 mg | ORAL | Q0180 |
| Dolophine HCl | up to 10 mg | IM, SC | J1230 |
| Dommanate | up to 50 mg | IM, IV | J1240 |
| Donbax | 10 mg |  | J1267 |
| Dopamine | 40 mg |  | J1265 |
| Dopamine HCl | 40 mg |  | J1265 |
| Doribax | 10 mg |  | J1267 |
| Doripenem | 10 mg | IV | J1267 |
| Dornase alpha, unit dose form | per mg | INH | J7639 |

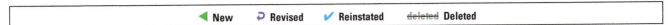

◄ New    ↻ Revised    ✔ Reinstated    ~~deleted~~ Deleted

| DRUG NAME | DOSAGE | METHOD OF ADMINISTRATION | HCPCS CODE |
|---|---|---|---|
| Dotarem | 0.1 ml | | A9575 |
| Doxercalciferol | 1 mcg | IV | J1270 |
| Doxil | 10 mg | IV | J9000, Q2050 |
| Doxorubicin HCL | 10 mg | IV | J9000 |
| Doxy | 100 mg | | J3490 |
| Dramamine | up to 50 mg | IM, IV | J1240 |
| Dramanate | up to 50 mg | IM, IV | J1240 |
| Dramilin | up to 50 mg | IM, IV | J1240 |
| Dramocen | up to 50 mg | IM, IV | J1240 |
| Dramoject | up to 50 mg | IM, IV | J1240 |
| Dronabinol | 2.5 mg | ORAL | Q0167 |
| Droperidol | up to 5 mg | IM, IV | J1790 |
| Droperidol and fentanyl citrate | up to 2 ml ampule | IM, IV | J1810 |
| Droxia | | ORAL | J8999 |
| Drug administered through a metered dose inhaler | | INH | J3535 |
| DTIC-Dome | 100 mg | IV | J9130 |
| Dua-Gen L.A. | 1 mg | IM | J3121 |
| DuoNeb | up to 2.5 mg | | J7620 |
| Duopa | 20 ml | | J7340 |
| Duoval P.A. | 1 mg | IM | J3121 |
| Durabolin | up to 50 mg | IM | J2320 |
| Duracillin A.S. | up to 600,000 units | IM, IV | J2510 |
| Duraclon | 1 mg | Epidural | J0735 |
| Dura-Estrin | up to 5 mg | IM | J1000 |
| Duragen-10 | up to 10 mg | IM | J1380 |
| Duragen-20 | up to 10 mg | IM | J1380 |
| Duragen-40 | up to 10 mg | IM | J1380 |
| Duralone-40 | 20 mg | IM | J1020 |
| | 40 mg | IM | J1030 |
| | 80 mg | IM | J1040 |
| Duralone-80 | 20 mg | IM | J1020 |
| | 40 mg | IM | J1030 |
| | 80 mg | IM | J1040 |
| Duralutin, *see* Hydroxyprogesterone Caproate | | | |
| Duramorph | up to 10 mg | IM, IV, SC | J2270, J2274 |
| Duratest-100 | 1 mg | | J1071 |
| Duratest-200 | 1 mg | | J1071 |
| Duratestrin | 1 mg | | J1071 |
| Durathate-200 | 1 mg | IM | J3121 |
| Durvalumab | 10 mg | IV | J9173 |

◄ **New**    ↻ **Revised**    ✔ **Reinstated**    ~~deleted~~ **Deleted**

| DRUG NAME | DOSAGE | METHOD OF ADMINISTRATION | HCPCS CODE |
|---|---|---|---|
| Dymenate | up to 50 mg | IM, IV | J1240 |
| Dyphylline | up to 500 mg | IM | J1180 |
| Dysport | 5 units | | J0586 |
| Dalvance | 5 mg | | J0875 |
| E | | | |
| Ecallantide | 1 mg | SC | J1290 |
| Eculizumab | 10 mg | IV | J1300 |
| Edaravone | 1 mg | IV | J1301 |
| Edetate calcium disodium | up to 1,000 mg | IV, SC, IM | J0600 |
| Edetate disodium | per 150 mg | IV | J3520 |
| Elaprase | 1 mg | | J1743 |
| Elavil | up to 20 mg | IM | J1320 |
| Elelyso | 10 units | | J3060 |
| Eligard | 7.5 mg | | J9217 |
| Elitek | 0.5 mg | | J2783 |
| Ellence | 2 mg | | J9178 |
| Elliotts B solution | 1 ml | OTH | J9175 |
| Eloctate | per IU | | J7205 |
| Elosulfase alfa | 1 mg | IV | J1322 |
| Elotuzumab | 1 mg | IV | J9176 |
| Eloxatin | 0.5 mg | | J9263 |
| Elspar | 10,000 units | IV, IM | J9020 |
| Emapalunab-lzsg | 1 mg | IV | J9210 ◄ |
| Emend | | | J1453, J8501 |
| Emete-Con, *see* Benzquinamide | | | |
| Eminase | 30 units | IV | J0350 |
| Empliciti | 1 mg | | J9176 |
| Enbrel | 25 mg | IM, IV | J1438 |
| Endrate ethylenediamine-tetra-acetic acid | per 150 mg | IV | J3520 |
| Enfuvirtide | 1 mg | SC | J1324 |
| Engerix-B | | | J3490 |
| Enovil | up to 20 mg | IM | J1320 |
| Enoxaparin sodium | 10 mg | SC | J1650 |
| Entyvio | | | J3380 |
| Eovist | 1 ml | | A9581 |
| Epinephrine | | | J7799 |
| Epinephrine, adrenalin | 0.1 mg | SC, IM | J0171 |
| Epirubicin hydrochloride | 2 mg | | J9178 |
| Epoetin alfa | 100 units | IV, SC | Q4081 |
| Epoetin alfa, non-ESRD use | 1000 units | IV | J0885 |

◄ New    ↻ Revised    ✔ Reinstated    ~~deleted~~ Deleted

| DRUG NAME | DOSAGE | METHOD OF ADMINISTRATION | HCPCS CODE | |
|---|---|---|---|---|
| Epoetin alfa, ESRD use | 100 mg | IV, SC | Q5105 | |
| Epoetin alfa, non-ESRD use | 1000 units | IV | Q5106 | |
| Epoetin alfa-epbx (Retacrit) non-ESRD use | 1000 units | IV | Q5106 | ◄ |
| Epoetin alfa-epbx (Retacrit) for-ESRD use | 100 units | IV | Q5105 | ◄ |
| Epoetin beta, ESRD use | 1 mcg | IV | J0887 | |
| Epoetin beta, non-ESRD use | 1 mcg | IV | J0888 | |
| Epogen | 1,000 units | | J0885 | |
| | | | Q4081 | |
| Epoprostenol | 0.5 mg | IV | J1325 | |
| Eptifibatide, injection | 5 mg | IM, IV | J1327 | |
| Eravacycline | 1 mg | IV | J0122 | ◄ |
| Eraxis | 1 mg | IV | J0348 | |
| Erbitux | 10 mg | | J9055 | |
| Ergonovine maleate | up to 0.2 mg | IM, IV | J1330 | |
| Eribulin mesylate | 0.1 mg | IV | J9179 | |
| Erivedge | 150 mg | | J8999 | |
| Ertapenem sodium | 500 mg | IM, IV | J1335 | |
| Erwinase | 1,000 units | IV, IM | J9019 | |
| | 10,000 units | IV, IM | J9020 | |
| Erythromycin lactobionate | 500 mg | IV | J1364 | |
| Estra-D | up to 5 mg | IM | J1000 | |
| Estradiol | | | | |
|    L.A. | up to 10 mg | IM | J1380 | |
|    L.A. 20 | up to 10 mg | IM | J1380 | |
|    L.A. 40 | up to 10 mg | IM | J1380 | |
| Estradiol Cypionate | up to 5 mg | IM | J1000 | |
| Estradiol valerate | up to 10 mg | IM | J1380 | |
| Estra-L 20 | up to 10 mg | IM | J1380 | |
| Estra-L 40 | up to 10 mg | IM | J1380 | |
| Estra-Testrin | 1 mg | IM | J3121 | |
| Estro-Cyp | up to 5 mg | IM | J1000 | |
| Estrogen, conjugated | per 25 mg | IV, IM | J1410 | |
| Estroject L.A. | up to 5 mg | IM | J1000 | |
| Estrone | per 1 mg | IM | J1435 | |
| Estrone 5 | per 1 mg | IM | J1435 | |
| Estrone Aqueous | per 1 mg | IM | J1435 | |
| Estronol | per 1 mg | IM | J1435 | |
| Estronol-L.A. | up to 5 mg | IM | J1000 | |
| Etanercept, injection | 25 mg | IM, IV | J1438 | |
| Etelcalcetide | 0.1 mg | IV | Q4078 | |

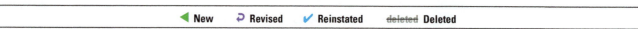

◄ New   ↻ Revised   ✔ Reinstated   ~~deleted~~ Deleted

| DRUG NAME | DOSAGE | METHOD OF ADMINISTRATION | HCPCS CODE |
|---|---|---|---|
| Eteplirsen | 10 mg | IV | J1428 |
| Ethamolin | 100 mg | | J1430 |
| Ethanolamine | 100 mg | | J1430, J3490 |
| Ethyol | 500 mg | IV | J0207 |
| Etidronate disodium | per 300 mg | IV | J1436 |
| Etonogestrel implant | | | J7307 |
| Etopophos | 10 mg | IV | J9181 |
| Etoposide | 10 mg | IV | J9181 |
| oral | 50 mg | ORAL | J8560 |
| Euflexxa | per dose | OTH | J7323 |
| Everolimus | 0.25 mg | ORAL | J7527 |
| Everone | 1 mg | IM | J3121 |
| Evomela | 50 mg | | J9245 |
| Eylea | 1 mg | OTH | J0178 |
| **F** | | | |
| Fabrazyme | 1 mg | IV | J0180 |
| Factor IX | | | |
| anti-hemophilic factor, purified, non-recombinant | per IU | IV | J7193 |
| anti-hemophilic factor, recombinant | per IU | IV | J7195, J7200-J7202 |
| complex | per IU | IV | J7194 |
| Factor VIIa (coagulation factor, recombinant) | 1 mcg | IV | J7189 |
| Factor VIII (anti-hemophilic factor) | per IU | IV | J7208 |
| human | per IU | IV | J7190 |
| porcine | per IU | IV | J7191 |
| recombinant | per IU | IV | J7182, J7185, J7192, J7188 |
| Factor VIII (anti-hemophilic factor recombinant) | | | |
| (Afstyla) | per IU | IV | J7210 |
| (Kovaltry) | per IU | IV | J7211 |
| Factor VIII Fc fusion (recombinant) | per IU | IV | J7205, J7207, J7209 |
| Factor X (human) | per IU | IV | J7175 |
| Factor XIII A-subunit (recombinant) | per IU | IV | J7181 |
| Factors, other hemophilia clotting | per IU | IV | J7196 |
| Factrel | per 100 mcg | SC, IV | J1620 |
| Famotidine | | | J3490 |
| Faslodex | 25 mg | | J9395 |
| Feiba NF | | | J7198 |
| Feiba VH Immuno | per IU | IV | J7196 |
| Fentanyl citrate | 0.1 mg | IM, IV | J3010 |

◄ New   ↻ Revised   ✔ Reinstated   ~~deleted~~ Deleted

| DRUG NAME | DOSAGE | METHOD OF ADMINISTRATION | HCPCS CODE |
|---|---|---|---|
| Feraheme | 1 mg | | Q0138, Q0139 |
| Ferric carboxymaltose | 1 mg | IV | J1439 |
| Ferric pyrophosphate citrate powder | 0.1 mg of iron | IV | J1444 ◄ |
| Ferric pyrophosphate citrate solution | 0.1 mg of iron | IV | J1443 |
| Ferrlecit | 12.5 mg | | J2916 |
| Ferumoxytol | 1 mg | | Q0138, Q0139 |
| Filgrastim-aafi | 1 mcg | IV | Q5110 |
| Filgrastim | | | |
|   (G-CSF) | 1 mcg | SC, IV | J1442, Q5101 |
|   (TBO) | 1 mcg | IV | J1447 |
| Firazyr | 1 mg | SC | J1744 |
| Firmagon | 1 mg | | J9155 |
| Flebogamma | 500 mg | IV | J1572 |
| | 1 cc | | J1460 |
| Flexoject | up to 60 mg | IV, IM | J2360 |
| Flexon | up to 60 mg | IV, IM | J2360 |
| Flolan | 0.5 mg | IV | J1325 |
| Flo-Pred | 5 mg | | J7510 |
| Florbetaben f18, diagnostic | per study dose | IV | Q9983 |
| Floxuridine | 500 mg | IV | J9200 |
| Fluconazole | 200 mg | IV | J1450 |
| Fludara | 1 mg | ORAL | J8562 |
| | 50 mg | IV | J9185 |
| Fludarabine phosphate | 1 mg | ORAL | J8562 |
| | 50 mg | IV | J9185 |
| Flunisolide inhalation solution, unit dose form | per mg | INH | J7641 |
| Fluocinolone | | OTH | J7311, J7313 |
| Fluocinolone acetonide (Yutiq) | 0.01 mg | OTH | J7314 ◄ |
| Fluorouracil | 500 mg | IV | J9190 |
| Fluphenazine decanoate | up to 25 mg | | J2680 |
| Flutamide | | | J8999 |
| Flutemetamol f18, diagnostic | per study dose | IV | Q9982 |
| Folex | 5 mg | IA, IM, IT, IV | J9250 |
| | 50 mg | IA, IM, IT, IV | J9260 |
| Folex PFS | 5 mg | IA, IM, IT, IV | J9250 |
| | 50 mg | IA, IM, IT, IV | J9260 |
| Follutein | per 1,000 USP units | IM | J0725 |
| Folotyn | 1 mg | | J9307 |
| Fomepizole | 15 mg | | J1451 |
| Fomivirsen sodium | 1.65 mg | Intraocular | J1452 |

◄ New    ↻ Revised    ✔ Reinstated    ~~deleted~~ Deleted

| DRUG NAME | DOSAGE | METHOD OF ADMINISTRATION | HCPCS CODE |
|---|---|---|---|
| Fondaparinux sodium | 0.5 mg | SC | J1652 |
| Formoterol | 12 mcg | INH | J7640 |
| Formoterol fumarate | 20 mcg | INH | J7606 |
| Fortaz | per 500 mg | IM, IV | J0713 |
| Fosaprepitant | 1 mg | IV | J1453 |
| Foscarnet sodium | per 1,000 mg | IV | J1455 |
| Foscavir | per 1,000 mg | IV | J1455 |
| Fosnetupitant 235 mg and palonosetron 0.25 mg | | IV | J1454 |
| Fosphenytoin | 50 mg | IV | Q2009 |
| Fragmin | per 2,500 IU | | J1645 |
| Fremanezumab-vfrm | 1 mg | IV | J3031 ◄ |
| FUDR | 500 mg | IV | J9200 |
| Fulvestrant | 25 mg | IM | J9395 |
| Fungizone intravenous | 50 mg | IV | J0285 |
| Furomide M.D. | up to 20 mg | IM, IV | J1940 |
| Furosemide | up to 20 mg | IM, IV | J1940 |
| **G** | | | |
| Gablofen | 10 mg | | J0475 |
| | 50 mcg | | J0476 |
| Gadavist | 0.1 ml | | A9585 |
| Gadoxetate disodium | 1 ml | IV | A9581 |
| Gallium nitrate | 1 mg | IV | J1457 |
| Galsulfase | 1 mg | IV | J1458 |
| Gamastan | 1 cc | IM | J1460 |
| | over 10 cc | IM | J1560 |
| Gamma globulin | 1 cc | IM | J1460 |
| | over 10 cc | IM | J1560 |
| Gammagard Liquid | 500 mg | IV | J1569 |
| Gammagard S/D | | | J1566 |
| GammaGraft | per square centimeter | | Q4111 |
| Gammaplex | 500 mg | IV | J1557 |
| Gammar | 1 cc | IM | J1460 |
| | over 10 cc | IM | J1560 |
| Gammar-IV, *see* Immune globin intravenous (human) | | | |
| Gamulin RH | | | |
|    immune globulin, human | 100 IU | | J2791 |
| | 1 dose package, 300 mcg | IM | J2790 |
|    immune globulin, human, solvent detergent | 100 IU | IV | J2792 |

◄ New    ↩ Revised    ✔ Reinstated    ~~deleted~~ Deleted

| DRUG NAME | DOSAGE | METHOD OF ADMINISTRATION | HCPCS CODE |
|---|---|---|---|
| Gamunex | 500 mg | IV | J1561 |
| Ganciclovir, implant | 4.5 mg | OTH | J7310 |
| Ganciclovir sodium | 500 mg | IV | J1570 |
| Ganirelix | | | J3490 |
| Garamycin, gentamicin | up to 80 mg | IM, IV | J1580 |
| Gastrografin | per ml | | Q9963 |
| Gatifloxacin | 10 mg | IV | J1590 |
| Gazyva | 10 mg | | J9301 |
| Gefitinib | 250 mg | ORAL | J8565 |
| Gel-One | per dose | OTH | J7326 |
| Gemcitabine HCl | 200 mg | IV | J9201 |
| Gemcitabine HCl, not otherwise specified | 200 mg | IV | J9201 ◄ |
| Gemcitabine HCl (Infugem) | 200 mg | IV | J9199 ◄ |
| Gemsar | 200 mg | IV | J9201 |
| Gemtuzumab ozogamicin | 5 mg | IV | J9300 |
| Gengraf | 100 mg | | J7502 |
| | 25 mg | ORAL | J7515 |
| Genotropin | 1 mg | | J2941 |
| Gentamicin Sulfate | up to 80 mg | IM, IV | J1580, J7699 |
| Gentran | 500 ml | IV | J7100 |
| Gentran 75 | 500 ml | IV | J7110 |
| Geodon | 10 mg | | J3486 |
| Gesterol 50 | per 50 mg | | J2675 |
| Glassia | 10 mg | IV | J0257 |
| Glatiramer Acetate | 20 mg | SC | J1595 |
| Gleevec (Film-Coated) | 400 mg | | J8999 |
| GlucaGen | per 1 mg | | J1610 |
| Glucagon HCl | per 1 mg | SC, IM, IV | J1610 |
| Glukor | per 1,000 USP units | IM | J0725 |
| Glycopyrrolate | | | |
|    concentrated form | per 1 mg | INH | J7642 |
|    unit dose form | per 1 mg | INH | J7643 |
| Gold sodium thiomalate | up to 50 mg | IM | J1600 |
| Golimumab | 1 mg | IV | J1602 |
| Gonadorelin HCl | per 100 mcg | SC, IV | J1620 |
| Gonal-F | | | J3490 |
| Gonic | per 1,000 USP units | IM | J0725 |
| Goserelin acetate implant | per 3.6 mg | SC | J9202 |
| Graftjacket | per square centimeter | | Q4107 |
| Graftjacket Xpress | 1 cc | | Q4113 |

| ◄ New | ↻ Revised | ✔ Reinstated | ~~deleted~~ Deleted |
|---|---|---|---|

| DRUG NAME | DOSAGE | METHOD OF ADMINISTRATION | HCPCS CODE |
|---|---|---|---|
| Granisetron HCl | | | |
| extended release | 0.1 mg | IV | J1627 |
| injection | 100 mcg | IV | J1626 |
| oral | 1 mg | ORAL | Q0166 |
| Guselkumab | 1 mg | IV | J1628 |
| Gynogen L.A. A10 | up to 10 mg | IM | J1380 |
| Gynogen L.A. A20 | up to 10 mg | IM | J1380 |
| Gynogen L.A. A40 | up to 10 mg | IM | J1380 |
| H | | | |
| Halaven | 0.1 mg | | J9179 |
| Haldol | up to 5 mg | IM, IV | J1630 |
| Haloperidol | up to 5 mg | IM, IV | J1630 |
| Haloperidol decanoate | per 50 mg | IM | J1631 |
| Haloperidol Lactate | up to 5 mg | | J1630 |
| Hectoral | 1 mcg | IV | J1270 |
| Helixate FS | per IU | | J7192 |
| Hemin | 1 mg | | J1640 |
| Hemofil M | per IU | IV | J7190 |
| Hemophilia clotting factors (e.g., anti-inhibitors) | per IU | IV | J7198 |
| NOC | per IU | IV | J7199 |
| Hepagam B | 0.5 ml | IM | J1571 |
| | 0.5 ml | IV | J1573 |
| Heparin sodium | 1,000 units | IV, SC | J1644 |
| Heparin sodium (heparin lock flush) | 10 units | IV | J1642 |
| Heparin Sodium (Procine) | per 1,000 units | | J1644 |
| Hep-Lock | 10 units | IV | J1642 |
| Hep-Lock U/P | 10 units | IV | J1642 |
| Herceptin | 10 mg | IV | J9355 |
| Hexabrix 320 | per ml | | Q9967 |
| Hexadrol Phosphate | 1 mg | IM, IV, OTH | J1100 |
| Hexaminolevulinate hydrochloride | 100 mg | IV | A9589 |
| Histaject | per 10 mg | IM, SC, IV | J0945 |
| Histerone 50 | up to 50 mg | IM | J3140 |
| Histerone 100 | up to 50 mg | IM | J3140 |
| Histrelin | | | |
| acetate | 10 mcg | | J1675 |
| implant | 50 mg | OTH | J9225, J9226 |
| Hizentra, see Immune globulin | | | |
| Humalog | per 5 units | | J1815 |
| | per 50 units | | J1817 |

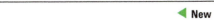

◄ New    ↻ Revised    ✔ Reinstated    ~~deleted~~ Deleted

| DRUG NAME | DOSAGE | METHOD OF ADMINISTRATION | HCPCS CODE |
|---|---|---|---|
| Human fibrinogen concentrate | 100 mg | IV | J7178 |
| Human fibrinogen concentrate (fibryga) | 1 mg | IV | J7177 |
| Humate-P | per IU | | J7187 |
| Humatrope | 1 mg | | J2941 |
| Humira | 20 mg | | J0135 |
| Humulin | per 5 units | | J1815 |
| | per 50 units | | J1817 |
| Hyalgan, Spurtaz or VISCO-3 | | IA | J7321 |
| Hyaluronan or derivative | per dose | IV | J7327 |
|    Durolane | 1 mg | IA | J7318 |
|    Gel-Syn | 0.1 mg | IA | J7328 |
|    Gelsyn-3 | 0.1 mg | IV | J7328 |
|    Gen Visc 850 | 1 mg | IA | J7320 |
|    Hymovis | 1 mg | IA | J7322 |
|    Synojoynt | 1 mg | VAR | J7331 ◀ |
|    Triluron | 1 mg | IV | J7332 ◀ |
|    Trivisc | 1 mg | IV | J7329 |
| Hyaluronic Acid | | | J3490 |
| Hyaluronidase | up to 150 units | SC, IV | J3470 |
| Hyaluronidase | | | |
|    ovine | up to 999 units | VAR | J3471 |
|    ovine | per 1000 units | VAR | J3472 |
|    recombinant | 1 usp | SC | J3473 |
| Hyate:C | per IU | IV | J7191 |
| Hybolin Decanoate | up to 50 mg | IM | J2320 |
| Hybolin Improved, *see* Nandrolone phenpropionate | | | |
| Hycamtin | 0.25 mg | ORAL | J8705 |
| | 4 mg | IV | J9351 |
| Hydralazine HCl | up to 20 mg | IV, IM | J0360 |
| Hydrate | up to 50 mg | IM, IV | J1240 |
| Hydrea | | | J8999 |
| Hydrocortisone acetate | up to 25 mg | IV, IM, SC | J1700 |
| Hydrocortisone sodium phosphate | up to 50 mg | IV, IM, SC | J1710 |
| Hydrocortisone succinate sodium | up to 100 mg | IV, IM, SC | J1720 |
| Hydrocortone Acetate | up to 25 mg | IV, IM, SC | J1700 |
| Hydrocortone Phosphate | up to 50 mg | IM, IV, SC | J1710 |
| Hydromorphone HCl | up to 4 mg | SC, IM, IV | J1170 |
| Hydroxyprogesterone Caproate | 1 mg | IM | J1725 |
|    (Makena) | 10 mg | IV | J1726 |
|    NOS | 10 mg | IV | J1729 |
| Hydroxyurea | | | J8999 |

◀ New    ↻ Revised    ✔ Reinstated    ~~deleted~~ Deleted

| DRUG NAME | DOSAGE | METHOD OF ADMINISTRATION | HCPCS CODE |
|---|---|---|---|
| Hydroxyzine HCl | up to 25 mg | IM | J3410 |
| Hydroxyzine Pamoate | 25 mg | ORAL | Q0177 |
| Hylan G-F 20 | | OTH | J7322 |
| Hylenex | 1 USP unit | | J3473 |
| Hyoscyamine sulfate | up to 0.25 mg | SC, IM, IV | J1980 |
| Hyperrho S/D | 300 mcg | | J2790 |
| | 100 IU | | J2792 |
| Hyperstat IV | up to 300 mg | IV | J1730 |
| Hyper-Tet | up to 250 units | IM | J1670 |
| HypRho-D | 300 mcg | IM | J2790 |
| | | | J2791 |
| | 50 mcg | | J2788 |
| Hyrexin-50 | up to 50 mg | IV, IM | J1200 |
| Hyzine-50 | up to 25 mg | IM | J3410 |
| **I** | | | |
| Ibalizumab-uiyk | 10 mg | IV | J1746 |
| Ibandronate sodium | 1 mg | IV | J1740 |
| Ibuprofen | 100 mg | IV | J1741 |
| Ibutilide fumarate | 1 mg | IV | J1742 |
| Icatibant | 1 mg | SC | J1744 |
| Idamycin | 5 mg | IV | J9211 |
| Idarubicin HCl | 5 mg | IV | J9211 |
| Idursulfase | 1 mg | IV | J1743 |
| Ifex | 1 g | IV | J9208 |
| Ifosfamide | 1 g | IV | J9208 |
| Ilaris | 1 mg | | J0638 |
| Iloprost | 20 mcg | INH | Q4074 |
| Ilotycin, *see* Erythromycin gluceptate | | | |
| Iluvien | 0.01 mg | | J7313 |
| Imferon | 50 mg | | J1750 |
| Imiglucerase | 10 units | IV | J1786 |
| Imitrex | 6 mg | SC | J3030 |
| Imlygic | per 1 million plaque forming units | | J9325, J9999 |
| Immune globulin | | | |
| Bivigam | 500 mg | IV | J1556 |
| Cuvitru | 100 mg | IV | J1555 |
| Flebogamma | 500 mg | IV | J1572 |
| Gammagard Liquid | 500 mg | IV | J1569 |
| Gammaplex | 500 mg | IV | J1557 |
| Gamunex | 500 mg | IV | J1561 |

◄ New    ↻ Revised    ✔ Reinstated    ~~deleted~~ Deleted

| DRUG NAME | DOSAGE | METHOD OF ADMINISTRATION | HCPCS CODE |
|---|---|---|---|
| Immune globulin *(Continued)* | | | |
| HepaGam B | 0.5 ml | IM | **J1571** |
| | 0.5 ml | IV | **J1573** |
| Hizentra | 100 mg | SC | **J1559** |
| Hyaluronidase, (HYQVIA) | 100 mg | IV | **J1575** |
| NOS | 500 mg | IV | **J1566, J1599** |
| Octagam | 500 mg | IV | **J1568** |
| Privigen | 500 mg | IV | **J1459** |
| Rhophylac | 100 IU | IM | **J2791** |
| Subcutaneous | 100 mg | SC | **J1562** |
| Immunosuppressive drug, not otherwise classified | | | **J7599** |
| Imuran | 50 mg | ORAL | J7500 |
| | 100 mg | IV | J7501 |
| Inapsine | up to 5 mg | IM, IV | J1790 |
| Incobotulinumtoxin type A | 1 unit | IM | **J0588** |
| Increlex | 1 mg | | J2170 |
| Inderal | up to 1 mg | IV | J1800 |
| Infed | 50 mg | | J1750 |
| Infergen | 1 mcg | SC | J9212 |
| Inflectra | | | Q5102 |
| Infliximab | | | |
| dyyb | 10 mg | IM, IV | **Q5103** |
| abda | 10 mg | IM, IV | **Q5104** |
| qbtx | 10 mg | IM, IV | **Q5109** |
| Infumorph | 10 mg | | J2274 |
| Injectafer | 1 mg | | J1439 |
| Injection factor ix, glycopegylated | 1 iu | IV | **J7203** |
| Injection sulfur hexafluoride lipid microspheres | per ml | IV | **Q9950** |
| Innohep | 1,000 iu | SC | J1655 |
| Innovar | up to 2 ml ampule | IM, IV | J1810 |
| Inotuzumab orogamicin | 0.1 mg | IV | **J9229** |
| Insulin | 5 units | SC | **J1815** |
| Insulin-Humalog | per 50 units | | J1817 |
| Insulin lispro | 50 units | SC | **J1817** |
| Intal | per 10 mg | INH | J7631, J7632 |
| Integra | | | |
| Bilayer Matrix Wound Dressing (BMWD) | per square centimeter | | Q4104 |
| Dermal Regeneration Template (DRT) | per square centimeter | | Q4105 |
| Flowable Wound Matrix | 1 cc | | Q4114 |
| Matrix | per square centimeter | | Q4108 |

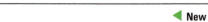  ◄ New  � Revised  ✔ Reinstated  ~~deleted~~ Deleted

| DRUG NAME | DOSAGE | METHOD OF ADMINISTRATION | HCPCS CODE |
|---|---|---|---|
| Integrilin | 5 mg | IM, IV | J1327 |
| Interferon alfa-2a, recombinant | 3 million units | SC, IM | J9213 |
| Interferon alfa-2b, recombinant | 1 million units | SC, IM | J9214 |
| Interferon alfa-n3 (human leukocyte derived) | 250,000 IU | IM | J9215 |
| Interferon alphacon-1, recombinant | 1 mcg | SC | J9212 |
| Interferon beta-1a | 30 mcg | IM | J1826 |
| | 1 mcg | IM | Q3027 |
| | 1 mcg | SC | Q3028 |
| Interferon beta-1b | 0.25 mg | SC | J1830 |
| Interferon gamma-1b | 3 million units | SC | J9216 |
| Intrauterine copper contraceptive | | OTH | J7300 |
| Intron-A | 1 million units | | J9214 |
| Invanz | 500 mg | | J1335 |
| Invega Sustenna | 1 mg | | J2426 |
| Ipilimumab | 1 mg | IV | J9228 |
| Ipratropium bromide, unit dose form | per mg | INH | J3535, J7620, J7644, J7645 |
| Iressa | 250 mg | | J8565 |
| Irinotecan | 20 mg | IV | J9206, J9205 |
| Iron dextran | 50 mg | IV, IM | J1750 |
| Iron sucrose | 1 mg | IV | J1756 |
| Irrigation solution for Tx of bladder calculi | per 50 ml | OTH | Q2004 |
| Isavuconazonium | 1 mg | IV | J1833 |
| Isocaine HCl | per 10 ml | VAR | J0670 |
| Isoetharine HCl | | | |
|    concentrated form | per mg | INH | J7647, J7648 |
|    unit dose form | per mg | INH | J7649, J7650 |
| Isoproterenol HCl | | | |
|    concentrated form | per mg | INH | J7657, J7658 |
|    unit dose form | per mg | INH | J7659, J7660 |
| Isovue | per ml | | Q9966, Q9967 |
| Istodax | 1 mg | | J9315 |
| Isuprel | | | |
|    concentrated form | per mg | INH | J7657, J7658 |
|    unit dose form | per mg | INH | J7659, J7660 |
| Itraconazole | 50 mg | IV | J1835 |
| Ixabepilone | 1 mg | IV | J9207 |
| Ixempra | 1 mg | | J9207 |

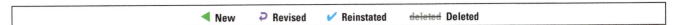

◄ New    ↻ Revised    ✔ Reinstated    ~~deleted~~ Deleted

| DRUG NAME | DOSAGE | METHOD OF ADMINISTRATION | HCPCS CODE |
|---|---|---|---|
| **J** | | | |
| Jenamicin | up to 80 mg | IM, IV | J1580 |
| Jetrea | 0.125 mg | | J7316 |
| Jevtana | 1 mg | | J9043 |
| **K** | | | |
| Kabikinase | per 250,000 IU | IV | J2995 |
| Kadcyla | 1 mg | | J9354 |
| Kalbitor | 1 mg | | J1290 |
| Kaleinate | per 10 ml | IV | J0610 |
| Kanamycin sulfate | up to 75 mg | IM, IV | **J1850** |
| | up to 500 mg | IM, IV | **J1840** |
| Kantrex | up to 75 mg | IM, IV | J1850 |
| | up to 500 mg | IM, IV | J1840 |
| Keflin | up to 1 g | IM, IV | J1890 |
| Kefurox | per 750 mg | | J0697 |
| Kefzol | 500 mg | IV, IM | J0690 |
| Kenaject-40 | 1 mg | | J3300 |
| | per 10 mg | IM | J3301 |
| Kenalog-10 | 1 mg | | J3300 |
| | per 10 mg | IM | J3301 |
| Kenalog-40 | 1 mg | | J3300 |
| | per 10 mg | IM | J3301 |
| Kepivance | 50 mcg | | J2425 |
| Keppra | 10 mg | | J1953 |
| Keroxx | 1 cc | IV | **Q4202** |
| Kestrone 5 | per 1 mg | IM | J1435 |
| Ketorolac tromethamine | per 15 mg | IM, IV | **J1885** |
| Key-Pred 25 | up to 1 ml | IM | J2650 |
| Key-Pred 50 | up to 1 ml | IM | J2650 |
| Key-Pred-SP, *see* Prednisolone sodium phosphate | | | |
| Keytruda | 1 mg | | J9271 |
| K-Flex | up to 60 mg | IV, IM | J2360 |
| Khapzory | 0.5 mg | IV | **J0642** ◀ |
| Kinevac | 5 mcg | IV | J2805 |
| Kitabis PAK | per 300 mg | | J7682 |
| Klebcil | up to 75 mg | IM, IV | J1850 |
| | up to 500 mg | IM, IV | J1840 |

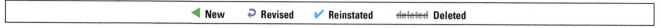

◀ New    ↻ Revised    ✔ Reinstated    ~~deleted~~ Deleted

| DRUG NAME | DOSAGE | METHOD OF ADMINISTRATION | HCPCS CODE |
|---|---|---|---|
| Koate-HP (anti-hemophilic factor) | | | |
| human | per IU | IV | J7190 |
| porcine | per IU | IV | J7191 |
| recombinant | per IU | IV | J7192 |
| Kogenate | | | |
| human | per IU | IV | J7190 |
| porcine | per IU | IV | J7191 |
| recombinant | per IU | IV | J7192 |
| Konakion | per 1 mg | IM, SC, IV | J3430 |
| Konyne-80 | per IU | IV | J7194 |
| Krystexxa | 1 mg | | J2507 |
| Kyleena | 19.5 mg | OTH | J7296 |
| Kyprolis | 1 mg | | J9047 |
| Kytril | 1 mg | ORAL | Q0166 |
| | 1 mg | IV | S0091 |
| | 100 mcg | IV | J1626 |
| **L** | | | |
| L.A.E. 20 | up to 10 mg | IM | J1380 |
| Laetrile, Amygdalin, vitamin B-17 | | | J3570 |
| Lanadelumab-flyo | 1 mg | IV | J0593 |
| Lanoxin | up to 0.5 mg | IM, IV | J1160 |
| Lanreotide | 1 mg | SC | J1930 |
| Lantus | per 5 units | | J1815 |
| Largon, *see* Propiomazine HCl | | | |
| Laronidase | 0.1 mg | IV | J1931 |
| Lasix | up to 20 mg | IM, IV | J1940 |
| L-Caine | 10 mg | IV | J2001 |
| Lemtrada | 1 mg | | J0202 |
| Lepirudin | 50 mg | | J1945 |
| Leucovorin calcium | per 50 mg | IM, IV | J0640 |
| Leukeran | | | J8999 |
| Leukine | 50 mcg | IV | J2820 |
| Leuprolide acetate | per 1 mg | IM | J9218 |
| Leuprolide acetate (for depot suspension) | per 3.75 mg | IM | J1950 |
| | 7.5 mg | IM | J9217 |
| Leuprolide acetate implant | 65 mg | OTH | J9219 |
| Leustatin | per mg | IV | J9065 |

◄ New    ↻ Revised    ✔ Reinstated    ~~deleted~~ Deleted

| DRUG NAME | DOSAGE | METHOD OF ADMINISTRATION | HCPCS CODE |
|---|---|---|---|
| Levalbuterol HCl | | | |
|    concentrated form | 0.5 mg | INH | J7607, J7612 |
|    unit dose form | 0.5 mg | INH | J7614, J7615 |
| Levaquin I.U. | 250 mg | IV | J1956 |
| Levetiracetam | 10 mg | IV | J1953 |
| Levocarnitine | per 1 gm | IV | J1955 |
| Levo-Dromoran | up to 2 mg | SC, IV | J1960 |
| Levofloxacin | 250 mg | IV | J1956 |
| Levoleucovorin NOS | 0.5 mg | IV | J0641 |
| Levonorgestrel implant | | OTH | J7306 |
| Levonorgestrel-releasing intrauterine contraceptive system | 52 mg | OTH | J7297, J7298 |
|    Kyleena | 19.5 mg | OTH | J7296 |
| Levorphanol tartrate | up to 2 mg | SC, IV | J1960 |
| Levsin | up to 0.25 mg | SC, IM, IV | J1980 |
| Levulan Kerastick | unit dose (354 mg) | OTH | J7308 |
| Lexiscan | 0.1 mg | | J2785 |
| Librium | up to 100 mg | IM, IV | J1990 |
| Lidocaine HCl | 10 mg | IV | J2001 |
| Lidoject-1 | 10 mg | IV | J2001 |
| Lidoject-2 | 10 mg | IV | J2001 |
| Liletta | 52 mg | OTH | J7297 |
| Lincocin | up to 300 mg | IV | J2010 |
| Lincomycin HCl | up to 300 mg | IV | J2010 |
| Linezolid | 200 mg | IV | J2020 |
| Lioresal | 10 mg | IT | J0475 |
| | | | J0476 |
| Liposomal | | | |
|    Cytarabine | 2.27 mg | IV | J9153 |
|    Daunorubicin | 1 mg | IV | J9153 |
| Liquaemin Sodium | 1,000 units | IV, SC | J1644 |
| LMD (10%) | 500 ml | IV | J7100 |
| Locort | 1.5 mg | | J8540 |
| Lorazepam | 2 mg | IM, IV | J2060 |
| Lovenox | 10 mg | SC | J1650 |
| Loxapine | 1 mg | OTH | J2062 |
| Lucentis | 0.1 mg | | J2778 |
| Lufyllin | up to 500 mg | IM | J1180 |
| Lumason | per ml | | Q9950 |
| Luminal Sodium | up to 120 mg | IM, IV | J2560 |
| Lumizyme | 10 mg | | J0221 |

◄ New    ↺ Revised    ✔ Reinstated    ~~deleted~~ Deleted

| DRUG NAME | DOSAGE | METHOD OF ADMINISTRATION | HCPCS CODE |
|---|---|---|---|
| Lupon Depot | 7.5 mg | | J9217 |
| | 3.75 mg | | J1950 |
| Lupron | per 1 mg | IM | J9218 |
| | per 3.75 mg | IM | J1950 |
| | 7.5 mg | IM | J9217 |
| Lyophilized, *see* Cyclophosphamide, lyophilized | | | |
| **M** | | | |
| Macugen | 0.3 mg | | J2503 |
| Magnesium sulfate | 500 mg | | **J3475** |
| Magnevist | per ml | | A9579 |
| Makena | 1 mg | | J1725 |
| Mannitol | 25% in 50 ml | IV | **J2150** |
| | 5 mg | INH | **J7665** |
| Marcaine | | | J3490 |
| Marinol | 2.5 mg | ORAL | Q0167 |
| Marmine | up to 50 mg | IM, IV | J1240 |
| Matulane | 50 mg | | J8999 |
| Maxipime | 500 mg | IV | J0692 |
| MD-76R | per ml | | Q9963 |
| MD Gastroview | per ml | | Q9963 |
| Mecasermin | 1 mg | SC | **J2170** |
| Mechlorethamine HCl (nitrogen mustard), HN2 | 10 mg | IV | **J9230** |
| Medralone 40 | 20 mg | IM | J1020 |
| | 40 mg | IM | J1030 |
| | 80 mg | IM | J1040 |
| Medralone 80 | 20 mg | IM | J1020 |
| | 40 mg | IM | J1030 |
| | 80 mg | IM | J1040 |
| Medrol | per 4 mg | ORAL | J7509 |
| Medroxyprogesterone acetate | 1 mg | IM | **J1050** |
| Mefoxin | 1 g | IV, IM | J0694 |
| Megestrol Acetate | | | J8999 |
| Melphalan HCl | 50 mg | IV | J9245 |
| Melphalan, oral | 2 mg | ORAL | J8600 |
| Menoject LA | 1 mg | | J1071 |
| Mepergan injection | up to 50 mg | IM, IV | J2180 |
| Meperidine and promethazine HCl | up to 50 mg | IM, IV | **J2180** |
| Meperidine HCl | per 100 mg | IM, IV, SC | **J2175** |
| Mepivacaine HCl | per 10 ml | VAR | **J0670** |
| Mepolizumab | 1 mg | IV | **J2182** |

◀ New   ↻ Revised   ✔ Reinstated   ~~deleted~~ **Deleted**

| DRUG NAME | DOSAGE | METHOD OF ADMINISTRATION | HCPCS CODE |
|---|---|---|---|
| Mercaptopurine | | | J8999 |
| Meropenem | 100 mg | IV | J2185 |
| Merrem | 100 mg | | J2185 |
| Mesna | 200 mg | IV | J9209 |
| Mesnex | 200 mg | IV | J9209 |
| Metaprel | | | |
| concentrated form | per 10 mg | INH | J7667, J7668 |
| unit dose form | per 10 mg | INH | J7669, J7670 |
| Metaproterenol sulfate | | | |
| concentrated form | per 10 mg | INH | J7667, J7668 |
| unit dose form | per 10 mg | INH | J7669, J7670 |
| Metaraminol bitartrate | per 10 mg | IV, IM, SC | J0380 |
| Metastron | per millicurie | | A9600 |
| Methacholine chloride | 1 mg | INH | J7674 |
| Methadone HCl | up to 10 mg | IM, SC | J1230 |
| Methergine | up to 0.2 mg | | J2210 |
| Methocarbamol | up to 10 ml | IV, IM | J2800 |
| Methotrexate LPF | 5 mg | IV, IM, IT, IA | J9250 |
| | 50 mg | IV, IM, IT, IA | J9260 |
| Methotrexate, oral | 2.5 mg | ORAL | J8610 |
| Methotrexate sodium | 5 mg | IV, IM, IT, IA | J9250 |
| | 50 mg | IV, IM, IT, IA | J9260 |
| Methyldopate HCl | up to 250 mg | IV | J0210 |
| Methylergonovine maleate | up to 0.2 mg | | J2210 |
| Methylnaltrexone | 0.1 mg | SC | J2212 |
| Methylprednisolone acetate | 20 mg | IM | J1020 |
| | 40 mg | IM | J1030 |
| | 80 mg | IM | J1040 |
| Methylprednisolone, oral | per 4 mg | ORAL | J7509 |
| Methylprednisolone sodium succinate | up to 40 mg | IM, IV | J2920 |
| | up to 125 mg | IM, IV | J2930 |
| Metoclopramide HCl | up to 10 mg | IV | J2765 |
| Metrodin | 75 IU | | J3355 |
| Metronidazole | | | J3490 |
| Metvixia | 1 g | OTH | J7309 |
| Miacalcin | up to 400 units | SC, IM | J0630 |
| Micafungin sodium | 1 mg | | J2248 |
| MicRhoGAM | 50 mcg | | J2788 |
| Midazolam HCl | per 1 mg | IM, IV | J2250 |
| Milrinone lactate | 5 mg | IV | J2260 |

 New     Revised    ✔ Reinstated    ~~deleted~~ Deleted

| DRUG NAME | DOSAGE | METHOD OF ADMINISTRATION | HCPCS CODE |
|---|---|---|---|
| Minocine | 1 mg | | J2265 |
| Minocycline Hydrochloride | 1 mg | IV | J2265 |
| Mircera | 1 mcg | | J0887, J0888 |
| Mirena | 52 mg | OTH | J7297, J7298 |
| Mithracin | 2,500 mcg | IV | J9270 |
| Mitomycin | 0.2 mg | Ophthalmic | J7315 |
| | 5 mg | IV | J9280 |
| Mitosol | 0.2 mg | Ophthalmic | J7315 |
| | 5 mg | IV | J9280 |
| Mitoxantrone HCl | per 5 mg | IV | J9293 |
| Mogamulizumab-kpkc | 1 mg | IV | J9204 ◄ |
| Monocid, *see* Cefonicic sodium | | | |
| Monoclate-P | | | |
|   human | per IU | IV | J7190 |
|   porcine | per IU | IV | J7191 |
| Monoclonal antibodies, parenteral | 5 mg | IV | J7505 |
| Mononine | per IU | IV | J7193 |
| Monovisc | | | J7327 |
| Morphine sulfate | up to 10 mg | IM, IV, SC | J2270 |
|   preservative-free | 10 mg | SC, IM, IV | J2274 |
| Moxetumomab Pasudotox-tdfk | 0.01 mg | IV | J9313 ◄ |
| Moxifloxacin | 100 mg | IV | J2280 |
| Mozobil | 1 mg | | J2562 |
| M-Prednisol-40 | 20 mg | IM | J1020 |
| | 40 mg | IM | J1030 |
| | 80 mg | IM | J1040 |
| M-Prednisol-80 | 20 mg | IM | J1020 |
| | 40 mg | IM | J1030 |
| | 80 mg | IM | J1040 |
| Mucomyst | | | |
|   unit dose form | per gram | INH | J7604, J7608 |
| Mucosol | | | |
|   injection | 100 mg | IV | J0132 |
|   unit dose | per gram | INH | J7604, J7608 |
| MultiHance | per ml | | A9577 |
| MultiHance Multipack | per ml | | A9578 |
| Muromonab-CD3 | 5 mg | IV | J7505 |
| Muse | | OTH | J0275 |
| | 1.25 mcg | OTH | J0270 |
| Mustargen | 10 mg | IV | J9230 |

◄ New    ↻ Revised    ✔ Reinstated    ~~deleted~~ Deleted

| DRUG NAME | DOSAGE | METHOD OF ADMINISTRATION | HCPCS CODE |
|---|---|---|---|
| Mutamycin | | | |
| | 0.2 mg | Ophthalmic | **J7315** |
| | 5 mg | IV | **J9280** |
| Mycamine | 1 mg | | J2248 |
| Mycophenolate Mofetil | 250 mg | ORAL | **J7517** |
| Mycophenolic acid | 180 mg | ORAL | **J7518** |
| Myfortic | 180 mg | | J7518 |
| Myleran | 1 mg | | J0594 |
| | 2 mg | ORAL | J8510 |
| Mylotarg | 5 mg | IV | J9300 |
| Myobloc | per 100 units | IM | J0587 |
| Myochrysine | up to 50 mg | IM | J1600 |
| Myolin | up to 60 mg | IV, IM | J2360 |
| **N** | | | |
| Nabilone | 1 mg | ORAL | **J8650** |
| Nafcillin | | | J3490 |
| Naglazyme | 1 mg | | J1458 |
| Nalbuphine HCl | per 10 mg | IM, IV, SC | **J2300** |
| Naloxone HCl | per 1 mg | IM, IV, SC | **J2310**, J3490 |
| Naltrexone | | | J3490 |
| Naltrexone, depot form | 1 mg | IM | **J2315** |
| Nandrobolic L.A. | up to 50 mg | IM | J2320 |
| Nandrolone decanoate | up to 50 mg | IM | **J2320** |
| Narcan | 1 mg | IM, IV, SC | J2310 |
| Naropin | 1 mg | | J2795 |
| Nasahist B | per 10 mg | IM, SC, IV | J0945 |
| Nasal vaccine inhalation | | INH | **J3530** |
| Natalizumab | 1 mg | IV | **J2323** |
| Natrecor | 0.1 mg | | J2325 |
| Navane, *see* Thiothixene | | | |
| Navelbine | per 10 mg | IV | J9390 |
| ND Stat | per 10 mg | IM, SC, IV | J0945 |
| Nebcin | up to 80 mg | IM, IV | J3260 |
| NebuPent | per 300 mg | INH | J2545, J7676 |
| Necitumumab | 1 mg | IV | **J9295** |
| Nelarabine | 50 mg | IV | **J9261** |
| Nembutal Sodium Solution | per 50 mg | IM, IV, OTH | J2515 |
| Neocyten | up to 60 mg | IV, IM | J2360 |
| Neo-Durabolic | up to 50 mg | IM | J2320 |
| Neoquess | up to 20 mg | IM | J0500 |

◄ New ↵ Revised ✔ Reinstated ~~deleted~~ Deleted

| DRUG NAME | DOSAGE | METHOD OF ADMINISTRATION | HCPCS CODE |
|---|---|---|---|
| Neoral | 100 mg | | J7502 |
| | 25 mg | | J7515 |
| Neosar | 100 mg | IV | J9070 |
| Neostigmine methylsulfate | up to 0.5 mg | IM, IV, SC | J2710 |
| Neo-Synephrine | up to 1 ml | SC, IM, IV | J2370 |
| Nervocaine 1% | 10 mg | IV | J2001 |
| Nervocaine 2% | 10 mg | IV | J2001 |
| Nesacaine | per 30 ml | VAR | J2400 |
| Nesacaine-MPF | per 30 ml | VAR | J2400 |
| Nesiritide | 0.1 mg | IV | J2325 |
| Netupitant 300 mg and palonosetron 0.5 mg | | ORAL | J8655 |
| Neulasta | 6 mg | | J2505 |
| Neumega | 5 mg | SC | J2355 |
| Neupogen | | | |
| (G-CSF) | 1 mcg | SC, IV | J1442 |
| Neutrexin | per 25 mg | IV | J3305 |
| Nipent | per 10 mg | IV | J9268 |
| Nivolumab | 1 mg | IV | J9299 |
| Nolvadex | | | J8999 |
| Nordryl | up to 50 mg | IV, IM | J1200 |
| | 50 mg | ORAL | Q0163 |
| Norflex | up to 60 mg | IV, IM | J2360 |
| Norzine | up to 10 mg | IM | J3280 |
| Not otherwise classified drugs | | | J3490 |
| other than inhalation solution administered through DME | | | J7799 |
| inhalation solution administered through DME | | | J7699 |
| anti-neoplastic | | | J9999 |
| chemotherapeutic | | ORAL | J8999 |
| immunosuppressive | | | J7599 |
| nonchemotherapeutic | | ORAL | J8499 |
| Novantrone | per 5 mg | IV | J9293 |
| Novarel | per 1,000 USP Units | | J0725 |
| Novolin | per 5 units | | J1815 |
| | per 50 units | | J1817 |
| Novolog | per 5 units | | J1815 |
| | per 50 units | | J1817 |
| Novo Seven | 1 mcg | IV | J7189 |
| Novoeight | | | J7182 |
| NPH | 5 units | SC | J1815 |

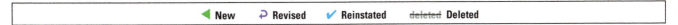
◄ New    ↻ Revised    ✔ Reinstated    deleted Deleted

| DRUG NAME | DOSAGE | METHOD OF ADMINISTRATION | HCPCS CODE |
|---|---|---|---|
| Nplate | 100 units | | J0587 |
| | 10 mcg | | J2796 |
| Nubain | per 10 mg | IM, IV, SC | J2300 |
| Nulecit | 12.5 mg | | J2916 |
| Nulicaine | 10 mg | IV | J2001 |
| Nulojix | 1 mg | IV | J0485 |
| Numorphan | up to 1 mg | IV, SC, IM | J2410 |
| Numorphan H.P. | up to 1 mg | IV, SC, IM | J2410 |
| Nusinersen | 0.1 mg | IV | J2326 |
| Nutropin | 1 mg | | J2941 |
| **O** | | | |
| Oasis Burn Matrix | per square centimeter | | Q4103 |
| Oasis Wound Matrix | per square centimeter | | Q4102 |
| Obinutuzumab | 10 mg | | J9301 |
| Ocriplasmin | 0.125 mg | IV | J7316 |
| Ocrelizumab | 1 mg | IV | J2350 |
| Octagam | 500 mg | IV | J1568 |
| Octreotide Acetate, injection | 1 mg | IM | J2353 |
| | 25 mcg | IV, SQ | J2354 |
| Oculinum | per unit | IM | J0585 |
| Ofatumumab | 10 mg | IV | J9302 |
| Ofev | | | J8499 |
| Ofirmev | 10 mg | IV | J0131 |
| O-Flex | up to 60 mg | IV, IM | J2360 |
| Oforta | 10 mg | | J8562 |
| Olanzapine | 1 mg | IM | J2358 |
| Olaratumab | 10 mg | IV | J9285 |
| Omadacycline | 1 mg | IV | J0121 |
| Omacetaxine Mepesuccinate | 0.01 mg | IV | J9262 |
| Omalizumab | 5 mg | SC | J2357 |
| Omnipaque | per ml | | Q9965, Q9966, Q9967 |
| Omnipen-N | up to 500 mg | IM, IV | J0290 |
| | per 1.5 gm | IM, IV | J0295 |
| Omniscan | per ml | | A9579 |
| Omnitrope | 1 mg | | J2941 |
| Omontys | 0.1 mg | IV, SC | J0890 |
| OnabotulinumtoxinA | 1 unit | IM | J0585 |
| Oncaspar | per single dose vial | IM, IV | J9266 |
| Oncovin | 1 mg | IV | J9370 |

◀ **New**    ↵ **Revised**    ✔ **Reinstated**    ~~deleted~~ **Deleted**

| DRUG NAME | DOSAGE | METHOD OF ADMINISTRATION | HCPCS CODE |
|---|---|---|---|
| Ondansetron HCl | 1 mg | IV | J2405 |
| | 1 mg | ORAL | Q0162 |
| Onivyde | 1 mg | | J9205 |
| Opana | up to 1 mg | | J2410 |
| Opdivo | 1 mg | | J9299 |
| Oprelvekin | 5 mg | SC | J2355 |
| Optimark | per ml | | A9579 |
| Optiray | per ml | | Q9966, Q9967 |
| Optison | per ml | | Q9956 |
| Oraminic II | per 10 mg | IM, SC, IV | J0945 |
| Orapred | per 5 mg | ORAL | J7510 |
| Orbactiv | 10 mg | | J2407 |
| Orencia | 10 mg | | J0129 |
| Oritavancin | 10 mg | IV | J2407 |
| Ormazine | up to 50 mg | IM, IV | J3230 |
| Orphenadrine citrate | up to 60 mg | IV, IM | J2360 |
| Orphenate | up to 60 mg | IV, IM | J2360 |
| Orthovisc | | OTH | J7324 |
| Or-Tyl | up to 20 mg | IM | J0500 |
| Osmitrol | | | J7799 |
| Ovidrel | | | J3490 |
| Oxacillin sodium | up to 250 mg | IM, IV | J2700 |
| Oxaliplatin | 0.5 mg | IV | J9263 |
| Oxilan | per ml | | Q9967 |
| Oxymorphone HCl | up to 1 mg | IV, SC, IM | J2410 |
| Oxytetracycline HCl | up to 50 mg | IM | J2460 |
| Oxytocin | up to 10 units | IV, IM | J2590 |
| Ozurdex | 0.1 mg | | J7312 |
| **P** | | | |
| Paclitaxel | 1 mg | IV | J9267 |
| Paclitaxel protein-bound particles | 1 mg | IV | J9264 |
| Palifermin | 50 mcg | IV | J2425 |
| Paliperidone Palmitate | 1 mg | IM | J2426 |
| Palonosetron HCl | 25 mcg | IV | J2469 |
|   Netupitant 300 mg and palonosetron 0.5 mg | | ORAL | J8655 |
| Pamidronate disodium | per 30 mg | IV | J2430 |
| Panhematin | 1 mg | | J1640 |
| Panitumumab | 10 mg | IV | J9303 |
| Papaverine HCl | up to 60 mg | IV, IM | J2440 |
| Paragard T 380 A | | OTH | J7300 |

◀ **New**  ↻ **Revised**  ✔ **Reinstated**  ~~deleted~~ **Deleted**

| DRUG NAME | DOSAGE | METHOD OF ADMINISTRATION | HCPCS CODE |
|---|---|---|---|
| Paraplatin | 50 mg | IV | J9045 |
| Paricalcitol, injection | 1 mcg | IV, IM | J2501 |
| Pasireotide, long acting | 1 mg | IV | J2502 |
| Pathogen(s) test for platelets | | OTH | P9100 |
| Patisiran | 0.1 mg | IV | J0222 |
| Peforomist | 20 mcg | | J7606 |
| Pegademase bovine | 25 IU | | J2504 |
| Pegaptinib | 0.3 mg | OTH | J2503 |
| Pegaspargase | per single dose vial | IM, IV | J9266 |
| Pegasys | | | J3490 |
| Pegfilgrastim | 0.5 mg | SC | J2505 |
| Pegfilgrastim-jmdb | 0.5 mg | SC | Q5108 |
| Peginesatide | 0.1 mg | IV, SC | J0890 |
| Peg-Intron | | | J3490 |
| Pegloticase | 1 mg | IV | J2507 |
| Pembrolizumab | 1 mg | IV | J9271 |
| Pemetrexed | 10 mg | IV | J9305 |
| Penicillin G Benzathine | 100,000 units | IM | J0561 |
| Penicillin G Benzathine and Penicillin G Procaine | 100,000 units | IM | J0558 |
| Penicillin G potassium | up to 600,000 units | IM, IV | J2540 |
| Penicillin G procaine, aqueous | up to 600,000 units | IM, IV | J2510 |
| Penicillin G Sodium | | | J3490 |
| Pentam | per 300 mg | | J7676 |
| Pentamidine isethionate | per 300 mg | INH, IM | J2545, J7676 |
| Pentastarch, 10% | 100 ml | | J2513 |
| Pentazocine HCl | 30 mg | IM, SC, IV | J3070 |
| Pentobarbital sodium | per 50 mg | IM, IV, OTH | J2515 |
| Pentostatin | per 10 mg | IV | J9268 |
| Peramivir | 1 mg | IV | J2547 |
| Perjeta | 1 mg | | J9306 |
| Permapen | up to 600,000 | IM | J0561 |
| Perphenazine | | | |
|    injection | up to 5 mg | IM, IV | J3310 |
|    tablets | 4 mg | ORAL | Q0175 |
| Persantine IV | per 10 mg | IV | J1245 |
| Pertuzumab | 1 mg | IV | J9306 |
| Pet Imaging | | | |
|    Fluciclovine F-18, diagnostic | 1 millcurie | IV | A9588 |
|    Gallium Ga-68, dotatate, diagnostic | 0.1 millicurie | IV | A9587 |
| Pfizerpen | up to 600,000 units | IM, IV | J2540 |

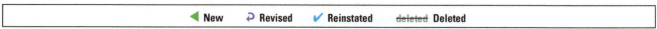

◄ New    ↻ Revised    ✔ Reinstated    ~~deleted~~ Deleted

| DRUG NAME | DOSAGE | METHOD OF ADMINISTRATION | HCPCS CODE | |
|---|---|---|---|---|
| Pfizerpen A.S. | up to 600,000 units | IM, IV | J2510 | |
| Phenadoz | | | J8498 | |
| Phenazine 25 | up to 50 mg | IM, IV | J2550 | |
| | 12.5 mg | ORAL | Q0169 | |
| Phenazine 50 | up to 50 mg | IM, IV | J2550 | |
| | 12.5 mg | ORAL | Q0169 | |
| Phenergan | 12.5 mg | ORAL | Q0169 | |
| | up to 50 mg | IM, IV | J2550 | |
| | | | J8498 | |
| Phenobarbital sodium | up to 120 mg | IM, IV | J2560 | |
| Phentolamine mesylate | up to 5 mg | IM, IV | J2760 | |
| Phenylephrine HCl | up to 1 ml | SC, IM, IV | J2370, J7799 | |
| Phenylephrine 10.16 mg/Ketorolac 2.88 | 1 ml | VAR | J1097 | ◄ |
| Phenytoin sodium | per 50 mg | IM, IV | J1165 | |
| Photofrin | 75 mg | IV | J9600 | |
| Phytonadione (Vitamin K) | per 1 mg | IM, SC, IV | J3430 | |
| Piperacillin/Tazobactam Sodium, injection | 1.125 g | IV | J2543 | |
| Pitocin | up to 10 units | IV, IM | J2590 | |
| Plantinol AQ | 10 mg | IV | J9060 | |
| Plasma | | | | |
|    cryoprecipitate reduced | each unit | IV | P9044 | |
|    pooled multiple donor, frozen | each unit | IV | P9023, P9070 | |
|    (single donor), pathogen reduced, frozen | each unit | IV | P9071 | |
| Plas+SD | each unit | IV | P9023 | |
| Platelets, pheresis, pathogen reduced | each unit | IV | P9073 | |
|    Pathogen(s) test for platelets | | OTH | P9100 | |
| Platinol | 10 mg | IV, IM | J9060 | |
| Plazomicin | 5 mg | IV | J0291 | ◄ |
| Plerixafor | 1 mg | SC | J2562 | |
| Plicamycin | 2,500 mcg | IV | J9270 | |
| Polatuzumab vedotin | 1 mg | IV | J9309 | ◄ |
| Polocaine | per 10 ml | VAR | J0670 | |
| Polycillin-N | up to 500 mg | IM, IV | J0290 | |
| | per 1.5 gm | IM, IV | J0295 | |
| Polygam | 500 mg | | J1566 | |
| Porfimer Sodium | 75 mg | IV | J9600 | |
| Portrazza | 1 mg | | J9295 | |
| Positron emission tomography radiopharmaceutical, diagnostic | | | | |
|    for non-tumor identification, NOC | | IV | A9598 | |
|    for tumor identification, NOC | | IV | A9597 | |

◄ **New**    ↩ **Revised**    ✔ **Reinstated**    ~~deleted~~ **Deleted**

| DRUG NAME | DOSAGE | METHOD OF ADMINISTRATION | HCPCS CODE |
|---|---|---|---|
| Potassium chloride | per 2 mEq | IV | J3480 |
| Potassium Chloride | up to 1,000 cc | | J7120 |
| Pralatrexate | 1 mg | IV | J9307 |
| Pralidoxime chloride | up to 1 g | IV, IM, SC | J2730 |
| Predalone-50 | up to 1 ml | IM | J2650 |
| Predcor-25 | up to 1 ml | IM | J2650 |
| Predcor-50 | up to 1 ml | IM | J2650 |
| Predicort-50 | up to 1 ml | IM | J2650 |
| Prednisolone acetate | up to 1 ml | IM | J2650 |
| Prednisolone, oral | 5 mg | ORAL | J7510 |
| Prednisone, immediate release or delayed release | 1 mg | ORAL | J7512 |
| Predoject-50 | up to 1 ml | IM | J2650 |
| Pregnyl | per 1,000 USP units | IM | J0725 |
| Premarin Intravenous | per 25 mg | IV, IM | J1410 |
| Prescription, chemotherapeutic, not otherwise specified | | ORAL | J8999 |
| Prescription, nonchemotherapeutic, not otherwise specified | | ORAL | J8499 |
| Prialt | 1 mcg | | J2278 |
| Primacor | 5 mg | IV | J2260 |
| Primatrix | per square centimeter | | Q4110 |
| Primaxin | per 250 mg | IV, IM | J0743 |
| Priscoline HCl | up to 25 mg | IV | J2670 |
| Privigen | 500 mg | IV | J1459 |
| Probuphine System Kit | | | J0570 |
| Procainamide HCl | up to 1 g | IM, IV | J2690 |
| Prochlorperazine | up to 10 mg | IM, IV | J0780 |
| | | | J8498 |
| Prochlorperazine maleate | 5 mg | ORAL | Q0164 |
| | 5 mg | | S0183 |
| Procrit | | | J0885 |
| | | | Q4081 |
| Pro-Depo, *see* Hydroxyprogesterone Caproate | | | |
| Profasi HP | per 1,000 USP units | IM | J0725 |
| Profilnine Heat-Treated | | | |
| non-recombinant | per IU | IV | J7193 |
| recombinant | per IU | IU | J7195, J7200-J7202 |
| complex | per IU | IV | J7194 |
| Profonol | 10 mg/ml | | J3490 |
| Progestaject | per 50 mg | | J2675 |
| Progesterone | per 50 mg | IM | J2675 |

◄ New    ↻ Revised    ✔ Reinstated    ~~deleted~~ Deleted

| DRUG NAME | DOSAGE | METHOD OF ADMINISTRATION | HCPCS CODE |
|---|---|---|---|
| Prograf | | | |
|   oral | 1 mg | ORAL | J7507 |
|   parenteral | 5 mg | | J7525 |
| Prohance Multipack | per ml | | A9576 |
| Prokine | 50 mcg | IV | J2820 |
| Prolastin | 10 mg | IV | J0256 |
| Proleukin | per single use vial | IM, IV | J9015 |
| Prolia | 1 mg | | J0897 |
| Prolixin Decanoate | up to 25 mg | IM, SC | J2680 |
| Promazine HCl | up to 25 mg | IM | J2950 |
| Promethazine | | | J8498 |
| Promethazine HCl | | | |
|   injection | up to 50 mg | IM, IV | J2550 |
|   oral | 12.5 mg | ORAL | Q0169 |
| Promethegan | | | J8498 |
| Pronestyl | up to 1 g | IM, IV | J2690 |
| Proplex SX-T | | | |
|   non-recombinant | per IU | IV | J7193 |
|   recombinant | per IU | | J7195, J7200-J7202 |
|   complex | per IU | IV | J7194 |
| Proplex T | | | |
|   non-recombinant | per IU | IV | J7193 |
|   recombinant | per IU | | J7195, J7200-J7202 |
|   complex | per IU | IV | J7194 |
| Propofol | 10 mg | IV | J2704 |
| Propranolol HCl | up to 1 mg | IV | J1800 |
| Prorex-25 | | | |
| | up to 50 mg | IM, IV | J2550 |
| | 12.5 mg | ORAL | Q0169 |
| Prorex-50 | up to 50 mg | IM, IV | J2550 |
| | 12.5 mg | ORAL | Q0169 |
| Prostaglandin E1 | per 1.25 mcg | | J0270 |
| Prostaphlin | up to 1 g | IM, IV | J2690 |
| Prostigmin | up to 0.5 mg | IM, IV, SC | J2710 |
| Prostin VR Pediatric | 0.5 mg | | J0270 |
| Protamine sulfate | per 10 mg | IV | J2720 |
| Protein C Concentrate | 10 IU | IV | J2724 |
| Prothazine | up to 50 mg | IM, IV | J2550 |
| | 12.5 mg | ORAL | Q0169 |

◄ New    ↻ Revised    ✔ Reinstated    ~~deleted~~ Deleted

| DRUG NAME | DOSAGE | METHOD OF ADMINISTRATION | HCPCS CODE |
|---|---|---|---|
| Protirelin | per 250 mcg | IV | J2725 |
| Protonix | | | J3490 |
| Protopam Chloride | up to 1 g | IV, IM, SC | J2730 |
| Provenge | | | Q2043 |
| Proventil | | | |
| concentrated form | 1 mg | INH | J7610, J7611 |
| unit dose form | 1 mg | INH | J7609, J7613 |
| Provocholine | per 1 mg | | J7674 |
| Prozine-50 | up to 25 mg | IM | J2950 |
| Pulmicort Respules | | | |
| concentrated form | 0.25 mg | INH | J7633, J7634 |
| unit does | 0.5 mg | INH | J7626, J7627 |
| Pulmozyme | per mg | | J7639 |
| Pyridoxine HCl | 100 mg | | J3415 |
| **Q** | | | |
| Quelicin | up to 20 mg | IV, IM | J0330 |
| Quinupristin/dalfopristin | 500 mg (150/350) | IV | J2770 |
| Qutenza | per square cm | | J7336 |
| **R** | | | |
| Ramucirumab | 5 mg | IV | J9308 |
| Ranibizumab | 0.1 mg | OTH | J2778 |
| Ranitidine HCl, injection | 25 mg | IV, IM | J2780 |
| Rapamune | 1 mg | ORAL | J7520 |
| Rasburicase | 0.5 mg | IV | J2783 |
| Ravulizumab-cwvz | 10 mg | IV | J1303 ◄ |
| Rebif | 11 mcg | | Q3026 |
| Reclast | 1 mg | | J3489 |
| Recombinate | | | |
| human | per IU | IV | J7190 |
| porcine | per IU | IV | J7191 |
| recombinant | per IU | IV | J7192 |
| Recombivax | | | J3490 |
| Redisol | up to 1,000 mcg | IM, SC | J3420 |
| Regadenoson | 0.1 mg | IV | J2785 |
| Regitine | up to 5 mg | IM, IV | J2760 |
| Reglan | up to 10 mg | IV | J2765 |
| Regular | 5 units | SC | J1815 |
| Relefact TRH | per 250 mcg | IV | J2725 |
| Relistor | 0.1 mg | SC | J2212 |
| Remicade | 10 mg | IM, IV | J1745 |

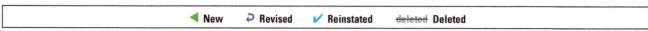

◄ New ↻ Revised ✔ Reinstated ~~deleted~~ Deleted

| DRUG NAME | DOSAGE | METHOD OF ADMINISTRATION | HCPCS CODE |
|---|---|---|---|
| Remodulin | 1 mg | | J3285 |
| Renflexis | | | Q5102 |
| ReoPro | 10 mg | IV | J0130 |
| Rep-Pred 40 | 20 mg | IM | J1020 |
| | 40 mg | IM | J1030 |
| | 80 mg | IM | J1040 |
| Rep-Pred 80 | 20 mg | IM | J1020 |
| | 40 mg | IM | J1030 |
| | 80 mg | IM | J1040 |
| Resectisol | | | J7799 |
| Reslizumab | 1 mg | IV | J2786 |
| Retavase | 18.1 mg | IV | J2993 |
| Reteplase | 18.8 mg | IV | J2993 |
| Retisert | | | J7311 |
| Retrovir | 10 mg | IV | J3485 |
| Revefenacin inhalation solution | — | INH | J7677 ◄ |
| Rheomacrodex | 500 ml | IV | J7100 |
| Rhesonativ | 300 mcg | IM | J2790 |
| | 50 mg | | J2788 |
| Rheumatrex Dose Pack | 2.5 mg | ORAL | J8610 |
| Rho(D) | | | |
| immune globulin | | IM, IV | J2791 |
| immune globulin, human | 1 dose package/ 300 mcg | IM | J2790 |
| | 50 mg | IM | J2788 |
| immune globulin, human, solvent detergent | 100 | IV, IU | J2792 |
| RhoGAM | 300 mcg | IM | J2790 |
| | 50 mg | | J2788 |
| Rhophylac | 100 IU | IM, IV | J2791 |
| Riastap | 100 mg | | J7178 |
| Rifadin | | | J3490 |
| Rifampin | | | J3490 |
| Rilonacept | 1 mg | SC | J2793 |
| RimabotulinumtoxinB | 100 units | IM | J0587 |
| Rimso-50 | 50 ml | | J1212 |
| Ringers lactate infusion | up to 1,000 cc | IV | J7120, J7121 |
| Risperdal Costa | 0.5 mg | | J2794 |
| Risperidone | 0.5 mg | IM | J2794 |
| Risperidone (perseris) | 0.5 mg | IV | J2798 ◄ |
| Rituxan | 100 mg | IV | J9310 |

◄ New    ↻ Revised    ✔ Reinstated    ~~deleted~~ Deleted

| DRUG NAME | DOSAGE | METHOD OF ADMINISTRATION | HCPCS CODE | |
|---|---|---|---|---|
| Rituximab | 100 mg | IV | J9310 | |
| Rituximab-abbs | 10 mg | IV | Q5115 | ◄ |
| Rixubis | | | J7200 | |
| Robaxin | up to 10 ml | IV, IM | J2800 | |
| Rocephin | per 250 mg | IV, IM | J0696 | |
| Roferon-A | 3 million units | SC, IM | J9213 | |
| Rolapitant | 0.5 mg | IV | J2797 | |
| Rolapitant, oral, 1 mg | 1 mg | ORAL | J8670 | |
| Romidepsin | 1 mg | IV | J9315 | |
| Romiplostim | 10 mcg | SC | J2796 | |
| Romosozumab-aqqg | 1 mg | IV | J3111 | ◄ |
| Ropivacaine Hydrochloride | 1 mg | OTH | J2795 | |
| Rubex | 10 mg | IV | J9000 | |
| Rubramin PC | up to 1,000 mcg | IM, SC | J3420 | |
| **S** | | | | |
| Saizen | 1 mg | | J2941 | |
| Saline solution | 10 ml | | A4216 | |
| 5% dextrose | 500 ml | IV | J7042 | |
| infusion | 250 cc | IV | J7050 | |
| | 1,000 cc | IV | J7030 | |
| sterile | 500 ml = 1 unit | IV, OTH | J7040 | |
| Sandimmune | 25 mg | ORAL | J7515 | |
| | 100 mg | ORAL | J7502 | |
| | 250 mg | OTH | J7516 | |
| Sandoglobulin, *see* Immune globin intravenous (human) | | | | |
| Sandostatin, Lar Depot | 25 mcg | | J2354 | |
| | 1 mg | IM | J2353 | |
| Sargramostim (GM-CSF) | 50 mcg | IV | J2820 | |
| Sculptra | 0.5 mg | IV | Q2028 | |
| Sebelelipase alfa | 1 mg | IV | J2840 | |
| Selestoject | per 4 mg | IM, IV | J0702 | |
| Sermorelin acetate | 1 mcg | SC | Q0515 | |
| Serostim | 1 mg | | J2941 | |
| Signifor LAR | 20 ml | | J2502 | |
| Siltuximab | 10 mg | IV | J2860 | |
| Simponi Aria | 1 mg | | J1602 | |
| Simulect | 20 mg | | J0480 | |
| Sincalide | 5 mcg | IV | J2805 | |
| Sinografin | per ml | | Q9963 | |
| Sinusol-B | per 10 mg | IM, SC, IV | J0945 | |

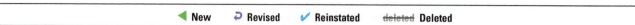

◄ New   ↻ Revised   ✔ Reinstated   ~~deleted~~ Deleted

| DRUG NAME | DOSAGE | METHOD OF ADMINISTRATION | HCPCS CODE |
|---|---|---|---|
| Sirolimus | 1 mg | ORAL | J7520 |
| Sivextro | 1 mg | | J3090 |
| Skyla | 13.5 mg | OTH | J7301 |
| Smz-TMP | | | J3490 |
| Sodium Chloride | 1,000 cc | | J7030 |
| | 500 ml = 1 unit | | J7040 |
| | 500 ml | | A4217 |
| | 250 cc | | J7050 |
|   Bacteriostatic | 10 ml | | A4216 |
| Sodium Chloride Concentrate | | | J7799 |
| Sodium ferricgluconate in sucrose | 12.5 mg | | J2916 |
| Sodium Hyaluronate | | | J3490 |
|   Euflexxa | | | J7323 |
|   Hyalgan | | | J7321 |
|   Orthovisc | | | J7324 |
| Solganal | up to 50 mg | IM | J2910 |
| Soliris | 10 mg | | J1300 |
| Solu-Cortef | up to 50 mg | IV, IM, SC | J1710 |
| | 100 mg | | J1720 |
| Solu-Medrol | up to 40 mg | IM, IV | J2920 |
| | up to 125 mg | IM, IV | J2930 |
| Solurex | 1 mg | IM, IV, OTH | J1100 |
| Solurex LA | 1 mg | IM | J1094 |
| Somatrem | 1 mg | SC | J2940 |
| Somatropin | 1 mg | SC | J2941 |
| Somatulin Depot | 1 mg | | J1930 |
| Sparine | up to 25 mg | IM | J2950 |
| Spasmoject | up to 20 mg | IM | J0500 |
| Spectinomycin HCl | up to 2 g | IM | J3320 |
| Sporanox | 50 mg | IV | J1835 |
| Staphcillin, *see* Methicillin sodium | | | |
| Stelara | 1 mg | | J3357 |
| Stilphostrol | 250 mg | IV | J9165 |
| Streptase | 250,000 IU | IV | J2995 |
| Streptokinase | per 250,000 | IU, IV | J2995 |
| Streptomycin | up to 1 g | IM | J3000 |
| Streptomycin Sulfate | up to 1 g | IM | J3000 |
| Streptozocin | 1 gm | IV | J9320 |
| Strontium-89 chloride | per millicurie | | A9600 |
| Sublimaze | 0.1 mg | IM, IV | J3010 |

◀ New    ↪ Revised    ✔ Reinstated    ~~deleted~~ Deleted

| DRUG NAME | DOSAGE | METHOD OF ADMINISTRATION | HCPCS CODE |
|---|---|---|---|
| Succinylcholine chloride | up to 20 mg | IV, IM | J0330 |
| Sufentanil Citrate | | | J3490 |
| Sumarel Dosepro | 6 mg | | J3030 |
| Sumatriptan succinate | 6 mg | SC | J3030 |
| Supartz | | OTH | J7321 |
| Supprelin LA | 50 mg | | J9226 |
| Surostrin | up to 20 mg | IV, IM | J0330 |
| Sus-Phrine | up to 1 ml ampule | SC, IM | J0171 |
| Synercid | 500 mg (150/350) | IV | J2770 |
| Synkavite | per 1 mg | IM, SC, IV | J3430 |
| Synribo | 0.01 mg | | J9262 |
| Syntocinon | up to 10 units | IV, IM | J2590 |
| Synvisc and Synvisc-One | 1 mg | OTH | J7325 |
| Syrex | 10 ml | | A4216 |
| Sytobex | 1,000 mcg | IM, SC | J3420 |
| **T** | | | |
| Tacrolimus | | | |
|   (Envarsus XR) | 0.25 mg | ORAL | J7503 |
|   oral, extended release | 0.1 mg | ORAL | J7508 |
|   oral, immediate release | 1 mg | ORAL | J7507 |
|   parenteral | 5 mg | IV | J7525 |
| Tagraxofusp-erzs | 10 mcg | IV | J9269 |
| Taliglucerase Alfa | 10 units | IV | J3060 |
| Talimogene laherparepvec | per 1 million plaque forming units | IV | J9325 |
| Talwin | 30 mg | IM, SC, IV | J3070 |
| Tamoxifen Citrate | | | J8999 |
| Taractan, *see* Chlorprothixene | | | |
| Taxol | 1 mg | IV | J9267 |
| Taxotere | 20 mg | IV | J9171 |
| Tazicef | per 500 mg | | J0713 |
| Tazidime, *see* Ceftazidime Technetium TC Sestambi | per dose | | A9500 |
| | | | J0713 |
| Tedizolid phosphate | 1 mg | IV | J3090 |
| TEEV | 1 mg | IM | J3121 |
| Teflaro | 1 mg | | J0712 |
| Telavancin | 10 mg | IV | J3095 |
| Temodar | 5 mg | ORAL | J8700, J9328 |
| Temozolomide | 1 mg | IV | J9328 |
| | 5 mg | ORAL | J8700 |

◀ New    ↩ Revised    ✔ Reinstated    ~~deleted~~ Deleted

| DRUG NAME | DOSAGE | METHOD OF ADMINISTRATION | HCPCS CODE |
|---|---|---|---|
| Temsirolimus | 1 mg | IV | J9330 |
| Tenecteplase | 1 mg | IV | J3101 |
| Teniposide | 50 mg | | Q2017 |
| Tepadina | 15 mg | | J9340 |
| Tequin | 10 mg | IV | J1590 |
| Terbutaline sulfate | up to 1 mg | SC, IV | J3105 |
|   concentrated form | per 1 mg | INH | J7680 |
|   unit dose form | per 1 mg | INH | J7681 |
| Teriparatide | 10 mcg | SC | J3110 |
| Terramycin IM | up to 50 mg | IM | J2460 |
| Testa-C | 1 mg | | J1071 |
| Testadiate | 1 mg | IM | J3121 |
| Testadiate-Depo | 1 mg | | J1071 |
| Testaject-LA | 1 mg | | J1071 |
| Testaqua | up to 50 mg | IM | J3140 |
| Test-Estro Cypionates | 1 mg | | J1071 |
| Test-Estro-C | 1 mg | | J1071 |
| Testex | up to 100 mg | IM | J3150 |
| Testo AQ | up to 50 mg | | J3140 |
| Testoject-50 | up to 50 mg | IM | J3140 |
| Testoject-LA | 1 mg | | J1071 |
| Testone | | | |
|   LA 100 | 1 mg | IM | J3121 |
|   LA 200 | 1 mg | IM | J3121 |
| Testopel Pellets | | | J3490 |
| Testosterone Aqueous | up to 50 mg | IM | J3140 |
| Testosterone cypionate | 1 mg | IM | J1071 |
| Testosterone enanthate | 1 mg | IM | J3121 |
| Testosterone undecanoate | 1 mg | IM | J3145 |
| Testradiol 90/4 | 1 mg | IM | J3121 |
| Testrin PA | 1 mg | IM | J3121 |
| Testro AQ | up to 50 mg | | J3140 |
| Tetanus immune globulin, human | up to 250 units | IM | J1670 |
| Tetracycline | up to 250 mg | IM, IV | J0120 |
| Thallous Chloride TI-201 | per MCI | | A9505 |
| Theelin Aqueous | per 1 mg | IM | J1435 |
| Theophylline | per 40 mg | IV | J2810 |
| ~~TheraCys~~ | ~~per vial~~ | ~~IV~~ | ~~J9031~~ ✖ |
| Thiamine HCl | 100 mg | | J3411 |

◀ **New**   ⤺ **Revised**   ✔ **Reinstated**   ~~deleted~~ **Deleted**

| DRUG NAME | DOSAGE | METHOD OF ADMINISTRATION | HCPCS CODE |
|---|---|---|---|
| Thiethylperazine maleate | | | |
|    injection | up to 10 mg | IM | J3280 |
|    oral | 10 mg | ORAL | Q0174 |
| Thiotepa | 15 mg | IV | J9340 |
| Thorazine | up to 50 mg | IM, IV | J3230 |
| Thrombate III | per IU | | J7197 |
| Thymoglobulin (*see also* Immune globin) | | | |
|    anti-thymocyte globulin, equine | 250 mg | IV | J7504 |
|    anti-thymocyte globulin, rabbit | 25 mg | IV | J7511 |
| Thypinone | per 250 mcg | IV | J2725 |
| Thyrogen | 0.9 mg | IM, SC | J3240 |
| Thyrotropin Alfa, injection | 0.9 mg | IM, SC | J3240 |
| ~~Tice BCG~~ | ~~per vial~~ | ~~IV~~ | ~~J9031~~ |
| Ticon | | | |
|    injection | up to 200 mg | IM | J3250 |
|    oral | 250 mg | ORAL | Q0173 |
| Tigan | | | |
|    injection | up to 200 mg | IM | J3250 |
|    oral | 250 mg | ORAL | Q0173 |
| Tigecycline | 1 mg | IV | J3243 |
| Tiject-20 | | | |
|    injection | up to 200 mg | IM | J3250 |
|    oral | 250 mg | ORAL | Q0173 |
| Tinzaparin | 1,000 IU | SC | J1655 |
| Tirofiban Hydrochloride, injection | 0.25 mg | IM, IV | J3246 |
| TNKase | 1 mg | IV | J3101 |
| Tobi | 300 mg | INH | J7682, J7685 |
| Tobramycin, inhalation solution | 300 mg | INH | J7682, J7685 |
| Tobramycin sulfate | up to 80 mg | IM, IV | J3260 |
| Tocilizumab | 1 mg | IV | J3262 |
| Tofranil, *see* Imipramine HCl | | | |
| Tolazoline HCl | up to 25 mg | IV | J2670 |
| Toposar | 10 mg | | J9181 |
| Topotecan | 0.25 mg | ORAL | J8705 |
| | 0.1 mg | IV | J9351 |
| Toradol | per 15 mg | IM, IV | J1885 |
| Torecan | | | |
|    injection | up to 10 mg | IM | J3280 |
|    oral | 10 mg | ORAL | Q0174 |
| Torisel | 1 mg | | J9330 |

◀ New    ↻ Revised    ✔ Reinstated    ~~deleted~~ Deleted

| DRUG NAME | DOSAGE | METHOD OF ADMINISTRATION | HCPCS CODE | |
|---|---|---|---|---|
| Tornalate | | | | |
| concentrated form | per mg | INH | J7628 | |
| unit dose | per mg | INH | J7629 | |
| Torsemide | 10 mg/ml | IV | J3265 | |
| Totacillin-N | up to 500 mg | IM, IV | J0290 | |
| | per 1.5 gm | IM, IV | J0295 | |
| Trabectedin | 0.1 mg | IV | J9352 | |
| Trastuzumab | 10 mg | IV | J9355 | |
| Trastuzumab-anns (kanjinti) | 10 mg | IV | Q5117 | ◄ |
| Trastuzumab-dkst | 10 mg | IV | Q5114 | ◄ |
| Trastuzumab-dttb | 10 mg | IV | Q5112 | ◄ |
| Trastuzumab-pkrb | 10 mg | IV | Q5113 | ◄ |
| Trastuzumab-qyyp (trazimera) | 10 mg | IV | Q5116 | ◄ |
| Trastuzumab and Hyaluronidase | 10 mg | IV | J9356 | ◄ |
| Treanda | 1 mg | IV | J3490, J9033 | |
| Trelstar | 3.75 mg | | J3315 | |
| Treprostinil | 1 mg | | J3285, J7686 | |
| Trexall | 2.5 mg | ORAL | J8610 | |
| Triam-A | 1 mg | | J3300 | |
| | per 10 mg | IM | J3301 | |
| Triamcinolone | | | | |
| concentrated form | per 1 mg | INH | J7683 | |
| unit dose | per 1 mg | INH | J7684 | |
| Triamcinolone acetonide | 1 mg | | J3300 | |
| | per 10 mg | IM | J3301 | |
| Triamcinolone acetonide XR | 1 mg | IM | J3304 | |
| Triamcinolone diacetate | per 5 mg | IM | J3302 | |
| Triamcinolone hexacetonide | per 5 mg | VAR | J3303 | |
| Triesence | 1 mg | | J3300 | |
| | per 10 mg | IM | J3301 | |
| Triethylene thio-Phosphoramide/T | 15 mg | | J9340 | |
| Triflupromazine HCl | up to 20 mg | IM, IV | J3400 | |
| Tri-Kort | 1 mg | | J3300 | |
| | per 10 mg | IM | J3301 | |
| Trilafon | 4 mg | ORAL | Q0175 | |
| | up to 5 mg | IM, IV | J3310 | |
| Trilog | 1 mg | | J3300 | |
| | per 10 mg | IM | J3301 | |
| Trilone | per 5 mg | | J3302 | |

| ◄ New | ↩ Revised | ✔ Reinstated | ~~deleted~~ Deleted |
|---|---|---|---|

| DRUG NAME | DOSAGE | METHOD OF ADMINISTRATION | HCPCS CODE |
|---|---|---|---|
| Trimethobenzamide HCl | | | |
|    injection | up to 200 mg | IM | J3250 |
|    oral | 250 mg | ORAL | Q0173 |
| Trimetrexate glucuronate | per 25 mg | IV | J3305 |
| Triptorelin Pamoate | 3.75 mg | SC | J3315 |
| Triptorelin XR | 3.75 mg | SC | J3316 |
| Trisenox | 1 mg | IV | J9017 |
| Trobicin | up to 2 g | IM | J3320 |
| Trovan | 100 mg | IV | J0200 |
| Tysabri | 1 mg | | J2323 |
| Tyvaso | 1.74 mg | | J7686 |
| **U** | | | |
| Ultravist 240 | per ml | | Q9966 |
| Ultravist 300 | per ml | | Q9967 |
| Ultravist 370 | per ml | | Q9967 |
| Ultrazine-10 | up to 10 mg | IM, IV | J0780 |
| Unasyn | per 1.5 gm | IM, IV | J0295 |
| Unclassified drugs (*see also* Not elsewhere classified) | | | J3490 |
| Unclassified drugs or biological used for ESRD on dialysis | | IV | J3591 |
| Unspecified oral antiemetic | | | Q0181 |
| Urea | up to 40 g | IV | J3350 |
| Ureaphil | up to 40 g | IV | J3350 |
| Urecholine | up to 5 mg | SC | J0520 |
| Urofollitropin | 75 IU | | J3355 |
| Urokinase | 5,000 IU vial | IV | J3364 |
| | 250,000 IU vial | IV | J3365 |
| Ustekinumab | 1 mg | SC | J3357 |
| | 1 mg | IV | J3358 |
| **V** | | | |
| Valcyte | | | J3490 |
| Valergen 10 | 10 mg | IM | J1380 |
| Valergen 20 | 10 mg | IM | J1380 |
| Valergen 40 | up to 10 mg | IM | J1380 |
| Valertest No. 1 | 1 mg | IM | J3121 |
| Valertest No. 2 | 1 mg | IM | J3121 |
| Valganciclovir HCL | | | J8499 |
| Valium | up to 5 mg | IM, IV | J3360 |
| Valrubicin, intravesical | 200 mg | OTH | J9357 |
| Valstar | 200 mg | OTH | J9357 |

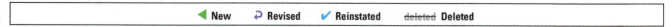

◀ New    ↩ Revised    ✔ Reinstated    ~~deleted~~ Deleted

| DRUG NAME | DOSAGE | METHOD OF ADMINISTRATION | HCPCS CODE |
|---|---|---|---|
| Vancocin | 500 mg | IV, IM | J3370 |
| Vancoled | 500 mg | IV, IM | J3370 |
| Vancomycin HCl | 500 mg | IV, IM | J3370 |
| Vantas | 50 mg | | J9226, J9225 |
| Varubi | 90 mg | | J8670 |
| Vasceze | per 10 mg | | J1642 |
| Vasoxyl, *see* Methoxamine HCl | | | |
| Vectibix | 10 mg | | J9303 |
| Vedolizumab | 1 mg | IV | J3380 |
| Velaglucerase alfa | 100 units | IV | J3385 |
| Velban | 1 mg | IV | J9360 |
| Velcade | 0.1 mg | | J9041 |
| Veletri | 0.5 mg | | J1325 |
| Velsar | 1 mg | IV | J9360 |
| Venofer | 1 mg | IV | J1756 |
| Ventavis | 20 mcg | | Q4074 |
| Ventolin | 0.5 mg | INH | J7620 |
| concentrated form | 1 mg | INH | J7610, J7611 |
| unit dose form | 1 mg | INH | J7609, J7613 |
| VePesid | 50 mg | ORAL | J8560 |
| Veritas Collagen Matrix | | | J3490 |
| Versed | per 1 mg | IM, IV | J2250 |
| Verteporfin | 0.1 mg | IV | J3396 |
| Vesprin | up to 20 mg | IM, IV | J3400 |
| Vestronidase alfa-vjbk | 1 mg | IV | J3397 |
| VFEND IV | 10 mg | IV | J3465 |
| V-Gan 25 | up to 50 mg | IM, IV | J2550 |
| | 12.5 mg | ORAL | Q0169 |
| V-Gan 50 | up to 50 mg | IM, IV | J2550 |
| | 12.5 mg | ORAL | Q0169 |
| Viadur | 65 mg | OTH | J9219 |
| Vibativ | 10 mg | | J3095 |
| Vinblastine sulfate | 1 mg | IV | J9360 |
| Vincasar PFS | 1 mg | IV | J9370 |
| Vincristine sulfate | 1 mg | IV | J9370 |
| Vincristine sulfate Liposome | 1 mg | IV | J9371 |
| Vinorelbine tartrate | per 10 mg | IV | J9390 |
| Vispaque | per ml | | Q9966, Q9967 |
| Vistaject-25 | up to 25 mg | IM | J3410 |

◀ New    ⟳ Revised    ✔ Reinstated    ~~deleted~~ Deleted

| DRUG NAME | DOSAGE | METHOD OF ADMINISTRATION | HCPCS CODE |
|---|---|---|---|
| Vistaril | up to 25 mg | IM | J3410 |
| | 25 mg | ORAL | Q0177 |
| Vistide | 375 mg | IV | J0740 |
| Visudyne | 0.1 mg | IV | J3396 |
| Vitamin B-12 cyanocobalamin | up to 1,000 mcg | IM, SC | J3420 |
| Vitamin K, phytonadione, menadione, menadiol sodium diphosphate | per 1 mg | IM, SC, IV | J3430 |
| Vitrase | per 1 USP unit | | J3471 |
| Vivaglobin | 100 mg | | J1562 |
| Vivitrol | 1 mg | | J2315 |
| Von Willebrand Factor Complex, human | per IU VWF:RCo | IV | J7187 |
| Wilate | per IU VWF | IV | J7183 |
| Vonvendi | per IU VWF | IV | J7179 |
| Voretigene neparvovec-rzyl | 1 billion vector genomes | IV | J3398 |
| Voriconazole | 10 mg | IV | J3465 |
| Vpriv | 100 units | | J3385 |
| **W** | | | |
| Wehamine | up to 50 mg | IM, IV | J1240 |
| Wehdryl | up to 50 mg | IM, IV | J1200 |
| | 50 mg | ORAL | Q0163 |
| Wellcovorin | per 50 mg | IM, IV | J0640 |
| Wilate | per IU | IV | J7183 |
| Win Rho SD | 100 IU | IV | J2792 |
| Wyamine Sulfate, *see* Mephentermine sulfate | | | |
| Wycillin | up to 600,000 units | IM, IV | J2510 |
| Wydase | up to 150 units | SC, IV | J3470 |
| **X** | | | |
| Xeloda | 150 mg | ORAL | J8520 |
| | 500 mg | ORAL | J8521 |
| Xeomin | 1 unit | | J0588 |
| Xgera | 1 mg | | J0987 |
| Xgeva | 1 mg | | J0897 |
| Xiaflex | 0.01 mg | | J0775 |
| Xolair | 5 mg | | J2357 |
| Xopenex | 0.5 mg | INH | J7620 |
| concentrated form | 1 mg | INH | J7610, J7611, J7612 |
| unit dose form | 1 mg | INH | J7609, J7613, J7614 |

◄ **New**    ⮌ **Revised**    ✔ **Reinstated**    ~~deleted~~ **Deleted**

| DRUG NAME | DOSAGE | METHOD OF ADMINISTRATION | HCPCS CODE |
|---|---|---|---|
| Xylocaine HCl | 10 mg | IV | J2001 |
| Xyntha | per IU | IV | J7185, J7192, J7182, J7188 |
| **Y** | | | |
| Yervoy, *see* Ipilimumab | | | |
| Yondelis | 0.1 mg | | J9352, J9999 |
| **Z** | | | |
| Zaltrap | 1 mg | | J9400 |
| Zanosar | 1 g | IV | J9320 |
| Zantac | 25 mg | IV, IM | J2780 |
| Zarxio | 1 mcg | | Q5101 |
| Zemaira | 10 mg | IV | J0256 |
| Zemplar | 1 mcg | IM, IV | J2501 |
| Zenapax | 25 mg | IV | J7513 |
| Zerbaxa | 1 gm | | J0695 |
| Zetran | up to 5 mg | IM, IV | J3360 |
| Ziconotide | 1 mcg | OTH | **J2278** |
| Zidovudine | 10 mg | IV | **J3485** |
| Zinacef | per 750 mg | IM, IV | J0697 |
| Zinecard | per 250 mg | | J1190 |
| Ziprasidone Mesylate | 10 mg | IM | **J3486** |
| Zithromax | 1 gm | ORAL | Q0144 |
| injection | 500 mg | IV | J0456 |
| Ziv-Aflibercept | 1 mg | IV | **J9400** |
| Zmax | 1 g | | Q0144 |
| Zofran | 1 mg | IV | J2405 |
| | 1 mg | ORAL | Q0162 |
| Zoladex | per 3.6 mg | SC | J9202 |
| Zoledronic Acid | 1 mg | IV | **J3489** |
| Zolicef | 500 mg | IV, IM | J0690 |
| Zometra | 1 mg | | J3489 |
| Zorbtive | 1 mg | | J2941 |
| Zortress | 0.25 mg | ORAL | J7527 |
| Zosyn | 1.125 g | IV | J2543 |
| Zovirax | 5 mg | | J8499 |
| Zyprexa Relprevv | 1 mg | | J2358 |
| Zyvox | 200 mg | IV | J2020 |

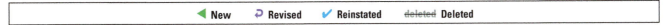

◄ New    ↩ Revised    ✔ Reinstated    ~~deleted~~ **Deleted**

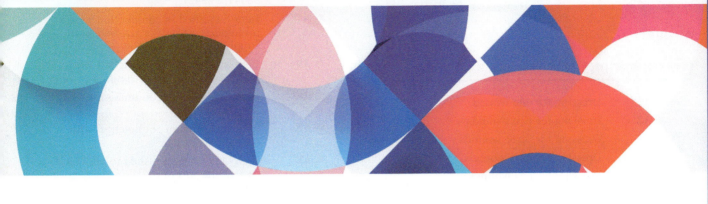

# HCPCS 2020

# LEVEL II NATIONAL CODES

2020 HCPCS quarterly updates available on the
companion website at: http://www.codingupdates.com

**DISCLAIMER**

Every effort has been made to make this text complete and accurate,
but no guarantee, warranty, or representation is made for its
accuracy or completeness. This text is based on the Centers for
Medicare and Medicaid Services Healthcare Common Procedure
Coding System (HCPCS).

Do not report HCPCS modifiers with MIPS CPT Category II codes, rather, use Performance Measurement Modifiers 1P, 2P, 3P, and 8P, as instructed in the CPT guidelines for Category II codes under 'Modifiers'.

## LEVEL II NATIONAL MODIFIERS

✳ **A1** Dressing for one wound

✳ **A2** Dressing for two wounds

✳ **A3** Dressing for three wounds

✳ **A4** Dressing for four wounds

✳ **A5** Dressing for five wounds

✳ **A6** Dressing for six wounds

✳ **A7** Dressing for seven wounds

✳ **A8** Dressing for eight wounds

✳ **A9** Dressing for nine or more wounds

⚙ **AA** Anesthesia services performed personally by anesthesiologist

*IOM: 100-04, 12, 90.4*

⚙ **AD** Medical supervision by a physician: more than four concurrent anesthesia procedures

*IOM: 100-04, 12, 90.4*

✳ **AE** Registered dietician

✳ **AF** Specialty physician

✳ **AG** Primary physician

⚙ **AH** Clinical psychologist

*IOM: 100-04, 12, 170*

✳ **AI** Principal physician of record

⚙ **AJ** Clinical social worker

*IOM: 100-04, 12, 170; 100-04, 12, 150*

✳ **AK** Nonparticipating physician

⚙ **AM** Physician, team member service

Not assigned for Medicare

*Cross Reference QM*

✳ **AO** Alternate payment method declined by provider of service

✳ **AP** Determination of refractive state was not performed in the course of diagnostic ophthalmological examination

✳ **AQ** Physician providing a service in an unlisted health professional shortage area (HPSA)

✳ **AR** Physician provider services in a physician scarcity area

✳ **AS** Physician assistant, nurse practitioner, or clinical nurse specialist services for assistant at surgery

✳ **AT** Acute treatment (this modifier should be used when reporting service 98940, 98941, 98942)

✳ **AU** Item furnished in conjunction with a urological, ostomy, or tracheostomy supply

✳ **AV** Item furnished in conjunction with a prosthetic device, prosthetic or orthotic

✳ **AW** Item furnished in conjunction with a surgical dressing

✳ **AX** Item furnished in conjunction with dialysis services

✳ **AY** Item or service furnished to an ESRD patient that is not for the treatment of ESRD

🚫 **AZ** Physician providing a service in a dental health professional shortage area for the purpose of an electronic health record incentive payment

✳ **BA** Item furnished in conjunction with parenteral enteral nutrition (PEN) services

✳ **BL** Special acquisition of blood and blood products

✳ **BO** Orally administered nutrition, not by feeding tube

✳ **BP** The beneficiary has been informed of the purchase and rental options and has elected to purchase the item

✳ **BR** The beneficiary has been informed of the purchase and rental options and has elected to rent the item

✳ **BU** The beneficiary has been informed of the purchase and rental options and after 30 days has not informed the supplier of his/her decision

✳ **CA** Procedure payable only in the inpatient setting when performed emergently on an outpatient who expires prior to admission

✳ **CB** Service ordered by a renal dialysis facility (RDF) physician as part of the ESRD beneficiary's dialysis benefit, is not part of the composite rate, and is separately reimbursable

✳ **CC** Procedure code change (Use CC when the procedure code submitted was changed either for administrative reasons or because an incorrect code was filed)

⚙ **CD** AMCC test has been ordered by an ESRD facility or MCP physician that is part of the composite rate and is not separately billable

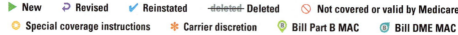

▶ New    ↩ Revised    ✔ Reinstated    ~~deleted~~ Deleted    🚫 Not covered or valid by Medicare
⚙ Special coverage instructions    ✳ Carrier discretion    🅑 Bill Part B MAC    🅑 Bill DME MAC

⚙ **CE** AMCC test has been ordered by an ESRD facility or MCP physician that is a composite rate test but is beyond the normal frequency covered under the rate and is separately reimbursable based on medical necessity

⚙ **CF** AMCC test has been ordered by an ESRD facility or MCP physician that is not part of the composite rate and is separately billable

✳ **CG** Policy criteria applied

⚙ **CH** 0 percent impaired, limited or restricted

⚙ **CI** At least 1 percent but less than 20 percent impaired, limited or restricted

⚙ **CJ** At least 20 percent but less than 40 percent impaired, limited or restricted

⚙ **CK** At least 40 percent but less than 60 percent impaired, limited or restricted

⚙ **CL** At least 60 percent but less than 80 percent impaired, limited or restricted

⚙ **CM** At least 80 percent but less than 100 percent impaired, limited or restricted

⚙ **CN** 100 percent impaired, limited or restricted

✳ **CO** Outpatient occupational therapy services furnished in whole or in part by an occupational therapy assistant

✳ **CR** Catastrophe/Disaster related

✳ **CS** Item or service related, in whole or in part, to an illness, injury, or condition that was caused by or exacerbated by the effects, direct or indirect, of the 2010 oil spill in the Gulf of Mexico, including but not limited to subsequent clean-up activities

✳ **CT** Computed tomography services furnished using equipment that does not meet each of the attributes of the national electrical manufacturers association (NEMA) XR-29-2013 standard

*Coding Clinic: 2017, Q1, P6*

✳ **CQ** Outpatient physical therapy services furnished in whole or in part by a physical therapist assistant

✳ **DA** Oral health assessment by a licensed health professional other than a dentist

✳ **E1** Upper left, eyelid

*Coding Clinic: 2016, Q3, P3*

✳ **E2** Lower left, eyelid

*Coding Clinic: 2016, Q3, P3*

✳ **E3** Upper right, eyelid

*Coding Clinic: 2011, Q3, P6*

✳ **E4** Lower right, eyelid

⚙ **EA** Erythropoetic stimulating agent (ESA) administered to treat anemia due to anti-cancer chemotherapy

CMS requires claims for non-ESRD ESAs (J0881 and J0885) to include one of three modifiers: EA, EB, EC.

⚙ **EB** Erythropoetic stimulating agent (ESA) administered to treat anemia due to anti-cancer radiotherapy

CMS requires claims for non-ESRD ESAs (J0881 and J0885) to include one of three modifiers: EA, EB, EC.

⚙ **EC** Erythropoetic stimulating agent (ESA) administered to treat anemia not due to anti-cancer radiotherapy or anti-cancer chemotherapy

CMS requires claims for non-ESRD ESAs (J0881 and J0885) to include one of three modifiers: EA, EB, EC.

⚙ **ED** Hematocrit level has exceeded 39% (or hemoglobin level has exceeded 13.0 g/dl) for 3 or more consecutive billing cycles immediately prior to and including the current cycle

⚙ **EE** Hematocrit level has not exceeded 39% (or hemoglobin level has not exceeded 13.0 g/dl) for 3 or more consecutive billing cycles immediately prior to and including the current cycle

⚙ **EJ** Subsequent claims for a defined course of therapy, e.g., EPO, sodium hyaluronate, infliximab

⚙ **EM** Emergency reserve supply (for ESRD benefit only)

✳ **EP** Service provided as part of Medicaid early periodic screening diagnosis and treatment (EPSDT) program

✳ **ER** Items and services furnished by a provider-based, off-campus emergency department

✳ **ET** Emergency services

✳ **EX** Expatriate beneficiary

✳ **EY** No physician or other licensed health care provider order for this item or service

Items billed before a signed and dated order has been received by the supplier must be submitted with an EY modifier added to each related HCPCS code.

✳ **F1** Left hand, second digit

✳ **F2** Left hand, third digit

🏷 MIPS    Qp Quantity Physician    Qh Quantity Hospital    ♀ Female only
♂ Male only    A Age    ♿ DMEPOS    A2-Z3 ASC Payment Indicator    A-Y ASC Status Indicator    Coding Clinic

| | | |
|---|---|---|
| ✳ **F3** | Left hand, fourth digit | |
| ✳ **F4** | Left hand, fifth digit | |
| ✳ **F5** | Right hand, thumb | |
| ✳ **F6** | Right hand, second digit | |
| ✳ **F7** | Right hand, third digit | |
| ✳ **F8** | Right hand, fourth digit | |
| ✳ **F9** | Right hand, fifth digit | |
| ✳ **FA** | Left hand, thumb | |
| ⊘ **FB** | Item provided without cost to provider, supplier or practitioner, or full credit received for replaced device (examples, but not limited to, covered under warranty, replaced due to defect, free samples) | |
| ✿ **FC** | Partial credit received for replaced device | |
| ✳ **FP** | Service provided as part of family planning program | |
| ✳ **FX** | X-ray taken using film | |
| | *Coding Clinic: 2017, Q1, P6* | |
| ✳ **FY** | X-ray taken using computed radiography technology/cassette-based imaging | |
| ✳ **G0** | Telehealth services for diagnosis, evaluation, or treatment, of symptoms of an acute stroke | |
| ✳ **G1** | Most recent URR reading of less than 60 | |
| | *IOM: 100-04, 8, 50.9* | |
| ✳ **G2** | Most recent URR reading of 60 to 64.9 | |
| | *IOM: 100-04, 8, 50.9* | |
| ✳ **G3** | Most recent URR reading of 65 to 69.9 | |
| | *IOM: 100-04, 8, 50.9* | |
| ✳ **G4** | Most recent URR reading of 70 to 74.9 | |
| | *IOM: 100-04, 8, 50.9* | |
| ✳ **G5** | Most recent URR reading of 75 or greater | |
| | *IOM: 100-04, 8, 50.9* | |
| ✳ **G6** | ESRD patient for whom less than six dialysis sessions have been provided in a month | |
| | *IOM: 100-04, 8, 50.9* | |
| ✿ **G7** | Pregnancy resulted from rape or incest or pregnancy certified by physician as life threatening | |
| | *IOM: 100-02, 15, 20.1; 100-03, 3, 170.3* | |
| ✳ **G8** | Monitored anesthesia care (MAC) for deep complex, complicated, or markedly invasive surgical procedure | |
| ✳ **G9** | Monitored anesthesia care for patient who has history of severe cardiopulmonary condition | |

✳ **GA** Waiver of liability statement issued as required by payer policy, individual case

An item/service is expected to be denied as not reasonable and necessary and an ABN is on file. Modifier GA can be used on either a specific or a miscellaneous HCPCS code. Modifiers GA and GY should never be reported together on the same line for the same HCPCS code.

✳ **GB** Claim being resubmitted for payment because it is no longer covered under a global payment demonstration

✿ **GC** This service has been performed in part by a resident under the direction of a teaching physician

*IOM: 100-04, 12, 90.4, 100*

~~**GD** Units of service exceeds medically unlikely edit value and represents reasonable and necessary services~~ ✖

✿ **GE** This service has been performed by a resident without the presence of a teaching physician under the primary care exception

✳ **GF** Non-physician (e.g., nurse practitioner (NP), certified registered nurse anesthetist (CRNA), certified registered nurse (CRN), clinical nurse specialist (CNS), physician assistant (PA)) services in a critical access hospital

✳ **GG** Performance and payment of a screening mammogram and diagnostic mammogram on the same patient, same day

✳ **GH** Diagnostic mammogram converted from screening mammogram on same day

✳ **GJ** "Opt out" physician or practitioner emergency or urgent service

✳ **GK** Reasonable and necessary item/service associated with a GA or GZ modifier

An upgrade is defined as an item that goes beyond what is medically necessary under Medicare's coverage requirements. An item can be considered an upgrade even if the physician has signed an order for it. When suppliers know that an item will not be paid in full because it does not meet the coverage criteria stated in the LCD, the supplier can still obtain partial payment at the time of initial determination if the claim is billed using one of the upgrade modifiers (GK or GL). (https://www.cms.gov/manuals/downloads/clm104c01.pdf)

| | | | | |
|---|---|---|---|---|
| ▶ New | ↻ Revised | ✔ Reinstated | ~~deleted~~ Deleted | ⊘ Not covered or valid by Medicare |
| ✿ Special coverage instructions | | ✳ Carrier discretion | Ⓑ Bill Part B MAC | Ⓑ Bill DME MAC |

✳ **GL** Medically unnecessary upgrade provided instead of non-upgraded item, no charge, no Advance Beneficiary Notice (ABN)

✳ **GM** Multiple patients on one ambulance trip

✳ **GN** Services delivered under an outpatient speech language pathology plan of care

✳ **GO** Services delivered under an outpatient occupational therapy plan of care

✳ **GP** Services delivered under an outpatient physical therapy plan of care

✳ **GQ** Via asynchronous telecommunications system

✳ **GR** This service was performed in whole or in part by a resident in a department of Veterans Affairs medical center or clinic, supervised in accordance with VA policy

⊛ **GS** Dosage of erythropoietin-stimulating agent has been reduced and maintained in response to hematocrit or hemoglobin level

⊛ **GT** Via interactive audio and video telecommunication systems

✳ **GU** Waiver of liability statement issued as required by payer policy, routine notice

⊛ **GV** Attending physician not employed or paid under arrangement by the patient's hospice provider

⊛ **GW** Service not related to the hospice patient's terminal condition

✳ **GX** Notice of liability issued, voluntary under payer policy

*GX modifier must be submitted with non-covered charges only. This modifier differentiates from the required uses in conjunction with ABN. (https://www.cms.gov/manuals/downloads/clm104c01.pdf)*

⊘ **GY** Item or service statutorily excluded, does not meet the definition of any Medicare benefit or, for non-Medicare insurers, is not a contract benefit

*Examples of "statutorily excluded" include: Infusion drug not administered using a durable infusion pump, a wheelchair that is for use for mobility outside the home or hearing aids. GA and GY should never be coded together on the same line for the same HCPCS code. (https://www.cms.gov/manuals/downloads/clm104c01.pdf)*

⊘ **GZ** Item or service expected to be denied as not reasonable or necessary

*Used when an ABN is not on file and can be used on either a specific or a miscellaneous HCPCS code. It would never be correct to place any combination of GY, GZ or GA modifiers on the same claim line and will result in rejected or denied claim for invalid coding. (https://www.cms.gov/manuals/downloads/clm104c01.pdf)*

⊘ **H9** Court-ordered

⊘ **HA** Child/adolescent program

⊘ **HB** Adult program, nongeriatric

⊘ **HC** Adult program, geriatric

⊘ **HD** Pregnant/parenting women's program

⊘ **HE** Mental health program

⊘ **HF** Substance abuse program

⊘ **HG** Opioid addiction treatment program

⊘ **HH** Integrated mental health/substance abuse program

⊘ **HI** Integrated mental health and intellectual disability/developmental disabilities program

⊘ **HJ** Employee assistance program

⊘ **HK** Specialized mental health programs for high-risk populations

⊘ **HL** Intern

⊘ **HM** Less than bachelor degree level

⊘ **HN** Bachelors degree level

⊘ **HO** Masters degree level

⊘ **HP** Doctoral level

⊘ **HQ** Group setting

⊘ **HR** Family/couple with client present

⊘ **HS** Family/couple without client present

⊘ **HT** Multi-disciplinary team

⊘ **HU** Funded by child welfare agency

⊘ **HV** Funded by state addictions agency

⊘ **HW** Funded by state mental health agency

⊘ **HX** Funded by county/local agency

⊘ **HY** Funded by juvenile justice agency

⊘ **HZ** Funded by criminal justice agency

✳ **J1** Competitive acquisition program no-pay submission for a prescription number

✳ **J2** Competitive acquisition program, restocking of emergency drugs after emergency administration

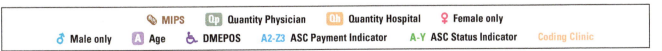

✳ **J3** Competitive acquisition program (CAP), drug not available through CAP as written, reimbursed under average sales price methodology

✳ **J4** DMEPOS item subject to DMEPOS competitive bidding program that is furnished by a hospital upon discharge

✳ **JA** Administered intravenously

This modifier is informational only (not a payment modifier) and may be submitted with all injection codes. According to Medicare, reporting this modifier is voluntary. (CMS Pub. 100-04, chapter 8, section 60.2.3.1 and Pub. 100-04, chapter 17, section 80.11)

✳ **JB** Administered subcutaneously

✳ **JC** Skin substitute used as a graft

✳ **JD** Skin substitute not used as a graft

✳ **JE** Administered via dialysate

✳ **JG** Drug or biological acquired with 340B drug pricing program discount

✳ **JW** Drug amount discarded/not administered to any patient

Use JW to identify unused drugs or biologicals from single use vial/package that are appropriately discarded. Bill on separate line for payment of discarded drug/biological.

*IOM: 100-4, 17, 40*

Coding Clinic: 2016, Q4, P4-7; 2010, Q3, P10

✳ **K0** Lower extremity prosthesis functional Level 0 - does not have the ability or potential to ambulate or transfer safely with or without assistance and a prosthesis does not enhance their quality of life or mobility.

✳ **K1** Lower extremity prosthesis functional Level 1 - has the ability or potential to use a prosthesis for transfers or ambulation on level surfaces at fixed cadence. Typical of the limited and unlimited household ambulator.

✳ **K2** Lower extremity prosthesis functional Level 2 - has the ability or potential for ambulation with the ability to traverse low level environmental barriers such as curbs, stairs or uneven surfaces. Typical of the limited community ambulator.

✳ **K3** Lower extremity prosthesis functional Level 3 - has the ability or potential for ambulation with variable cadence. Typical of the community ambulator who has the ability to traverse most environmental barriers and may have vocational, therapeutic, or exercise activity that demands prosthetic utilization beyond simple locomotion.

✳ **K4** Lower extremity prosthesis functional Level 4 - has the ability or potential for prosthetic ambulation that exceeds the basic ambulation skills, exhibiting high impact, stress, or energy levels, typical of the prosthetic demands of the child, active adult, or athlete.

✳ **KA** Add on option/accessory for wheelchair

✳ **KB** Beneficiary requested upgrade for ABN, more than 4 modifiers identified on claim

✳ **KC** Replacement of special power wheelchair interface

✳ **KD** Drug or biological infused through DME

✳ **KE** Bid under round one of the DMEPOS competitive bidding program for use with non-competitive bid base equipment

✳ **KF** Item designated by FDA as Class III device

✳ **KG** DMEPOS item subject to DMEPOS competitive bidding program number 1

✳ **KH** DMEPOS item, initial claim, purchase or first month rental

✳ **KI** DMEPOS item, second or third month rental

✳ **KJ** DMEPOS item, parenteral enteral nutrition (PEN) pump or capped rental, months four to fifteen

✳ **KK** DMEPOS item subject to DMEPOS competitive bidding program number 2

✳ **KL** DMEPOS item delivered via mail

✳ **KM** Replacement of facial prosthesis including new impression/moulage

✳ **KN** Replacement of facial prosthesis using previous master model

✳ **KO** Single drug unit dose formulation

✳ **KP** First drug of a multiple drug unit dose formulation

✳ **KQ** Second or subsequent drug of a multiple drug unit dose formulation

✳ **KR** Rental item, billing for partial month

✿ **KS** Glucose monitor supply for diabetic beneficiary not treated with insulin

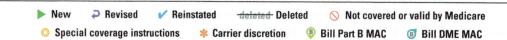

▶ New   ↻ Revised   ✔ Reinstated   ~~deleted~~ Deleted   ⊘ Not covered or valid by Medicare
✿ Special coverage instructions   ✳ Carrier discretion   Ⓑ Bill Part B MAC   ⓑ Bill DME MAC

\* **KT**    Beneficiary resides in a competitive bidding area and travels outside that competitive bidding area and receives a competitive bid item

\* **KU**    DMEPOS item subject to DMEPOS competitive bidding program number 3

\* **KV**    DMEPOS item subject to DMEPOS competitive bidding program that is furnished as part of a professional service

\* **KW**    DMEPOS item subject to DMEPOS competitive bidding program number 4

\* **KX**    Requirements specified in the medical policy have been met

Used for physical, occupational, or speech-language therapy to request an exception to therapy payment caps and indicate the services are reasonable and necessary and that there is documentation of medical necessity in the patient's medical record. (Pub 100-04 Attachment - Business Requirements Centers for Medicare and Medicaid Services, Transmittal 2457, April 27, 2012)

Medicare requires modifier KX for implanted permanent cardiac pacemakers, single chamber or duel chamber, for one of the following CPT codes: 33206, 33207, 33208.

\* **KY**    DMEPOS item subject to DMEPOS competitive bidding program number 5

\* **KZ**    New coverage not implemented by managed care

\* **LC**    Left circumflex coronary artery

\* **LD**    Left anterior descending coronary artery

\* **LL**    Lease/rental (use the LL modifier when DME equipment rental is to be applied against the purchase price)

\* **LM**    Left main coronary artery

\* **LR**    Laboratory round trip

○ **LS**    FDA-monitored intraocular lens implant

\* **LT**    Left side (used to identify procedures performed on the left side of the body)

Modifiers LT and RT identify procedures which can be performed on paired organs. Used for procedures performed on one side only. Should also be used when the procedures are similar but not identical and are performed on paired body parts.

Coding Clinic: 2016, Q3, P5

\* **M2**    Medicare secondary payer (MSP)

▶\* **MA**    Ordering professional is not required to consult a clinical decision support mechanism due to service being rendered to a patient with a suspected or confirmed emergency medical condition

▶\* **MB**    Ordering professional is not required to consult a clinical decision support mechanism due to the significant hardship exception of insufficient internet access

▶\* **MC**    Ordering professional is not required to consult a clinical decision support mechanism due to the significant hardship exception of electronic health record or clinical decision support mechanism vendor issues

▶\* **MD**    Ordering professional is not required to consult a clinical decision support mechanism due to the significant hardship exception of extreme and uncontrollable circumstances

▶\* **ME**    The order for this service adheres to appropriate use criteria in the clinical decision support mechanism consulted by the ordering professional

▶\* **MF**    The order for this service does not adhere to the appropriate use criteria in the clinical decision support mechanism consulted by the ordering professional

▶\* **MG**    The order for this service does not have applicable appropriate use criteria in the qualified clinical decision support mechanism consulted by the ordering professional

▶\* **MH**    Unknown if ordering professional consulted a clinical decision support mechanism for this service, related information was not provided to the furnishing professional or provider

\* **MS**    Six month maintenance and servicing fee for reasonable and necessary parts and labor which are not covered under any manufacturer or supplier warranty

\* **NB**    Nebulizer system, any type, FDA-cleared for use with specific drug

\* **NR**    New when rented (use the NR modifier when DME which was new at the time of rental is subsequently purchased)

\* **NU**    New equipment

\* **P1**    A normal healthy patient

\* **P2**    A patient with mild systemic disease

\* **P3**    A patient with severe systemic disease

---

| 🏷 MIPS | Qp Quantity Physician | Qh Quantity Hospital | ♀ Female only |
|---|---|---|---|
| ♂ Male only | A Age | ♿ DMEPOS | A2-Z3 ASC Payment Indicator | A-Y ASC Status Indicator | Coding Clinic |

✳ **P4** A patient with severe systemic disease that is a constant threat to life

✳ **P5** A moribund patient who is not expected to survive without the operation

✳ **P6** A declared brain-dead patient whose organs are being removed for donor purposes

⊘ **PA** Surgical or other invasive procedure on wrong body part

⊘ **PB** Surgical or other invasive procedure on wrong patient

⊘ **PC** Wrong surgery or other invasive procedure on patient

✳ **PD** Diagnostic or related non diagnostic item or service provided in a wholly owned or operated entity to a patient who is admitted as an inpatient within 3 days

✳ **PI** Positron emission tomography (PET) or PET/computed tomography (CT) to inform the initial treatment strategy of tumors that are biopsy proven or strongly suspected of being cancerous based on other diagnostic testing

✳ **PL** Progressive addition lenses

✳ **PM** Post mortem

✳ **PN** Non-excepted service provided at an off-campus, outpatient, provider-based department of a hospital

✳ **PO** Expected services provided at off-campus, outpatient, provider-based department of a hospital

✳ **PS** Positron emission tomography (PET) or PET/computed tomography (CT) to inform the subsequent treatment strategy of cancerous tumors when the beneficiary's treating physician determines that the PET study is needed to inform subsequent anti-tumor strategy

✳ **PT** Colorectal cancer screening test; converted to diagnostic text or other procedure

Assign this modifier with the appropriate CPT procedure code for colonoscopy, flexible sigmoidoscopy, or barium enema when the service is initiated as a colorectal cancer screening service but then becomes a diagnostic service. MLN Matters article MM7012 (PDF, 75 KB) Reference Medicare Transmittal 3232 April 3, 2015.

Coding Clinic: 2011, Q1, P10

⊛ **Q0** Investigational clinical service provided in a clinical research study that is in an approved clinical research study

⊛ **Q1** Routine clinical service provided in a clinical research study that is in an approved clinical research study

✳ **Q2** Demonstration procedure/service

✳ **Q3** Live kidney donor surgery and related services

✳ **Q4** Service for ordering/referring physician qualifies as a service exemption

⊛ **Q5** Service furnished under a reciprocal billing arrangement by a substitute physician or by a substitute physical therapist furnishing outpatient physical therapy services in a health professional shortage area, a medically underserved area, or a rural area

*IOM: 100-04, 1, 30.2.10*

⊛ **Q6** Service furnished under a fee-for-time compensation arrangement by a substitute physician or by a substitute physical therapist furnishing outpatient physical therapy services in a health professional shortage area, a medically underserved area, or a rural area

*IOM: 100-04, 1, 30.2.11*

✳ **Q7** One Class A finding

✳ **Q8** Two Class B findings

✳ **Q9** One Class B and two Class C findings

✳ **QA** Prescribed amounts of stationary oxygen for daytime use while at rest and nighttime use differ and the average of the two amounts is less than 1 liter per minute (lpm)

✳ **QB** Prescribed amounts of stationary oxygen for daytime use while at rest and nighttime use differ and the average of the two amounts exceeds 4 liters per minute (lpm) and portable oxygen is prescribed

✳ **QC** Single channel monitoring

✳ **QD** Recording and storage in solid state memory by a digital recorder

✳ **QE** Prescribed amount of stationary oxygen while at rest is less than 1 liter per minute (LPM)

✳ **QF** Prescribed amount of stationary oxygen while at rest exceeds 4 liters per minute (LPM) and portable oxygen is prescribed

---

▶ **New**   ⇄ **Revised**   ✔ **Reinstated**   ~~deleted~~ **Deleted**   ⊘ **Not covered or valid by Medicare**
⊛ **Special coverage instructions**   ✳ **Carrier discretion**   Ⓑ **Bill Part B MAC**   Ⓑ **Bill DME MAC**

✳ **QG**    Prescribed amount of stationary oxygen while at rest is greater than 4 liters per minute (LPM)

✳ **QH**    Oxygen conserving device is being used with an oxygen delivery system

⚙ **QJ**    Services/items provided to a prisoner or patient in state or local custody, however, the state or local government, as applicable, meets the requirements in 42 CFR 411.4 (B)

⚙ **QK**    Medical direction of two, three, or four concurrent anesthesia procedures involving qualified individuals

*IOM: 100-04, 12, 50K, 90*

✳ **QL**    Patient pronounced dead after ambulance called

✳ **QM**    Ambulance service provided under arrangement by a provider of services

✳ **QN**    Ambulance service furnished directly by a provider of services

⚙ **QP**    Documentation is on file showing that the laboratory test(s) was ordered individually or ordered as a CPT-recognized panel other than automated profile codes 80002-80019, G0058, G0059, and G0060

✳ **QQ**    Ordering professional consulted a qualified clinical decision support mechanism for this service and the related data was provided to the furnishing professional

✳ **QR**    Prescribed amounts of stationary oxygen for daytime use while at rest and nighttime use differ and the average of the two amounts is greater than 4 liters per minute (lpm)

⚙ **QS**    Monitored anesthesia care service

*IOM: 100-04, 12, 30.6, 501*

✳ **QT**    Recording and storage on tape by an analog tape recorder

✳ **QW**    CLIA-waived test

✳ **QX**    CRNA service: with medical direction by a physician

⚙ **QY**    Medical direction of one certified registered nurse anesthetist (CRNA) by an anesthesiologist

*IOM: 100-04, 12, 50K, 90*

✳ **QZ**    CRNA service: without medical direction by a physician

✳ **RA**    Replacement of a DME, orthotic or prosthetic item

Contractors will deny claims for replacement parts when furnished in conjunction with the repair of a capped rental item and billed with modifier RB, including claims for parts submitted using code E1399, that are billed during the capped rental period (i.e., the last day of the 13th month of continuous use or before). Repair includes all maintenance, servicing, and repair of capped rental DME because it is included in the allowed rental payment amounts. (Pub 100-20 One-Time Notification Centers for Medicare & Medicaid Services, Transmittal: 901, May 13, 2011)

✳ **RB**    Replacement of a part of a DME, orthotic or prosthetic item furnished as part of a repair

✳ **RC**    Right coronary artery

✳ **RD**    Drug provided to beneficiary, but not administered "incident-to"

✳ **RE**    Furnished in full compliance with FDA-mandated risk evaluation and mitigation strategy (REMS)

✳ **RI**    Ramus intermedius coronary artery

✳ **RR**    Rental (use the 'RR' modifier when DME is to be rented)

✳ **RT**    Right side (used to identify procedures performed on the right side of the body)

Modifiers LT and RT identify procedures which can be performed on paired organs. Used for procedures performed on one side only. Should also be used when the procedures are similar but not identical and are performed on paired body parts.

Coding Clinic: 2016, Q3, P5

⊘ **SA**    Nurse practitioner rendering service in collaboration with a physician

⊘ **SB**    Nurse midwife

✳ **SC**    Medically necessary service or supply

⊘ **SD**    Services provided by registered nurse with specialized, highly technical home infusion training

⊘ **SE**    State and/or federally funded programs/services

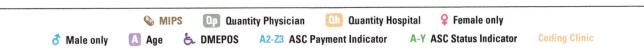

🐾 MIPS    ⓠ Quantity Physician    ⓠ Quantity Hospital    ♀ Female only
♂ Male only    Ⓐ Age    ♿ DMEPOS    A2-Z3 ASC Payment Indicator    A-Y ASC Status Indicator    Coding Clinic

LEVEL II NATIONAL MODIFIERS   QG – SE

**109**

✳ **SF**     Second opinion ordered by a professional review organization (PRO) per Section 9401, P.L. 99-272 (100% reimbursement – no Medicare deductible or coinsurance)

✳ **SG**     Ambulatory surgical center (ASC) facility service

Only valid for surgical codes. After 1/1/08 not required for ASC facility charges.

⊘ **SH**     Second concurrently administered infusion therapy

⊘ **SJ**     Third or more concurrently administered infusion therapy

⊘ **SK**     Member of high risk population (use only with codes for immunization)

⊘ **SL**     State supplied vaccine

⊘ **SM**     Second surgical opinion

⊘ **SN**     Third surgical opinion

⊘ **SQ**     Item ordered by home health

⊘ **SS**     Home infusion services provided in the infusion suite of the IV therapy provider

⊘ **ST**     Related to trauma or injury

⊘ **SU**     Procedure performed in physician's office (to denote use of facility and equipment)

⊘ **SV**     Pharmaceuticals delivered to patient's home but not utilized

✳ **SW**     Services provided by a certified diabetic educator

⊘ **SY**     Persons who are in close contact with member of high-risk population (use only with codes for immunization)

✳ **T1**     Left foot, second digit

✳ **T2**     Left foot, third digit

✳ **T3**     Left foot, fourth digit

✳ **T4**     Left foot, fifth digit

✳ **T5**     Right foot, great toe

✳ **T6**     Right foot, second digit

✳ **T7**     Right foot, third digit

✳ **T8**     Right foot, fourth digit

✳ **T9**     Right foot, fifth digit

✳ **TA**     Left foot, great toe

✳ **TB**     Drug or biological acquired with 340B drug pricing program discount, reported for informational purposes

✳ **TC**     Technical component; under certain circumstances, a charge may be made for the technical component alone; under those circumstances the technical component charge is identified by adding modifier TC to the usual procedure number; technical component charges are institutional charges and not billed separately by physicians; however, portable x-ray suppliers only bill for technical component and should utilize modifier TC; the charge data from portable x-ray suppliers will then be used to build customary and prevailing profiles.

⊘ **TD**     RN

⊘ **TE**     LPN/LVN

⊘ **TF**     Intermediate level of care

⊘ **TG**     Complex/high tech level of care

⊘ **TH**     Obstetrical treatment/services, prenatal or postpartum

⊘ **TJ**     Program group, child and/or adolescent

⊘ **TK**     Extra patient or passenger, non-ambulance

⊘ **TL**     Early intervention/individualized family service plan (IFSP)

⊘ **TM**     Individualized education program (IEP)

⊘ **TN**     Rural/outside providers' customary service area

⊘ **TP**     Medical transport, unloaded vehicle

⊘ **TQ**     Basic life support transport by a volunteer ambulance provider

⊘ **TR**     School-based individual education program (IEP) services provided outside the public school district responsible for the student

✳ **TS**     Follow-up service

⊘ **TT**     Individualized service provided to more than one patient in same setting

⊘ **TU**     Special payment rate, overtime

⊘ **TV**     Special payment rates, holidays/weekends

⊘ **TW**     Back-up equipment

⊘ **U1**     Medicaid Level of Care 1, as defined by each State

⊘ **U2**     Medicaid Level of Care 2, as defined by each State

⊘ **U3**     Medicaid Level of Care 3, as defined by each State

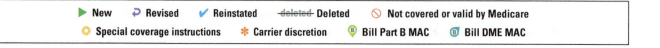

▶ New     ↻ Revised     ✔ Reinstated     ~~deleted~~ Deleted     ⊘ Not covered or valid by Medicare     ⊙ Special coverage instructions     ✳ Carrier discretion     Ⓑ Bill Part B MAC     Ⓓ Bill DME MAC

⊘ **U4**  Medicaid Level of Care 4, as defined by each State

⊘ **U5**  Medicaid Level of Care 5, as defined by each State

⊘ **U6**  Medicaid Level of Care 6, as defined by each State

⊘ **U7**  Medicaid Level of Care 7, as defined by each State

⊘ **U8**  Medicaid Level of Care 8, as defined by each State

⊘ **U9**  Medicaid Level of Care 9, as defined by each State

⊘ **UA**  Medicaid Level of Care 10, as defined by each State

⊘ **UB**  Medicaid Level of Care 11, as defined by each State

⊘ **UC**  Medicaid Level of Care 12, as defined by each State

⊘ **UD**  Medicaid Level of Care 13, as defined by each State

✳ **UE**  Used durable medical equipment

⊘ **UF**  Services provided in the morning

⊘ **UG**  Services provided in the afternoon

⊘ **UH**  Services provided in the evening

✳ **UJ**  Services provided at night

⊘ **UK**  Services provided on behalf of the client to someone other than the client (collateral relationship)

✳ **UN**  Two patients served

✳ **UP**  Three patients served

✳ **UQ**  Four patients served

✳ **UR**  Five patients served

✳ **US**  Six or more patients served

✳ **V1**  Demonstration Modifier 1

✳ **V2**  Demonstration Modifier 2

✳ **V3**  Demonstration Modifier 3

✳ **V5**  Vascular catheter (alone or with any other vascular access)

✳ **V6**  Arteriovenous graft (or other vascular access not including a vascular catheter)

✳ **V7**  Arteriovenous fistula only (in use with two needles)

✳ **VM**  Medicare diabetes prevention program (MDPP) virtual make-up session

✳ **VP**  Aphakic patient

✳ **X1**  Continuous/broad services: for reporting services by clinicians, who provide the principal care for a patient, with no planned endpoint of the relationship; services in this category represent comprehensive care, dealing with the entire scope of patient problems, either directly or in a care coordination role; reporting clinician service examples include, but are not limited to: primary care, and clinicians providing comprehensive care to patients in addition to specialty care

✳ **X2**  Continuous/focused services: for reporting services by clinicians whose expertise is needed for the ongoing management of a chronic disease or a condition that needs to be managed and followed with no planned endpoint to the relationship; reporting clinician service examples include but are not limited to: a rheumatologist taking care of the patient's rheumatoid arthritis longitudinally but not providing general primary care services

✳ **X3**  Episodic/broad services: for reporting services by clinicians who have broad responsibility for the comprehensive needs of the patient that is limited to a defined period and circumstance such as a hospitalization; reporting clinician service examples include but are not limited to the hospitalist's services rendered providing comprehensive and general care to a patient while admitted to the hospital

✳ **X4**  Episodic/focused services: for reporting services by clinicians who provide focused care on particular types of treatment limited to a defined period and circumstance; the patient has a problem, acute or chronic, that will be treated with surgery, radiation, or some other type of generally time-limited intervention; reporting clinician service examples include but are not limited to, the orthopedic surgeon performing a knee replacement and seeing the patient through the postoperative period

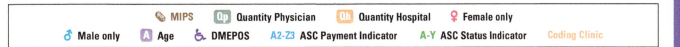

🐾 **MIPS**  **Op** Quantity Physician  **Oh** Quantity Hospital  ♀ **Female only**
♂ **Male only**  **A** Age  ♿ **DMEPOS**  **A2-Z3** ASC Payment Indicator  **A-Y** ASC Status Indicator  *Coding Clinic*

* **X5**    Diagnostic services requested by another clinician: for reporting services by a clinician who furnishes care to the patient only as requested by another clinician or subsequent and related services requested by another clinician; this modifier is reported for patient relationships that may not be adequately captured by the above alternative categories; reporting clinician service examples include but are not limited to, the radiologist's interpretation of an imaging study requested by another clinician

* **XE**    Separate encounter, a service that is distinct because it occurred during a separate encounter

* **XP**    Separate practitioner, a service that is distinct because it was performed by a different practitioner

* **XS**    Separate structure, a service that is distinct because it was performed on a separate organ/structure

* **XU**    Unusual non-overlapping service, the use of a service that is distinct because it does not overlap usual components of the main service

## Ambulance Modifiers

Modifiers that are used on claims for ambulance services are created by combining two alpha characters. Each alpha character, with the exception of X, represents an origin (source) code or a destination code. The pair of alpha codes creates one modifier. The first position alpha-code = origin; the second position alpha-code = destination. On form CMS-1491, used to report ambulance services, Item 12 should contain the origin code and Item 13 should contain the destination code. Origin and destination codes and their descriptions are as follows:

| | |
|---|---|
| D | Diagnostic or therapeutic site other than P or H when these are used as origin codes |
| E | Residential, domiciliary, custodial facility (other than an 1819 facility) |
| G | Hospital-based ESRD facility |
| H | Hospital |
| I | Site of transfer (e.g., airport or helicopter pad) between modes of ambulance transport |
| J | Freestanding ESRD facility |
| N | Skilled nursing facility |
| P | Physician's office |
| R | Residence |
| S | Scene of accident or acute event |
| X | Intermediate stop at physician's office on way to hospital (destination code only) |

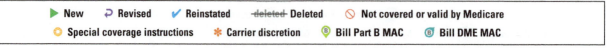

▶ New    ↩ Revised    ✔ Reinstated    ~~deleted~~ Deleted    ⊘ Not covered or valid by Medicare
✪ Special coverage instructions    ✳ Carrier discretion    Ⓑ Bill Part B MAC    Ⓑ Bill DME MAC

## TRANSPORT SERVICES INCLUDING AMBULANCE (A0000-A0999)

⊘ **A0021** Ambulance service, outside state per mile, transport (Medicaid only) Ⓑ Qp Qh      E1

*Cross Reference A0030*

⊘ **A0080** Non-emergency transportation, per mile - vehicle provided by volunteer (individual or organization), with no vested interest Ⓑ Qp Qh    E1

⊘ **A0090** Non-emergency transportation, per mile - vehicle provided by individual (family member, self, neighbor) with vested interest Ⓑ Qp Qh   E1

⊘ **A0100** Non-emergency transportation; taxi Ⓑ Qp Qh      E1

⊘ **A0110** Non-emergency transportation and bus, intra- or interstate carrier Ⓑ Qp Qh      E1

⊘ **A0120** Non-emergency transportation: mini-bus, mountain area transports, or other transportation systems Ⓑ Qp Qh      E1

⊘ **A0130** Non-emergency transportation: wheelchair van Ⓑ Qp Qh      E1

⊘ **A0140** Non-emergency transportation and air travel (private or commercial), intra- or interstate Ⓑ Qp Qh      E1

⊘ **A0160** Non-emergency transportation: per mile - caseworker or social worker Ⓑ Qp Qh      E1

⊘ **A0170** Transportation: ancillary: parking fees, tolls, other Ⓑ Qp Qh      E1

⊘ **A0180** Non-emergency transportation: ancillary: lodging - recipient Ⓑ Qp Qh      E1

⊘ **A0190** Non-emergency transportation: ancillary: meals - recipient Ⓑ Qp Qh      E1

⊘ **A0200** Non-emergency transportation: ancillary: lodging - escort Ⓑ Qp Qh      E1

⊘ **A0210** Non-emergency transportation: ancillary: meals - escort Ⓑ Qp Qh      E1

⊘ **A0225** Ambulance service, neonatal transport, base rate, emergency transport, one way Ⓑ Qp Qh      E1

⊘ **A0380** BLS mileage (per mile) Ⓑ Qp Qh   E1

*Cross Reference A0425*

⊘ **A0382** BLS routine disposable supplies Ⓑ Qp Qh      E1

⊘ **A0384** BLS specialized service disposable supplies; defibrillation (used by ALS ambulances and BLS ambulances in jurisdictions where defibrillation is permitted in BLS ambulances) Ⓑ Qp Qh   E1

⊘ **A0390** ALS mileage (per mile) Ⓑ Qp Qh   E1

*Cross Reference A0425*

⊘ **A0392** ALS specialized service disposable supplies; defibrillation (to be used only in jurisdictions where defibrillation cannot be performed in BLS ambulances) Ⓑ Qp Qh   E1

⊘ **A0394** ALS specialized service disposable supplies; IV drug therapy Ⓑ Qp Qh E1

⊘ **A0396** ALS specialized service disposable supplies; esophageal intubation Ⓑ Qp Qh      E1

⊘ **A0398** ALS routine disposable supplies Ⓑ Qp Qh      E1

⊘ **A0420** Ambulance waiting time (ALS or BLS), one half (½) hour increments Ⓑ Qp Qh      E1

| Waiting Time Table | | | |
|---|---|---|---|
| UNITS | TIME | UNITS | TIME |
| 1 | ½ to 1 hr. | 6 | 3 to 3½ hrs. |
| 2 | 1 to 1½ hrs. | 7 | 3½ to 4 hrs. |
| 3 | 1½ to 2 hrs. | 8 | 4 to 4½ hrs. |
| 4 | 2 to 2½ hrs. | 9 | 4½ to 5 hrs. |
| 5 | 2½ to 3 hrs. | 10 | 5 to 5½ hrs. |

⊘ **A0422** Ambulance (ALS or BLS) oxygen and oxygen supplies, life sustaining situation Ⓑ Qp Qh      E1

⊘ **A0424** Extra ambulance attendant, ground (ALS or BLS) or air (fixed or rotary winged); (requires medical review) Ⓑ Qp Qh      E1

✳ **A0425** Ground mileage, per statute mile Ⓑ Qp Qh      A

✳ **A0426** Ambulance service, advanced life support, non-emergency transport, Level 1 (ALS 1) Ⓑ Qp Qh      A

✳ **A0427** Ambulance service, advanced life support, emergency transport, Level 1 (ALS 1-Emergency) Ⓑ Qp Qh   A

✳ **A0428** Ambulance service, basic life support, non-emergency transport (BLS) Ⓑ Qp Qh      A

✳ **A0429** Ambulance service, basic life support, emergency transport (BLS-Emergency) Ⓑ Qp Qh      A

🖐 MIPS    Qp Quantity Physician    Qh Quantity Hospital    ♀ Female only    ♂ Male only    Ⓐ Age    ♿ DMEPOS    A2-Z3 ASC Payment Indicator    A-Y ASC Status Indicator    Coding Clinic

* **A0430** Ambulance service, conventional air services, transport, one way (fixed wing) 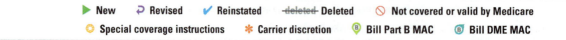 Qp Qh    A

* **A0431** Ambulance service, conventional air services, transport, one way (rotary wing) 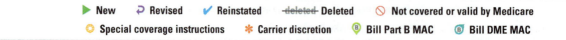 Qp Qh    A

* **A0432** Paramedic intercept (PI), rural area, transport furnished by a volunteer ambulance company, which is prohibited by state law from billing third party payers B Qp Qh    A

* **A0433** Advanced life support, Level 2 (ALS2) B Qp Qh    A

* **A0434** Specialty care transport (SCT) B Qp Qh    A

* **A0435** Fixed wing air mileage, per statute mile B Qp Qh    A

* **A0436** Rotary wing air mileage, per statute mile B Qp Qh    A

⊘ **A0888** Noncovered ambulance mileage, per mile (e.g., for miles traveled beyond closest appropriate facility) B Qp Qh    E1
  *MCM: 2125*

⊘ **A0998** Ambulance response and treatment, no transport B Qp Qh    E1
  *IOM: 100-02, 10, 20*

✪ **A0999** Unlisted ambulance service B    A
  *IOM: 100-02, 10, 20*

## MEDICAL AND SURGICAL SUPPLIES (A4000-A8004)

### Injection and Infusion

* **A4206** Syringe with needle, sterile 1 cc or less, each B B    N

* **A4207** Syringe with needle, sterile 2 cc, each B B    N

* **A4208** Syringe with needle, sterile 3 cc, each B B    N

* **A4209** Syringe with needle, sterile 5 cc or greater, each B B    N

⊘ **A4210** Needle-free injection device, each B Qp Qh    E1
  *IOM: 100-03, 4, 280.1*

✪ **A4211** Supplies for self-administered injections B B Qp Qh    N
  *IOM: 100-02, 15, 50*

* **A4212** Non-coring needle or stylet with or without catheter B Qp Qh    N

* **A4213** Syringe, sterile, 20 cc or greater, each B B    N

* **A4215** Needle, sterile, any size, each B B    N

✪ **A4216** Sterile water, saline and/or dextrose diluent/flush, 10 ml B B ♿    N
  *Other: Sodium Chloride, Bacteriostatic, Syrex*
  *IOM: 100-02, 15, 50*

✪ **A4217** Sterile water/saline, 500 ml B B ♿    N
  *Other: Sodium Chloride*
  *IOM: 100-02, 15, 50*

✪ **A4218** Sterile saline or water, metered dose dispenser, 10 ml B B    N
  *Other: Sodium Chloride*

✪ **A4220** Refill kit for implantable infusion pump B Qp Qh    N
  Do not report with 95990 or 95991 since Medicare payment for these codes includes the refill kit.
  *IOM: 100-03, 4, 280.1*

* **A4221** Supplies for maintenance of non-insulin drug infusion catheter, per week (list drugs separately) B Qp Qh ♿    N
  Includes dressings for catheter site and flush solutions not directly related to drug infusion.

* **A4222** Infusion supplies for external drug infusion pump, per cassette or bag (list drug separately) B Qp Qh ♿    N
  Includes cassette or bag, diluting solutions, tubing and/or administration supplies, port cap changes, compounding charges, and preparation charges.

* **A4223** Infusion supplies not used with external infusion pump, per cassette or bag (list drugs separately) B    N
  *IOM: 100-03, 4, 280.1*

* **A4224** Supplies for maintenance of insulin infusion catheter, per week B Qp Qh ♿    N

✪ **A4225** Supplies for external insulin infusion pump, syringe type cartridge, sterile, each B Qp Qh ♿    N
  *IOM: 100-03, 1, 50.3*

▶ * **A4226** Supplies for maintenace of insulin infusion pump with dosage rate adjustment using therapeutic continuous glucose sensing, per week N

---

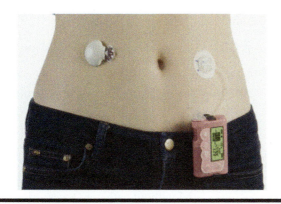

**Figure 1**   Insulin pump.

○ **A4230**   Infusion set for external insulin pump, non-needle cannula type Ⓑ    N

Requires prior authorization and copy of invoice.

*IOM: 100-03, 4, 280.1*

○ **A4231**   Infusion set for external insulin pump, needle type Ⓑ    N

Requires prior authorization and copy of invoice.

*IOM: 100-03, 4, 280.1*

⊘ **A4232**   Syringe with needle for external insulin pump, sterile, 3 cc Ⓑ Ⓠp Ⓠh    E1

Reports insulin reservoir for use with external insulin infusion pump (E0784); may be glass or plastic; includes needle for drawing up insulin. Does not include insulin for use in reservoir.

*IOM: 100-03, 4, 280.1*

## Replacement Batteries

✱ **A4233**   Replacement battery, alkaline (other than J cell), for use with medically necessary home blood glucose monitor owned by patient, each Ⓑ Ⓠh ♿    E1

✱ **A4234**   Replacement battery, alkaline, J cell, for use with medically necessary home blood glucose monitor owned by patient, each Ⓑ Ⓠh ♿    E1

✱ **A4235**   Replacement battery, lithium, for use with medically necessary home blood glucose monitor owned by patient, each Ⓑ Ⓠp Ⓠh ♿    E1

✱ **A4236**   Replacement battery, silver oxide, for use with medically necessary home blood glucose monitor owned by patient, each Ⓑ Ⓠh ♿    E1

## Miscellaneous Supplies

✱ **A4244**   Alcohol or peroxide, per pint Ⓑ Ⓑ    N

✱ **A4245**   Alcohol wipes, per box Ⓑ Ⓑ    N

✱ **A4246**   Betadine or pHisoHex solution, per pint Ⓑ Ⓑ    N

✱ **A4247**   Betadine or iodine swabs/wipes, per box Ⓑ Ⓑ    N

✱ **A4248**   Chlorhexidine containing antiseptic, 1 ml Ⓑ Ⓑ    N

⊘ **A4250**   Urine test or reagent strips or tablets (100 tablets or strips) Ⓑ Ⓑ Ⓠp Ⓠh    E1

*IOM: 100-02, 15, 110*

⊘ **A4252**   Blood ketone test or reagent strip, each Ⓑ Ⓠp Ⓠh    E1

*Medicare Statute 1861(n)*

○ **A4253**   Blood glucose test or reagent strips for home blood glucose monitor, per 50 strips Ⓑ Ⓠp Ⓠh ♿    N

Test strips (1 unit = 50 strips); non-insulin treated (every 3 months) 100 test strips (1×/day testing), 100 lancets (1×/day testing); modifier KS

*IOM: 100-03, 1, 40.2*

○ **A4255**   Platforms for home blood glucose monitor, 50 per box Ⓑ Ⓠp Ⓠh ♿    N

*IOM: 100-03, 1, 40.2*

○ **A4256**   Normal, low and high calibrator solution/chips Ⓑ Ⓠp Ⓠh ♿    N

*IOM: 100-03, 1, 40.2*

✱ **A4257**   Replacement lens shield cartridge for use with laser skin piercing device, each Ⓑ Ⓠp Ⓠh ♿    E1

○ **A4258**   Spring-powered device for lancet, each Ⓑ Ⓠp Ⓠh ♿    N

*IOM: 100-03, 1, 40.2*

○ **A4259**   Lancets, per box of 100 Ⓑ Ⓠp Ⓠh ♿ N

*IOM: 100-03, 1, 40.2*

⊘ **A4261**   Cervical cap for contraceptive use Ⓑ Ⓠp Ⓠh ♀    E1

*Medicare Statute 1862A1*

○ **A4262**   Temporary, absorbable lacrimal duct implant, each Ⓑ Ⓠp Ⓠh    N

*IOM: 100-04, 12, 20.3, 30.4*

○ **A4263**   Permanent, long term, non-dissolvable lacrimal duct implant, each Ⓑ Ⓠp Ⓠh    N

Bundled with insertion if performed in physician office.

*IOM: 100-04, 12, 30.4*

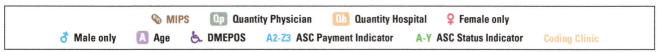

| 🖉 MIPS | Ⓠp Quantity Physician | Ⓠh Quantity Hospital | ♀ Female only |
| --- | --- | --- | --- |
| ♂ Male only | Ⓐ Age | ♿ DMEPOS | A2-Z3 ASC Payment Indicator | A-Y ASC Status Indicator | Coding Clinic |

⊘ **A4264** Permanent implantable contraceptive intratubal occlusion device(s) and delivery system Ⓑ Qp Qh ♀    E1

   *Reports the Essure device.*

✪ **A4265** Paraffin, per pound Ⓑ Ⓑ Qp Qh ♿    N

   *IOM: 100-03, 4, 280.1*

⊘ **A4266** Diaphragm for contraceptive use Ⓑ Qp Qh ♀    E1

⊘ **A4267** Contraceptive supply, condom, male, each Ⓑ Qp Qh ♂    E1

⊘ **A4268** Contraceptive supply, condom, female, each Ⓑ Qp Qh ♀    E1

⊘ **A4269** Contraceptive supply, spermicide (e.g., foam, gel), each ⑨ Qp Qh    E1

✱ **A4270** Disposable endoscope sheath, each Ⓑ Qp Qh    N

✱ **A4280** Adhesive skin support attachment for use with external breast prosthesis, each Ⓑ Qh ♀ ♿    N

✱ **A4281** Tubing for breast pump, replacement Ⓑ ♀    E1

✱ **A4282** Adapter for breast pump, replacement Ⓑ ♀    E1

✱ **A4283** Cap for breast pump bottle, replacement Ⓑ ♀    E1

✱ **A4284** Breast shield and splash protector for use with breast pump, replacement Ⓑ ♀    E1

✱ **A4285** Polycarbonate bottle for use with breast pump, replacement Ⓑ ♀    E1

✱ **A4286** Locking ring for breast pump, replacement Ⓑ ♀    E1

✱ **A4290** Sacral nerve stimulation test lead, each Ⓑ    N

   *Service not separately priced by Part B (e.g., services not covered, bundled, used by Part A only)*

## Implantable Catheters

✪ **A4300** Implantable access catheter, (e.g., venous, arterial, epidural subarachnoid, or peritoneal, etc.) external access Ⓑ Qp Qh    N

   *IOM: 100-02, 15, 120*

✱ **A4301** Implantable access total; catheter, port/reservoir (e.g., venous, arterial, epidural, subarachnoid, peritoneal, etc.) Ⓑ Qp Qh    N

## Disposable Drug Delivery System

✱ **A4305** Disposable drug delivery system, flow rate of 50 ml or greater per hour ⑨ Ⓑ Qp Qh    N

✱ **A4306** Disposable drug delivery system, flow rate of less than 50 ml per hour ⑨ Ⓑ Qp Qh    N

## Incontinence Appliances and Care Supplies

✪ **A4310** Insertion tray without drainage bag and without catheter (accessories only) Ⓑ Ⓑ Qp Qh ♿    N

   *IOM: 100-02, 15, 120*

✪ **A4311** Insertion tray without drainage bag with indwelling catheter, Foley type, two-way latex with coating (Teflon, silicone, silicone elastomer, or hydrophilic, etc.) ⑨ Ⓑ Qp Qh ♿    N

   *IOM: 100-02, 15, 120*

✪ **A4312** Insertion tray without drainage bag with indwelling catheter, Foley type, two-way, all silicone Ⓑ Ⓑ Qp Qh ♿ N

   Must meet criteria for indwelling catheter and medical record must justify need for:

   • Recurrent encrustation

   • Inability to pass a straight catheter

   • Sensitivity to latex

   Must be medically necessary.

   *IOM: 100-02, 15, 120*

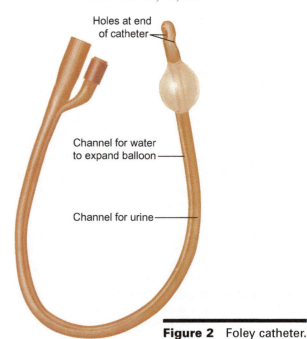

Holes at end of catheter

Channel for water to expand balloon

Channel for urine

**Figure 2**   Foley catheter.

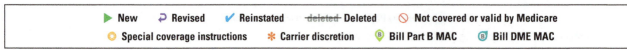

▶ New    ⟲ Revised    ✔ Reinstated    ~~deleted~~ Deleted    ⊘ Not covered or valid by Medicare
✪ Special coverage instructions    ✱ Carrier discretion    ⑨ Bill Part B MAC    Ⓑ Bill DME MAC

**A4313** Insertion tray without drainage bag with indwelling catheter, Foley type, three-way, for continuous irrigation Ⓑ Ⓖ Qp Qh    N

Must meet criteria for indwelling catheter and medical record must justify need for:

• Recurrent encrustation

• Inability to pass a straight catheter

• Sensitivity to latex

Must be medically necessary.

*IOM: 100-02, 15, 120*

**A4314** Insertion tray with drainage bag with indwelling catheter, Foley type, two-way latex with coating (Teflon, silicone, silicone elastomer or hydrophilic, etc.) Ⓑ Ⓖ Qp Qh    N

*IOM: 100-02, 15, 120*

**A4315** Insertion tray with drainage bag with indwelling catheter, Foley type, two-way, all silicone Ⓑ Ⓖ Qp Qh    N

*IOM: 100-02, 15, 120*

**A4316** Insertion tray with drainage bag with indwelling catheter, Foley type, three-way, for continuous irrigation Ⓑ Ⓖ Qp Qh    N

*IOM: 100-02, 15, 120*

**A4320** Irrigation tray with bulb or piston syringe, any purpose Ⓑ Ⓖ Qp Qh    N

*IOM: 100-02, 15, 120*

**A4321** Therapeutic agent for urinary catheter irrigation Ⓑ Ⓖ    N

*IOM: 100-02, 15, 120*

**A4322** Irrigation syringe, bulb, or piston, each Ⓑ Ⓖ Qp Qh    N

*IOM: 100-02, 15, 120*

**A4326** Male external catheter with integral collection chamber, any type, each Ⓑ Ⓖ Qp Qh ♂    N

*IOM: 100-02, 15, 120*

**A4327** Female external urinary collection device; meatal cup, each Ⓑ Ⓖ Qp Qh ♀    N

*IOM: 100-02, 15, 120*

**A4328** Female external urinary collection device; pouch, each Ⓑ Ⓖ Qp Qh ♀    N

*IOM: 100-02, 15, 120*

**A4330** Perianal fecal collection pouch with adhesive, each Ⓑ Ⓖ Qp Qh    N

*IOM: 100-02, 15, 120*

**A4331** Extension drainage tubing, any type, any length, with connector/adaptor, for use with urinary leg bag or urostomy pouch, each Ⓑ Ⓖ Qh    N

*IOM: 100-02, 15, 120*

**A4332** Lubricant, individual sterile packet, each Ⓑ Ⓖ Qp Qh    N

*IOM: 100-02, 15, 120*

**A4333** Urinary catheter anchoring device, adhesive skin attachment, each Ⓑ Ⓖ    N

*IOM: 100-02, 15, 120*

**A4334** Urinary catheter anchoring device, leg strap, each Ⓑ Ⓖ    N

*IOM: 100-02, 15, 120*

**A4335** Incontinence supply; miscellaneous Ⓑ Ⓖ Qp Qh    N

*IOM: 100-02, 15, 120*

**A4336** Incontinence supply, urethral insert, any type, each Ⓑ Ⓖ    N

*IOM: 100-02, 15, 120*

**A4337** Incontinence supply, rectal insert, any type, each Ⓑ Ⓖ Qp Qh    N

*IOM: 100-02, 15, 120*

**A4338** Indwelling catheter; Foley type, two-way latex with coating (Teflon, silicone, silicone elastomer, or hydrophilic, etc.), each Ⓑ Ⓖ Qp Qh    N

*IOM: 100-02, 15, 120*

**A4340** Indwelling catheter; specialty type (e.g., coude, mushroom, wing, etc.), each Ⓑ Ⓖ Qp Qh    N

Must meet criteria for indwelling catheter and medical record must justify need for:

• Recurrent encrustation

• Inability to pass a straight catheter

• Sensitivity to latex

Must be medically necessary.

*IOM: 100-02, 15, 120*

**A4344** Indwelling catheter, Foley type, two-way, all silicone, each Ⓑ Ⓖ Qp Qh    N

Must meet criteria for indwelling catheter and medical record must justify need for:

• Recurrent encrustation

• Inability to pass a straight catheter

• Sensitivity to latex

Must be medically necessary.

*IOM: 100-02, 15, 120*

---

| 🖐 MIPS | Qp Quantity Physician | Qh Quantity Hospital | ♀ Female only |
| ♂ Male only | Ⓐ Age | & DMEPOS | A2-Z3 ASC Payment Indicator | A-Y ASC Status Indicator | Coding Clinic |

⚙ **A4346** Indwelling catheter; Foley type, three way for continuous irrigation, each Ⓑ Ⓓ Qp Qh ♿ N

*IOM: 100-02, 15, 120*

⚙ **A4349** Male external catheter, with or without adhesive, disposable, each Ⓟ Ⓓ ♂ ♿ N

*IOM: 100-02, 15, 120*

⚙ **A4351** Intermittent urinary catheter; straight tip, with or without coating (Teflon, silicone, silicone elastomer, or hydrophilic, etc.), each Ⓟ Ⓑ Qp Qh ♿ N

*IOM: 100-02, 15, 120*

⚙ **A4352** Intermittent urinary catheter; coude (curved) tip, with or without coating (Teflon, silicone, silicone elastomeric, or hydrophilic, etc.), each Ⓟ Ⓑ Qp Qh ♿ N

*IOM: 100-02, 15, 120*

⚙ **A4353** Intermittent urinary catheter, with insertion supplies Ⓟ Ⓑ Qh ♿ N

*IOM: 100-02, 15, 120*

⚙ **A4354** Insertion tray with drainage bag but without catheter Ⓑ Ⓓ Qp Qh ♿ N

*IOM: 100-02, 15, 120*

⚙ **A4355** Irrigation tubing set for continuous bladder irrigation through a three-way indwelling Foley catheter, each Ⓑ Ⓓ Qp Qh ♿ N

*IOM: 100-02, 15, 120*

## External Urinary Supplies

⚙ **A4356** External urethral clamp or compression device (not to be used for catheter clamp), each Ⓟ Ⓓ Qp Qh ♿ N

*IOM: 100-02, 15, 120*

⚙ **A4357** Bedside drainage bag, day or night, with or without anti-reflux device, with or without tube, each Ⓟ Ⓑ Qp Qh ♿ N

*IOM: 100-02, 15, 120*

⚙ **A4358** Urinary drainage bag, leg or abdomen, vinyl, with or without tube, with straps, each Ⓟ Ⓓ Qp ♿ N

*IOM: 100-02, 15, 120*

⚙ **A4360** Disposable external urethral clamp or compression device, with pad and/or pouch, each Ⓟ Ⓓ ♿ N

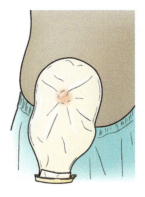

**Figure 3** Ostomy pouch.

## Ostomy Supplies

⚙ **A4361** Ostomy faceplate, each Ⓑ Ⓓ Qp Qh ♿ N

*IOM: 100-02, 15, 120*

⚙ **A4362** Skin barrier; solid, 4 × 4 or equivalent; each Ⓟ Ⓓ Qp Qh ♿ N

*IOM: 100-02, 15, 120*

⚙ **A4363** Ostomy clamp, any type, replacement only, each Ⓟ Ⓓ Qp Qh ♿ E1

⚙ **A4364** Adhesive, liquid or equal, any type, per oz Ⓟ Ⓓ Qp Qh ♿ N

Fee schedule category: Ostomy, tracheostomy, and urologicals items.

*IOM: 100-02, 15, 120*

✳ **A4366** Ostomy vent, any type, each Ⓟ Ⓓ Qh ♿ N

⚙ **A4367** Ostomy belt, each Ⓟ Ⓓ Qp Qh ♿ N

*IOM: 100-02, 15, 120*

✳ **A4368** Ostomy filter, any type, each Ⓟ Ⓓ Qp Qh ♿ N

⚙ **A4369** Ostomy skin barrier, liquid (spray, brush, etc.), per oz Ⓓ Ⓓ ♿ N

*IOM: 100-02, 15, 120*

⚙ **A4371** Ostomy skin barrier, powder, per oz Ⓟ Ⓓ Ⓓ N

*IOM: 100-02, 15, 120*

⚙ **A4372** Ostomy skin barrier, solid 4 × 4 or equivalent, standard wear, with built-in convexity, each Ⓑ Ⓓ Qh ♿ N

*IOM: 100-02, 15, 120*

⚙ **A4373** Ostomy skin barrier, with flange (solid, flexible, or accordion), with built-in convexity, any size, each Ⓑ Ⓓ Qh ♿ N

*IOM: 100-02, 15, 120*

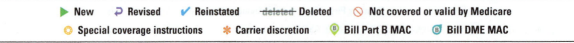

▶ New ⤺ Revised ✔ Reinstated ~~deleted~~ Deleted ⊘ Not covered or valid by Medicare
⚙ Special coverage instructions ✳ Carrier discretion Ⓑ Bill Part B MAC Ⓓ Bill DME MAC

**A4375** Ostomy pouch, drainable, with faceplate attached, plastic, each ⑨ Ⓑ Qp Qh ♿     N

*IOM: 100-02, 15, 120*

**A4376** Ostomy pouch, drainable, with faceplate attached, rubber, each Ⓑ Ⓑ Qp Qh ♿     N

*IOM: 100-02, 15, 120*

**A4377** Ostomy pouch, drainable, for use on faceplate, plastic, each ⑨ Ⓑ Qp Qh ♿     N

*IOM: 100-02, 15, 120*

**A4378** Ostomy pouch, drainable, for use on faceplate, rubber, each Ⓑ Ⓑ Qp Qh ♿     N

*IOM: 100-02, 15, 120*

**A4379** Ostomy pouch, urinary, with faceplate attached, plastic, each Ⓑ Ⓑ Qp Qh ♿     N

*IOM: 100-02, 15, 120*

**A4380** Ostomy pouch, urinary, with faceplate attached, rubber, each ⑨ Ⓑ Qp Qh ♿     N

*IOM: 100-02, 15, 120*

**A4381** Ostomy pouch, urinary, for use on faceplate, plastic, each ⑨ Ⓑ Qp Qh ♿     N

*IOM: 100-02, 15, 120*

**A4382** Ostomy pouch, urinary, for use on faceplate, heavy plastic, each ⑨ Ⓑ Qp Qh ♿     N

*IOM: 100-02, 15, 120*

**A4383** Ostomy pouch, urinary, for use on faceplate, rubber, each ⑨ Ⓑ Qp Qh ♿     N

*IOM: 100-02, 15, 120*

**A4384** Ostomy faceplate equivalent, silicone ring, each ⑨ Ⓑ Qp Qh ♿     N

*IOM: 100-02, 15, 120*

**A4385** Ostomy skin barrier, solid 4 × 4 or equivalent, extended wear, without built-in convexity, each ⑨ Ⓑ Qp Qh ♿     N

*IOM: 100-02, 15, 120*

**A4387** Ostomy pouch closed, with barrier attached, with built-in convexity (1 piece), each ⑨ Ⓑ Qh ♿     N

*IOM: 100-02, 15, 120*

**A4388** Ostomy pouch, drainable, with extended wear barrier attached (1 piece), each ⑨ Ⓑ Qh ♿     N

*IOM: 100-02, 15, 120*

**A4389** Ostomy pouch, drainable, with barrier attached, with built-in convexity (1 piece), each ⑨ Ⓑ Qp Qh ♿     N

*IOM: 100-02, 15, 120*

**A4390** Ostomy pouch, drainable, with extended wear barrier attached, with built-in convexity (1 piece), each ⑨ Ⓒ Qh ♿     N

*IOM: 100-02, 15, 120*

**A4391** Ostomy pouch, urinary, with extended wear barrier attached (1 piece), each ⑨ Ⓑ Qh ♿     N

*IOM: 100-02, 15, 120*

**A4392** Ostomy pouch, urinary, with standard wear barrier attached, with built-in convexity (1 piece), each ⑨ Ⓑ Qp Qh ♿     N

*IOM: 100-02, 15, 120*

**A4393** Ostomy pouch, urinary, with extended wear barrier attached, with built-in convexity (1 piece), each ⑨ Ⓑ Qh ♿ N

*IOM: 100-02, 15, 120*

**A4394** Ostomy deodorant, with or without lubricant, for use in ostomy pouch, per fluid ounce Ⓑ Ⓒ ♿     N

*IOM: 100-02, 15, 20*

**A4395** Ostomy deodorant for use in ostomy pouch, solid, per tablet ⑨ Ⓒ ♿     N

*IOM: 100-02, 15, 20*

**A4396** Ostomy belt with peristomal hernia support ⑨ Ⓑ Qh ♿     N

*IOM: 100-02, 15, 120*

**A4397** Irrigation supply; sleeve, each ⑨ Ⓑ Qp Qh ♿     N

*IOM: 100-02, 15, 120*

**A4398** Ostomy irrigation supply; bag, each ⑨ Ⓒ Qp Qh ♿     N

*IOM: 100-02, 15, 120*

**A4399** Ostomy irrigation supply; cone/catheter, with or without brush Ⓑ Ⓒ Qp Qh ♿     N

*IOM: 100-02, 15, 120*

**A4400** Ostomy irrigation set ⑨ Ⓑ Qp Qh ♿ N

*IOM: 100-02, 15, 120*

**A4402** Lubricant, per ounce ⑨ Ⓑ Qp Qh ♿ N

*IOM: 100-02, 15, 120*

**A4404** Ostomy ring, each ⑨ Ⓒ Qp Qh ♿ N

*IOM: 100-02, 15, 120*

**A4405** Ostomy skin barrier, non-pectin based, paste, per ounce ⑨ Ⓒ ♿     N

*IOM: 100-02, 15, 120*

---

    🖐 **MIPS**     Qp **Quantity Physician**     Qh **Quantity Hospital**     ♀ **Female only**

♂ **Male only**     Ⓐ **Age**     ♿ **DMEPOS**     A2-Z3 **ASC Payment Indicator**     A-Y **ASC Status Indicator**     Coding Clinic

⊛ **A4406** Ostomy skin barrier, pectin-based, paste, per ounce Ⓑ Ⓓ ♿    N

*IOM: 100-02, 15, 120*

⊛ **A4407** Ostomy skin barrier, with flange (solid, flexible, or accordion), extended wear, with built-in convexity, 4 × 4 inches or smaller, each Ⓑ Ⓓ Qp Qh ♿    N

*IOM: 100-02, 15, 120*

⊛ **A4408** Ostomy skin barrier, with flange (solid, flexible, or accordion), extended wear, with built-in convexity, larger than 4 × 4 inches, each Ⓑ Ⓓ Qh ♿    N

*IOM: 100-02, 15, 120*

⊛ **A4409** Ostomy skin barrier, with flange (solid, flexible, or accordion), extended wear, without built-in convexity, 4 × 4 inches or smaller, each Ⓑ Ⓓ Qh ♿    N

*IOM: 100-02, 15, 120*

⊛ **A4410** Ostomy skin barrier, with flange (solid, flexible, or accordion), extended wear, without built-in convexity, larger than 4 × 4 inches, each Ⓑ Ⓓ Qp Qh ♿    N

*IOM: 100-02, 15, 120*

⊛ **A4411** Ostomy skin barrier, solid 4 × 4 or equivalent, extended wear, with built-in convexity, each Ⓑ Ⓓ Qh ♿    N

⊛ **A4412** Ostomy pouch, drainable, high output, for use on a barrier with flange (2 piece system), without filter, each Ⓑ Ⓓ Qh ♿    N

*IOM: 100-02, 15, 120*

⊛ **A4413** Ostomy pouch, drainable, high output, for use on a barrier with flange (2 piece system), with filter, each Ⓑ Ⓓ Qp Qh ♿    N

*IOM: 100-02, 15, 120*

⊛ **A4414** Ostomy skin barrier, with flange (solid, flexible, or accordion), without built-in convexity, 4 × 4 inches or smaller, each Ⓑ Ⓓ Qh ♿    N

*IOM: 100-02, 15, 120*

⊛ **A4415** Ostomy skin barrier, with flange (solid, flexible, or accordion), without built-in convexity, larger than 4 × 4 inches, each Ⓑ Ⓓ Qh ♿    N

*IOM: 100-02, 15, 120*

✳ **A4416** Ostomy pouch, closed, with barrier attached, with filter (1 piece), each Ⓑ Ⓑ Qp Qh ♿    N

✳ **A4417** Ostomy pouch, closed, with barrier attached, with built-in convexity, with filter (1 piece), each Ⓑ Ⓓ Qh ♿    N

✳ **A4418** Ostomy pouch, closed; without barrier attached, with filter (1 piece), each Ⓑ Ⓑ Qh ♿    N

✳ **A4419** Ostomy pouch, closed; for use on barrier with non-locking flange, with filter (2 piece), each Ⓑ Ⓑ Qp Qh ♿    N

✳ **A4420** Ostomy pouch, closed; for use on barrier with locking flange (2 piece), each Ⓑ Ⓑ Qh ♿    N

✳ **A4421** Ostomy supply; miscellaneous Ⓑ Ⓓ    N

⊛ **A4422** Ostomy absorbent material (sheet/pad/crystal packet) for use in ostomy pouch to thicken liquid stomal output, each Ⓑ Ⓑ ♿    N

*IOM: 100-02, 15, 120*

✳ **A4423** Ostomy pouch, closed; for use on barrier with locking flange, with filter (2 piece), each Ⓑ Ⓑ Qp Qh ♿    N

✳ **A4424** Ostomy pouch, drainable, with barrier attached, with filter (1 piece), each Ⓑ Ⓑ Qh ♿    N

✳ **A4425** Ostomy pouch, drainable; for use on barrier with non-locking flange, with filter (2 piece system), each Ⓑ Ⓑ Qh ♿    N

✳ **A4426** Ostomy pouch, drainable; for use on barrier with locking flange (2 piece system), each Ⓑ Ⓑ Qp Qh ♿    N

✳ **A4427** Ostomy pouch, drainable; for use on barrier with locking flange, with filter (2 piece system), each Ⓑ Ⓑ Qh ♿    N

✳ **A4428** Ostomy pouch, urinary, with extended wear barrier attached, with faucet-type tap with valve (1 piece), each Ⓑ Ⓑ Qh ♿    N

✳ **A4429** Ostomy pouch, urinary, with barrier attached, with built-in convexity, with faucet-type tap with valve (1 piece), each Ⓑ Ⓑ Qp Qh ♿    N

✳ **A4430** Ostomy pouch, urinary, with extended wear barrier attached, with built-in convexity, with faucet-type tap with valve (1 piece), each Ⓑ Ⓑ Qh ♿    N

✳ **A4431** Ostomy pouch, urinary; with barrier attached, with faucet-type tap with valve (1 piece), each Ⓑ Ⓑ Qh ♿    N

✳ **A4432** Ostomy pouch, urinary; for use on barrier with non-locking flange, with faucet-type tap with valve (2 piece), each Ⓑ Ⓑ Qp Qh ♿    N

✳ **A4433** Ostomy pouch, urinary; for use on barrier with locking flange (2 piece), each Ⓑ Ⓑ Qh ♿    N

---

▶ New    ↺ Revised    ✔ Reinstated    ~~deleted~~ Deleted    ⊘ Not covered or valid by Medicare
⊛ Special coverage instructions    ✳ Carrier discretion    Ⓑ Bill Part B MAC    Ⓓ Bill DME MAC

✳ **A4434** Ostomy pouch, urinary; for use on barrier with locking flange, with faucet-type tap with valve (2 piece), each Ⓑ Ⓑ Qh ♿     N

✳ **A4435** Ostomy pouch, drainable, high output, with extended wear barrier (one-piece system), with or without filter, each Ⓥ Ⓑ Qp Qh ♿     N

## Miscellaneous Supplies

✿ **A4450** Tape, non-waterproof, per 18 square inches Ⓥ Ⓑ ♿     N

If used with surgical dressings, billed with AW modifier (in addition to appropriate A1-A9 modifier).

*IOM: 100-02, 15, 120*

✿ **A4452** Tape, waterproof, per 18 square inches Ⓥ Ⓑ ♿     N

If used with surgical dressings, billed with AW modifier (in addition to appropriate A1-A9 modifier).

*IOM: 100-02, 15, 120*

✿ **A4455** Adhesive remover or solvent (for tape, cement or other adhesive), per ounce Ⓑ Ⓑ Qp Qh ♿     N

*IOM: 100-02, 15, 120*

✿ **A4456** Adhesive remover, wipes, any type, each Ⓥ Ⓑ ♿     N

May be reimbursed for male or female clients to home health DME providers and DME medical suppliers in the home setting.

*IOM: 100-02, 15, 120*

✳ **A4458** Enema bag with tubing, reusable Ⓑ     N

✳ **A4459** Manual pump-operated enema system, includes balloon, catheter and all accessories, reusable, any type Ⓑ Qp Qh     N

✳ **A4461** Surgical dressing holder, non-reusable, each Ⓥ Ⓑ Qp Qh ♿     N

✳ **A4463** Surgical dressing holder, reusable, each Ⓥ Ⓑ Qh ♿     N

✳ **A4465** Non-elastic binder for extremity Ⓑ Qp Qh     N

⊘ **A4467** Belt, strap, sleeve, garment, or covering, any type Ⓑ Qp Qh     E1

✿ **A4470** Gravlee jet washer Ⓥ Qp Qh     N

Symptoms suggestive of endometrial disease must be present for this disposable diagnostic tool to be covered.

*IOM: 100-02, 16, 90; 100-03, 4, 230.5*

✿ **A4480** VABRA aspirator Ⓥ Qp Qh     N

Symptoms suggestive of endometrial disease must be present for this disposable diagnostic tool to be covered.

*IOM: 100-02, 16, 90; 100-03, 4, 230.6*

✿ **A4481** Tracheostoma filter, any type, any size, each Ⓑ Ⓑ Qh ♿     N

*IOM: 100-02, 15, 120*

✿ **A4483** Moisture exchanger, disposable, for use with invasive mechanical ventilation Ⓑ ♿     N

*IOM: 100-02, 15, 120*

⊘ **A4490** Surgical stockings above knee length, each Ⓑ Qp Qh     E1

*IOM: 100-02, 15, 100; 100-02, 15, 110; 100-03, 4, 280.1*

⊘ **A4495** Surgical stockings thigh length, each Ⓑ Qp Qh     E1

*IOM: 100-02, 15, 100; 100-02, 15, 110; 100-03, 4, 280.1*

⊘ **A4500** Surgical stockings below knee length, each Ⓑ Qp Qh     E1

*IOM: 100-02, 15, 100; 100-02, 15, 110; 100-03, 4, 280.1*

⊘ **A4510** Surgical stockings full length, each Ⓑ Qp Qh     E1

*IOM: 100-02, 15, 100; 100-02, 15, 110; 100-03, 4, 280.1*

⊘ **A4520** Incontinence garment, any type (e.g., brief, diaper), each Ⓑ Qp Qh     E1

*IOM: 100-03, 4, 280.1*

✿ **A4550** Surgical trays Ⓥ Qp Qh     B

No longer payable by Medicare; included in practice expense for procedures. Some private payers may pay, most private payers follow Medicare guidelines.

*IOM: 100-04, 12, 20.3, 30.4*

⊘ **A4553** Non-disposable underpads, all sizes Ⓑ Qp Qh     E1

*IOM: 100-03, 4, 280.1*

⊘ **A4554** Disposable underpads, all sizes Ⓑ Qp Qh     E1

*IOM: 100-03, 4, 280.1*

⊘ **A4555** Electrode/transducer for use with electrical stimulation device used for cancer treatment, replacement only Ⓥ Qp Qh     E1

✳ **A4556** Electrodes (e.g., apnea monitor), per pair Ⓥ Ⓑ Qp Qh ♿     N

---

🖐 MIPS    Qp Quantity Physician    Qh Quantity Hospital    ♀ Female only

♂ Male only    Ⓐ Age    ♿ DMEPOS    A2-Z3 ASC Payment Indicator    A-Y ASC Status Indicator    Coding Clinic

✳ **A4557** Lead wires (e.g., apnea monitor), per pair Ⓑ Ⓓ Qp Qh ⚇     N

✳ **A4558** Conductive gel or paste, for use with electrical device (e.g., TENS, NMES), per oz Ⓥ Ⓑ Qp Qh ⚇     N

✳ **A4559** Coupling gel or paste, for use with ultrasound device, per oz Ⓥ Ⓑ ⚇     N

✳ **A4561** Pessary, rubber, any type Ⓑ Qp Qh ♀ ⚇     N

✳ **A4562** Pessary, non-rubber, any type Ⓑ Qp Qh ♀ ⚇     N

✳ **A4563** Rectal control system for vaginal insertion, for long term use, includes pump and all supplies and accessories, any type each Ⓑ     N

✳ **A4565** Slings Ⓑ Qp Qh ⚇     N

⊘ **A4566** Shoulder sling or vest design, abduction restrainer, with or without swathe control, prefabricated, includes fitting and adjustment Ⓑ Qp Qh     E1

⊘ **A4570** Splint Ⓑ Qp Qh     E1

    *IOM: 100-02, 6, 10; 100-02, 15, 100; 100-04, 4, 240*

✳ **A4575** Topical hyperbaric oxygen chamber, disposable Ⓑ Qp Qh     A

⊘ **A4580** Cast supplies (e.g., plaster) Ⓥ Qp Qh     E1

    *IOM: 100-02, 6, 10; 100-02, 15, 100; 100-04, 4, 240*

⊘ **A4590** Special casting material (e.g., fiberglass) Ⓥ Qp Qh     E1

    *IOM: 100-02, 6, 10; 100-02, 15, 100; 100-04, 4, 240*

❂ **A4595** Electrical stimulator supplies, 2 lead, per month (e.g., TENS, NMES) Ⓥ Ⓑ Qp Qh ⚇     N

    *IOM: 100-03, 2, 160.13*

✳ **A4600** Sleeve for intermittent limb compression device, replacement only, each Ⓑ     E1

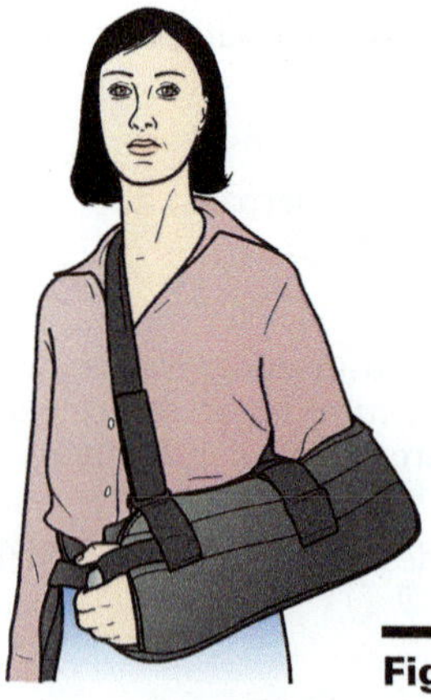

✳ **A4601** Lithium ion battery, rechargeable, for non-prosthetic use, replacement Ⓑ     E1

✳ **A4602** Replacement battery for external infusion pump owned by patient, lithium, 1.5 volt, each Ⓥ Qp Qh ⚇     N

✳ **A4604** Tubing with integrated heating element for use with positive airway pressure device Ⓑ Qh     N

✳ **A4605** Tracheal suction catheter, closed system, each Ⓑ Qh ⚇     N

✳ **A4606** Oxygen probe for use with oximeter device, replacement Ⓑ Qp Qh     N

✳ **A4608** Transtracheal oxygen catheter, each Ⓑ ⚇     N

## Supplies for Respiratory and Oxygen Equipment

⊘ **A4611** Battery, heavy duty; replacement for patient owned ventilator Ⓑ Qp Qh     E1

    *Medicare Statute 1834(a)(3)(a)*

⊘ **A4612** Battery cables; replacement for patient-owned ventilator Ⓑ Qh     E1

    *Medicare Statute 1834(a)(3)(a)*

⊘ **A4613** Battery charger; replacement for patient-owned ventilator Ⓑ Qh     E1

    *Medicare Statute 1834(a)(3)(a)*

✳ **A4614** Peak expiratory flow rate meter, hand held Ⓥ Ⓑ Qp Qh ⚇     N

❂ **A4615** Cannula, nasal Ⓥ Ⓑ ⚇     N

    *IOM: 100-03, 2, 160.6; 100-04, 20, 100.2*

❂ **A4616** Tubing (oxygen), per foot Ⓑ Ⓥ ⚇     N

    *IOM: 100-03, 2, 160.6; 100-04, 20, 100.2*

**Figure 4**   Arm sling.

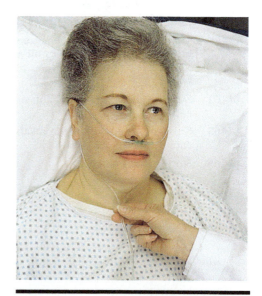

**Figure 5**   Nasal cannula.

---

▶ New    ↻ Revised    ✔ Reinstated    ~~deleted~~ Deleted    ⊘ Not covered or valid by Medicare

❂ Special coverage instructions    ✳ Carrier discretion    Ⓑ Bill Part B MAC    Ⓥ Bill DME MAC

○ **A4617**  Mouth piece ⑧ ⑧ ♿  N

*IOM: 100-03, 2, 160.6; 100-04, 20, 100.2*

○ **A4618**  Breathing circuits ⑧ ⑧ ⓆⓅ ⓆⒽ ♿  N

*IOM: 100-03, 2, 160.6; 100-04, 20, 100.2*

○ **A4619**  Face tent ⑧ ⑧ ♿  N

*IOM: 100-03, 2, 160.6; 100-04, 20, 100.2*

○ **A4620**  Variable concentration mask ⑧ ⑧ ♿  N

*IOM: 100-03, 2, 160.6; 100-04, 20, 100.2*

○ **A4623**  Tracheostomy, inner cannula ⑧ ⑧ ⓆⒽ ♿  N

*IOM: 100-02, 15, 120; 100-03, 1, 20.9*

✳ **A4624**  Tracheal suction catheter, any type, other than closed system, each ⑧ ⑧ ⓆⒽ ♿  N

Sterile suction catheters are medically necessary only for tracheostomy suctioning. Limitations include three suction catheters per day when covered for medically necessary tracheostomy suctioning. Assign DX V44.0 or V55.0 on the claim form. (CMS Manual System, Pub. 100-3, NCD manual, Chapter 1, Section 280-1)

○ **A4625**  Tracheostomy care kit for new tracheostomy ⑧ ⑧ ⓆⓅ ⓆⒽ ♿  N

Dressings used with tracheostomies are included in the allowance for the code. This starter kit is covered after a surgical tracheostomy. (https://www.noridianmedicare.com/dme/coverage/docs/lcds/current_lcds/tracheostomy_care_supplies.htm)

*IOM: 100-02, 15, 120*

○ **A4626**  Tracheostomy cleaning brush, each ⑧ ⑧ ♿  N

*IOM: 100-02, 15, 120*

⊘ **A4627**  Spacer, bag, or reservoir, with or without mask, for use with metered dose inhaler ⑧ ⑧ ⓆⓅ ⓆⒽ  E1

*IOM: 100-02, 15, 110*

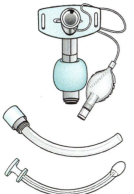

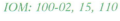

**Figure 6** Tracheostomy cannula.

✳ **A4628**  Oropharyngeal suction catheter, each ⑧ ⑧ ⓆⒽ ♿  N

No more than three catheters per week are covered for medically necessary oropharyngeal suctioning because the catheters can be reused if cleansed and disinfected. (MS Manual System, Pub. 100-3, NCD manual, Chapter 1, Section 280-1)

○ **A4629**  Tracheostomy care kit for established tracheostomy ⑧ ⑧ ⓆⒽ ♿  N

*IOM: 100-02, 15, 120*

## Replacement Parts

○ **A4630**  Replacement batteries, medically necessary, transcutaneous electrical stimulator, owned by patient ⑧ ♿  E1

*IOM: 100-03, 3, 160.7*

✳ **A4633**  Replacement bulb/lamp for ultraviolet light therapy system, each ⑧ ⓆⓅ ⓆⒽ ♿  E1

✳ **A4634**  Replacement bulb for therapeutic light box, tabletop model ⑧  N

○ **A4635**  Underarm pad, crutch, replacement, each ⑧ ⓆⓅ ⓆⒽ ♿  E1

*IOM: 100-03, 4, 280.1*

○ **A4636**  Replacement, handgrip, cane, crutch, or walker, each ⑧ ⓆⒽ ♿  E1

*IOM: 100-03, 4, 280.1*

○ **A4637**  Replacement, tip, cane, crutch, walker, each ⑧ ⓆⒽ ♿  E1

*IOM: 100-03, 4, 280.1*

✳ **A4638**  Replacement battery for patient-owned ear pulse generator, each ⑧ ⓆⓅ ⓆⒽ ♿  E1

✳ **A4639**  Replacement pad for infrared heating pad system, each ⑧ ♿  E1

○ **A4640**  Replacement pad for use with medically necessary alternating pressure pad owned by patient ⑧ ⓆⓅ ⓆⒽ ♿  E1

*IOM: 100-03, 4, 280.1; 100-08, 5, 5.2.3*

## Supplies for Radiological Procedures

✳ **A4641**  Radiopharmaceutical, diagnostic, not otherwise classified ⑧  N

Is not an applicable tracer for PET scans

✳ **A4642**  Indium In-111 satumomab pendetide, diagnostic, per study dose, up to 6 millicuries ⑧ ⓆⓅ ⓆⒽ  N

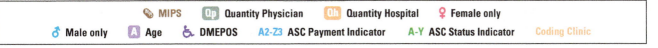

🖐 MIPS   ⓆⓅ Quantity Physician   ⓆⒽ Quantity Hospital   ♀ Female only

♂ Male only   Ⓐ Age   ♿ DMEPOS   A2-Z3 ASC Payment Indicator   A-Y ASC Status Indicator   Coding Clinic

## Miscellaneous Supplies

**✳ A4648** Tissue marker, implantable, any type, each ⑬ **Qp** **Qh**          N

*Coding Clinic: 2018, Q2, P4,5; 2013, Q3, P9*

**✳ A4649** Surgical supply miscellaneous ⑬ ⑬ **Qp**          N

**✳ A4650** Implantable radiation dosimeter, each ⑬ **Qp** **Qh**          N

**⚙ A4651** Calibrated microcapillary tube, each ⑬          N

*IOM: 100-04, 3, 40.3*

**⚙ A4652** Microcapillary tube sealant ⑬          N

*IOM: 100-04, 3, 40.3*

## Supplies for Dialysis

**✳ A4653** Peritoneal dialysis catheter anchoring device, belt, each ⑬ **Qp** **Qh**          N

**⚙ A4657** Syringe, with or without needle, each ⑬ **Qp** **Qh**          N

*IOM: 100-04, 8, 90.3.2*

**⚙ A4660** Sphygmomanometer/blood pressure apparatus with cuff and stethoscope ⑬ **Qp** **Qh**          N

*IOM: 100-04, 8, 90.3.2*

**⚙ A4663** Blood pressure cuff only ⑬ **Qp** **Qh**          N

*IOM: 100-04, 8, 90.3.2*

**⊘ A4670** Automatic blood pressure monitor ⑬ **Qp** **Qh**          E1

*IOM: 100-04, 8, 90.3.2*

**⚙ A4671** Disposable cycler set used with cycler dialysis machine, each ⑬ **Qp** **Qh**          B

*IOM: 100-04, 8, 90.3.2*

**⚙ A4672** Drainage extension line, sterile, for dialysis, each ⑬ **Qp** **Qh**          B

*IOM: 100-04, 8, 90.3.2*

**⚙ A4673** Extension line with easy lock connectors, used with dialysis ⑬ **Qp** **Qh**          B

*IOM: 100-04, 8, 90.3.2*

**⚙ A4674** Chemicals/antiseptics solution used to clean/sterilize dialysis equipment, per 8 oz ⑬ **Qp** **Qh**          B

*IOM: 100-04, 8, 90.3.2*

**⚙ A4680** Activated carbon filters for hemodialysis, each ⑬ **Qp** **Qh**          N

*IOM: 100-04, 8, 90.3.2*

**⚙ A4690** Dialyzers (artificial kidneys), all types, all sizes, for hemodialysis, each ⑬ **Qp** **Qh**          N

*IOM: 100-04, 8, 90.3.2*

**⚙ A4706** Bicarbonate concentrate, solution, for hemodialysis, per gallon ⑬ **Qp** **Qh**          N

*IOM: 100-04, 8, 90.3.2*

**⚙ A4707** Bicarbonate concentrate, powder, for hemodialysis, per packet ⑬ **Qp** **Qh**          N

*IOM: 100-04, 8, 90.3.2*

**⚙ A4708** Acetate concentrate solution, for hemodialysis, per gallon ⑬ **Qp** **Qh**          N

*IOM: 100-04, 8, 90.3.2*

**⚙ A4709** Acid concentrate, solution, for hemodialysis, per gallon ⑬ **Qp** **Qh**          N

*IOM: 100-04, 8, 90.3.2*

**⚙ A4714** Treated water (deionized, distilled, or reverse osmosis) for peritoneal dialysis, per gallon ⑬ **Qp** **Qh**          N

*IOM: 100-03, 4, 230.7; 100-04, 3, 40.3*

**⚙ A4719** "Y set" tubing for peritoneal dialysis ⑬ **Qp** **Qh**          N

*IOM: 100-04, 8, 90.3.2*

**⚙ A4720** Dialysate solution, any concentration of dextrose, fluid volume greater than 249 cc, but less than or equal to 999 cc, for peritoneal dialysis ⑬ **Qp** **Qh**          N

Do not use AX modifier.

*IOM: 100-04, 8, 90.3.2*

**⚙ A4721** Dialysate solution, any concentration of dextrose, fluid volume greater than 999 cc but less than or equal to 1999 cc, for peritoneal dialysis ⑬ **Qp** **Qh**          N

*IOM: 100-04, 8, 90.3.2*

**⚙ A4722** Dialysate solution, any concentration of dextrose, fluid volume greater than 1999 cc but less than or equal to 2999 cc, for peritoneal dialysis ⑬ **Qp** **Qh**          N

*IOM: 100-04, 8, 90.3.2*

**⚙ A4723** Dialysate solution, any concentration of dextrose, fluid volume greater than 2999 cc but less than or equal to 3999 cc, for peritoneal dialysis ⑬ **Qp** **Qh**          N

*IOM: 100-04, 8, 90.3.2*

**⚙ A4724** Dialysate solution, any concentration of dextrose, fluid volume greater than 3999 cc but less than or equal to 4999 cc for peritoneal dialysis ⑬ **Qp** **Qh**          N

*IOM: 100-04, 8, 90.3.2*

---

▶ New   ↻ Revised   ✔ Reinstated   ~~deleted~~ Deleted   ⊘ Not covered or valid by Medicare
⚙ Special coverage instructions   ✳ Carrier discretion   ⑬ Bill Part B MAC   ⑬ Bill DME MAC

⚙ **A4725** Dialysate solution, any concentration of dextrose, fluid volume greater than 4999 cc but less than or equal to 5999 cc, for peritoneal dialysis Ⓑ Qp Qh N

*IOM: 100-04, 8, 90.3.2*

⚙ **A4726** Dialysate solution, any concentration of dextrose, fluid volume greater than 5999 cc, for peritoneal dialysis Ⓑ Qp Qh N

*IOM: 100-04, 8, 90.3.2*

✳ **A4728** Dialysate solution, non-dextrose containing, 500 ml Ⓑ Qp Qh B

⚙ **A4730** Fistula cannulation set for hemodialysis, each Ⓑ Qp Qh N

⚙ **A4736** Topical anesthetic, for dialysis, per gram Ⓑ Qp Qh N

*IOM: 100-04, 8, 90.3.2*

⚙ **A4737** Injectable anesthetic, for dialysis, per 10 ml Ⓑ Qp Qh N

*IOM: 100-04, 8, 90.3.2*

⚙ **A4740** Shunt accessory, for hemodialysis, any type, each Ⓑ Qp Qh N

*IOM: 100-04, 8, 90.3.2*

⚙ **A4750** Blood tubing, arterial or venous, for hemodialysis, each Ⓑ Qp Qh N

*IOM: 100-04, 8, 90.3.2*

⚙ **A4755** Blood tubing, arterial and venous combined, for hemodialysis, each Ⓑ Qp Qh N

*IOM: 100-04, 8, 90.3.2*

⚙ **A4760** Dialysate solution test kit, for peritoneal dialysis, any type, each Ⓑ Qp Qh N

*IOM: 100-04, 8, 90.3.2*

⚙ **A4765** Dialysate concentrate, powder, additive for peritoneal dialysis, per packet Ⓑ Qp Qh N

*IOM: 100-04, 8, 90.3.2*

⚙ **A4766** Dialysate concentrate, solution, additive for peritoneal dialysis, per 10 ml Ⓑ Qp Qh N

*IOM: 100-04, 8, 90.3.2*

⚙ **A4770** Blood collection tube, vacuum, for dialysis, per 50 Ⓑ Qp Qh N

*IOM: 100-04, 8, 90.3.2*

⚙ **A4771** Serum clotting time tube, for dialysis, per 50 Ⓑ Qp Qh N

*IOM: 100-04, 8, 90.3.2*

⚙ **A4772** Blood glucose test strips, for dialysis, per 50 Ⓑ Qp Qh N

*IOM: 100-04, 8, 90.3.2*

⚙ **A4773** Occult blood test strips, for dialysis, per 50 Ⓑ Qp Qh N

*IOM: 100-04, 8, 90.3.2*

⚙ **A4774** Ammonia test strips, for dialysis, per 50 Ⓑ Qp Qh N

⚙ **A4802** Protamine sulfate, for hemodialysis, per 50 mg Ⓑ Qp Qh N

*IOM: 100-04, 8, 90.3.2*

⚙ **A4860** Disposable catheter tips for peritoneal dialysis, per 10 Ⓑ Qp Qh N

*IOM: 100-04, 8, 90.3.2*

⚙ **A4870** Plumbing and/or electrical work for home hemodialysis equipment Ⓑ Qp Qh N

*IOM: 100-04, 8, 90.3.2*

⚙ **A4890** Contracts, repair and maintenance, for hemodialysis equipment Ⓑ Qp Qh N

*IOM: 100-02, 15, 110.2*

⚙ **A4911** Drain bag/bottle, for dialysis, each Ⓑ Qp Qh N

⚙ **A4913** Miscellaneous dialysis supplies, not otherwise specified Ⓑ Qp Qh N

Items not related to dialysis must not be billed with the miscellaneous codes A4913 or E1699.

⚙ **A4918** Venous pressure clamp, for hemodialysis, each Ⓑ Qp Qh N

⚙ **A4927** Gloves, non-sterile, per 100 Ⓑ Qp Qh N

⚙ **A4928** Surgical mask, per 20 Ⓑ Qp Qh N

⚙ **A4929** Tourniquet for dialysis, each Ⓑ Qp Qh N

⚙ **A4930** Gloves, sterile, per pair Ⓑ Qp Qh N

✳ **A4931** Oral thermometer, reusable, any type, each Ⓑ Qp Qh N

✳ **A4932** Rectal thermometer, reusable, any type, each Ⓑ Qp Qh N

## Additional Ostomy Supplies

⚙ **A5051** Ostomy pouch, closed; with barrier attached (1 piece), each ⊙ Ⓑ Qp Qh ♿ N

*IOM: 100-02, 15, 120*

⚙ **A5052** Ostomy pouch, closed; without barrier attached (1 piece), each ⊙ Ⓑ Qp Qh ♿ N

*IOM: 100-02, 15, 120*

---

🖐 MIPS   Qp Quantity Physician   Qh Quantity Hospital   ♀ Female only

♂ Male only   Ⓐ Age   ♿ DMEPOS   A2-Z3 ASC Payment Indicator   A-Y ASC Status Indicator   Coding Clinic

⚙ **A5053** Ostomy pouch, closed; for use on faceplate, each Ⓑ Ⓓ Qp Qh ♿  N
*IOM: 100-02, 15, 120*

⚙ **A5054** Ostomy pouch, closed; for use on barrier with flange (2 piece), each Ⓑ Ⓓ Qp ♿  N
*IOM: 100-02, 15, 120*

⚙ **A5055** Stoma cap Ⓑ Ⓓ Qp Qh ♿  N
*IOM: 100-02, 15, 120*

⚙ **A5056** Ostomy pouch, drainable, with extended wear barrier attached, with filter (1 piece), each Ⓑ Ⓓ Qp Qh ♿  N
*IOM: 100-02, 15, 120*

⚙ **A5057** Ostomy pouch, drainable, with extended wear barrier attached, with built in convexity, with filter (1 piece), each Ⓑ Ⓓ Qp Qh ♿  N
*IOM: 100-02, 15, 120*

✳ **A5061** Ostomy pouch, drainable; with barrier attached (1 piece), each Ⓑ Ⓓ Qp Qh ♿  N
*IOM: 100-02, 15, 120*

⚙ **A5062** Ostomy pouch, drainable; without barrier attached (1 piece), each Ⓑ Ⓓ Qp Qh ♿  N
*IOM: 100-02, 15, 120*

⚙ **A5063** Ostomy pouch, drainable; for use on barrier with flange (2 piece system), each Ⓑ Ⓓ Qp Qh ♿  N
*IOM: 100-02, 15, 120*

⚙ **A5071** Ostomy pouch, urinary; with barrier attached (1 piece), each Ⓑ Ⓓ Qp Qh ♿  N
*IOM: 100-02, 15, 120*

⚙ **A5072** Ostomy pouch, urinary; without barrier attached (1 piece), each Ⓑ Ⓓ Qp Qh ♿  N
*IOM: 100-02, 15, 120*

⚙ **A5073** Ostomy pouch, urinary; for use on barrier with flange (2 piece), each Ⓑ Ⓓ Qp Qh ♿  N
*IOM: 100-02, 15, 120*

⚙ **A5081** Stoma plug or seal, any type Ⓑ Ⓓ Qp Qh ♿  N
*IOM: 100-02, 15, 120*

⚙ **A5082** Continent device; catheter for continent stoma Ⓑ Ⓓ Qp Qh ♿  N
*IOM: 100-02, 15, 120*

✳ **A5083** Continent device, stoma absorptive cover for continent stoma Ⓑ Ⓓ Qh ♿  N

⚙ **A5093** Ostomy accessory; convex insert Ⓑ Ⓓ Qp Qh ♿  N
*IOM: 100-02, 15, 120*

## Additional Incontinence and Ostomy Supplies

⚙ **A5102** Bedside drainage bottle with or without tubing, rigid or expandable, each Ⓑ Ⓓ Qp Qh ♿  N
*IOM: 100-02, 15, 120*

⚙ **A5105** Urinary suspensory, with leg bag, with or without tube, each Ⓑ Ⓓ Qp Qh ♿  N
*IOM: 100-02, 15, 120*

⚙ **A5112** Urinary drainage bag, leg bag, leg or abdomen, latex, with or without tube, with straps, each Ⓑ Ⓓ Qp Qh ♿  N
*IOM: 100-02, 15, 120*

⚙ **A5113** Leg strap; latex, replacement only, per set Ⓑ Ⓓ Qp Qh ♿  E1
*IOM: 100-02, 15, 120*

⚙ **A5114** Leg strap; foam or fabric, replacement only, per set Ⓑ Ⓓ Qp Qh ♿  E1
*IOM: 100-02, 15, 120*

⚙ **A5120** Skin barrier, wipes or swabs, each Ⓑ Ⓓ Qp Qh ♿  N
*IOM: 100-02, 15, 120*

⚙ **A5121** Skin barrier; solid, 6 × 6 or equivalent, each Ⓑ Ⓓ Qp Qh ♿  N
*IOM: 100-02, 15, 120*

⚙ **A5122** Skin barrier; solid, 8 × 8 or equivalent, each Ⓑ Ⓓ Qp Qh ♿  N
*IOM: 100-02, 15, 120*

⚙ **A5126** Adhesive or non-adhesive; disk or foam pad Ⓑ Ⓓ Qp Qh ♿  N
*IOM: 100-02, 15, 120*

⚙ **A5131** Appliance cleaner, incontinence and ostomy appliances, per 16 oz Ⓑ Ⓓ Qp Qh ♿  N
*IOM: 100-02, 15, 120*

⚙ **A5200** Percutaneous catheter/tube anchoring device, adhesive skin attachment Ⓑ Ⓓ Qh ♿  N
*IOM: 100-02, 15, 120*

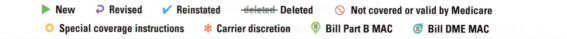

▶ New    ↻ Revised    ✔ Reinstated    ~~deleted~~ Deleted    ⊘ Not covered or valid by Medicare
⚙ Special coverage instructions    ✳ Carrier discretion    Ⓑ Bill Part B MAC    Ⓓ Bill DME MAC

## Diabetic Shoes, Fitting, and Modifications

**A5500** For diabetics only, fitting (including follow-up), custom preparation and supply of off-the-shelf depth-inlay shoe manufactured to accommodate multi-density insert(s), per shoe ⒷⓆpⓆh ♿  Y

*IOM: 100-02, 15, 140*

**A5501** For diabetics only, fitting (including follow-up), custom preparation and supply of shoe molded from cast(s) of patient's foot (custom-molded shoe), per shoe ⒷⓆpⓆh ♿  Y

The diabetic patient must have at least one of the following conditions: peripheral neuropathy with evidence of callus formation, pre-ulcerative calluses, previous ulceration, foot deformity, previous amputation or poor circulation.

*IOM: 100-02, 15, 140*

**A5503** For diabetics only, modification (including fitting) of off-the-shelf depth-inlay shoe or custom-molded shoe with roller or rigid rocker bottom, per shoe ⒷⓆpⓆh ♿  Y

*IOM: 100-02, 15, 140*

**A5504** For diabetics only, modification (including fitting) of off-the-shelf depth-inlay shoe or custom-molded shoe with wedge(s), per shoe ⒷⓆpⓆh ♿  Y

*IOM: 100-02, 15, 140*

**A5505** For diabetics only, modification (including fitting) of off-the-shelf depth-inlay shoe or custom-molded shoe with metatarsal bar, per shoe ⒷⓆpⓆh ♿  Y

*IOM: 100-02, 15, 140*

**A5506** For diabetics only, modification (including fitting) of off-the-shelf depth-inlay shoe or custom-molded shoe with off-set heel(s), per shoe ⒷⓆpⓆh ♿  Y

*IOM: 100-02, 15, 140*

**A5507** For diabetics only, not otherwise specified modification (including fitting) of off-the-shelf depth-inlay shoe or custom-molded shoe, per shoe ⒷⓆpⓆh ♿  Y

Only used for not otherwise specified therapeutic modifications to shoe or for repairs to a diabetic shoe(s)

*IOM: 100-02, 15, 140*

**A5508** For diabetics only, deluxe feature of off-the-shelf depth-inlay shoe or custom-molded shoe, per shoe ⒷⓆpⓆh  Y

*IOM: 100-02, 15, 40*

**A5510** For diabetics only, direct formed, compression molded to patient's foot without external heat source, multiple-density insert(s) prefabricated, per shoe ⒷⓆpⓆh  N

*IOM: 100-02, 15, 140*

**✳ A5512** For diabetics only, multiple density insert, direct formed, molded to foot after external heat source of 230 degrees Fahrenheit or higher, total contact with patient's foot, including arch, base layer minimum of 1/4 inch material of shore a 35 durometer or 3/16 inch material of shore a 40 durometer (or higher), prefabricated, each ⒷⓆpⓆh ♿  Y

**✳ A5513** For diabetics only, multiple density insert, custom molded from model of patient's foot, total contact with patient's foot, including arch, base layer minimum of 3/16 inch material of shore a 35 durometer (or higher), includes arch filler and other shaping material, custom fabricated, each ⒷⓆpⓆh ♿  Y

**A5514** For diabetics only, multiple density insert, made by direct carving with cam technology from a rectified CAD model created from a digitized scan of the patient, total contact with patient's foot, including arch, base layer minimum of 3/16 inch material of shore a 35 durometer (or higher), includes arch filler and other shaping material, custom fabricated, each Ⓑ  Y

## Dressings

**⊘ A6000** Non-contact wound warming wound cover for use with the non-contact wound warming device and warming card ⒷⓆpⓆh  E1

*IOM: 100-02, 16, 20*

**A6010** Collagen based wound filler, dry form, sterile, per gram of collagen ♐Ⓑ♿  N

*IOM: 100-02, 15, 100*

**A6011** Collagen based wound filler, gel/paste, per gram of collagen ⒷⓄ♿  N

*IOM: 100-02, 15, 100*

**A6021** Collagen dressing, sterile, size 16 sq. in. or less, each ♐Ⓑ♿  N

*IOM: 100-02, 15, 100*

**A6022** Collagen dressing, sterile, size more than 16 sq. in. but less than or equal to 48 sq. in., each ♐ⒷⓆp♿  N

*IOM: 100-02, 15, 100*

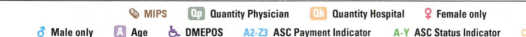

♚ MIPS  Ⓠp Quantity Physician  Ⓠh Quantity Hospital  ♀ Female only  ♂ Male only  Ⓐ Age  ♿ DMEPOS  A2-Z3 ASC Payment Indicator  A-Y ASC Status Indicator  Coding Clinic

✿ **A6023** Collagen dressing, sterile, size more than 48 sq. in., each 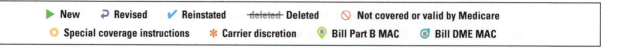 N

*IOM: 100-02, 15, 100*

✿ **A6024** Collagen dressing wound filler, sterile, per 6 inches 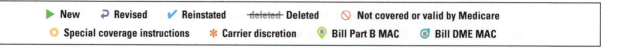 N

*IOM: 100-02, 15, 100*

✱ **A6025** Gel sheet for dermal or epidermal application (e.g., silicone, hydrogel, other), each 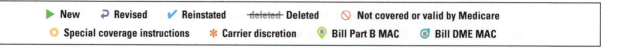 N

If used for the treatment of keloids or other scars, a silicone gel sheet will not meet the definition of the surgical dressing benefit and will be denied as noncovered.

✿ **A6154** Wound pouch, each 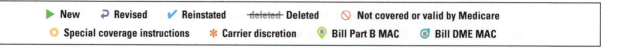 N

Waterproof collection device with drainable port that adheres to skin around wound. Usual dressing change is up to 3 times per week.

*IOM: 100-02, 15, 100*

✿ **A6196** Alginate or other fiber gelling dressing, wound cover, sterile, pad size 16 sq. in. or less, each dressing 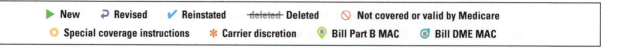 N

*IOM: 100-02, 15, 100*

✿ **A6197** Alginate or other fiber gelling dressing, wound cover, sterile, pad size more than 16 sq. in., but less than or equal to 48 sq. in., each dressing 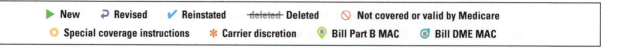 N

*IOM: 100-02, 15, 100*

✿ **A6198** Alginate or other fiber gelling dressing, wound cover, sterile, pad size more than 48 sq. in., each dressing 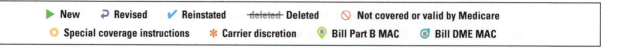 N

*IOM: 100-02, 15, 100*

✿ **A6199** Alginate or other fiber gelling dressing, wound filler, sterile, per 6 inches 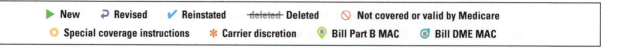 N

*IOM: 100-02, 15, 100*

✿ **A6203** Composite dressing, sterile, pad size 16 sq. in. or less, with any size adhesive border, each dressing 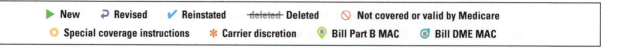 N

Usual composite dressing change is up to 3 times per week, one wound cover per dressing change.

*IOM: 100-02, 15, 100*

✿ **A6204** Composite dressing, sterile, pad size more than 16 sq. in. but less than or equal to 48 sq. in., with any size adhesive border, each dressing 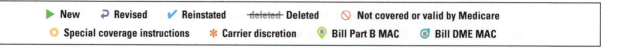 N

Usual composite dressing change is up to 3 times per week, one wound cover per dressing change.

*IOM: 100-02, 15, 100*

✿ **A6205** Composite dressing, sterile, pad size more than 48 sq. in., with any size adhesive border, each dressing 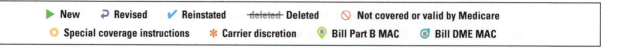 N

Usual composite dressing change is up to 3 times per week, one wound cover per dressing change.

*IOM: 100-02, 15, 100*

✿ **A6206** Contact layer, sterile, 16 sq. in. or less, each dressing 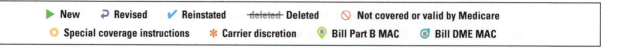 N

Contact layers are porous to allow wound fluid to pass through for absorption by separate overlying dressing and are not intended to be changed with each dressing change. Usual dressing change is up to once per week.

*IOM: 100-02, 15, 100*

✿ **A6207** Contact layer, sterile, more than 16 sq. in. but less than or equal to 48 sq. in., each dressing 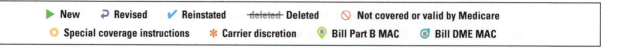 N

Contact layer dressings are used to line the entire wound; they are not intended to be changed with each dressing change. Usual dressing change is up to once per week.

*IOM: 100-02, 15, 100*

✿ **A6208** Contact layer, sterile, more than 48 sq. in., each dressing 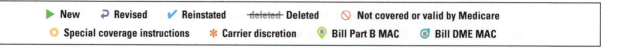 N

Contact layer dressings are used to line the entire wound; they are not intended to be changed with each dressing change. Usual dressing change is up to once per week.

*IOM: 100-02, 15, 100*

✿ **A6209** Foam dressing, wound cover, sterile, pad size 16 sq. in. or less, without adhesive border, each dressing 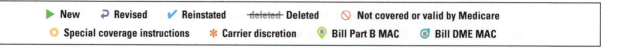 N

Made of open cell, medical grade expanded polymer; with nonadherent property over wound site.

*IOM: 100-02, 15, 100*

▶ New ⤴ Revised ✔ Reinstated ~~deleted~~ Deleted ⊘ Not covered or valid by Medicare
✿ Special coverage instructions ✱ Carrier discretion Ⓑ Bill Part B MAC Ⓑ Bill DME MAC

A6023 – A6209   MEDICAL AND SURGICAL SUPPLIES

128

**A6210** Foam dressing, wound cover, sterile, pad size more than 16 sq. in. but less than or equal to 48 sq. in., without adhesive border, each dressing ⑧ ⑧ Qp ♿ N

Foam dressings are covered items when used on full thickness wounds (e.g., stage III or IV ulcers) with moderate to heavy exudates. Usual dressing change for a foam wound cover when used as primary dressing is up to 3 times per week. When foam wound cover is used as a secondary dressing for wounds with very heavy exudates, dressing change may be up to 3 times per week. Usual dressing change for foam wound fillers is up to once per day (A6209-A6215).

*IOM: 100-02, 15, 100*

**A6211** Foam dressing, wound cover, sterile, pad size more than 48 sq. in., without adhesive border, each dressing ⑧ ⑧ Qp ♿ N

*IOM: 100-02, 15, 100*

**A6212** Foam dressing, wound cover, sterile, pad size 16 sq. in. or less, with any size adhesive border, each dressing ⑧ ⑧ Qp ♿ N

*IOM: 100-02, 15, 100*

**A6213** Foam dressing, wound cover, sterile, pad size more than 16 sq. in. but less than or equal to 48 sq. in., with any size adhesive border, each dressing ⑧ ⑧ Qp N

*IOM: 100-02, 15, 100*

**A6214** Foam dressing, wound cover, sterile, pad size more than 48 sq. in., with any size adhesive border, each dressing ⑧ ⑧ Qp ♿ N

*IOM: 100-02, 15, 100*

**A6215** Foam dressing, wound filler, sterile, per gram ⑧ ⑧ Qp N

*IOM: 100-02, 15, 100*

**A6216** Gauze, non-impregnated, non-sterile, pad size 16 sq. in. or less, without adhesive border, each dressing ⑧ ⑧ Qp ♿ N

*IOM: 100-02, 15, 100*

**A6217** Gauze, non-impregnated, non-sterile, pad size more than 16 sq. in. but less than or equal to 48 sq. in., without adhesive border, each dressing ⑧ ⑧ Qp ♿ N

*IOM: 100-02, 15, 100*

**A6218** Gauze, non-impregnated, non-sterile, pad size more than 48 sq. in., without adhesive border, each dressing ⑧ ⑧ Qp N

*IOM: 100-02, 15, 100*

**A6219** Gauze, non-impregnated, sterile, pad size 16 sq. in. or less, with any size adhesive border, each dressing ⑧ ⑧ Qp ♿ N

*IOM: 100-02, 15, 100*

**A6220** Gauze, non-impregnated, sterile, pad size more than 16 sq. in. but less than or equal to 48 sq. in., with any size adhesive border, each dressing ⑧ ⑧ Qp ♿ N

*IOM: 100-02, 15, 100*

**A6221** Gauze, non-impregnated, sterile, pad size more than 48 sq. in., with any size adhesive border, each dressing ⑧ ⑧ N

*IOM: 100-02, 15, 100*

**A6222** Gauze, impregnated with other than water, normal saline, or hydrogel, sterile, pad size 16 sq. in. or less, without adhesive border, each dressing ⑧ ⑧ Qp ♿ N

Substances may have been incorporated into dressing material (i.e., iodinated agents, petrolatum, zinc paste, crystalline sodium chloride, chlorhexadine gluconate [CHG], bismuth tribromophenate [BTP], water, aqueous saline, hydrogel, or agents).

*IOM: 100-02, 15, 100*

**A6223** Gauze, impregnated with other than water, normal saline, or hydrogel, sterile, pad size more than 16 sq. in. but less than or equal to 48 sq. in., without adhesive border, each dressing ⑧ ⑧ Qp ♿ N

*IOM: 100-02, 15, 100*

**A6224** Gauze, impregnated with other than water, normal saline, or hydrogel, sterile, pad size more than 48 sq. in., without adhesive border, each dressing ⑧ ⑧ Qp ♿ N

*IOM: 100-02, 15, 100*

**A6228** Gauze, impregnated, water or normal saline, sterile, pad size 16 sq. in. or less, without adhesive border, each dressing ⑧ ⑧ Qp Qh N

*IOM: 100-02, 15, 100*

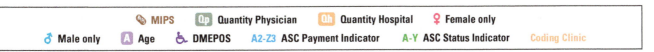

🏷 MIPS   Qp Quantity Physician   Qh Quantity Hospital   ♀ Female only   ♂ Male only   Ⓐ Age   ♿ DMEPOS   A2-Z3 ASC Payment Indicator   A-Y ASC Status Indicator   Coding Clinic

⚙ **A6229** Gauze, impregnated, water or normal saline, sterile, pad size more than 16 sq. in. but less than or equal to 48 sq. in., without adhesive border, each dressing Ⓑ Ⓑ Qp ♿  N

*IOM: 100-02, 15, 100*

⚙ **A6230** Gauze, impregnated, water or normal saline, sterile, pad size more than 48 sq. in., without adhesive border, each dressing Ⓑ Ⓑ Qp Qh  N

*IOM: 100-02, 15, 100*

⚙ **A6231** Gauze, impregnated, hydrogel, for direct wound contact, sterile, pad size 16 sq. in. or less, each dressing Ⓑ Ⓑ Qp  N

*IOM: 100-02, 15, 100*

⚙ **A6232** Gauze, impregnated, hydrogel, for direct wound contact, sterile, pad size greater than 16 sq. in., but less than or equal to 48 sq. in., each dressing Ⓑ Ⓑ ♿  N

*IOM: 100-02, 15, 100*

⚙ **A6233** Gauze, impregnated, hydrogel, for direct wound contact, sterile, pad size more than 48 sq. in., each dressing Ⓑ Ⓑ ♿  N

*IOM: 100-02, 15, 100*

⚙ **A6234** Hydrocolloid dressing, wound cover, sterile, pad size 16 sq. in. or less, without adhesive border, each dressing Ⓑ Ⓑ Qp ♿  N

This type of dressing is usually used on wounds with light to moderate exudate with an average of three dressing changes per week.

*IOM: 100-02, 15, 100*

⚙ **A6235** Hydrocolloid dressing, wound cover, sterile, pad size more than 16 sq. in. but less than or equal to 48 sq. in., without adhesive border, each dressing Ⓑ Ⓑ Qp ♿  N

*IOM: 100-02, 15, 100*

⚙ **A6236** Hydrocolloid dressing, wound cover, sterile, pad size more than 48 sq. in., without adhesive border, each dressing Ⓑ Ⓑ Qp Qh ♿  N

*IOM: 100-02, 15, 100*

⚙ **A6237** Hydrocolloid dressing, wound cover, sterile, pad size 16 sq. in. or less, with any size adhesive border, each dressing Ⓑ Ⓑ Qp ♿  N

*IOM: 100-02, 15, 100*

⚙ **A6238** Hydrocolloid dressing, wound cover, sterile, pad size more than 16 sq. in. but less than or equal to 48 sq. in., with any size adhesive border, each dressing Ⓑ Ⓑ Qp Qh ♿  N

*IOM: 100-02, 15, 100*

⚙ **A6239** Hydrocolloid dressing, wound cover, sterile, pad size more than 48 sq. in., with any size adhesive border, each dressing Ⓑ Ⓑ Qp Qh  N

*IOM: 100-02, 15, 100*

⚙ **A6240** Hydrocolloid dressing, wound filler, paste, sterile, per ounce Ⓑ Ⓑ Qp Qh ♿  N

*IOM: 100-02, 15, 100*

⚙ **A6241** Hydrocolloid dressing, wound filler, dry form, sterile, per gram Ⓑ Ⓑ Qp Qh ♿  N

*IOM: 100-02, 15, 100*

⚙ **A6242** Hydrogel dressing, wound cover, sterile, pad size 16 sq. in. or less, without adhesive border, each dressing Ⓑ Ⓑ Qp ♿  N

Considered medically necessary when used on full thickness wounds with minimal or no exudate (e.g., stage III or IV ulcers).

Usually up to one dressing change per day is considered medically necessary, but if well documented and medically necessary, the payer may allow more frequent dressing changes.

*IOM: 100-02, 15, 100*

⚙ **A6243** Hydrogel dressing, wound cover, sterile, pad size more than 16 sq. in. but less than or equal to 48 sq. in., without adhesive border, each dressing Ⓑ Ⓑ Qp ♿  N

*IOM: 100-02, 15, 100*

⚙ **A6244** Hydrogel dressing, wound cover, sterile, pad size more than 48 sq. in., without adhesive border, each dressing Ⓑ Ⓑ Qp Qh ♿  N

*IOM: 100-02, 15, 100*

⚙ **A6245** Hydrogel dressing, wound cover, sterile, pad size 16 sq. in. or less, with any size adhesive border, each dressing Ⓑ Ⓑ Qp ♿  N

Coverage of a non-elastic gradient compression wrap is limited to one per 6 months per leg.

*IOM: 100-02, 15, 100*

▶ New   ↻ Revised   ✔ Reinstated   ~~deleted~~ Deleted   ⊘ Not covered or valid by Medicare   ⚙ Special coverage instructions   ✳ Carrier discretion   Ⓑ Bill Part B MAC   Ⓑ Bill DME MAC

**A6246** Hydrogel dressing, wound cover, sterile, pad size more than 16 sq. in. but less than or equal to 48 sq. in., with any size adhesive border, each dressing ⑬ ⑬ **Qp** **Qh**   N

*IOM: 100-02, 15, 100*

**A6247** Hydrogel dressing, wound cover, sterile, pad size more than 48 sq. in., with any size adhesive border, each dressing ⑬ ⑬ **Qp** **Qh**   N

*IOM: 100-02, 15, 100*

**A6248** Hydrogel dressing, wound filler, gel, per fluid ounce ⑬ ⑬ **Qp**   N

*IOM: 100-02, 15, 100*

**A6250** Skin sealants, protectants, moisturizers, ointments, any type, any size ⑬ ⑬ **Qp** **Qh**   N

*IOM: 100-02, 15, 100*

**A6251** Specialty absorptive dressing, wound cover, sterile, pad size 16 sq. in. or less, without adhesive border, each dressing ⑬ ⑬ **Qp**   N

*IOM: 100-02, 15, 100*

**A6252** Specialty absorptive dressing, wound cover, sterile, pad size more than 16 sq. in. but less than or equal to 48 sq. in., without adhesive border, each dressing ⑬ ⑬ **Qp**   N

*IOM: 100-02, 15, 100*

**A6253** Specialty absorptive dressing, wound cover, sterile, pad size more than 48 sq. in., without adhesive border, each dressing ⑬ ⑬ **Qp**   N

*IOM: 100-02, 15, 100*

**A6254** Specialty absorptive dressing, wound cover, sterile, pad size 16 sq. in. or less, with any size adhesive border, each dressing ⑬ ⑬ **Qp**   N

*IOM: 100-02, 15, 100*

**A6255** Specialty absorptive dressing, wound cover, sterile, pad size more than 16 sq. in. but less than or equal to 48 sq. in., with any size adhesive border, each dressing ⑬ ⑬ **Qp**   N

*IOM: 100-02, 15, 100*

**A6256** Specialty absorptive dressing, wound cover, sterile, pad size more than 48 sq. in., with any size adhesive border, each dressing ⑬ ⑬ **Qp** **Qh**   N

Considered medically necessary when used for moderately or highly exudative wounds (e.g., stage III or IV ulcers).

*IOM: 100-02, 15, 100*

**A6257** Transparent film, sterile, 16 sq. in. or less, each dressing ⑬ ⑬ **Qp**   N

Considered medically necessary when used on open partial thickness wounds with minimal exudate or closed wounds.

*IOM: 100-02, 15, 100*

**A6258** Transparent film, sterile, more than 16 sq. in. but less than or equal to 48 sq. in., each dressing ⑬ ⑬ **Qp**   N

*IOM: 100-02, 15, 100*

**A6259** Transparent film, sterile, more than 48 sq. in., each dressing ⑬ ⑬ **Qp** **Qh**   N

*IOM: 100-02, 15, 100*

**A6260** Wound cleansers, any type, any size ⑬ ⑬ **Qp**   N

*IOM: 100-02, 15, 100*

**A6261** Wound filler, gel/paste, per fluid ounce, not otherwise specified ⑬ ⑬ **Qp** **Qh** N

Units of service for wound fillers are 1 gram, 1 fluid ounce, 6 inch length, or 1 yard depending on product.

*IOM: 100-02, 15, 100*

**A6262** Wound filler, dry form, per gram, not otherwise specified ⑬ ⑬ **Qp** **Qh**   N

Dry forms (e.g., powder, granules, beads) are used to eliminate dead space in an open wound.

*IOM: 100-02, 15, 100*

**A6266** Gauze, impregnated, other than water, normal saline, or zinc paste, sterile, any width, per linear yard ⑬ ⑬ **Qp**   N

*IOM: 100-02, 15, 100*

**A6402** Gauze, non-impregnated, sterile, pad size 16 sq. in. or less, without adhesive border, each dressing ⑬ ⑬ **Qp**   N

*IOM: 100-02, 15, 100*

**A6403** Gauze, non-impregnated, sterile, pad size more than 16 sq. in., less than or equal to 48 sq. in., without adhesive border, each dressing ⑬ ⑬ **Qp**   N

*IOM: 100-02, 15, 100*

**A6404** Gauze, non-impregnated, sterile, pad size more than 48 sq. in., without adhesive border, each dressing ⑬ ⑬ **Qp** **Qh**   N

*IOM: 100-02, 15, 100*

**✳ A6407** Packing strips, non-impregnated, sterile, up to 2 inches in width, per linear yard ⑬ ⑬   N

*IOM: 100-02, 15, 100*

**A6410** Eye pad, sterile, each ⑬ ⑬ **Qp** **Qh** & N

*IOM: 100-02, 15, 100*

🐾 MIPS    **Qp** Quantity Physician    **Qh** Quantity Hospital    ♀ Female only

♂ Male only    Ⓐ Age    & DMEPOS    A2-Z3 ASC Payment Indicator    A-Y ASC Status Indicator    Coding Clinic

○ **A6411** Eye pad, non-sterile, each Ⓑ Ⓓ Qh ♿     **N**

*IOM: 100-02, 15, 100*

\* **A6412** Eye patch, occlusive, each Ⓑ Ⓓ     **N**

## Bandages

⊘ **A6413** Adhesive bandage, first-aid type, any size, each Ⓑ Ⓓ Qp Qh     **E1**

First aid type bandage is a wound cover with a pad size of less than 4 sq. in. Does not meet the definition of the surgical dressing benefit and will be denied as non-covered.

*Medicare Statute 1861(s)(5)*

\* **A6441** Padding bandage, non-elastic, non-woven/non-knitted, width greater than or equal to three inches and less than five inches, per yard Ⓑ Ⓓ ♿     **N**

\* **A6442** Conforming bandage, non-elastic, knitted/woven, non-sterile, width less than three inches, per yard Ⓑ Ⓓ ♿     **N**

Non-elastic, moderate or high compression that is typically sustained for one week

\* **A6443** Conforming bandage, non-elastic, knitted/woven, non-sterile, width greater than or equal to three inches and less than five inches, per yard Ⓑ Ⓓ ♿     **N**

\* **A6444** Conforming bandage, non-elastic, knitted/woven, non-sterile, width greater than or equal to five inches, per yard Ⓑ Ⓓ ♿     **N**

\* **A6445** Conforming bandage, non-elastic, knitted/woven, sterile, width less than three inches, per yard Ⓑ Ⓓ ♿     **N**

\* **A6446** Conforming bandage, non-elastic, knitted/woven, sterile, width greater than or equal to three inches and less than five inches, per yard Ⓑ Ⓓ ♿     **N**

\* **A6447** Conforming bandage, non-elastic, knitted/woven, sterile, width greater than or equal to five inches, per yard Ⓑ Ⓓ ♿     **N**

\* **A6448** Light compression bandage, elastic, knitted/woven, width less than three inches, per yard Ⓑ Ⓓ ♿     **N**

Used to hold wound cover dressings in place over a wound. Example is an ACE type elastic bandage.

\* **A6449** Light compression bandage, elastic, knitted/woven, width greater than or equal to three inches and less than five inches, per yard Ⓑ Ⓓ ♿     **N**

\* **A6450** Light compression bandage, elastic, knitted/woven, width greater than or equal to five inches, per yard Ⓑ Ⓓ ♿     **N**

\* **A6451** Moderate compression bandage, elastic, knitted/woven, load resistance of 1.25 to 1.34 foot pounds at 50% maximum stretch, width greater than or equal to three inches and less than five inches, per yard Ⓑ Ⓓ ♿     **N**

Elastic bandages that produce moderate compression that is typically sustained for one week

Medicare considers coverage if part of a multi-layer compression bandage system for the treatment of a venous stasis ulcer. Do not assign for strains or sprains.

\* **A6452** High compression bandage, elastic, knitted/woven, load resistance greater than or equal to 1.35 foot pounds at 50% maximum stretch, width greater than or equal to three inches and less than five inches, per yard Ⓑ Ⓓ ♿     **N**

Elastic bandages that produce high compression that is typically sustained for one week

\* **A6453** Self-adherent bandage, elastic, non-knitted/non-woven, width less than three inches, per yard Ⓑ Ⓓ ♿     **N**

\* **A6454** Self-adherent bandage, elastic, non-knitted/non-woven, width greater than or equal to three inches and less than five inches, per yard Ⓑ Ⓓ ♿     **N**

\* **A6455** Self-adherent bandage, elastic, non-knitted/non-woven, width greater than or equal to five inches, per yard Ⓑ Ⓓ ♿     **N**

\* **A6456** Zinc paste impregnated bandage, non-elastic, knitted/woven, width greater than or equal to three inches and less than five inches, per yard Ⓑ Ⓓ ♿     **N**

\* **A6457** Tubular dressing with or without elastic, any width, per linear yard Ⓑ Ⓓ ♿     **N**

\* **A6460** Synthetic resorbable wound dressing, sterile, pad size 16 sq. in. or less, without adhesive border, each dressing Ⓓ     **N**

\* **A6461** Synthetic resorbable wound dressing, sterile, pad size more than 16 sq. in. but less than or equal to 48 sq. in., without adhesive border, each dressing Ⓓ     **N**

---

▶ New    ↻ Revised    ✔ Reinstated    ~~deleted~~ Deleted    ⊘ Not covered or valid by Medicare

○ Special coverage instructions    \* Carrier discretion    Ⓑ Bill Part B MAC    Ⓓ Bill DME MAC

## Compression Garments

⚙ **A6501** Compression burn garment, bodysuit (head to foot), custom fabricated ⓥ Ⓑ Qp Qh ♿    N

*Garments used to reduce hypertrophic scarring and joint contractures following burn injury*

*IOM: 100-02, 15, 100*

⚙ **A6502** Compression burn garment, chin strap, custom fabricated ⓥ Ⓑ Qp Qh ♿   N

*IOM: 100-02, 15, 100*

⚙ **A6503** Compression burn garment, facial hood, custom fabricated ⓥ Ⓑ Qp Qh ♿   N

*IOM: 100-02, 15, 100*

⚙ **A6504** Compression burn garment, glove to wrist, custom fabricated ⓥ Ⓑ Qp Qh ♿   N

*IOM: 100-02, 15, 100*

⚙ **A6505** Compression burn garment, glove to elbow, custom fabricated ⓥ Ⓑ Qp Qh ♿   N

*IOM: 100-02, 15, 100*

⚙ **A6506** Compression burn garment, glove to axilla, custom fabricated ⓥ Ⓑ Qp Qh ♿   N

*IOM: 100-02, 15, 100*

⚙ **A6507** Compression burn garment, foot to knee length, custom fabricated ⓥ Ⓑ Qp Qh ♿   N

*IOM: 100-02, 15, 100*

⚙ **A6508** Compression burn garment, foot to thigh length, custom fabricated ⓥ Ⓑ Qp Qh ♿   N

*IOM: 100-02, 15, 100*

⚙ **A6509** Compression burn garment, upper trunk to waist including arm openings (vest), custom fabricated ⓥ Ⓑ Qp Qh ♿   N

*IOM: 100-02, 15, 100*

⚙ **A6510** Compression burn garment, trunk, including arms down to leg openings (leotard), custom fabricated ⓥ Ⓑ Qp Qh ♿   N

*IOM: 100-02, 15, 100*

⚙ **A6511** Compression burn garment, lower trunk including leg openings (panty), custom fabricated ⓥ Ⓑ Qp Qh ♿   N

*IOM: 100-02, 15, 100*

⚙ **A6512** Compression burn garment, not otherwise classified ⓥ Ⓑ   N

*IOM: 100-02, 15, 100*

✱ **A6513** Compression burn mask, face and/or neck, plastic or equal, custom fabricated Ⓑ Qp Qh ♿   B

⊘ **A6530** Gradient compression stocking, below knee, 18-30 mmHg, each Ⓑ Qp Qh   E1

*IOM: 100-03, 4, 280.1*

⚙ **A6531** Gradient compression stocking, below knee, 30-40 mmHg, each ⓥ Qp Qh ♿   N

*Covered when used in treatment of open venous stasis ulcer. Modifiers A1-A9 are not assigned. Must be billed with AW, RT, or LT.*

*IOM: 100-02, 15, 100*

⚙ **A6532** Gradient compression stocking, below knee, 40-50 mmHg, each Ⓑ Qp Qh ♿   N

*Covered when used in treatment of open venous stasis ulcer. Modifiers A1-A9 are not assigned. Must be billed with AW, RT, or LT.*

*IOM: 100-02, 15, 100*

⊘ **A6533** Gradient compression stocking, thigh length, 18-30 mmHg, each Ⓑ Qp Qh   E1

*IOM: 100-02, 15, 130; 100-03, 4, 280.1*

⊘ **A6534** Gradient compression stocking, thigh length, 30-40 mmHg, each Ⓑ Qp Qh   E1

*IOM: 100-02, 15, 130; 100-03, 4, 280.1*

⊘ **A6535** Gradient compression stocking, thigh length, 40-50 mmHg, each Ⓑ Qp Qh   E1

*IOM: 100-02, 15, 130; 100-03, 4, 280.1*

⊘ **A6536** Gradient compression stocking, full length/chap style, 18-30 mmHg, each Ⓑ Qp Qh   E1

*IOM: 100-02, 15, 130; 100-03, 4, 280.1*

⊘ **A6537** Gradient compression stocking, full length/chap style, 30-40 mmHg, each Ⓑ Qp Qh   E1

*IOM: 100-02, 15, 130; 100-03, 4, 280.1*

⊘ **A6538** Gradient compression stocking, full length/chap style, 40-50 mmHg, each Ⓑ Qp Qh   E1

*IOM: 100-02, 15, 130; 100-03, 4, 280.1*

⊘ **A6539** Gradient compression stocking, waist length, 18-30 mmHg, each Ⓑ Qp Qh   E1

*IOM: 100-02, 15, 130; 100-03, 4, 280.1*

⊘ **A6540** Gradient compression stocking, waist length, 30-40 mmHg, each Ⓑ Qp Qh   E1

*IOM: 100-02, 15, 130; 100-03, 4, 280.1*

🖱 MIPS   Qp Quantity Physician   Qh Quantity Hospital   ♀ Female only   ♂ Male only   Ⓐ Age   ♿ DMEPOS   A2-Z3 ASC Payment Indicator   A-Y ASC Status Indicator   Coding Clinic

⊘ **A6541** Gradient compression stocking, waist length, 40-50 mmHg, each Ⓑ Qp Qh  E1

*IOM: 100-02, 15, 130; 100-03, 4, 280.1*

⊘ **A6544** Gradient compression stocking, garter belt Ⓑ Qp Qh  E1

*IOM: 100-02, 15, 130; 100-03, 4, 280.1*

⊙ **A6545** Gradient compression wrap, non-elastic, below knee, 30-50 mm hg, each Ⓑ Qp Qh ♿  N

Modifiers RT and/or LT must be appended. When assigned for bilateral items (left/right) on the same date of service, bill both items on the same claim line using RT/LT modifiers and 2 units of service.

*IOM: 10-02, 15, 100*

⊘ **A6549** Gradient compression stocking/sleeve, not otherwise specified Ⓑ Qp Qh  E1

*IOM: 100-02, 15, 130; 100-03, 4, 280.1*

## Wound Care

✳ **A6550** Wound care set, for negative pressure wound therapy electrical pump, includes all supplies and accessories Ⓑ Qh ♿  N

## Respiratory Supplies

✳ **A7000** Canister, disposable, used with suction pump, each Ⓑ Qp Qh ♿  Y

✳ **A7001** Canister, non-disposable, used with suction pump, each Ⓑ Qh ♿  Y

✳ **A7002** Tubing, used with suction pump, each Ⓑ Qh ♿  Y

✳ **A7003** Administration set, with small volume nonfiltered pneumatic nebulizer, disposable Ⓑ Qp Qh ♿  Y

✳ **A7004** Small volume nonfiltered pneumatic nebulizer, disposable Ⓑ Qh ♿  Y

✳ **A7005** Administration set, with small volume nonfiltered pneumatic nebulizer, non-disposable Ⓑ Qp Qh ♿  Y

✳ **A7006** Administration set, with small volume filtered pneumatic nebulizer Ⓑ Qp Qh ♿  Y

✳ **A7007** Large volume nebulizer, disposable, unfilled, used with aerosol compressor Ⓑ Qh ♿  Y

✳ **A7008** Large volume nebulizer, disposable, prefilled, used with aerosol compressor Ⓑ ♿  Y

✳ **A7009** Reservoir bottle, nondisposable, used with large volume ultrasonic nebulizer Ⓑ ♿  Y

✳ **A7010** Corrugated tubing, disposable, used with large volume nebulizer, 100 feet Ⓑ Qh ♿  Y

✳ **A7012** Water collection device, used with large volume nebulizer Ⓑ Qh ♿  Y

✳ **A7013** Filter, disposable, used with aerosol compressor or ultrasonic generator Ⓑ Qp Qh ♿  Y

✳ **A7014** Filter, non-disposable, used with aerosol compressor or ultrasonic generator Ⓑ Qp Qh  Y

✳ **A7015** Aerosol mask, used with DME nebulizer Ⓑ Qh ♿  Y

✳ **A7016** Dome and mouthpiece, used with small volume ultrasonic nebulizer Ⓑ Qp Qh ♿  Y

⊙ **A7017** Nebulizer, durable, glass or autoclavable plastic, bottle type, not used with oxygen Ⓑ Qp Qh ♿  Y

*IOM: 100-03, 4, 280.1*

✳ **A7018** Water, distilled, used with large volume nebulizer, 1000 ml Ⓑ Qh ♿  Y

✳ **A7020** Interface for cough stimulating device, includes all components, replacement only Ⓑ Qp Qh ♿  Y

✳ **A7025** High frequency chest wall oscillation system vest, replacement for use with patient owned equipment, each Ⓑ Qp Qh ♿  N

✳ **A7026** High frequency chest wall oscillation system hose, replacement for use with patient owned equipment, each Ⓑ Qp Qh  Y

✳ **A7027** Combination oral/nasal mask, used with continuous positive airway pressure device, each Ⓑ Qp Qh  Y

✳ **A7028** Oral cushion for combination oral/nasal mask, replacement only, each Ⓑ Qp Qh ♿  Y

✳ **A7029** Nasal pillows for combination oral/nasal mask, replacement only, pair Ⓑ Qp Qh ♿  Y

✳ **A7030** Full face mask used with positive airway pressure device, each Ⓑ Qh ♿  Y

✳ **A7031** Face mask interface, replacement for full face mask, each Ⓑ Qh ♿  Y

✳ **A7032** Cushion for use on nasal mask interface, replacement only, each Ⓑ Qp Qh ♿  Y

---

▶ New   ⤻ Revised   ✔ Reinstated   ~~deleted~~ Deleted   ⊘ Not covered or valid by Medicare
⊙ Special coverage instructions   ✳ Carrier discretion   Ⓑ Bill Part B MAC   Ⓑ Bill DME MAC

* **A7033** Pillow for use on nasal cannula type interface, replacement only, pair ⑧ Qh ♿    Y

* **A7034** Nasal interface (mask or cannula type) used with positive airway pressure device, with or without head strap ⑧ Qh ♿    Y

* **A7035** Headgear used with positive airway pressure device ⑧ Qp Qh ♿    Y

* **A7036** Chinstrap used with positive airway pressure device ⑧ Qp Qh ♿    Y

* **A7037** Tubing used with positive airway pressure device ⑧ Qp Qh ♿    Y

* **A7038** Filter, disposable, used with positive airway pressure device ⑧ Qh ♿    Y

* **A7039** Filter, non disposable, used with positive airway pressure device ⑧ Qp Qh ♿    Y

* **A7040** One way chest drain valve ⑧ Qp Qh ♿    N

* **A7041** Water seal drainage container and tubing for use with implanted chest tube ⑨ Qp Qh ♿    N

* **A7044** Oral interface used with positive airway pressure device, each ⑧ Qp Qh ♿    Y

○ **A7045** Exhalation port with or without swivel used with accessories for positive airway devices, replacement only ⑧ Qh ♿    Y

*IOM: 100-03, 4, 230.17*

○ **A7046** Water chamber for humidifier, used with positive airway pressure device, replacement, each ⑧ Qh ♿    Y

*IOM: 100-03, 4, 230.17*

* **A7047** Oral interface used with respiratory suction pump, each ⑧ Qp Qh ♿    N

* **A7048** Vacuum drainage collection unit and tubing kit, including all supplies needed for collection unit change, for use with implanted catheter, each ⑧ Qp Qh ♿    N

## Tracheostomy Supplies

○ **A7501** Tracheostoma valve, including diaphragm, each ⑧ Qp Qh ♿    N

*IOM: 100-02, 15, 120*

○ **A7502** Replacement diaphragm/faceplate for tracheostoma valve, each ⑧ Qh ♿    N

*IOM: 100-02, 15, 120*

○ **A7503** Filter holder or filter cap, reusable, for use in a tracheostoma heat and moisture exchange system, each ⑧ Qh ♿    N

*IOM: 100-02, 15, 120*

○ **A7504** Filter for use in a tracheostoma heat and moisture exchange system, each ⑧ Qp Qh ♿    N

*IOM: 100-02, 15, 120*

○ **A7505** Housing, reusable without adhesive, for use in a heat and moisture exchange system and/or with a tracheostoma valve, each ⑧ Qh ♿    N

*IOM: 100-02, 15, 120*

○ **A7506** Adhesive disc for use in a heat and moisture exchange system and/or with tracheostoma valve, any type, each ⑧ Qh ♿    N

*IOM: 100-02, 15, 120*

○ **A7507** Filter holder and integrated filter without adhesive, for use in a tracheostoma heat and moisture exchange system, each ⑧ Qp Qh ♿    N

*IOM: 100-02, 15, 120*

○ **A7508** Housing and integrated adhesive, for use in a tracheostoma heat and moisture exchange system and/or with a tracheostoma valve, each ⑧ Qh ♿    N

*IOM: 100-02, 15, 120*

○ **A7509** Filter holder and integrated filter housing, and adhesive, for use as a tracheostoma heat and moisture exchange system, each ⑧ Qh ♿    N

*IOM: 100-02, 15, 120*

* **A7520** Tracheostomy/laryngectomy tube, non-cuffed, polyvinylchloride (PVC), silicone or equal, each ⑧ Qp Qh ♿    N

* **A7521** Tracheostomy/laryngectomy tube, cuffed, polyvinylchloride (PVC), silicone or equal, each ⑧ Qh ♿    N

* **A7522** Tracheostomy/laryngectomy tube, stainless steel or equal (sterilizable and reusable), each ⑧ Qh ♿    N

* **A7523** Tracheostomy shower protector, each ⑧    N

* **A7524** Tracheostoma stent/stud/button, each ⑧ Qp Qh ♿    N

* **A7525** Tracheostomy mask, each ⑧ Qh ♿    N

* **A7526** Tracheostomy tube collar/holder, each ⑧ Qh ♿    N

* **A7527** Tracheostomy/laryngectomy tube plug/stop, each ⑧ Qp Qh ♿    N

🖐 MIPS   Qp Quantity Physician   Qh Quantity Hospital   ♀ Female only   ♂ Male only   A Age   ♿ DMEPOS   A2-Z3 ASC Payment Indicator   A-Y ASC Status Indicator   Coding Clinic

**135**

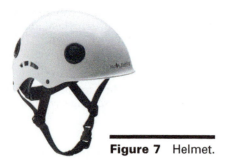

**Figure 7** Helmet.

## Helmets

* **A8000** Helmet, protective, soft, prefabricated, includes all components and accessories Ⓑ ♿    **Y**

* **A8001** Helmet, protective, hard, prefabricated, includes all components and accessories Ⓑ ♿    **Y**

* **A8002** Helmet, protective, soft, custom fabricated, includes all components and accessories Ⓑ ♿    **Y**

* **A8003** Helmet, protective, hard, custom fabricated, includes all components and accessories Ⓑ ♿    **Y**

* **A8004** Soft interface for helmet, replacement only Ⓑ ♿    **Y**

# ADMINISTRATIVE, MISCELLANEOUS, AND INVESTIGATIONAL (A9000-A9999)

**NOTE:** The following codes do not imply that codes in other sections are necessarily covered.

## Miscellaneous Supplies

⚙ **A9150** Non-prescription drugs Ⓑ    **B**
    *IOM: 100-02, 15, 50*

⊘ **A9152** Single vitamin/mineral/trace element, oral, per dose, not otherwise specified ⦿ Qp Qh    **E1**

⊘ **A9153** Multiple vitamins, with or without minerals and trace elements, oral, per dose, not otherwise specified ⦿ Qp Qh    **E1**

* **A9155** Artificial saliva, 30 ml ⦿ Qp Qh    **B**

⊘ **A9180** Pediculosis (lice infestation) treatment, topical, for administration by patient/caretaker Ⓑ Qp Qh    **E1**

⊘ **A9270** Non-covered item or service Ⓑ Qp Qh    **E1**
    *IOM: 100-02, 16, 20*

⊘ **A9272** Wound suction, disposable, includes dressing, all accessories and components, any type, each Ⓑ Qp Qh    **E1**
    *Medicare Statute 1861(n)*

⊘ **A9273** Cold or hot water bottle, ice cap or collar, heat and/or cold wrap, any type Ⓑ Qp Qh    **E1**

⊘ **A9274** External ambulatory insulin delivery system, disposable, each, includes all supplies and accessories Ⓑ Qp Qh    **E1**
    *Medicare Statute 1861(n)*

⊘ **A9275** Home glucose disposable monitor, includes test strips Ⓑ Qp Qh    **E1**

⊘ **A9276** Sensor; invasive (e.g., subcutaneous), disposable, for use with interstitial continuous glucose monitoring system, one unit = 1 day supply Ⓑ Qp Qh    **E1**
    *Medicare Statute 1861(n)*

⊘ **A9277** Transmitter; external, for use with interstitial continuous glucose monitoring system Ⓑ Qp Qh    **E1**
    *Medicare Statute 1861(n)*

⊘ **A9278** Receiver (monitor); external, for use with interstitial continuous glucose monitoring system Ⓑ Qp Qh    **E1**
    *Medicare Statute 1861(n)*

⊘ **A9279** Monitoring feature/device, stand-alone or integrated, any type, includes all accessories, components and electronics, not otherwise classified Ⓑ Qp Qh    **E1**
    *Medicare Statute 1861(n)*

⊘ **A9280** Alert or alarm device, not otherwise classified Ⓑ Qp Qh    **E1**
    *Medicare Statute 1861*

⊘ **A9281** Reaching/grabbing device, any type, any length, each Ⓑ Qp Qh    **E1**
    *Medicare Statute 1862 SSA*

⊘ **A9282** Wig, any type, each Ⓑ Qp Qh    **E1**
    *Medicare Statute 1862 SSA*

⊘ **A9283** Foot pressure off loading/supportive device, any type, each Ⓑ Qp Qh    **E1**
    *Medicare Statute 1862A(i)13*

⚙ **A9284** Spirometer, non-electronic, includes all accessories Ⓑ Qp Qh    **N**

* **A9285** Inversion/eversion correction device Ⓑ Qp Qh    **A**

⊘ **A9286** Hygienic item or device, disposable or non-disposable, any type, each Ⓑ Qp Qh    **E1**
    *Medicare Statute 1834*

---

▶ New    ↻ Revised    ✔ Reinstated    ~~deleted~~ Deleted    ⊘ Not covered or valid by Medicare

⚙ Special coverage instructions    * Carrier discretion    Ⓑ Bill Part B MAC    Ⓑ Bill DME MAC

⊘ **A9300** Exercise equipment Ⓑ Qp Qh E1

*IOM: 100-02, 15, 110.1; 100-03, 4, 280.1*

## Supplies for Radiology Procedures (Radiopharmaceuticals)

✳ **A9500** Technetium Tc-99m sestamibi, diagnostic, per study dose Ⓑ Qp Qh N1 N

Should be filed on same claim as procedure code reporting radiopharmaceutical. Verify with payer definition of a "study."

Coding Clinic: 2006, Q2, P5

✳ **A9501** Technetium Tc-99m teboroxime, diagnostic, per study dose Ⓑ Qp Qh N1 N

✳ **A9502** Technetium Tc-99m tetrofosmin, diagnostic, per study dose Ⓑ Qp Qh N1 N

Coding Clinic: 2006, Q2, P5

✳ **A9503** Technetium Tc-99m medronate, diagnostic, per study dose, up to 30 millicuries Ⓑ Qp Qh N1 N

✳ **A9504** Technetium Tc-99m apcitide, diagnostic, per study dose, up to 20 millicuries Ⓑ Qp Qh N1 N

✳ **A9505** Thallium Tl-201 thallous chloride, diagnostic, per millicurie Ⓑ Qp Qh N1 N

✳ **A9507** Indium In-111 capromab pendetide, diagnostic, per study dose, up to 10 millicuries Ⓑ Qp Qh N1 N

✳ **A9508** Iodine I-131 iobenguane sulfate, diagnostic, per 0.5 millicurie Ⓑ Qp Qh N1 N

✳ **A9509** Iodine I-123 sodium iodide, diagnostic, per millicurie Ⓑ Qp Qh N1 N

✳ **A9510** Technetium Tc-99m disofenin, diagnostic, per study dose, up to 15 millicuries Ⓑ Qp Qh N1 N

✳ **A9512** Technetium Tc-99m pertechnetate, diagnostic, per millicurie Ⓑ Qp Qh N1 N

✿ **A9513** Lutetium lu 177, dotatate, therapeutic, 1 millicurie G

✳ **A9515** Choline C-11, diagnostic, per study dose up to 20 millicuries Qp Qh K2 G

✳ **A9516** Iodine I-123 sodium iodide, diagnostic, per 100 microcuries, up to 999 microcuries Ⓑ Qp Qh N1 N

✳ **A9517** Iodine I-131 sodium iodide capsule(s), therapeutic, per millicurie Ⓑ Qp Qh K

✳ **A9520** Technetium Tc-99m tilmanocept, diagnostic, up to 0.5 millicuries Ⓑ Qp Qh N1 N

✳ **A9521** Technetium Tc-99m exametazime, diagnostic, per study dose, up to 25 millicuries Ⓑ Qp Qh N1 N

✳ **A9524** Iodine I-131 iodinated serum albumin, diagnostic, per 5 microcuries Ⓑ Qp Qh N1 N

✳ **A9526** Nitrogen N-13 ammonia, diagnostic, per study dose, up to 40 millicuries Ⓑ Qp Qh N1 N

✳ **A9527** Iodine I-125, sodium iodide solution, therapeutic, per millicurie Ⓑ Qp Qh H2 U

✳ **A9528** Iodine I-131 sodium iodide capsule(s), diagnostic, per millicurie Ⓑ Qp Qh N1 N

✳ **A9529** Iodine I-131 sodium iodide solution, diagnostic, per millicurie Ⓑ Qp Qh N1 N

✳ **A9530** Iodine I-131 sodium iodide solution, therapeutic, per millicurie Ⓑ Qp Qh K

✳ **A9531** Iodine I-131 sodium iodide, diagnostic, per microcurie (up to 100 microcuries) Ⓑ Qp Qh N1 N

✳ **A9532** Iodine I-125 serum albumin, diagnostic, per 5 microcuries Ⓑ Qp Qh N1 N

✳ **A9536** Technetium Tc-99m depreotide, diagnostic, per study dose, up to 35 millicuries Ⓑ Qp Qh N1 N

✳ **A9537** Technetium Tc-99m mebrofenin, diagnostic, per study dose, up to 15 millicuries Ⓑ Qp Qh N1 N

✳ **A9538** Technetium Tc-99m pyrophosphate, diagnostic, per study dose, up to 25 millicuries Ⓑ Qp Qh N1 N

✳ **A9539** Technetium Tc-99m pentetate, diagnostic, per study dose, up to 25 millicuries Ⓑ Qp Qh N1 N

✳ **A9540** Technetium Tc-99m macroaggregated albumin, diagnostic, per study dose, up to 10 millicuries Ⓑ Qp Qh N1 N

✳ **A9541** Technetium Tc-99m sulfur colloid, diagnostic, per study dose, up to 20 millicuries Ⓑ Qp Qh N1 N

✳ **A9542** Indium In-111 ibritumomab tiuxetan, diagnostic, per study dose, up to 5 millicuries Ⓑ Qp Qh N1 N

Specifically for diagnostic use.

✳ **A9543** Yttrium Y-90 ibritumomab tiuxetan, therapeutic, per treatment dose, up to 40 millicuries Ⓑ Qp Qh K

Specifically for therapeutic use.

---

🖐 MIPS    Qp Quantity Physician    Qh Quantity Hospital    ♀ Female only
♂ Male only    Ⓐ Age    ♿ DMEPOS    A2-Z3 ASC Payment Indicator    A-Y ASC Status Indicator    Coding Clinic

* **A9546** Cobalt Co-57/58, cyanocobalamin, diagnostic, per study dose, up to 1 microcurie Ⓑ Qp Qh    N1 N

* **A9547** Indium In-111 oxyquinoline, diagnostic, per 0.5 millicurie Ⓑ Qp Qh    N1 N

* **A9548** Indium In-111 pentetate, diagnostic, per 0.5 millicurie Ⓑ Qp Qh    N1 N

* **A9550** Technetium Tc-99m sodium glucceptate, diagnostic, per study dose, up to 25 millicuries Ⓑ Qp Qh    N1 N

* **A9551** Technetium Tc-99m succimer, diagnostic, per study dose, up to 10 millicuries Ⓑ Qp Qh    N1 N

* **A9552** Fluorodeoxyglucose F-18 FDG, diagnostic, per study dose, up to 45 millicuries Ⓑ Qp Qh    N1 N

    *Coding Clinic: 2008, Q3, P7*

* **A9553** Chromium Cr-51 sodium chromate, diagnostic, per study dose, up to 250 microcuries Ⓑ Qp Qh    N1 N

* **A9554** Iodine I-125 sodium Iothalamate, diagnostic, per study dose, up to 10 microcuries Ⓑ Qp Qh    N1 N

* **A9555** Rubidium Rb-82, diagnostic, per study dose, up to 60 millicuries Ⓑ Qp Qh    N1 N

* **A9556** Gallium Ga-67 citrate, diagnostic, per millicurie Ⓑ Qp Qh    N1 N

* **A9557** Technetium Tc-99m bicisate, diagnostic, per study dose, up to 25 millicuries Ⓑ Qp Qh    N1 N

* **A9558** Xenon Xe-133 gas, diagnostic, per 10 millicuries Ⓑ Qp Qh    N1 N

* **A9559** Cobalt Co-57 cyanocobalamin, oral, diagnostic, per study dose, up to 1 microcurie Ⓑ Qp Qh    N1 N

* **A9560** Technetium Tc-99m labeled red blood cells, diagnostic, per study dose, up to 30 millicuries Ⓑ Qp Qh    N1 N

    *Coding Clinic: 2008, Q3, P7*

* **A9561** Technetium Tc-99m oxidronate, diagnostic, per study dose, up to 30 millicuries Ⓑ Qp Qh    N1 N

* **A9562** Technetium Tc-99m mertiatide, diagnostic, per study dose, up to 15 millicuries Ⓑ Qp Qh    N1 N

* **A9563** Sodium phosphate P-32, therapeutic, per millicurie Ⓑ Qp Qh    K

* **A9564** Chromic phosphate P-32 suspension, therapeutic, per millicurie Ⓑ Qp Qh    E1

* **A9566** Technetium Tc-99m fanolesomab, diagnostic, per study dose, up to 25 millicuries Ⓑ Qp Qh    N1 N

* **A9567** Technetium Tc-99m pentetate, diagnostic, aerosol, per study dose, up to 75 millicuries Ⓑ Qp Qh    N1 N

* **A9568** Technetium TC-99m arcitumomab, diagnostic, per study dose, up to 45 millicuries Ⓑ Qp Qh    N1 N

* **A9569** Technetium Tc-99m exametazime labeled autologous white blood cells, diagnostic, per study dose Ⓑ Qp Qh    N1 N

* **A9570** Indium In-111 labeled autologous white blood cells, diagnostic, per study dose Ⓑ Qp Qh    N1 N

* **A9571** Indium In-111 labeled autologous platelets, diagnostic, per study dose Ⓑ Qp Qh    N1 N

* **A9572** Indium In-111 pentetreotide, diagnostic, per study dose, up to 6 millicuries Ⓑ Qp Qh    N1 N

* **A9575** Injection, gadoterate meglumine, 0.1 ml Ⓑ Qp Qh    N1 N

    *Other: Dotarem*

* **A9576** Injection, gadoteridol, (ProHance Multipack), per ml Ⓑ Qp Qh    N1 N

* **A9577** Injection, gadobenate dimeglumine (MultiHance), per ml Ⓑ Qp Qh    N1 N

* **A9578** Injection, gadobenate dimeglumine (MultiHance Multipack), per ml Ⓑ Qp Qh    N1 N

* **A9579** Injection, gadolinium-based magnetic resonance contrast agent, not otherwise specified (NOS), per ml Ⓑ Qp Qh    N1 N

    *Other: Magnevist, Omniscan, Optimark, Prohance*

* **A9580** Sodium fluoride F-18, diagnostic, per study dose, up to 30 millicuries Ⓑ Qp Qh    N1 N

* **A9581** Injection, gadoxetate disodium, 1 ml Ⓑ Qp Qh    N1 N

    Local Medicare contractors may require the use of modifier JW to identify unused product from single-dose vials that are appropriately discarded.

    *Other: Eovist*

* **A9582** Iodine I-123 iobenguane, diagnostic, per study dose, up to 15 millicuries Ⓑ Qp Qh    N1 N

    Molecular imaging agent that assists in the identification of rare neuroendocrine tumors.

---

▶ New    ↻ Revised    ✔ Reinstated    ~~deleted~~ Deleted    ⊘ Not covered or valid by Medicare
◉ Special coverage instructions    * Carrier discretion    Ⓑ Bill Part B MAC    Ⓓ Bill DME MAC

✳ **A9583** Injection, gadofosveset trisodium, 1 ml Ⓑ Qp Qh      **N1 N**

✳ **A9584** Iodine 1-123 ioflupane, diagnostic, per study dose, up to 5 millicuries Ⓑ Qp Qh    **N1 N**

    *Coding Clinic: 2012, Q1, P9*

✳ **A9585** Injection, gadobutrol, 0.1 ml Ⓑ Qp Qh      **N1 N**

    *Other: Gadavist*

    *Coding Clinic: 2012, Q1, P8*

✿ **A9586** Florbetapir F18, diagnostic, per study dose, up to 10 millicuries Ⓑ Qp Qh    **N1 N**

✳ **A9587** Gallium Ga-68, dotatate, diagnostic, 0.1 millicurie Qp Qh       **K2 G**

    *Coding Clinic: 2017, Q1, P9*

✳ **A9589** Instillation, hexaminolevulinate hydrochloride, 100 mg      **N1 N**

✳ **A9588** Fluciclovine F-18, diagnostic, 1 millicurie Qp Qh      **K2 G**

    *Coding Clinic: 2017, Q1, P9*

▶ ✳ **A9590** Iodine I-131, iobenguane, 1 millicurie           **N**

✳ **A9597** Positron emission tomography radiopharmaceutical, diagnostic, for tumor identification, not otherwise classified      **N1 N**

    *Coding Clinic: 2017, Q1, P8-9*

✳ **A9598** Positron emission tomography radiopharmaceutical, diagnostic, for non-tumor identification, not otherwise classified      **N1 N**

    *Coding Clinic: 2017, Q1, P8-9*

✳ **A9600** Strontium Sr-89 chloride, therapeutic, per millicurie Ⓑ Qp Qh      **K**

✳ **A9604** Samarium SM-153 lexidronam, therapeutic, per treatment dose, up to 150 millicuries Ⓑ Qp Qh    **K**

✳ **A9606** Radium Ra-223 dichloride, therapeutic, per microcurie Qp Qh      **K**

✿ **A9698** Non-radioactive contrast imaging material, not otherwise classified, per study Ⓑ      **N1 N**

    *IOM: 100-04, 12, 70; 100-04, 13, 20*

    *Coding Clinic: 2017, Q1, P8*

✳ **A9699** Radiopharmaceutical, therapeutic, not otherwise classified Ⓑ      **N**

✿ **A9700** Supply of injectable contrast material for use in echocardiography, per study Ⓑ Qp Qh    **N1 N**

    *IOM: 100-04, 12, 30.4*

    *Coding Clinic: 2017, Q1, P8*

## Miscellaneous Service Component

✳ **A9900** Miscellaneous DME supply, accessory, and/or service component of another HCPCS code Ⓑ Ⓑ      **Y**

    On DMEPOS fee schedule as a payable replacement for miscellaneous implanted or non-implanted items.

✳ **A9901** DME delivery, set up, and/or dispensing service component of another HCPCS code Ⓑ      **A**

✳ **A9999** Miscellaneous DME supply or accessory, not otherwise specified Ⓑ Ⓑ      **Y**

    On DMEPOS fee schedule as a payable replacement for miscellaneous implanted or non-implanted items.

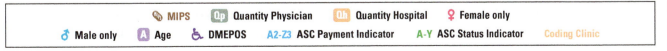

🄼 MIPS     Qp Quantity Physician     Qh Quantity Hospital     ♀ Female only
♂ Male only     A Age     ♿ DMEPOS     A2-Z3 ASC Payment Indicator     A-Y ASC Status Indicator     Coding Clinic

# ENTERAL AND PARENTERAL THERAPY
## (B4000-B9999)

## Enteral Feeding Supplies

⚙ **B4034** Enteral feeding supply kit; syringe fed, per day, includes but not limited to feeding/flushing syringe, administration set tubing, dressings, tape ⓑ Qh    Y

Dressings used with gastrostomy tubes for enteral nutrition (covered under the prosthetic device benefit) are included in the payment.

*IOM: 100-02, 15, 120; 100-03, 3, 180.2; 100-04, 20, 100.2.2*

PEN: On Fee Schedule

⚙ **B4035** Enteral feeding supply kit; pump fed, per day, includes but not limited to feeding/flushing syringe, administration set tubing, dressings, tape ⓑ Qh    Y

*IOM: 100-02, 15, 120; 100-03, 3, 180.2; 100-04, 20, 100.2.2*

PEN: On Fee Schedule

⚙ **B4036** Enteral feeding supply kit; gravity fed, per day, includes but not limited to feeding/flushing syringe, administration set tubing, dressings, tape ⓑ Qh    Y

*IOM: 100-02, 15, 120; 100-03, 3, 180.2; 100-04, 20, 100.2.2*

PEN: On Fee Schedule

⚙ **B4081** Nasogastric tubing with stylet ⓑ Qp Qh    Y

More than 3 nasogastric tubes (B4081-B4083), or 1 gastrostomy/jejunostomy tube (B4087-B4088) every three months is rarely medically necessary.

*IOM: 100-02, 15, 120; 100-03, 3, 180.2; 100-04, 20, 100.2.2*

PEN: On Fee Schedule

⚙ **B4082** Nasogastric tubing without stylet ⓑ Qp Qh    Y

*IOM: 100-02, 15, 120; 100-03, 3, 180.2; 100-04, 20, 100.2.2*

PEN: On Fee Schedule

⚙ **B4083** Stomach tube - Levine type ⓑ Qp Qh    Y

*IOM: 100-02, 15, 120; 100-03, 3, 180.2; 100-04, 20, 100.2.2*

PEN: On Fee Schedule

✱ **B4087** Gastrostomy/jejunostomy tube, standard, any material, any type, each ⓑ Qp Qh    A

PEN: On Fee Schedule

✱ **B4088** Gastrostomy/jejunostomy tube, low-profile, any material, any type, each ⓑ Qp Qh    A

PEN: On Fee Schedule

## Enteral Formulas and Additives

⊘ **B4100** Food thickener, administered orally, per ounce ⓑ    E1

⚙ **B4102** Enteral formula, for adults, used to replace fluids and electrolytes (e.g., clear liquids), 500 ml = 1 unit ⓑ A    Y

*IOM: 100-03, 3, 180.2*

⚙ **B4103** Enteral formula, for pediatrics, used to replace fluids and electrolytes (e.g., clear liquids), 500 ml = 1 unit ⓑ A    Y

*IOM: 100-03, 3, 180.2*

⚙ **B4104** Additive for enteral formula (e.g., fiber) ⓑ    E1

*IOM: 100-03, 3, 180.2*

⚙ **B4105** In-line cartridge containing digestive enzyme(s) for enteral feeding, each    Y

*Cross Reference Q9994*

⚙ **B4149** Enteral formula, manufactured blenderized natural foods with intact nutrients, includes proteins, fats, carbohydrates, vitamins and minerals, may include fiber, administered through an enteral feeding tube, 100 calories = 1 unit ⓑ Qp Qh    Y

Produced to meet unique nutrient needs for specific disease conditions; medical record must document specific condition and need for special nutrient.

*IOM: 100-02, 15, 120; 100-03, 3, 180.2; 100-04, 20, 100.2.2*

PEN: On Fee Schedule

⚙ **B4150** Enteral formulae, nutritionally complete with intact nutrients, includes proteins, fats, carbohydrates, vitamins, and minerals, may include fiber, administered through an enteral feeding tube, 100 calories = 1 unit ⓑ Qh    Y

*IOM: 100-02, 15, 120; 100-03, 3, 180.2; 100-04, 20, 100.2.2*

PEN: On Fee Schedule

| ▶ New | ↩ Revised | ✔ Reinstated | deleted Deleted | ⊘ Not covered or valid by Medicare |
|---|---|---|---|---|
| ⚙ Special coverage instructions | | ✱ Carrier discretion | ⓑ Bill Part B MAC | ⓑ Bill DME MAC |

⚙ **B4152** Enteral formula, nutritionally complete, calorically dense (equal to or greater than 1.5 kcal/ml) with intact nutrients, includes proteins, fats, carbohydrates, vitamins and minerals, may include fiber, administered through an enteral feeding tube, 100 calories = 1 unit Ⓑ Qh     Y

*IOM: 100-02, 15, 120; 100-03, 3, 180.2; 100-04, 20, 100.2.2*

PEN: On Fee Schedule

⚙ **B4153** Enteral formula, nutritionally complete, hydrolyzed proteins (amino acids and peptide chain), includes fats, carbohydrates, vitamins and minerals, may include fiber, administered through an enteral feeding tube, 100 calories = 1 unit Ⓑ Qp Qh     Y

If 2 enteral nutrition products described by same HCPCS code and provided at same time billed on single claim line with units of service reflecting total calories of both nutrients

*IOM: 100-02, 15, 120; 100-03, 3, 180.2; 100-04, 20, 100.2.2*

PEN: On Fee Schedule

⚙ **B4154** Enteral formula, nutritionally complete, for special metabolic needs, excludes inherited disease of metabolism, includes altered composition of proteins, fats, carbohydrates, vitamins and/or minerals, may include fiber, administered through an enteral feeding tube, 100 calories = 1 unit Ⓑ Qh     Y

*IOM: 100-02, 15, 120; 100-03, 3, 180.2; 100-04, 20, 100.2.2*

PEN: On Fee Schedule

⚙ **B4155** Enteral formula, nutritionally incomplete/modular nutrients, includes specific nutrients, carbohydrates (e.g., glucose polymers), proteins/amino acids (e.g., glutamine, arginine), fat (e.g., medium chain triglycerides) or combination, administered through an enteral feeding tube, 100 calories = 1 unit Ⓑ Qh     Y

*IOM: 100-02, 15, 120; 100-03, 3, 180.2; 100-04, 20, 100.2.2*

PEN: On Fee Schedule

⚙ **B4157** Enteral formula, nutritionally complete, for special metabolic needs for inherited disease of metabolism, includes proteins, fats, carbohydrates, vitamins and minerals, may include fiber, administered through an enteral feeding tube, 100 calories = 1 unit Ⓑ Qp Qh     Y

*IOM: 100-03, 3, 180.2*

⚙ **B4158** Enteral formula, for pediatrics, nutritionally complete with intact nutrients, includes proteins, fats, carbohydrates, vitamins and minerals, may include fiber and/or iron, administered through an enteral feeding tube, 100 calories = 1 unit Ⓑ Qh A     Y

*IOM: 100-03, 3, 180.2*

⚙ **B4159** Enteral formula, for pediatrics, nutritionally complete soy based with intact nutrients, includes proteins, fats, carbohydrates, vitamins and minerals, may include fiber and/or iron, administered through an enteral feeding tube, 100 calories = 1 unit Ⓑ Qh A     Y

*IOM: 100-03, 3, 180.2*

⚙ **B4160** Enteral formula, for pediatrics, nutritionally complete calorically dense (equal to or greater than 0.7 kcal/ml) with intact nutrients, includes proteins, fats, carbohydrates, vitamins and minerals, may include fiber, administered through an enteral feeding tube, 100 calories = 1 unit Ⓑ Qp Qh A     Y

*IOM: 100-03, 3, 180.2*

⚙ **B4161** Enteral formula, for pediatrics, hydrolyzed/amino acids and peptide chain proteins, includes fats, carbohydrates, vitamins and minerals, may include fiber, administered through an enteral feeding tube, 100 calories = 1 unit Ⓑ Qh A     Y

*IOM: 100-03, 3, 180.2*

⚙ **B4162** Enteral formula, for pediatrics, special metabolic needs for inherited disease of metabolism, includes proteins, fats, carbohydrates, vitamins and minerals, may include fiber, administered through an enteral feeding tube, 100 calories = 1 unit Ⓑ Qh A     Y

*IOM: 100-03, 3, 180.2*

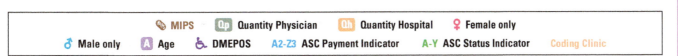

🔗 MIPS    Qp Quantity Physician    Qh Quantity Hospital    ♀ Female only    ♂ Male only    A Age    ♿ DMEPOS    A2-Z3 ASC Payment Indicator    A-Y ASC Status Indicator    Coding Clinic

ENTERAL AND PARENTERAL THERAPY    B4152 — B4162

141

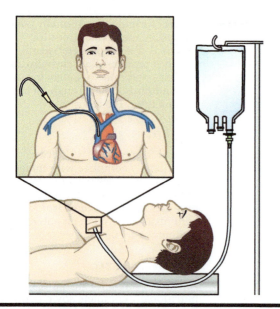

**Figure 8** Total Parenteral Nutrition (TPN) involves percutaneous placement of central venous catheter into vena cava or right atrium.

## Parenteral Nutritional Solutions and Supplies

**B4164** Parenteral nutrition solution: carbohydrates (dextrose), 50% or less (500 ml = 1 unit) - home mix Ⓑ Qp Qh  Y

*IOM: 100-02, 15, 120; 100-03, 3, 180.2; 100-04, 20, 100.2.2*

PEN: On Fee Schedule

**B4168** Parenteral nutrition solution; amino acid, 3.5%, (500 ml = 1 unit) - home mix Ⓑ Qp Qh  Y

*IOM: 100-02, 15, 120; 100-03, 3, 180.2; 100-04, 20, 100.2.2*

PEN: On Fee Schedule

**B4172** Parenteral nutrition solution; amino acid, 5.5% through 7%, (500 ml = 1 unit) - home mix Ⓑ Qp Qh  Y

*IOM: 100-02, 15, 120; 100-03, 3, 180.2; 100-04, 20, 100.2.2*

**B4176** Parenteral nutrition solution; amino acid, 7% through 8.5%, (500 ml = 1 unit) - home mix Ⓑ Qp Qh  Y

*IOM: 100-02, 15, 120; 100-03, 3, 180.2; 100-04, 20, 100.2.2*

PEN: On Fee Schedule

**B4178** Parenteral nutrition solution: amino acid, greater than 8.5% (500 ml = 1 unit) - home mix Ⓑ Qp Qh  Y

*IOM: 100-02, 15, 120; 100-03, 3, 180.2; 100-04, 20, 100.2.2*

PEN: On Fee Schedule

**B4180** Parenteral nutrition solution; carbohydrates (dextrose), greater than 50% (500 ml = 1 unit) - home mix Ⓑ Qp Qh  Y

*IOM: 100-02, 15, 120; 100-03, 3, 180.2; 100-04, 20, 100.2.2*

PEN: On Fee Schedule

**B4185** Parenteral nutrition solution, not otherwise specified, 10 grams lipids Ⓑ  B

PEN: On Fee Schedule

**B4187** Omegaven, 10 grams lipids  Y

**B4189** Parenteral nutrition solution; compounded amino acid and carbohydrates with electrolytes, trace elements, and vitamins, including preparation, any strength, 10 to 51 grams of protein - premix Ⓑ Qp Qh  Y

*IOM: 100-02, 15, 120; 100-03, 3, 180.2; 100-04, 20, 100.2.2*

PEN: On Fee Schedule

**B4193** Parenteral nutrition solution; compounded amino acid and carbohydrates with electrolytes, trace elements, and vitamins, including preparation, any strength, 52 to 73 grams of protein - premix Ⓑ Qh  Y

*IOM: 100-02, 15, 120; 100-03, 3, 180.2; 100-04, 20, 100.2.2*

PEN: On Fee Schedule

**B4197** Parenteral nutrition solution; compounded amino acid and carbohydrates with electrolytes, trace elements and vitamins, including preparation, any strength, 74 to 100 grams of protein - premix Ⓑ Qh  Y

*IOM: 100-02, 15, 120; 100-03, 3, 180.2; 100-04, 20, 100.2.2*

PEN: On Fee Schedule

**B4199** Parenteral nutrition solution; compounded amino acid and carbohydrates with electrolytes, trace elements and vitamins, including preparation, any strength, over 100 grams of protein - premix Ⓑ Qp Qh  Y

*IOM: 100-02, 15, 120; 100-03, 3, 180.2; 100-04, 20, 100.2.2*

PEN: On Fee Schedule

▶ New  ↻ Revised  ✔ Reinstated  ~~deleted~~ Deleted  ⊘ Not covered or valid by Medicare

✪ Special coverage instructions  ✳ Carrier discretion  Ⓑ Bill Part B MAC  Ⓑ Bill DME MAC

✿ **B4216** Parenteral nutrition; additives (vitamins, trace elements, heparin, electrolytes) home mix per day Ⓑ Qh                                  Y

*IOM: 100-02, 15, 120; 100-03, 3, 180.2; 100-04, 20, 100.2.2*

PEN: On Fee Schedule

✿ **B4220** Parenteral nutrition supply kit; premix, per day Ⓑ Qh                    Y

*IOM: 100-02, 15, 120; 100-03, 3, 180.2; 100-04, 20, 100.2.2*

PEN: On Fee Schedule

✿ **B4222** Parenteral nutrition supply kit; home mix, per day Ⓑ Qh                  Y

*IOM: 100-02, 15, 120; 100-03, 3, 180.2; 100-04, 20, 100.2.2*

PEN: On Fee Schedule

✿ **B4224** Parenteral nutrition administration kit, per day Ⓑ Qh                    Y

Dressings used with parenteral nutrition (covered under the prosthetic device benefit) are included in the payment. (www.cms.gov/medicare-coverage-database/)

*IOM: 100-02, 15, 120; 100-03, 3, 180.2; 100-04, 20, 100.2.2*

PEN: On Fee Schedule

✿ **B5000** Parenteral nutrition solution compounded amino acid and carbohydrates with electrolytes, trace elements, and vitamins, including preparation, any strength, renal - Aminosyn-RF, NephrAmine, RenAmine - premix Ⓑ Qp Qh          Y

*IOM: 100-02, 15, 120; 100-03, 3, 180.2; 100-04, 20, 100.2.2*

PEN: On Fee Schedule

✿ **B5100** Parenteral nutrition solution compounded amino acid and carbohydrates with electrolytes, trace elements, and vitamins, including preparation, any strength, hepatic, HepatAmine - premix Ⓑ Qp Qh          Y

*IOM: 100-02, 15, 120; 100-03, 3, 180.2; 100-04, 20, 100.2.2*

PEN: On Fee Schedule

✿ **B5200** Parenteral nutrition solution compounded amino acid and carbohydrates with electrolytes, trace elements, and vitamins, including preparation, any strength, stress-branch chain amino acids-FreAmine-HBC - premix Ⓑ Qp Qh          Y

*IOM: 100-02, 15, 120; 100-03, 3, 180.2; 100-04, 20, 100.2.2*

## Enteral and Parenteral Pumps

✿ **B9002** Enteral nutrition infusion pump, any type Ⓑ Qh                            Y

*IOM: 100-02, 15, 120; 100-03, 3, 180.2; 100-04, 20, 100.2.2*

PEN: On Fee Schedule

✿ **B9004** Parenteral nutrition infusion pump, portable Ⓑ Qh                        Y

*IOM: 100-02, 15, 120; 100-03, 3, 180.2; 100-04, 20, 100.2.2*

PEN: On Fee Schedule

✿ **B9006** Parenteral nutrition infusion pump, stationary Ⓑ Qh                      Y

*IOM: 100-02, 15, 120; 100-03, 3, 180.2; 100-04, 20, 100.2.2*

PEN: On Fee Schedule

✿ **B9998** NOC for enteral supplies Ⓑ              Y

*IOM: 100-02, 15, 120; 100-03, 3, 180.2; 100-04, 20, 100.2.2*

✿ **B9999** NOC for parenteral supplies Ⓑ          Y

Determine if an alternative HCPCS Level II or a CPT code better describes the service being reported. This code should be reported only if a more specific code is unavailable.

*IOM: 100-02, 15, 120; 100-03, 3, 180.2; 100-04, 20, 100.2.2*

---

🔊 MIPS   Qp Quantity Physician   Qh Quantity Hospital   ♀ Female only

♂ Male only   Ⓐ Age   ♿ DMEPOS   A2-Z3 ASC Payment Indicator   A-Y ASC Status Indicator   Coding Clinic

# CMS HOSPITAL OUTPATIENT PAYMENT SYSTEM (C1000-C9999)

**NOTE:** C-codes are used on Medicare Ambulatory Surgical Center (ASC) and Hospital Outpatient Prospective Payment System (OPPS) claims, but may also be recognized on claims from other providers or by other payment systems. As of 10/01/2006, the following non-OPPS providers have been able to bill Medicare using the C-codes, or an appropriate CPT code on Types of Bill (TOBs) 12X, 13X, or 85X:

- Critical Access Hospitals (CAHs);
- Indian Health Service Hospitals (IHS);
- Hospitals located in American Samoa, Guam, Saipan or the Virgin Islands; and
- Maryland waiver hospitals.

The billing of C-codes by Method I and Method II Critical Access Hospitals (CAHs) is limited to the billing for facility (technical) services. The C-codes shall not be billed by Method II CAHs for professional services with revenue codes (RCs) 96X, 97X, or 98X.

C codes are updated quarterly by the Centers for Medicare and Medicaid Services (CMS).

## Devices and Supplies

✪ **C1713** Anchor/Screw for opposing bone-to-bone or soft tissue-to-bone (implantable) **Qh**   N1  N

*Medicare Statute 1833(t)*

Coding Clinic: 2018, Q2, P5; Q1, P4; 2016, Q3, P16; 2015, Q3, P2; 2010, Q2, P3

✪ **C1714** Catheter, transluminal atherectomy, directional **Qh**   N1  N

*Medicare Statute 1833(t)*

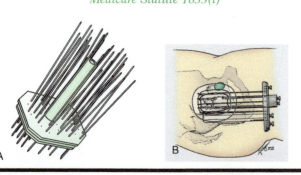

**Figure 9** (A) Brachytherapy device, (B) Brachytherapy device inserted.

✪ **C1715** Brachytherapy needle **Qh**   N1  N

*Medicare Statute 1833(t)*

## Brachytherapy Sources

✪ **C1716** Brachytherapy source, non-stranded, gold-198, per source **Qp** **Qh**   H2  U

*Medicare Statute 1833(t)*

✪ **C1717** Brachytherapy source, non-stranded, high dose rate iridium 192, per source **Qp** **Qh**   H2  U

*Medicare Statute 1833(t)*

✪ **C1719** Brachytherapy source, non-stranded, non-high dose rate iridium-192, per source **Qp** **Qh**   H2  U

*Medicare Statute 1833(t)*

## Cardioverter-Defibrilators

✪ **C1721** Cardioverter-defibrillator, dual chamber (implantable) **Qp** **Qh**   N1  N

Related CPT codes: 33224, 33240, 33249.

*Medicare Statute 1833(t)*

✪ **C1722** Cardioverter-defibrillator, single chamber (implantable) **Qp** **Qh**   N1  N

Related CPT codes: 33240, 33249.

*Medicare Statute 1833(t)*

Coding Clinic: 2017, Q2, P5; 2006, Q2, P9

## Catheters

✪ **C1724** Catheter, transluminal atherectomy, rotational **Qh**   N1  N

*Medicare Statute 1833(t)*

Coding Clinic: 2016, Q3, P9

✪ **C1725** Catheter, transluminal angioplasty, non-laser (may include guidance, infusion/perfusion capability) **Qh**   N1  N

*Medicare Statute 1833(t)*

Coding Clinic: 2016, Q3, P16, P19

✪ **C1726** Catheter, balloon dilatation, non-vascular **Qh**   N1  N

*Medicare Statute 1833(t)*

Coding Clinic: 2016, Q3, P16, P19

✪ **C1727** Catheter, balloon tissue dissector, non-vascular (insertable) **Qh**   N1  N

*Medicare Statute 1833(t)*

Coding Clinic: 2016, Q3, P16

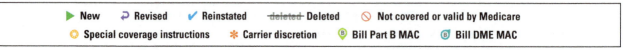

▶ New   ↻ Revised   ✔ Reinstated   ~~deleted~~ Deleted   ⊘ Not covered or valid by Medicare   ✪ Special coverage instructions   ✱ Carrier discretion   Ⓑ Bill Part B MAC   Ⓑ Bill DME MAC

⚙ **C1728** Catheter, brachytherapy seed administration [Qh]  N1 N
*Medicare Statute 1833(t)*

⚙ **C1729** Catheter, drainage [Qh]  N1 N
*Medicare Statute 1833(t)*
Coding Clinic: 2016, Q3, P17

⚙ **C1730** Catheter, electrophysiology, diagnostic, other than 3D mapping (19 or fewer electrodes) [Qp] [Qh]  N1 N
*Medicare Statute 1833(t)*
Coding Clinic: 2016, Q3, P17

⚙ **C1731** Catheter, electrophysiology, diagnostic, other than 3D mapping (20 or more electrodes) [Qp] [Qh]  N1 N
*Medicare Statute 1833(t)*
Coding Clinic: 2016, Q3, P17

⚙ **C1732** Catheter, electrophysiology, diagnostic/ablation, 3D or vector mapping [Qp] [Qh]  N1 N
*Medicare Statute 1833(t)*
Coding Clinic: 2016, Q3, P15, P17, P19

⚙ **C1733** Catheter, electrophysiology, diagnostic/ablation, other than 3D or vector mapping, other than cool-tip [Qp] [Qh]  N1 N
*Medicare Statute 1833(t)*
Coding Clinic: 2016, Q3, P17

▶⚙ **C1734** Orthopedic/device/drug matrix for opposing bone-to-bone or soft tissue-to-bone (implantable)  N1

⚙ **C1749** Endoscope, retrograde imaging/illumination colonoscope device (implantable) [Qp] [Qh]  N1 N

⚙ **C1750** Catheter, hemodialysis/peritoneal, long-term [Qh]  N1 N
*Medicare Statute 1833(t)*
Coding Clinic: 2015, Q4, P6

⚙ **C1751** Catheter, infusion, inserted peripherally, centrally, or midline (other than hemodialysis) [Qh]  N1 N
*Medicare Statute 1833(t)*

⚙ **C1752** Catheter, hemodialysis/peritoneal, short-term [Qh]  N1 N
*Medicare Statute 1833(t)*

⚙ **C1753** Catheter, intravascular ultrasound [Qh]  N1 N
*Medicare Statute 1833(t)*

⚙ **C1754** Catheter, intradiscal [Qh]  N1 N
*Medicare Statute 1833(t)*

⚙ **C1755** Catheter, instraspinal [Qh]  N1 N
*Medicare Statute 1833(t)*

⚙ **C1756** Catheter, pacing, transesophageal [Qh]  N1 N
*Medicare Statute 1833(t)*

⚙ **C1757** Catheter, thrombectomy/embolectomy [Qh]  N1 N
*Medicare Statute 1833(t)*

⚙ **C1758** Catheter, ureteral [Qh]  N1 N
*Medicare Statute 1833(t)*

⚙ **C1759** Catheter, intracardiac echocardiography [Qh]  N1 N
*Medicare Statute 1833(t)*

## Devices

⚙ **C1760** Closure device, vascular (implantable/insertable) [Qh]  N1 N
*Medicare Statute 1833(t)*
Coding Clinic: 2016, Q3, P19

⚙ **C1762** Connective tissue, human (includes fascia lata) [Qh]  N1 N
*Medicare Statute 1833(t)*
Coding Clinic: 2016, Q3, P9, P16, P19; 2015, Q3, P2; 2003, Q3, P12

⚙ **C1763** Connective tissue, non-human (includes synthetic) [Qh]  N1 N
*Medicare Statute 1833(t)*
Coding Clinic: 2016, Q3, P9, P17, P19; 2010, Q4, P3; Q2, P3; 2003, Q3, P12

⚙ **C1764** Event recorder, cardiac (implantable) [Qp] [Qh]  N1 N
*Medicare Statute 1833(t)*
Coding Clinic: 2015, Q2, P8

⚙ **C1765** Adhesion barrier [Qh]  N1 N
*Medicare Statute 1833(t)*
Coding Clinic: 2016, Q3, P16

⚙ **C1766** Introducer/sheath, guiding, intracardiac electrophysiological, steerable, other than peel-away [Qh]  N1 N
*Medicare Statute 1833(t)*

⚙ **C1767** Generator, neurostimulator (implantable), nonrechargeable [Qp] [Qh]  N1 N
Related CPT codes: 61885, 61886, 63685, 64590.
*Medicare Statute 1833(t)*
Coding Clinic: 2007, Q1, P8

⚙ **C1768** Graft, vascular [Qh]  N1 N
*Medicare Statute 1833(t)*

---

🖐 MIPS  [Qp] Quantity Physician  [Qh] Quantity Hospital  ♀ Female only
♂ Male only  [A] Age  ♿ DMEPOS  A2-Z3 ASC Payment Indicator  A-Y ASC Status Indicator  Coding Clinic

✿ **C1769**　Guide wire  Qh　　　　N1 N

*Medicare Statute 1833(t)*

Coding Clinic: 2019, Q3, P10; 2016, Q3, P3; 2007, Q2, P7-8

✿ **C1770**　Imaging coil, magnetic reasonance (insertable)  Qh　　　N1 N

*Medicare Statute 1833(t)*

✿ **C1771**　Repair device, urinary, incontinence, with sling graft  Qp  Qh　　N1 N

*Medicare Statute 1833(t)*

Coding Clinic: 2016, Q3, P19; 2008, Q3, P7

✿ **C1772**　Infusion pump, programmable (implantable)  Qp  Qh　　N1 N

*Medicare Statute 1833(t)*

✿ **C1773**　Retrieval device, insertable (used to retrieve fractured medical devices)  Qh　　　　N1 N

*Medicare Statute 1833(t)*

Coding Clinic: 2016, Q3, P19

✿ **C1776**　Joint device (implantable)  Qp  Qh  N1 N

*Medicare Statute 1833(t)*

Coding Clinic: 2018, Q3, P6; 2016, Q3, P3, P18; 2010, Q3, P6; 2008, Q4, P10

✿ **C1777**　Lead, cardioverter-defibrillator, endocardial single coil (implantable)  Qh　　　　N1 N

Related CPT codes: 33216, 33217, 33249.

*Medicare Statute 1833(t)*

Coding Clinic: 2017, Q2, P5; 2006, Q2, P9

✿ **C1778**　Lead, neurostimulator (implantable)  Qp  Qh　　N1 N

Related CPT codes: 43647, 63650, 63655, 63663, 63664, 64553, 64555, 64560, 64561, 64565, 64573, 64575, 64577, 64580, 64581.

*Medicare Statute 1833(t)*

Coding Clinic: 2019, Q1, P5; 2007, Q1, P8

✿ **C1779**　Lead, pacemaker, trasvenous VDD single pass  Qh　　　N1 N

Related CPT codes: 33206, 33207, 33208, 33210, 33211, 33214, 33216, 33217, 33249.

*Medicare Statute 1833(t)*

Coding Clinic: 2016, Q3, P19

✿ **C1780**　Lens, intraocular (new technology)  Qh　　　N1 N

*Medicare Statute 1833(t)*

Coding Clinic: 2016, Q3, P18

✿ **C1781**　Mesh (implantable)  Qh　　N1 N

*Medicare Statute 1833(t)*

Coding Clinic: 2019, Q1, P5; 2016, Q3, P18-19; 2012, Q2, P3; 2010, Q2, P2-3

✿ **C1782**　Morcellator  Qp  Qh　　N1 N

*Medicare Statute 1833(t)*

Coding Clinic: 2016, Q3, P18

✿ **C1783**　Ocular implant, aqueous drainage assist device  Qh　　　N1 N

*Medicare Statute 1833(t)*

Coding Clinic: 2017, Q1, P5

✿ **C1784**　Ocular device, intraoperative, detached retina  Qh　　　N1 N

*Medicare Statute 1833(t)*

Coding Clinic: 2016, Q3, P18

✿ **C1785**　Pacemaker, dual chamber, rate-responsive (implantable)  Qp  Qh  N1 N

Related CPT codes: 33206, 33207, 33208, 33213, 33214, 33224.

*Medicare Statute 1833(t)*

✿ **C1786**　Pacemaker, single chamber, rate-responsive (implantable)  Qp  Qh  N1 N

Related CPT codes: 33206, 33207, 33212.

*Medicare Statute 1833(t)*

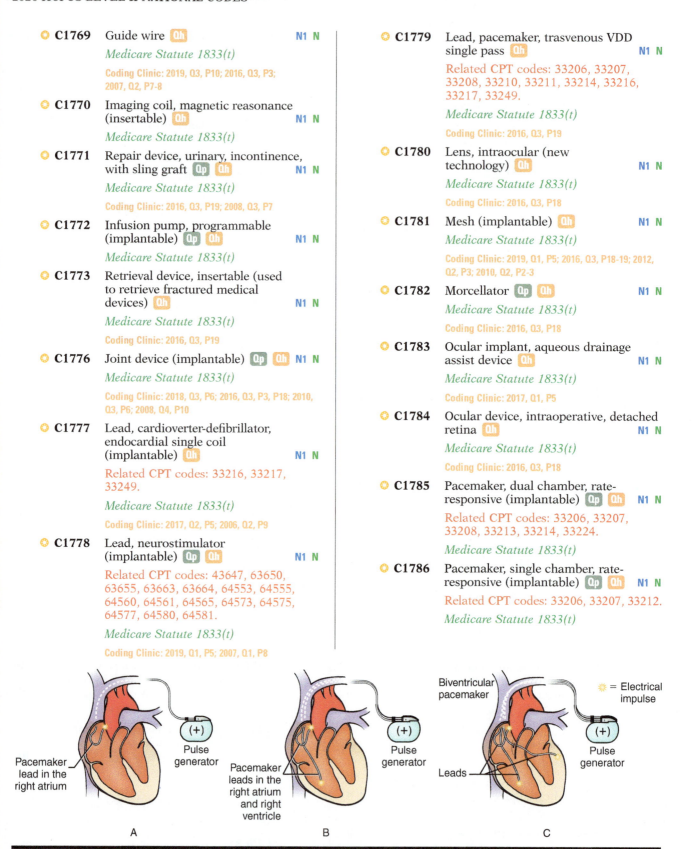

**Figure 10**　(A) Single pacemaker, (B) Dual pacemaker, (C) Biventricular pacemaker.

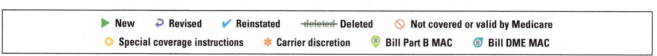

▶ New　↻ Revised　✓ Reinstated　~~deleted~~ Deleted　⊘ Not covered or valid by Medicare
✿ Special coverage instructions　✱ Carrier discretion　Ⓑ Bill Part B MAC　Ⓓ Bill DME MAC

✿ **C1787** Patient programmer, neurostimulator `Qh`  N1 N

*Medicare Statute 1833(t)*

Coding Clinic: 2016, Q3, P19

✿ **C1788** Port, indwelling (implantable) `Qh` N1 N

*Medicare Statute 1833(t)*

✿ **C1789** Prosthesis, breast (implantable) `Qh`  N1 N

*Medicare Statute 1833(t)*

✿ **C1813** Prosthesis, penile, inflatable `Qp` `Qh` ♂  N1 N

*Medicare Statute 1833(t)*

✿ **C1814** Retinal tamponade device, silicone oil `Qh`  N1 N

*Medicare Statute 1833(t)*

Coding Clinic: 2016, Q3, P19; 2006, Q2, P9

✿ **C1815** Prosthesis, urinary sphincter (implantable) `Qp` `Qh`  N1 N

*Medicare Statute 1833(t)*

✿ **C1816** Receiver and/or transmitter, neurostimulator (implantable) `Qh` N1 N

*Medicare Statute 1833(t)*

✿ **C1817** Septal defect implant system, intracardiac `Qp` `Qh`  N1 N

*Medicare Statute 1833(t)*

Coding Clinic: 2016, Q3, P19

✿ **C1818** Integrated keratoprosthesic `Qh`  N1 N

*Medicare Statute 1833(t)*

Coding Clinic: 2016, Q3, P18

✿ **C1819** Surgical tissue localization and excision device (implantable) `Qh`  N1 N

*Medicare Statute 1833(t)*

✿ **C1820** Generator, neurostimulator (implantable), with rechargeable battery and charging system `Qp` `Qh`  N1 N

Related CPT codes: 61885, 61886, 63685, 64590.

*Medicare Statute 1833(t)*

Coding Clinic: 2016, Q2, P7

✿ **C1821** Interspinous process distraction device (implantable) `Qh`  N1 N

*Medicare Statute 1833(t)*

✿ **C1822** Generator, neurostimulator (implantable), high frequency, with rechargeable battery and charging system `Qp` `Qh`  N1 N

*Medicare Statute 1833(T)*

Coding Clinic: 2016, Q2, P7

✿ **C1823** Generator, neurostimulator (implantable), non-rechargeable, with transvenous sensing and stimulation leads  H

*Medicare Statute 1833(t)*

▶ ✿ **C1824** Generator, cardiac contractility modulation (implantable)  N1

✿ **C1830** Powered bone marrow biopsy needle `Qp` `Qh`  N1 N

*Medicare Statute 1833(t)*

▶ ✿ **C1839** Iris prosthesis  N1

✿ **C1840** Lens, intraocular (telescopic) `Qp` `Qh`  N1 N

*Medicare Statute 1833(t)*

Coding Clinic: 2012, Q3, P10

✿ **C1841** Retinal prosthesis, includes all internal and external components `Qp` `Qh`  J7 N

*Medicare Statute 1833(t)*

✿ **C1842** Retinal prosthesis, includes all internal and external components; add-on to C1841 `Qp` `Qh`  J7 E1

*Medicare Statute 1833(t)*

Coding Clinic: 2017, Q1, P6

✿ **C1874** Stent, coated/covered, with delivery system `Qh`  N1 N

*Medicare Statute 1833(t)*

Coding Clinic: 2016, Q3, P16-17, P19

✿ **C1875** Stent, coated/covered, without delivery system `Qh`  N1 N

*Medicare Statute 1833(t)*

Coding Clinic: 2016, Q3, P16-17

✿ **C1876** Stent, non-coated/non-covered, with delivery system `Qh`  N1 N

*Medicare Statute 1833(t)*

Coding Clinic: 2016, Q3, P19

✿ **C1877** Stent, non-coated/non-covered, without delivery system `Qh`  N1 N

*Medicare Statute 1833(t)*

✿ **C1878** Material for vocal cord medialization, synthetic (implantable) `Qh`  N1 N

*Medicare Statute 1833(t)*

Coding Clinic: 2016, Q3, P18

✿ **C1880** Vena cava filter `Qh`  N1 N

*Medicare Statute 1833(t)*

✿ **C1881** Dialysis access system (implantable) `Qh`  N1 N

*Medicare Statute 1833(t)*

🖐 MIPS   `Qp` Quantity Physician   `Qh` Quantity Hospital   ♀ Female only   ♂ Male only   A Age   ♿ DMEPOS   A2-Z3 ASC Payment Indicator   A-Y ASC Status Indicator   Coding Clinic

○ **C1882** Cardioverter-defibrillator, other than single or dual chamber (implantable) `Qp` `Qh`  N1 N

Related CPT codes: 33224, 33240, 33249.

*Medicare Statute 1833(t)*

Coding Clinic: 2016, Q3, P16; 2012, Q2, P9; 2006, Q2, P9

○ **C1883** Adapter/Extension, pacing lead or neurostimulator lead (implantable) `Qh`  N1 N

*Medicare Statute 1833(t)*

Coding Clinic: 2016, Q3, P15, P17; 2007, Q1, P8

○ **C1884** Embolization protective system `Qh`  N1 N

*Medicare Statute 1833(t)*

Coding Clinic: 2016, Q3, P17

○ **C1885** Catheter, transluminal angioplasty, laser `Qh`  N1 N

*Medicare Statute 1833(t)*

Coding Clinic: 2016, Q3, p16, Q1, P5

○ **C1886** Catheter, extravascular tissue ablation, any modality (insertable) `Qp` `Qh` N1 N

*Medicare Statute 1833(t)*

○ **C1887** Catheter, guiding (may include infusion/perfusion capability) `Qh` N1 N

*Medicare Statute 1833(t)*

Coding Clinic: 2016, Q3, P17

○ **C1888** Catheter, ablation, non-cardiac, endovascular (implantable) `Qh` N1 N

*Medicare Statute 1833(t)*

Coding Clinic: 2016, Q3, P16

○ **C1889** Implantable/insertable device, not otherwise classified  N1 N

*Medicare Statute 1833(T)*

○ **C1891** Infusion pump, non-programmable, permanent (implantable) `Qp` `Qh` N1 N

*Medicare Statute 1833(t)*

○ **C1892** Introducer/sheath, guiding, intracardiac electrophysiological, fixed-curve, peel-away `Qh`  N1 N

*Medicare Statute 1833(t)*

Coding Clinic: 2016, Q3, P19

○ **C1893** Introducer/sheath, guiding, intracardiac electrophysiological, fixed-curve, other than peel-away `Qh`  N1 N

*Medicare Statute 1833(t)*

○ **C1894** Introducer/sheath, other than guiding, other than intracardiac electrophysiological, non-laser `Qh`  N1 N

*Medicare Statute 1833(t)*

○ **C1895** Lead, cardioverter-defibrillator, endocardial dual coil (implantable) `Qh`  N1 N

Related CPT codes: 33216, 33217, 33249.

*Medicare Statute 1833(t)*

Coding Clinic: 2006, Q2, P9

○ **C1896** Lead, cardioverter-defibrillator, other than endocardial single or dual coil (implantable) `Qh`  N1 N

Related CPT codes: 33216, 33217, 33249.

*Medicare Statute 1833(t)*

○ **C1897** Lead, neurostimulator test kit (implantable) `Qh`  N1 N

Related CPT codes: 43647, 63650, 63655, 63663, 63664, 64553, 64555, 64560, 64561, 64565, 64575, 64577, 64580, 64581.

*Medicare Statute 1833(t)*

Coding Clinic: 2007, Q1, P8

○ **C1898** Lead, pacemaker, other than transvenous VDD single pass `Qh`  N1 N

Related CPT codes: 33206, 33207, 33208, 33210, 33211, 33214, 33216, 33217, 33249.

*Medicare Statute 1833(t)*

Coding Clinic: 2002, Q3, P8

○ **C1899** Lead, pacemaker/cardioverter-defibrillator combination (implantable) `Qh` N1 N

Related CPT codes: 33216, 33217, 33249.

*Medicare Statute 1833(t)*

○ **C1900** Lead, left ventricular coronary venous system `Qp` `Qh` N1 N

Related CPT codes: 33224, 33225.

*Medicare Statute 1833(t)*

Coding Clinic: 2016, Q3, P18

▶ ○ **C1982** Catheter, pressure-generating, one-way valve, intermittently occlusive  N1

▶ ○ **C2596** Probe, image-guided, robotic, waterjet ablation  N1 H

○ **C2613** Lung biopsy plug with delivery system `Qp` `Qh`  N1 H

*Medicare Statute 1833(t)*

Coding Clinic: 2015, Q2, P11

○ **C2614** Probe, percutaneous lumbar discectomy `Qh`  N1 N

*Medicare Statute 1833(t)*

○ **C2615** Sealant, pulmonary, liquid `Qh`  N1 N

*Medicare Statute 1833(t)*

Coding Clinic: 2016, Q3, P18

---

▶ New　↻ Revised　✔ Reinstated　deleted Deleted　⊘ Not covered or valid by Medicare
○ Special coverage instructions　✳ Carrier discretion　Ⓑ Bill Part B MAC　Ⓓ Bill DME MAC

## Brachytherapy Source

⚙ **C2616**  Brachytherapy source, non-stranded, yttrium-90, per source `Qp` `Qh`  H2 U

*Medicare Statute 1833(t)*

## Cardiovascular and Genitourinary Devices

⚙ **C2617**  Stent, non-coronary, temporary, without delivery system `Qh`  N1 N

*Medicare Statute 1833(t)*

Coding Clinic: 2018, Q1, P4; 2016, Q3, P3, P19

⚙ **C2618**  Probe/needle, cryoablation `Qh`  N1 N

*Medicare Statute 1833(t)*

⚙ **C2619**  Pacemaker, dual chamber, non rate-responsive (implantable) `Qp` `Qh`  N1 N

Related CPT codes: 33206, 33207, 33208, 33213, 33214, 33224.

*Medicare Statute 1833(t)*

⚙ **C2620**  Pacemaker, single chamber, non rate-responsive (implantable) `Qp` `Qh`  N1 N

Related CPT codes: 33206, 33207, 33212, 33224.

*Medicare Statute 1833(t)*

⚙ **C2621**  Pacemaker, other than single or dual chamber (implantable) `Qp` `Qh`  N1 N

Related CPT codes: 33206, 33207, 33208, 33212, 33213, 33214, 33224.

*Medicare Statute 1833(t)*

Coding Clinic: 2016, Q3, P18; 2002, Q3, P8

⚙ **C2622**  Prosthesis, penile, non-inflatable `Qp` `Qh` ♂  N1 N

*Medicare Statute 1833(t)*

⚙ **C2623**  Catheter, transluminal angioplasty, drug-coated, non-laser `Qp` `Qh`  N1 N

*Medicare Statute 1833(t)*

⚙ **C2624**  Implantable wireless pulmonary artery pressure sensor with delivery catheter, including all system components `Qp` `Qh`  N1 N

*Medicare Statute 1833(t)*

Coding Clinic: 2015, Q3, P2

⚙ **C2625**  Stent, non-coronary, temporary, with delivery system `Qh`  N1 N

*Medicare Statute 1833(t)*

Coding Clinic: 2016, Q3, P19; 2015, Q2, P9

⚙ **C2626**  Infusion pump, non-programmable, temporary (implantable) `Qp` `Qh`  N1 N

*Medicare Statute 1833(t)*

Coding Clinic: 2016, Q3, P18

⚙ **C2627**  Catheter, suprapubic/cystoscopic `Qh`  N1 N

*Medicare Statute 1833(t)*

⚙ **C2628**  Catheter, occlusion `Qh`  N1 N

*Medicare Statute 1833(t)*

⚙ **C2629**  Introducer/Sheath, other than guiding, other than intracardiac electrophysiological, laser `Qh`  N1 N

*Medicare Statute 1833(t)*

⚙ **C2630**  Catheter, electrophysiology, diagnostic/ablation, other than 3D or vector mapping, cool-tip `Qp` `Qh`  N1 N

*Medicare Statute 1833(t)*

Coding Clinic: 2016, Q3, P17

⚙ **C2631**  Repair device, urinary, incontinence, without sling graft `Qp` `Qh`  N1 N

*Medicare Statute 1833(t)*

## Brachytherapy Sources

⚙ **C2634**  Brachytherapy source, non-stranded, high activity, iodine-125, greater than 1.01 mci (NIST), per source `Qp` `Qh`  H2 U

*Medicare Statute 1833(t)*

⚙ **C2635**  Brachytherapy source, non-stranded, high activity, palladium-103, greater than 2.2 mci (NIST), per source `Qp` `Qh`  H2 U

*Medicare Statute 1833(t)*

⚙ **C2636**  Brachytherapy linear source, non-stranded, palladium-103, per 1 mm `Qp` `Qh`  H2 U

⚙ **C2637**  Brachytherapy source, non-stranded, Ytterbium-169, per source `Qp` `Qh`  B

*Medicare Statute 1833(t)*

⚙ **C2638**  Brachytherapy source, stranded, iodine-125, per source `Qp` `Qh`  H2 U

*Medicare Statute 1833(t)(2)*

⚙ **C2639**  Brachytherapy source, non-stranded, iodine-125, per source `Qp` `Qh`  H2 U

*Medicare Statute 1833(t)(2)*

⚙ **C2640**  Brachytherapy source, stranded, palladium-103, per source `Qp` `Qh`  H2 U

*Medicare Statute 1833(t)(2)*

⚙ **C2641**  Brachytherapy source, non-stranded, palladium-103, per source `Qp` `Qh`  H2 U

*Medicare Statute 1833(t)(2)*

---

🐾 MIPS  `Qp` Quantity Physician  `Qh` Quantity Hospital  ♀ Female only
♂ Male only  A Age  ♿ DMEPOS  A2-Z3 ASC Payment Indicator  A-Y ASC Status Indicator  Coding Clinic

◎ **C2642** Brachytherapy source, stranded, cesium-131, per source `Qp` `Qh` H2 U

*Medicare Statute 1833(t)(2)*

◎ **C2643** Brachytherapy source, non-stranded, cesium-131, per source `Qp` `Qh` H2 U

*Medicare Statute 1833(t)(2)*

◎ **C2644** Brachytherapy source, Cesium-131 chloride solution, per millicurie `Qp` `Qh` H2 U

*Medicare Statute 1833(t)*

◎ **C2645** Brachytherapy planar source, palladium-103, per square millimeter `Qp` `Qh` H2 U

*Medicare Statute 1833(T)*

◎ **C2698** Brachytherapy source, stranded, not otherwise specified, per source H2 U

*Medicare Statute 1833(t)(2)*

◎ **C2699** Brachytherapy source, non-stranded, not otherwise specified, per source H2 U

*Medicare Statute 1833(t)(2)*

## Skin Substitute Graft Application

◎ **C5271** Application of low cost skin substitute graft to trunk, arms, legs, total wound surface area up to 100 sq cm; first 25 sq cm or less wound surface area `Qp` `Qh` T

*Medicare Statute 1833(t)*

◎ **C5272** Application of low cost skin substitute graft to trunk, arms, legs, total wound surface area up to 100 sq cm; each additional 25 sq cm wound surface area, or part thereof (list separately in addition to code for primary procedure) `Qp` `Qh` N

*Medicare Statute 1833(t)*

◎ **C5273** Application of low cost skin substitute graft to trunk, arms, legs, total wound surface area greater than or equal to 100 sq cm; first 100 sq cm wound surface area, or 1% of body area of infants and children `Qp` `Qh` `A` T

*Medicare Statute 1833(t)*

◎ **C5274** Application of low cost skin substitute graft to trunk, arms, legs, total wound surface area greater than or equal to 100 sq cm; each additional 100 sq cm wound surface area, or part thereof, or each additional 1% of body area of infants and children, or part thereof (list separately in addition to code for primary procedure) `Qp` `Qh` `A` N

*Medicare Statute 1833(t)*

◎ **C5275** Application of low cost skin substitute graft to face, scalp, eyelids, mouth, neck, ears, orbits, genitalia, hands, feet, and/or multiple digits, total wound surface area up to 100 sq cm; first 25 sq cm or less wound surface area `Qp` `Qh` T

*Medicare Statute 1833(t)*

◎ **C5276** Application of low cost skin substitute graft to face, scalp, eyelids, mouth, neck, ears, orbits, genitalia, hands, feet, and/or multiple digits, total wound surface area up to 100 sq cm; each additional 25 sq cm wound surface area, or part thereof (list separately in addition to code for primary procedure) `Qp` `Qh` N

*Medicare Statute 1833(t)*

◎ **C5277** Application of low cost skin substitute graft to face, scalp, eyelids, mouth, neck, ears, orbits, genitalia, hands, feet, and/or multiple digits, total wound surface area greater than or equal to 100 sq cm; first 100 sq cm wound surface area, or 1% of body area of infants and children `Qp` `Qh` `A` T

*Medicare Statute 1833(t)*

◎ **C5278** Application of low cost skin substitute graft to face, scalp, eyelids, mouth, neck, ears, orbits, genitalia, hands, feet, and/or multiple digits, total wound surface area greater than or equal to 100 sq cm; each additional 100 sq cm wound surface area, or part thereof, or each additional 1% of body area of infants and children, or part thereof (list separately in addition to code for primary procedure) `Qp` `Qh` `A` N

*Medicare Statute 1833(t)*

## Magnetic Resonance Angiography: Trunk and Lower Extremities

◎ **C8900** Magnetic resonance angiography with contrast, abdomen `Qp` `Qh` Z2 Q3

*Medicare Statute 1833(t)(2)*

◎ **C8901** Magnetic resonance angiography without contrast, abdomen `Qp` `Qh` Z2 Q3

*Medicare Statute 1833(t)(2)*

◎ **C8902** Magnetic resonance angiography without contrast followed by with contrast, abdomen `Qp` `Qh` Z2 Q3

*Medicare Statute 1833(t)(2)*

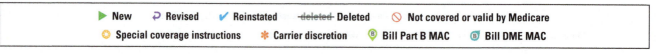

▶ New　↵ Revised　✔ Reinstated　<del>deleted</del> Deleted　⊘ Not covered or valid by Medicare
◎ Special coverage instructions　✱ Carrier discretion　Ⓑ Bill Part B MAC　Ⓑ Bill DME MAC

**C8903** Magnetic resonance imaging with contrast, breast; unilateral **Qp** **Qh** Z2 Q3

*Medicare Statute 1833(t)(2)*

**C8905** Magnetic resonance imaging without contrast followed by with contrast, breast; unilateral **Qp** **Qh** Z2 Q3

*Medicare Statute 1833(t)(2)*

**C8906** Magnetic resonance imaging with contrast, breast; bilateral **Qp** **Qh** Z2 Q3

*Medicare Statute 1833(t)(2)*

**C8908** Magnetic resonance imaging without contrast followed by with contrast, breast; bilateral **Qp** **Qh** Z2 Q3

*Medicare Statute 1833(t)(2)*

**C8909** Magnetic resonance angiography with contrast, chest (excluding myocardium) **Qp** **Qh** Z2 Q3

*Medicare Statute 1833(t)(2)*

**C8910** Magnetic resonance angiography without contrast, chest (excluding myocardium) **Qp** **Qh** Z2 Q3

*Medicare Statute 1833(t)(2)*

**C8911** Magnetic resonance angiography without contrast followed by with contrast, chest (excluding myocardium) **Qp** **Qh** Z2 Q3

*Medicare Statute 1833(t)(2)*

**C8912** Magnetic resonance angiography with contrast, lower extremity **Qp** **Qh** Z2 Q3

*Medicare Statute 1833(t)(2)*

**C8913** Magnetic resonance angiography without contrast, lower extremity **Qp** **Qh** Z2 Q3

*Medicare Statute 1833(t)(2)*

**C8914** Magnetic resonance angiography without contrast followed by with contrast, lower extremity **Qp** **Qh** Z2 Q3

*Medicare Statute 1833(t)(2)*

**C8918** Magnetic resonance angiography with contrast, pelvis **Qp** **Qh** Z2 Q3

*Medicare Statute 1833(t)(2)*

**C8919** Magnetic resonance angiography without contrast, pelvis **Qp** **Qh** Z2 Q3

*Medicare Statute 1833(t)(2)*

**C8920** Magnetic resonance angiography without contrast followed by with contrast, pelvis **Qp** **Qh** Z2 Q3

*Medicare Statute 1833(t)(2)*

## Transthoracic and Transesophageal Echocardiography

**C8921** Transthoracic echocardiography with contrast, or without contrast followed by with contrast, for congenital cardiac anomalies; complete **Qp** **Qh** S

*Medicare Statute 1833(t)(2)*

Coding Clinic: 2012, Q3, P8

**C8922** Transthoracic echocardiography with contrast, or without contrast followed by with contrast, for congenital cardiac anomalies; follow-up or limited study **Qp** **Qh** S

*Medicare Statute 1833(t)(2)*

Coding Clinic: 2012, Q3, P8

**C8923** Transthoracic echocardiography with contrast, or without contrast followed by with contrast, real-time with image documentation (2D), includes M-mode recording, when performed, complete, without spectral or color Doppler echocardiography **Qp** **Qh** S

*Medicare Statute 1833(t)(2)*

Coding Clinic: 2012, Q3, P8

**C8924** Transthoracic echocardiography with contrast, or without contrast followed by with contrast, real-time with image documentation (2D), includes M-mode recording, when performed, follow-up or limited study **Qp** **Qh** S

*Medicare Statute 1833(t)(2)*

Coding Clinic: 2012, Q3, P8

**C8925** Transesophageal echocardiography (TEE) with contrast, or without contrast followed by with contrast, real time with image documentation (2D) (with or without M-mode recording); including probe placement, image acquisition, interpretation and report **Qp** **Qh** S

*Medicare Statute 1833(t)(2)*

Coding Clinic: 2012, Q3, P8

**C8926** Transesophageal echocardiography (TEE) with contrast, or without contrast followed by with contrast, for congenital cardiac anomalies; including probe placement, image acquisition, interpretation and report **Qp** **Qh** S

*Medicare Statute 1833(t)(2)*

Coding Clinic: 2012, Q3, P8

| 🏷 MIPS | **Qp** Quantity Physician | **Qh** Quantity Hospital | ♀ Female only |
| ♂ Male only | A Age | 🦽 DMEPOS | A2-Z3 ASC Payment Indicator | A-Y ASC Status Indicator | Coding Clinic |

⚙ **C8927** Transesophageal echocardiography (TEE) with contrast, or without contrast followed by with contrast, for monitoring purposes, including probe placement, real time 2-dimensional image acquisition and interpretation leading to ongoing (continuous) assessment of (dynamically changing) cardiac pumping function and to therapeutic measures on an immediate time basis **Qp** **Qh**     S

*Medicare Statute 1833(t)(2)*

Coding Clinic: 2012, Q3, P8

⚙ **C8928** Transthoracic echocardiography with contrast, or without contrast followed by with contrast, real-time with image documentation (2D), includes M-mode recording, when performed, during rest and cardiovascular stress test using treadmill, bicycle exercise and/or pharmacologically induced stress, with interpretation and report **Qp** **Qh**     S

*Medicare Statute 1833(t)(2)*

Coding Clinic: 2012, Q3, P8

⚙ **C8929** Transthoracic echocardiography with contrast, or without contrast followed by with contrast, real-time with image documentation (2D), includes M-mode recording, when performed, complete, with spectral Doppler echocardiography, and with color flow Doppler echocardiography **Qp** **Qh**     S

*Medicare Statute 1833(t)(2)*

Coding Clinic: 2012, Q3, P8

⚙ **C8930** Transthoracic echocardiography, with contrast, or without contrast followed by with contrast, real-time with image documentation (2D), includes M-mode recording, when performed, during rest and cardiovascular stress test using treadmill, bicycle exercise and/or pharmacologically induced stress, with interpretation and report; including performance of continuous electrocardiographic monitoring, with physician supervision **Qp** **Qh**     S

*Medicare Statute 1833(t)(2)*

Coding Clinic: 2012, Q3, P8

## Magnetic Resonance Angiography: Spine and Upper Extremities

⚙ **C8931** Magnetic resonance angiography with contrast, spinal canal and contents **Qp** **Qh**     Z2 Q3

*Medicare Statute 1833(t)*

⚙ **C8932** Magnetic resonance angiography without contrast, spinal canal and contents **Qp** **Qh**     Z2 Q3

*Medicare Statute 1833(t)*

⚙ **C8933** Magnetic resonance angiography without contrast followed by with contrast, spinal canal and contents **Qp** **Qh**     Z2 Q3

*Medicare Statute 1833(t)*

⚙ **C8934** Magnetic resonance angiography with contrast, upper extremity **Qh**     Z2 Q3

*Medicare Statute 1833(t)*

⚙ **C8935** Magnetic resonance angiography without contrast, upper extremity **Qh**     Z2 Q3

*Medicare Statute 1833(t)*

⚙ **C8936** Magnetic resonance angiography without contrast followed by with contrast, upper extremity **Qh**     Z2 Q3

*Medicare Statute 1833(t)*

⚙ **C8937** Computer-aided detection, including computer algorithm analysis of breast MRI image data for lesion detection/ characterization, pharmacokinetic analysis, with further physician review for interpretation (list separately in addition to code for primary procedure)     N

*Medicare Statute 1833(t)*

## Drugs and Biologicals

⚙ **C8957** Intravenous infusion for therapy/ diagnosis; initiation of prolonged infusion (more than 8 hours), requiring use of portable or implantable pump **Qp** **Qh**     S

*Medicare Statute 1833(t)*

Coding Clinic: 2008, Q3, P8

⚙ **C9034** Injection, dexamethasone 9%, intraocular, 1 mcg     G

*Medicare Statute 1833(t)*

~~C9035~~ ~~Injection, aripiprazole lauroxil (aristada initio), 1 mg~~     ✖

~~C9036~~ ~~Injection, patisiran, 0.1 mg~~     ✖

~~C9037~~ ~~Injection, risperidone (perseris), 0.5 mg~~     ✖

~~C9038~~ ~~Injection, mogamulizumab-kpkc, 1 mg~~     ✖

~~C9039~~ ~~Injection, plazomicin, 5 mg~~     ✖

▶ ⚙ **C9041** Injection, coagulation factor Xa (recombinant), inactivated (Andexxa), 10 mg     K2 G

▶ ⚙ **C9046** Cocaine hydrochloride nasal solution for topical administration, 1 mg     K2 G

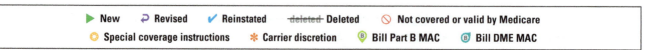

▶ New     ↩ Revised     ✔ Reinstated     ~~deleted~~ Deleted     ⊘ Not covered or valid by Medicare
⚙ Special coverage instructions     ✳ Carrier discretion     Ⓑ Bill Part B MAC     Ⓑ Bill DME MAC

▶ ⊛ **C9047** Injection, caplacizumab-yhdp, 1 mg      K2 G

▶ ⊛ **C9054** Injection, lefamulin (Xenleta), 1 mg      N1 G

▶ ⊛ **C9055** Injection, brexanolone, 1mg    N1 G G

⊛ **C9113** Injection, pantoprazole sodium, per vial Qp Qh    N1 N

*Medicare Statute 1833(t)*

⊛ **C9132** Prothrombin complex concentrate (human), Kcentra, per i.u. of Factor IX activity Qp Qh    K2 K

*Medicare Statute 1833(t)*

⊛ **C9248** Injection, clevidipine butyrate, 1 mg Qp Qh    N1 N

*Medicare Statute 1833(t)*

⊛ **C9250** Human plasma fibrin sealant, vapor-heated, solvent-detergent (ARTISS), 2 ml Qp Qh    K2 K

Example of diagnosis codes to be reported with C9250: T20.00-T25.799.

*Medicare Statute 621MMA*

⊛ **C9254** Injection, lacosamide, 1 mg Qp Qh    N1 N

*Medicare Statute 621MMA*

⊛ **C9257** injection, bevacizumab, 0.25 mg Qp Qh    K2 K

*Medicare Statute 1833(t)*

⊛ **C9285** Lidocaine 70 mg/tetracaine 70 mg, per patch Qp Qh    N1 N

*Medicare Statute 1833(t)*

Coding Clinic: 2011, Q3, P9

⊛ **C9290** Injection, bupivacine liposome, 1 mg Qp Qh    N1 N

*Medicare Statute 1833(t)*

⊛ **C9293** Injection, glucarpidase, 10 units Qp Qh    K2 K

*Medicare Statute 1833(t)*

⊛ **C9352** Microporous collagen implantable tube (NeuraGen Nerve Guide), per centimeter length Qp Qh    N1 N

*Medicare Statute 621MMA*

⊛ **C9353** Microporous collagen implantable slit tube (NeuraWrap Nerve Protector), per centimeter length Qp Qh    N1 N

*Medicare Statute 621MMA*

⊛ **C9354** Acellular pericardial tissue matrix of non-human origin (Veritas), per square centimeter Qp Qh    N1 N

*Medicare Statute 621MMA*

⊛ **C9355** Collagen nerve cuff (NeuroMatrix), per 0.5 centimeter length Qp Qh    N1 N

*Medicare Statute 621MMA*

⊛ **C9356** Tendon, porous matrix of cross-linked collagen and glycosaminoglycan matrix (TenoGlide Tendon Protector Sheet), per square centimeter Qp Qh    N1 N

*Medicare Statute 621MMA*

⊛ **C9358** Dermal substitute, native, non-denatured collagen, fetal bovine origin (SurgiMend Collagen Matrix), per 0.5 square centimeters Qp Qh    N1 N

*Medicare Statute 621MMA*

Coding Clinic: 2013, Q3, P9; 2012, Q2, P7

⊛ **C9359** Porous purified collagen matrix bone void filler (Integra Mozaik Osteoconductive Scaffold Putty, Integra OS Osteoconductive Scaffold Putty), per 0.5 cc Qp Qh    N1 N

*Medicare Statute 1833(t)*

Coding Clinic: 2015, Q3, P2

⊛ **C9360** Dermal substitute, native, non-denatured collagen, neonatal bovine origin (SurgiMend Collagen Matrix), per 0.5 square centimeters Qp Qh    N1 N

*Medicare Statute 621MMA*

Coding Clinic: 2012, Q2, P7

⊛ **C9361** Collagen matrix nerve wrap (NeuroMend Collagen Nerve Wrap), per 0.5 centimeter length Qp Qh   N1 N

*Medicare Statute 621MMA*

⊛ **C9362** Porous purified collagen matrix bone void filler (Integra Mozaik Osteoconductive Scaffold Strip), per 0.5 cc Qp Qh    N1 N

*Medicare Statute 621MMA*

Coding Clinic: 2010, Q2, P8

⊛ **C9363** Skin substitute, Integra Meshed Bilayer Wound Matrix, per square centimeter Qp Qh    N1 N

*Medicare Statute 621MMA*

Coding Clinic: 2012, Q2, P7; 2010, Q2, P8

⊛ **C9364** Porcine implant, Permacol, per square centimeter Qp Qh    N1 N

*Medicare Statute 621MMA*

⊛ **C9399** Unclassified drugs or biologicals    K7 A

*Medicare Statute 621MMA*

Coding Clinic: 2017, Q1, P1-3, P8; 2016, Q4, P10; 2014, Q2, P8; 2013, Q2, P3; 2010, Q3, P8

---

🐾 MIPS    Qp Quantity Physician    Qh Quantity Hospital    ♀ Female only

♂ Male only    A Age    ♿ DMEPOS    A2-Z3 ASC Payment Indicator    A-Y ASC Status Indicator    Coding Clinic

~~C9407    Iodine i-131 iobenguane, diagnostic,~~ ✖
~~1 millicurie~~ G

~~C9408    Iodine i-131 iobenguane, therapeutic,~~ ✖
~~1 millicurie~~

~~C9447    Injection, phenylephrine and~~ ✖
~~ketorolac, 4 ml vial~~

⚙ **C9460**    Injection, cangrelor, 1 mg  `Qp` `Qh`  **K2 G**

*Medicare Statute 1833(t)*

⚙ **C9462**    Injection, delafloxacin, 1 mg  **K2 G**

*Medicare Statute 1833(t)*

⚙ **C9482**    Injection, sotalol hydrochloride,
1 mg  `Qp` `Qh`  **K2 G**

*Medicare Statute 1833(t)*

**Coding Clinic: 2016, Q4, P9**

⚙ **C9488**    Injection, conivaptan
hydrochloride, 1 mg  **K2 G**

*Medicare Statute 1833(t)*

## Percutaneous Transcatheter and Transluminal Coronary Procedures

⚙ **C9600**    Percutaneous transcatheter placement
of drug eluting intracoronary stent(s),
with coronary angioplasty when
performed; a single major coronary
artery or branch  `Qp` `Qh`  **J1**

*Medicare Statute 1833(t)*

⚙ **C9601**    Percutaneous transcatheter placement
of drug-eluting intracoronary stent(s),
with coronary angioplasty when
performed; each additional branch of a
major coronary artery (list separately in
addition to code for primary
procedure)  `Qp` `Qh`  **N**

*Medicare Statute 1833(t)*

⚙ **C9602**    Percutaneous transluminal coronary
atherectomy, with drug eluting
intracoronary stent, with coronary
angioplasty when performed; a single
major coronary artery or
branch  `Qp` `Qh`  **J1**

*Medicare Statute 1833(t)*

⚙ **C9603**    Percutaneous transluminal coronary
atherectomy, with drug-eluting
intracoronary stent, with coronary
angioplasty when performed; each
additional branch of a major coronary
artery (list separately in addition to
code for primary procedure)  `Qp` `Qh`  **N**

*Medicare Statute 1833(t)*

⚙ **C9604**    Percutaneous transluminal
revascularization of or through
coronary artery bypass graft (internal
mammary, free arterial, venous), any
combination of drug-eluting
intracoronary stent, atherectomy and
angioplasty, including distal protection
when performed; a single
vessel  `Qp` `Qh`  **J1**

⚙ **C9605**    Percutaneous transluminal
revascularization of or through coronary
artery bypass graft (internal mammary,
free arterial, venous), any combination of
drug-eluting intracoronary stent,
atherectomy and angioplasty, including
distal protection when performed; each
additional branch subtended by the
bypass graft (list separately in addition to
code for primary procedure)  `Qp` `Qh`  **N**

*Medicare Statute 1833(t)*

⚙ **C9606**    Percutaneous transluminal
revascularization of acute total/subtotal
occlusion during acute myocardial
infarction, coronary artery or coronary
artery bypass graft, any combination of
drug-eluting intracoronary stent,
atherectomy and angioplasty, including
aspiration thrombectomy when
performed, single vessel  `Qp` `Qh`  **J1**

*Medicare Statute 1833(t)*

⚙ **C9607**    Percutaneous transluminal
revascularization of chronic total
occlusion, coronary artery, coronary
artery branch, or coronary artery bypass
graft, any combination of drug-eluting
intracoronary stent, atherectomy and
angioplasty; single vessel  `Qp` `Qh`  **J1**

*Medicare Statute 1833(t)*

⚙ **C9608**    Percutaneous transluminal
revascularization of chronic total
occlusion, coronary artery, coronary
artery branch, or coronary artery bypass
graft, any combination of drug-eluting
intracoronary stent, atherectomy and
angioplasty; each additional coronary
artery, coronary artery branch, or bypass
graft (list separately in addition to code
for primary procedure)  `Qp` `Qh`  **N**

*Medicare Statute 1833(t)*

## Therapeutic Services and Supplies

⚙ **C9725**    Placement of endorectal intracavitary
applicator for high intensity
brachytherapy  `Qp` `Qh`  **T**

*Medicare Statute 1833(t)*

---

▶ New    ↻ Revised    ✔ Reinstated    ~~deleted~~ Deleted    ⊘ Not covered or valid by Medicare
⚙ Special coverage instructions    ✳ Carrier discretion    Ⓑ Bill Part B MAC    Ⓓ Bill DME MAC

⚙ **C9726** Placement and removal (if performed) of applicator into breast for intraoperative radiation therapy, add-on to primary breast procedure Ⓠ**h** **N**

*Medicare Statute 1833(t)*

⚙ **C9727** Insertion of implants into the soft palate; minimum of three implants Ⓠ**p** Ⓠ**h** **T**

*Medicare Statute 1833(t)*

⚙ **C9728** Placement of interstitial device(s) for radiation therapy/surgery guidance (e.g., fiducial markers, dosimeter), for other than the following sites (any approach): abdomen, pelvis, prostate, retroperitoneum, thorax, single or multiple Ⓠ**p** Ⓠ**h** **S**

*Medicare Statute 1833(t)*

Coding Clinic: 2018, Q2, P4

⚙ **C9733** Non-ophthalmic fluorescent vascular angiography Ⓠ**p** Ⓠ**h** **Q2**

*Medicare Statute 1833(t)*

Coding Clinic: 2012, Q1, P7

⚙ **C9734** Focused ultrasound ablation/therapeutic intervention, other than uterine leiomyomata, with magnetic resonance (MR) guidance Ⓠ**p** Ⓠ**h** **J1**

*Medicare Statute 1833(t)*

⚙ **C9738** Adjunctive blue light cystoscopy with fluorescent imaging agent (list separately in addition to code for primary procedure) **N1** **N**

*Medicare Statute 1833(t)*

⚙ **C9739** Cystourethroscopy, with insertion of transprostatic implant; 1 to 3 implants Ⓠ**p** Ⓠ**h** **J1**

*Medicare Statute 1833(t)*

Coding Clinic: 2014, Q2, P6

⚙ **C9740** Cystourethroscopy, with insertion of transprostatic implant; 4 or more implants Ⓠ**p** Ⓠ**h** **J1**

*Medicare Statute 1833(t)*

Coding Clinic: 2014, Q2, P6

⚙ **C9745** Nasal endoscopy, surgical; balloon dilation of eustachian tube **J1**

*Medicare Statute 1833(t)*

~~C9746~~ ~~Transperineal implantation of permanent adjustable balloon continence device, with cystourethroscopy, when performed and/or fluoroscopy, when performed~~ ✖

⚙ **C9747** Ablation of prostate, transrectal, high intensity focused ultrasound (HIFU), including imaging guidance **J1**

*Medicare Statute 1833(t)*

⚙ **C9749** Repair of nasal vestibular lateral wall stenosis with implant(s) **J1**

*Medicare Statute 1833(t)*

⚙ **C9751** Bronchoscopy, rigid or flexible, transbronchial ablation of lesion(s) by microwave energy, including fluoroscopic guidance, when performed, with computed tomography acquisition(s) and 3-D rendering, computer-assisted, image-guided navigation, and endobronchial ultrasound (EBUS) guided transtracheal and/or transbronchial sampling (e.g., aspiration[s]/biopsy[ies]) and all mediastinal and/or hilar lymph node stations or structures and therapeutic intervention(s) **T**

*Medicare Statute 1833(t)*

⚙ **C9752** Destruction of intraosseous basivertebral nerve, first two vertebral bodies, including imaging guidance (e.g., fluoroscopy), lumbar/sacrum **J1**

*Medicare Statute 1833(t)*

⚙ **C9753** Destruction of intraosseous basivertebral nerve, each additional vertebral body, including imaging guidance (e.g., fluoroscopy), lumbar/sacrum (list separately in addition to code for primary procedure) **N**

*Medicare Statute 1833(t)*

⚙ **C9754** Creation of arteriovenous fistula, percutaneous; direct, any site, including all imaging and radiologic supervision and interpretation, when performed and secondary procedures to redirect blood flow (e.g., transluminal balloon angioplasty, coil embolization, when performed) **J1**

*Medicare Statute 1833(t)*

⚙ **C9755** Creation of arteriovenous fistula, percutaneous using magnetic-guided arterial and venous catheters and radiofrequency energy, including flow-directing procedures (e.g., vascular coil embolization with radiologic supervision and interpretation, when performed) and fistulogram(s), angiography, venography, and/or ultrasound, with radiologic supervision and interpretation, when performed **J1**

*Medicare Statute 1833(t)*

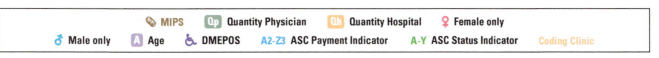

🐾 MIPS    ⓆⓅ Quantity Physician    Ⓠⓗ Quantity Hospital    ♀ Female only

♂ Male only    Ⓐ Age    ♿ DMEPOS    A2-Z3 ASC Payment Indicator    A-Y ASC Status Indicator    Coding Clinic

▶ ✪ **C9756** Intraoperative near-infrared fluorescence lymphatic mapping of lymph node(s) (sentinel or tumor draining) with administration of indocyanine green (ICG) (list separately in addition to code for primary procedure)   N

▶ ✪ **C9757** Laminotomy (hemilaminectomy), with decompression of nerve root(s), including partial facetectomy, foraminotomy and excision of herniated intervertebral disc, and repair of annular defect with implantation of bone anchored annular closure device, including annular defect measurement, alignment and sizing assessment, and image guidance; 1 interspace, lumbar   J1

▶ ✪ **C9758** Blinded procedure for NYHA class III/IV heart failure; transcatheter implantation of interatrial shunt or placebo control, including right heart catheterization, trans-esophageal echocardiography (TEE)/intracardiac echocardiography (ICE), and all imaging with or without guidance (e.g., ultrasound, fluoroscopy), performed in an approved investigational device exemption (IDE) study   T

✪ **C9898** Radiolabeled product provided during a hospital inpatient stay  Qh   N

✪ **C9899** Implanted prosthetic device, payable only for inpatients who do not have inpatient coverage   A

*Medicare Statute 1833(t)*

**New** ▶  **Revised** ⮌  **Reinstated** ✔  ~~deleted~~ **Deleted**  ⊘ **Not covered or valid by Medicare**  ✪ **Special coverage instructions**  ✳ **Carrier discretion**  Ⓑ **Bill Part B MAC**  Ⓓ **Bill DME MAC**

**156**

C9756 – C9899   CMS HOSPITAL OUTPATIENT PAYMENT SYSTEM

# DENTAL PROCEDURES (D0000-D9999)

## Diagnostic (D0120-D0999)
### Clinical Oral Evaluations

**D0120** Periodic oral evaluation - established patient Ⓑ  E1

An evaluation performed on a patient of record to determine any changes in the patient's dental and medical health status since a previous comprehensive or periodic evaluation. This includes an oral cancer evaluation and periodontal screening where indicated, and may require interpretation of information acquired through additional diagnostic procedures. Report additional diagnostic procedures separately.

**D0140** Limited oral evaluation - problem focused Ⓑ  E1

An evaluation limited to a specific oral health problem or complaint. This may require interpretation of information acquired through additional diagnostic procedures. Report additional diagnostic procedures separately. Definitive procedures may be required on the same date as the evaluation. Typically, patients receiving this type of evaluation present with a specific problem and/or dental emergencies, trauma, acute infections, etc.

**D0145** Oral evaluation for a patient under three years of age and counseling with primary caregiver Ⓑ Ⓐ  E1

Diagnostic services performed for a child under the age of three, preferably within the first six months of the eruption of the first primary tooth, including recording the oral and physical health history, evaluation of caries susceptibility, development of an appropriate preventive oral health regimen and communication with and counseling of the child's parent, legal guardian and/or primary caregiver.

**D0150** Comprehensive oral evaluation - new or established patient Ⓑ  S

Used by a general dentist and/or a specialist when evaluating a patient comprehensively. This applies to new patients; established patients who have had a significant change in health conditions or other unusual circumstances, by report, or established patients who have been absent from active treatment for three or more years. It is a thorough evaluation and recording of the extraoral and intraoral hard and soft tissues. It may require interpretation of information acquired through additional diagnostic procedures. Additional diagnostic procedures should be reported separately. This includes an evaluation for oral cancer where indicated, the evaluation and recording of the patient's dental and medical history and a general health assessment. It may include the evaluation and recording of dental caries, missing or unerupted teeth, restorations, existing prostheses, occlusal relationships, periodontal conditions (including periodontal screening and/or charting), hard and soft tissue anomalies, etc.

**D0160** Detailed and extensive oral evaluation - problem focused, by report Ⓑ  E1

A detailed and extensive problem focused evaluation entails extensive diagnostic and cognitive modalities based on the findings of a comprehensive oral evaluation. Integration of more extensive diagnostic modalities to develop a treatment plan for a specific problem is required. The condition requiring this type of evaluation should be described and documented. Examples of conditions requiring this type of evaluation may include dentofacial anomalies, complicated perio-prosthetic conditions, complex temporomandibular dysfunction, facial pain of unknown origin, conditions requiring multi-disciplinary consultation, etc.

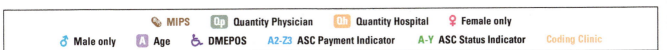

🐾 MIPS   Qp Quantity Physician   Qh Quantity Hospital   ♀ Female only
♂ Male only   Ⓐ Age   ♿ DMEPOS   A2-Z3 ASC Payment Indicator   A-Y ASC Status Indicator   Coding Clinic

**D0170** Re-evaluation - limited, problem focused (established patient; not post-operative visit) Ⓑ    E1

Assessing the status of a previously existing condition. For example: - a traumatic injury where no treatment was rendered but patient needs follow-up monitoring; - evaluation for undiagnosed continuing pain; - soft tissue lesion requiring follow-up evaluation.

**D0171** Re-evaluation - post-operative office visit Ⓑ    E1

**D0180** Comprehensive periodontal evaluation - new or established patient Ⓑ    E1

This procedure is indicated for patients showing signs or symptoms of periodontal disease and for patients with risk factors such as smoking or diabetes. It includes evaluation of periodontal conditions, probing and charting, evaluation and recording of the patient's dental and medical history and general health assessment. It may include the evaluation and recording of dental caries, missing or unerupted teeth, restorations, occlusal relationships and oral cancer evaluation.

## Pre-Diagnostic Services

**D0190** Screening of a patient Ⓑ    E1

A screening, including state or federally mandated screenings, to determine an individual's need to be seen by a dentist for diagnosis.

**D0191** Assessment of a patient Ⓑ    E1

A limited clinical inspection that is performed to identify possible signs of oral or systemic disease, malformation, or injury, and the potential need for referral for diagnosis and treatment.

## Diagnostic Imaging

**D0210** Intraoral - complete series of radiographic image Ⓑ    E1

A radiographic survey of the whole mouth, usually consisting of 14-22 periapical and posterior bitewing images intended to display the crowns and roots of all teeth, periapical areas and alveolar bone.

*Cross Reference 70320*

**D0220** Intraoral - periapical first radiographic image Ⓑ    E1

*Cross Reference 70300*

**D0230** Intraoral - periapical each additional radiographic image Ⓑ    E1

*Cross Reference 70310*

**D0240** Intraoral - occlusal radiographic image Ⓑ    S

**D0250** Extra-oral — 2D projection radiographic image created using a stationary radiation source, detector Ⓑ    S

These images include, but are not limited to: Lateral Skull; Posterior-Anterior Skull; Submentovertex; Waters; Reverse Tomes; Oblique Mandibular Body; Lateral Ramus.

**D0251** Extra-oral posterior dental radiographic image Ⓑ    Q1

Image limited to exposure of complete posterior teeth in both dental arches. This is a unique image that is not derived from another image.

**D0270** Bitewing - single radiographic image Ⓑ    S

**D0272** Bitewings - two radiographic images Ⓑ    S

**D0273** Bitewings - three radiographic images Ⓑ    E1

**D0274** Bitewings - four radiographic images Ⓑ    S

**D0277** Vertical bitewings - 7 to 8 radiographic images Ⓑ    S

This does not constitute a full mouth intraoral radiographic series.

**D0310** Sialography Ⓑ    E1

*Cross Reference 70390*

**D0320** Temporomandibular joint arthrogram, including injection Ⓑ    E1

*Cross Reference 70332*

**D0321** Other temporomandibular joint radiographic image, by report Ⓑ    E1

*Cross Reference 76499*

**D0322** Tomographic survey Ⓑ    E1

**D0330** Panoramic radiographic image Ⓑ    E1

*Cross Reference 70320*

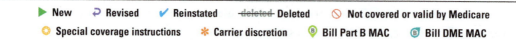

▶ New    ↻ Revised    ✔ Reinstated    ~~deleted~~ Deleted    ⊘ Not covered or valid by Medicare
🔅 Special coverage instructions    ✳ Carrier discretion    Ⓑ Bill Part B MAC    Ⓑ Bill DME MAC

**D0340** 2D cephalometric radiographic image - acquisition, measurement and analysis ⑧  E1

Image of the head made using a cephalostat to standardize anatomic positioning, and with reproducible x-ray beam geometry.

*Cross Reference 70350*

**D0350** 2D oral/facial photographic image obtained intra-orally or extra-orally ⑧  E1

**D0351** 3D photographic image ⑧  E1

This procedure is for dental or maxillofacial diagnostic purposes. Not applicable for a CAD-CAM procedure.

**D0364** Cone beam CT capture and interpretation with limited field of view - less than one whole jaw ⑧  E1

**D0365** Cone beam CT capture and interpretation with field of view of one full dental arch - mandible ⑧  E1

**D0366** Cone beam CT capture and interpretation with field of view of one full dental arch - maxilla, with or without cranium ⑧  E1

**D0367** Cone beam CT capture and interpretation with field of view of both jaws, with or without cranium ⑧  E1

**D0368** Cone beam CT capture and interpretation for TMJ series including two or more exposures ⑧  E1

**D0369** Maxillofacial MRI capture and interpretation ⑧  E1

**D0370** Maxillofacial ultrasound capture and interpretation ⑧  E1

**D0371** Sialoendoscopy capture and interpretation ⑧  E1

**D0380** Cone beam CT image capture with limited field of view - less than one whole jaw ⑧  E1

**D0381** Cone beam CT image capture with field of view of one full dental arch - mandible ⑧  E1

**D0382** Cone beam CT image capture with field of view of one full dental arch - maxilla, with or without cranium ⑧  E1

**D0383** Cone beam CT image capture with field of view of both jaws, with or without cranium ⑧  E1

**D0384** Cone beam CT image capture for TMJ series including two or more exposures ⑧  E1

**D0385** Maxillofacial MRI image capture ⑧  E1

**D0386** Maxillofacial ultrasound image capture ⑧  E1

**D0391** Interpretation of diagnostic image by a practitioner not associated with capture of the image, including report ⑧  E1

**D0393** Treatment simulation using 3D image volume ⑧  E1

The use of 3D image volumes for simulation of treatment including, but not limited to, dental implant placement, orthognathic surgery and orthodontic tooth movement.

**D0394** Digital subtraction of two or more images or image volumes of the same modality ⑧  E1

To demonstrate changes that have occurred over time.

**D0395** Fusion of two or more 3D image volumes of one or more modalities ⑧  E1

## Tests and Examinations

**D0411** HbA1c in-office point of service testing ⑧  E1

**D0412** Blood gucose level test - in-office using a glucose meter ⑧  E1

**D0414** Laboratory processing of microbial specimen to include culture and sensitivity studies, preparation and transmission of written report ⑧  E1

**D0415** Collection of microorganisms for culture and sensitivity ⑧  E1

*Cross Reference D0410*

**D0416** Viral culture ⑧  B

A diagnostic test to identify viral organisms, most often herpes virus.

**D0417** Collection and preparation of saliva sample for laboratory diagnostic testing ⑧  E1

**D0418** Analysis of saliva sample ⑧  E1

Chemical or biological analysis of saliva sample for diagnostic purposes.

▶ **D0419** Assessment of salivary flow by measurement  E1

**D0422** Collection and preparation of genetic sample material for laboratory analysis and report ⑧  E1

**D0423** Genetic test for susceptibility to diseases - specimen analysis ⑧  E1

Certified laboratory analysis to detect specific genetic variations associated with increased susceptibility for diseases.

---

🖐 **MIPS**   Qp **Quantity Physician**   Qh **Quantity Hospital**   ♀ **Female only**

♂ **Male only**   A **Age**   ♿ **DMEPOS**   A2-Z3 **ASC Payment Indicator**   A-Y **ASC Status Indicator**   *Coding Clinic*

**D0425** Caries susceptibility tests Ⓑ      E1

Not to be used for carious dentin staining.

**D0431** Adjunctive pre-diagnostic test that aids in detection of mucosal abnormalities including premalignant and malignant lesions, not to include cytology or biopsy procedures Ⓑ      B

**D0460** Pulp vitality tests Ⓑ      S

Includes multiple teeth and contra lateral comparison(s), as indicated.

**D0470** Diagnostic casts Ⓑ      E1

Also known as diagnostic models or study models.

### Oral Pathology Laboratory (Use Codes D0472 – D0502)

**D0472** Accession of tissue, gross examination, preparation and transmission of written report Ⓑ      B

To be used in reporting architecturally intact tissue obtained by invasive means.

**D0473** Accession of tissue, gross and microscopic examination, preparation and transmission of written report Ⓑ   B

To be used in reporting architecturally intact tissue obtained by invasive means.

**D0474** Accession of tissue, gross and microscopic examination, including assessment of surgical margins for presence of disease, preparation and transmission of written report Ⓑ      B

To be used in reporting architecturally intact tissue obtained by invasive means.

**D0475** Decalcification procedure Ⓑ      B

Procedure in which hard tissue is processed in order to allow sectioning and subsequent microscopic examination.

**D0476** Special stains for microorganisms Ⓑ   B

Procedure in which additional stains are applied to biopsy or surgical specimen in order to identify microorganisms.

**D0477** Special stains, not for microorganisms Ⓑ      B

Procedure in which additional stains are applied to a biopsy or surgical specimen in order to identify such things as melanin, mucin, iron, glycogen, etc.

**D0478** Immunohistochemical stains Ⓑ      B

A procedure in which specific antibody based reagents are applied to tissue samples in order to facilitate diagnosis.

**D0479** Tissue in-situ hybridization, including interpretation Ⓑ      B

A procedure which allows for the identification of nucleic acids, DNA and RNA, in the tissue sample in order to aid in the diagnosis of microorganisms and tumors.

**D0480** Accession of exfoliative cytologic smears, microscopic examination, preparation and transmission of written report Ⓑ      B

To be used in reporting disaggregated, non-transepithelial cell cytology sample via mild scraping of the oral mucosa.

**D0481** Electron microscopy Ⓑ      B

**D0482** Direct immunofluorescence Ⓑ      B

A technique used to identify immunoreactants which are localized to the patient's skin or mucous membranes.

**D0483** Indirect immunofluorescence Ⓑ      B

A technique used to identify circulating immunoreactants.

**D0484** Consultation on slides prepared elsewhere Ⓑ      B

A service provided in which microscopic slides of a biopsy specimen prepared at another laboratory are evaluated to aid in the diagnosis of a difficult case or to offer a consultative opinion at the patient's request. The findings are delivered by written report.

**D0485** Consultation, including preparation of slides from biopsy material supplied by referring source Ⓑ      B

A service that requires the consulting pathologist to prepare the slides as well as render a written report. The slides are evaluated to aid in the diagnosis of a difficult case or to offer a consultative opinion at the patient's request.

**D0486** Laboratory accession of transepithelial cytologic sample, microscopic examination, preparation and transmission of written report Ⓑ      E1

Analysis, and written report of findings, of cytologic sample of disaggregated transepithelial cells.

**D0502** Other oral pathology procedures, by report Ⓑ      B

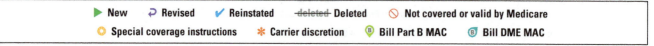

▶ New    ⮌ Revised    ✔ Reinstated    ~~deleted~~ Deleted    ⊘ Not covered or valid by Medicare
⊛ Special coverage instructions    ✳ Carrier discretion    Ⓑ Bill Part B MAC    Ⓑ Bill DME MAC

## Tests and Examinations

**D0600** Non-ionizing diagnostic procedure capable of quantifying, monitoring, and recording changes in structure of enamel, dentin, and cementum Ⓑ   **S**

**D0601** Caries risk assessment and documentation, with a finding of low risk Ⓑ   **E1**

Using recognized assessment tools.

**D0602** Caries risk assessment and documentation, with a finding of moderate risk Ⓑ   **E1**

Using recognized assessment tools.

**D0603** Caries risk assessment and documentation, with a finding of high risk Ⓑ   **E1**

Using recognized assessment tools.

## None

**D0999** Unspecified diagnostic procedure, by report Ⓑ   **B**

Used for procedure that is not adequately described by a code. Describe procedure.

## Preventative (D1110-D1999)
## Dental Prophylaxis

**D1110** Prophylaxis - adult Ⓑ Ⓐ   **E1**

Removal of plaque, calculus and stains from the tooth structures in the permanent and transitional dentition. It is intended to control local irritational factors.

**D1120** Prophylaxis - child Ⓑ Ⓐ   **E1**

Removal of plaque, calculus and stains from the tooth structures in the primary and transitional dentition. It is intended to control local irritational factors.

## Topical Fluoride Treatment (Office Procedure)

**D1206** Topical application of fluoride varnish Ⓑ   **E1**

**D1208** Topical application of fluoride — excluding varnish Ⓑ   **E1**

## Other Preventative Services

**D1310** Nutritional counseling for the control of dental disease Ⓑ   **E1**

Counseling on food selection and dietary habits as a part of treatment and control of periodontal disease and caries.

**D1320** Tobacco counseling for the control and prevention of oral disease Ⓑ   **E1**

Tobacco prevention and cessation services reduce patient risks of developing tobacco-related oral diseases and conditions and improves prognosis for certain dental therapies.

**D1330** Oral hygiene instruction Ⓑ   **E1**

This may include instructions for home care. Examples include tooth brushing technique, flossing, use of special oral hygiene aids.

**D1351** Sealant - per tooth Ⓑ   **E1**

Mechanically and/or chemically prepared enamel surface sealed to prevent decay.

**D1352** Preventive resin restoration in a moderate to high caries risk patient — permanent tooth Ⓑ   **E1**

Conservative restoration of an active cavitated lesion in a pit or fissure that does not extend into dentin; includes placement of a sealant in any radiating non-carious fissures or pits.

**D1353** Sealant repair — per tooth Ⓑ   **E1**

**D1354** Interim caries arresting medicament application — per tooth Ⓑ   **E1**

Conservative treatment of an active, non-symptomatic carious lesion by topical application of a caries arresting or inhibiting medicament and without mechanical removal of sound tooth structure.

## Space Maintenance (Passive Appliances)

↻ **D1510** Space maintainer - fixed - unilateral - per quadrant Ⓑ   **S**

Excludes a distal shoe space maintainer.

**D1516** Space Maintainer - fixed - bilateral, maxillary Ⓑ   **S**

**D1517** Space Maintainer - fixed - bilateral, mandibular Ⓑ   **S**

↻ **D1520** Space maintainer - removable - unilateral - per quadrant Ⓑ   **S**

**D1526** Space maintainer - removable - bilateral, maxillary Ⓑ   **S**

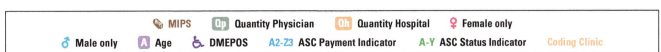

🐾 MIPS    **Qp** Quantity Physician    **Qh** Quantity Hospital    ♀ Female only

♂ **Male only**    Ⓐ Age    ♿ DMEPOS    **A2-Z3** ASC Payment Indicator    **A-Y** ASC Status Indicator    Coding Clinic

▶ **D1527** Space maintainer - removable - bilateral, mandibular Ⓑ  S

▶ **D1551** Re-cement or re-bond bilateral space maintainer - maxillary  S

▶ **D1552** Re-cement or re-bond bilateral space maintainer - mandibular  S

▶ **D1553** Re-cement or re-bond unilateral space maintainer - per quadrant  S

▶ **D1556** Removal of fixed unilateral space maintainer - per quadrant  E1

▶ **D1557** Removal of fixed bilateral space maintainer - maxillary  E1

▶ **D1558** Removal of fixed bilateral space maintainer - mandibular  E1

~~D1550~~ ~~Re-cement or re-bond space maintainer~~  ✖

~~D1555~~ ~~Removal of fixed space maintainer~~  ✖

## Space Maintainers

↻ **D1575** Distal shoe space maintainer - fixed - unilateral - per quadrant Ⓑ  S

Fabrication and delivery of fixed appliance extending subgingivally and distally to guide the eruption of the first permanent molar. Does not include ongoing follow-up or adjustments, or replacement appliances, once the tooth has erupted.

## None

**D1999** Unspecified preventive procedure, by report Ⓑ  E1

Used for procedure that is not adequately described by another CDT Code. Describe procedure.

## Restorative (D2140-D2999)
## Amalgam Restorations (Including Polishing)

**D2140** Amalgam - one surface, primary or permanent Ⓑ  E1

**D2150** Amalgam - two surfaces, primary or permanent Ⓑ  E1

**D2160** Amalgam - three surfaces, primary or permanent Ⓑ  E1

**D2161** Amalgam - four or more surfaces, primary or permanent Ⓑ  E1

## Resin-Based Composite Restorations – Direct

**D2330** Resin-based composite - one surface, anterior Ⓑ  E1

**D2331** Resin-based composite - two surfaces, anterior Ⓑ  E1

**D2332** Resin-based composite - three surfaces, anterior Ⓑ  E1

**D2335** Resin-based composite - four or more surfaces or involving incisal angle (anterior) Ⓑ  E1

Incisal angle to be defined as one of the angles formed by the junction of the incisal and the mesial or distal surface of an anterior tooth.

**D2390** Resin-based composite crown, anterior Ⓑ  E1

Full resin-based composite coverage of tooth.

**D2391** Resin-based composite - one surface, posterior Ⓑ  E1

Used to restore a carious lesion into the dentin or a deeply eroded area into the dentin. Not a preventive procedure.

**D2392** Resin-based composite - two surfaces, posterior Ⓑ  E1

**D2393** Resin-based composite - three surfaces, posterior Ⓑ  E1

**D2394** Resin-based composite - four or more surfaces, posterior Ⓑ  E1

## Gold Foil Restorations

**D2410** Gold foil - one surface Ⓑ  E1

**D2420** Gold foil - two surfaces Ⓑ  E1

**D2430** Gold foil - three surfaces Ⓑ  E1

## Inlay/Onlay Restorations

**D2510** Inlay - metallic - one surface Ⓑ  E1

**D2520** Inlay - metallic - two surfaces Ⓑ  E1

**D2530** Inlay - metallic - three or more surfaces Ⓑ  E1

**D2542** Onlay - metallic - two surfaces Ⓑ  E1

**D2543** Onlay - metallic - three surfaces Ⓑ  E1

**D2544** Onlay - metallic - four or more surfaces Ⓑ  E1

**D2610** Inlay - porcelain/ceramic - one surface Ⓑ  E1

**D2620** Inlay - porcelain/ceramic - two surfaces Ⓑ  E1

**D2630** Inlay - porcelain/ceramic - three or more surfaces Ⓑ  E1

**D2642** Onlay - porcelain/ceramic - two surfaces Ⓑ  E1

**D2643** Onlay - porcelain/ceramic - three surfaces Ⓑ  E1

---

▶ New  ↻ Revised  ✔ Reinstated  ~~deleted~~ Deleted  ⊘ Not covered or valid by Medicare
⊙ Special coverage instructions  ✳ Carrier discretion  Ⓑ Bill Part B MAC  Ⓓ Bill DME MAC

**D2644** Onlay - porcelain/ceramic - four or more surfaces Ⓑ    E1

**D2650** Inlay - resin-based composite - one surface Ⓑ    E1

**D2651** Inlay - resin-based composite - two surfaces Ⓑ    E1

**D2652** Inlay - resin-based composite - three or more surfaces Ⓑ    E1

**D2662** Onlay - resin-based composite - two surfaces Ⓑ    E1

**D2663** Onlay - resin-based composite - three surfaces Ⓑ    E1

**D2664** Onlay - resin-based composite - four or more surfaces Ⓑ    E1

## Crowns – Single Restoration Only

**D2710** Crown - resin-based composite (indirect) Ⓑ    E1

**D2712** Crown - 3/4 resin-based composite (indirect) Ⓑ    E1

> This procedure does not include facial veneers.

**D2720** Crown - resin with high noble metal Ⓑ    E1

**D2721** Crown - resin with predominantly base metal Ⓑ    E1

**D2722** Crown - resin with noble metal Ⓑ    E1

**D2740** Crown - porcelain/ceramic Ⓑ    E1

**D2750** Crown - porcelain fused to high noble metal Ⓑ    E1

**D2751** Crown - porcelain fused to predominantly base metal Ⓑ    E1

**D2752** Crown - porcelain fused to noble metal Ⓑ    E1

▶ **D2753** Crown - porcelain fused to titanium and titanium alloys    E1

**D2780** Crown - 3/4 cast high noble metal Ⓑ    E1

**D2781** Crown - 3/4 cast predominantly base metal Ⓑ    E1

**D2782** Crown - 3/4 cast noble metal Ⓑ    E1

**D2783** Crown - 3/4 porcelain/ceramic Ⓑ    E1

> This procedure does not include facial veneers.

**D2790** Crown - full cast high noble metal Ⓑ E1

**D2791** Crown - full cast predominantly base metal Ⓑ    E1

**D2792** Crown - full cast noble metal Ⓑ    E1

↻ **D2794** Crown - titanium and titanium alloys Ⓑ    E1

**D2799** Provisional crown - further treatment or completion of diagnosis necessary prior to final impression Ⓑ    E1

> Not to be used as a temporary crown for a routine prosthetic restoration.

## Other Restorative Services

**D2910** Re-cement or re-bond inlay, onlay, veneer or partial coverage restoration Ⓑ    E1

**D2915** Re-cement or re-bond indirectly fabricated cast or prefabricated post and core Ⓑ    E1

**D2920** Re-cement or re-bond crown Ⓑ    E1

**D2921** Reattachment of tooth fragment, incisal edge or cusp Ⓑ    E1

**D2929** Prefabricated porcelain/ceramic crown - primary tooth Ⓑ    E1

**D2930** Prefabricated stainless steel crown - primary tooth Ⓑ    E1

**D2931** Prefabricated stainless steel crown - permanent tooth Ⓑ    E1

**D2932** Prefabricated resin crown Ⓑ    E1

**D2933** Prefabricated stainless steel crown with resin window Ⓑ    E1

> Open-face stainless steel crown with aesthetic resin facing or veneer.

**D2934** Prefabricated esthetic coated stainless steel crown - primary tooth Ⓑ    E1

> Stainless steel primary crown with exterior esthetic coating.

**D2940** Protective restoration Ⓑ    E1

> Direct placement of a restorative material to protect tooth and/or tissue form. This procedure may be used to relieve pain, promote healing, or prevent further deterioration. Not to be used for endodontic access closure, or as a base or liner under a restoration.

**D2941** Interim therapeutic restoration - primary dentition Ⓑ    E1

> Placement of an adhesive restorative material following caries debridement by hand or other method for the management of early childhood caries. Not considered a definitive restoration.

**D2949** Restorative foundation for an indirect restoration Ⓑ    E1

> Placement of restorative material to yield a more ideal form, including elimination of undercuts.

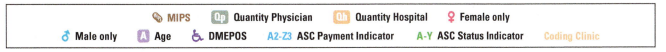

🐾 MIPS    **Qp** Quantity Physician    **Qh** Quantity Hospital    ♀ Female only

♂ **Male only**    Ⓐ **Age**    ♿ **DMEPOS**    **A2-Z3** ASC Payment Indicator    **A-Y** ASC Status Indicator    Coding Clinic

**D2950** Core build-up, including any pins when required Ⓑ                    **E1**

Refers to building up of coronal structure when there is insufficient retention for a separate extracoronal restorative procedure. A core build-up is not a filler to eliminate any undercut, box form, or concave irregularity in a preparation.

**D2951** Pin retention - per tooth, in addition to restoration Ⓑ                    **E1**

**D2952** Post and core in addition to crown, indirectly fabricated Ⓑ                    **E1**

Post and core are custom fabricated as a single unit.

**D2953** Each additional indirectly fabricated post - same tooth Ⓑ                    **E1**

To be used with D2952.

**D2954** Prefabricated post and core in addition to crown Ⓑ                    **E1**

Core is built around a prefabricated post. This procedure includes the core material.

**D2955** Post removal Ⓑ                    **E1**

**D2957** Each additional prefabricated post - same tooth Ⓑ                    **E1**

To be used with D2954.

**D2960** Labial veneer (laminate) - chairside Ⓑ **E1**

Refers to labial/facial direct resin bonded veneers.

**D2961** Labial veneer (resin laminate) - laboratory Ⓑ                    **E1**

Refers to labial/facial indirect resin bonded veneers.

**D2962** Labial veneer (porcelain laminate) - laboratory Ⓑ                    **E1**

Refers also to facial veneers that extend interproximally and/or cover the incisal edge. Porcelain/ceramic veneers presently include all ceramic and porcelain veneers.

**D2971** Additional procedures to construct new crown under existing partial denture framework Ⓑ                    **E1**

To be reported in addition to a crown code.

**D2975** Coping Ⓑ                    **E1**

A thin covering of the coronal portion of a tooth, usually devoid of anatomic contour, that can be used as a definitive restoration.

**D2980** Crown repair, necessitated by restorative material failure Ⓑ                    **E1**

**D2981** Inlay repair necessitated by restorative material failure Ⓑ                    **E1**

**D2982** Onlay repair necessitated by restorative material failure Ⓑ                    **E1**

**D2983** Veneer repair necessitated by restorative material failure Ⓑ                    **E1**

**D2990** Resin infiltration of incipient smooth surface lesions Ⓑ                    **E1**

Placement of an infiltrating resin restoration for strengthening, stabilizing and/or limiting the progression of the lesion.

### *None*

**D2999** Unspecified restorative procedure, by report Ⓑ                    **S**

Use for procedure that is not adequately described by a code. Describe procedure.

## Endodontics (D3110-D3999)
### *Pulp Capping*

**D3110** Pulp cap - direct (excluding final restoration) Ⓑ                    **E1**

Procedure in which the exposed pulp is covered with a dressing or cement that protects the pulp and promotes healing and repair.

**D3120** Pulp cap - indirect (excluding final restoration) Ⓑ                    **E1**

Procedure in which the nearly exposed pulp is covered with a protective dressing to protect the pulp from additional injury and to promote healing and repair via formation of secondary dentin. This code is not to be used for bases and liners when all caries has been removed.

### *Pulpotomy*

**D3220** Therapeutic pulpotomy (excluding final restoration) removal of pulp coronal to the dentinocemental junction and application of medicament Ⓑ                    **E1**

Pulpotomy is the surgical removal of a portion of the pulp with the aim of maintaining the vitality of the remaining portion by means of an adequate dressing.

– To be performed on primary or permanent teeth.

– This is not to be construed as the first stage of root canal therapy.

– Not to be used for apexogenesis.

▶ New   ↪ Revised   ✔ Reinstated   ~~deleted~~ Deleted   ⊘ Not covered or valid by Medicare
✳ Special coverage instructions   ✳ Carrier discretion   Ⓑ Bill Part B MAC   Ⓑ Bill DME MAC

**D3221** Pulpal debridement, primary and permanent teeth Ⓑ     E1

Pulpal debridement for the relief of acute pain prior to conventional root canal therapy. This procedure is not to be used when endodontic treatment is completed on the same day.

**D3222** Partial pulpotomy for apexogenesis - permanent tooth with incomplete root development Ⓑ     E1

Removal of a portion of the pulp and application of a medicament with the aim of maintaining the vitality of the remaining portion to encourage continued physiological development and formation of the root. This procedure is not to be construed as the first stage of root canal therapy.

## Endodontic Therapy on Primary Teeth

**D3230** Pulpal therapy (resorbable filling) - anterior, primary tooth (excluding final restoration) Ⓑ     E1

Primary incisors and cuspids.

**D3240** Pulpal therapy (resorbable filling) - posterior, primary tooth (excluding final restoration) Ⓑ     E1

Primary first and second molars.

## Endodontic Therapy (Including Treatment Plan, Clinical Procedures and Follow-Up Care)

**D3310** Endodontic therapy, anterior tooth (excluding final restoration) Ⓑ     E1

**D3320** Endodontic therapy, premolar tooth (excluding final restoration) Ⓑ     E1

**D3330** Endodontic therapy, molar (excluding final restoration) Ⓑ     E1

**D3331** Treatment of root canal obstruction; non-surgical access Ⓑ     E1

In lieu of surgery, the formation of a pathway to achieve an apical seal without surgical intervention because of a non-negotiable root canal blocked by foreign bodies, including but not limited to separated instruments, broken posts or calcification of 50% or more of the length of the tooth root.

**D3332** Incomplete endodontic therapy; inoperable, unrestorable or fractured tooth Ⓑ     E1

Considerable time is necessary to determine diagnosis and/or provide initial treatment before the fracture makes the tooth unretainable.

**D3333** Internal root repair of perforation defects Ⓑ     E1

Non-surgical seal of perforation caused by resorption and/or decay but not iatrogenic by provider filing claim.

## Endodontic Retreatment

**D3346** Retreatment of previous root canal therapy - anterior Ⓑ     E1

**D3347** Retreatment of previous root canal therapy - premolar Ⓑ     E1

**D3348** Retreatment of previous root canal therapy - molar Ⓑ     E1

## Apexification/Recalcification

**D3351** Apexification/recalcification - initial visit (apical closure/calcific repair of perforations, root resorption, etc.) Ⓑ E1

Includes opening tooth, preparation of canal spaces, first placement of medication and necessary radiographs. (This procedure may include first phase of complete root canal therapy.)

**D3352** Apexification/recalcification - interim medication replacement (apical closure/ calcific repair of perforations, root resorption, pulp space disinfection, etc.) Ⓑ     E1

For visits in which the intra-canal medication is replaced with new medication. Includes any necessary radiographs.

**D3353** Apexification/recalcification - final visit (includes completed root canal therapy - apical closure/calcific repair of perforations, root resorption, etc.) Ⓑ E1

Includes removal of intra-canal medication and procedures necessary to place final root canal filling material including necessary radiographs. (This procedure includes last phase of complete root canal therapy.)

## Pulpal Regeneration

**D3355** Pulpal regeneration - initial visit Ⓑ E1

Includes opening tooth, preparation of canal spaces, placement of medication.

**D3356** Pulpal regeneration - interim medication replacement Ⓑ     E1

**D3357** Pulpal regeneration - completion of treatment Ⓑ     E1

Does not include final restoration.

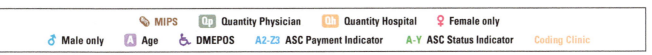

🐾 MIPS    Qp Quantity Physician    Qh Quantity Hospital    ♀ Female only

♂ Male only    A Age    ♿ DMEPOS    A2-Z3 ASC Payment Indicator    A-Y ASC Status Indicator    Coding Clinic

## Apicoectomy/Periradicular Services

**D3410** Apicoectomy - anterior Ⓑ    E1

For surgery on root of anterior tooth. Does not include placement of retrograde filling material.

**D3421** Apicoectomy - premolar (first root) ⒷE1

For surgery on one root of a premolar. Does not include placement of retrograde filling material. If more than one root is treated, see D3426.

**D3425** Apicoectomy - molar (first root) Ⓑ    E1

For surgery on one root of a molar tooth. Does not include placement of retrograde filling material. If more than one root is treated, see D3426.

**D3426** Apicoectomy (each additional root) ⒷE1

Typically used for premolar and molar surgeries when more than one root is treated during the same procedure. This does not include retrograde filling material placement.

**D3427** Periradicular surgery without apicoectomy Ⓑ    E1

**D3428** Bone graft in conjunction with periradicular surgery - per tooth, single site Ⓑ    E1

Includes non-autogenous graft material.

**D3429** Bone graft in conjunction with periradicular surgery - each additional contiguous tooth in the same surgical site Ⓑ    E1

Includes non-autogenous graft material.

**D3430** Retrograde filling - per root Ⓑ    E1

For placement of retrograde filling material during periradicular surgery procedures. If more than one filling is placed in one root - report as D3999 and describe.

**D3431** Bologic materials to aid in soft and osseous tissue regeneration in conjunction with periradicular surgery Ⓑ    E1

**D3432** Guided tissue regeneration, resorbable barrier, per site, in conjunction with periradicular surgery Ⓑ    E1

**D3450** Root amputation - per root Ⓑ    E1

Root resection of a multi-rooted tooth while leaving the crown. If the crown is sectioned, see D3920.

**D3460** Endodontic endosseous implant Ⓑ    S

Placement of implant material, which extends from a pulpal space into the bone beyond the end of the root.

**D3470** Intentional replantation (including necessary splinting) Ⓑ    E1

For the intentional removal, inspection and treatment of the root and replacement of a tooth into its own socket. This does not include necessary retrograde filling material placement.

## Other Endodontic Procedures

**D3910** Surgical procedure for isolation of tooth with rubber dam Ⓑ    E1

**D3920** Hemisection (including any root removal), not including root canal therapy Ⓑ    E1

Includes separation of a multi-rooted tooth into separate sections containing the root and the overlying portion of the crown. It may also include the removal of one or more of those sections.

**D3950** Canal preparation and fitting of preformed dowel or post Ⓑ    E1

Should not be reported in conjunction with D2952, D2953, D2954 or D2957 by the same practitioner.

## None

**D3999** Unspecified endodontic procedure, by report Ⓑ    S

Used for procedure that is not adequately described by a code. Describe procedure.

## Periodontics (D4210-D4999)
## Surgical Services (Including Usual Postoperative Care)

**D4210** Gingivectomy or gingivoplasty - four or more contiguous teeth or tooth bounded spaces per quadrant Ⓑ    E1

It is performed to eliminate suprabony pockets or to restore normal architecture when gingival enlargements or asymmetrical or unaesthetic topography is evident with normal bony configuration.

*Cross Reference 41820*

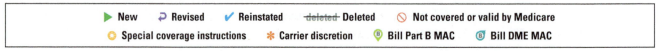

▶ New    ↺ Revised    ✔ Reinstated    ~~deleted~~ Deleted    ⊘ Not covered or valid by Medicare
✲ Special coverage instructions    ✳ Carrier discretion    Ⓑ Bill Part B MAC    Ⓑ Bill DME MAC

**D4211** Gingivectomy or gingivoplasty - one to three contiguous teeth or tooth bounded spaces per quadrant Ⓑ    E1

It is performed to eliminate suprabony pockets or to restore normal architecture when gingival enlargements or asymmetrical or unaesthetic topography is evident with normal bony configuration.

**D4212** Gingivectomy or gingivoplasty to allow access for restorative procedure, per tooth Ⓑ    E1

**D4230** Anatomical crown exposure - four or more contiguous teeth or bounded tooth spaces per quadrant Ⓑ    E1

This procedure is utilized in an otherwise periodontally healthy area to remove enlarged gingival tissue and supporting bone (ostectomy) to provide an anatomically correct gingival relationship.

**D4231** Anatomical crown exposure - one to three teeth or bounded tooth spaces per quadrant Ⓑ    E1

This procedure is utilized in an otherwise periodontally healthy area to remove enlarged gingival tissue and supporting bone (ostectomy) to provide an anatomically correct gingival relationship.

**D4240** Gingival flap procedure, including root planing - four or more contiguous teeth or tooth bounded spaces per quadrant Ⓑ    E1

A soft tissue flap is reflected or resected to allow debridement of the root surface and the removal of granulation tissue. Osseous recontouring is not accomplished in conjunction with this procedure. May include open flap curettage, reverse bevel flap surgery, modified Kirkland flap procedure, and modified Widman surgery. This procedure is performed in the presence of moderate to deep probing depths, loss of attachment, need to maintain esthetics, need for increased access to the root surface and alveolar bone, or to determine the presence of a cracked tooth, fractured root, or external root resorption. Other procedures may be required concurrent to D4240 and should be reported separately using their own unique codes.

**D4241** Gingival flap procedure, including root planing - one to three contiguous teeth or tooth bounded spaces per quadrant Ⓑ    E1

A soft tissue flap is reflected or resected to allow debridement of the root surface and the removal of granulation tissue. Osseous recontouring is not accomplished in conjunction with this procedure. May include open flap curettage, reverse bevel flap surgery, modified Kirkland flap procedure, and modified Widman surgery. This procedure is performed in the presence of moderate to deep probing depths, loss of attachment, need to maintain esthetics, need for increased access to the root surface and alveolar bone, or to determine the presence of a cracked tooth, fractured root, or external root resorption. Other procedures may be required concurrent to D4241 and should be reported separately using their own unique codes.

**D4245** Apically positioned flap Ⓑ    E1

Procedure is used to preserve keratinized gingiva in conjunction with osseous resection and second stage implant procedure. Procedure may also be used to preserve keratinized/ attached gingiva during surgical exposure of labially impacted teeth, and may be used during treatment of peri-implantitis.

**D4249** Clinical crown lengthening - hard tissue Ⓑ    E1

This procedure is employed to allow a restorative procedure on a tooth with little or no tooth structure exposed to the oral cavity. Crown lengthening requires reflection of a full thickness flap and removal of bone, altering the crown to root ratio. It is performed in a healthy periodontal environment, as opposed to osseous surgery, which is performed in the presence of periodontal disease.

🦢 MIPS    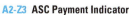 Quantity Physician     Quantity Hospital    ♀ Female only

♂ Male only    Ⓐ Age    ♿ DMEPOS    A2-Z3 ASC Payment Indicator    A-Y ASC Status Indicator    Coding Clinic

**D4260** Osseous surgery (including elevation of a full thickness flap and closure) - four or more contiguous teeth or tooth bounded spaces per quadrant Ⓑ  **S**

This procedure modifies the bony support of the teeth by reshaping the alveolar process to achieve a more physiologic form during the surgical procedure. This must include the removal of supporting bone (ostectomy) and/or non-supporting bone (osteoplasty). Other procedures may be required concurrent to D4260 and should be reported using their own unique codes.

**D4261** Osseous surgery (including elevation of a full thickness flap and closure) - one to three contiguous teeth or tooth bounded spaces per quadrant Ⓑ  **E1**

This procedure modifies the bony support of the teeth by reshaping the alveolar process to achieve a more physiologic form during the surgical procedure. This must include the removal of supporting bone (ostectomy) and/or non-supporting bone (osteoplasty). Other procedures may be required concurrent to D4261 and should be reported using their own unique codes.

**D4263** Bone replacement graft - retained natural tooth - first site in quadrant Ⓑ **S**

This procedure involves the use of grafts to stimulate periodontal regeneration when the disease process has led to a deformity of the bone. This procedure does not include flap entry and closure, wound debridement, osseous contouring, or the placement of biologic materials to aid in osseous tissue regeneration or barrier membranes. Other separate procedures delivered concurrently are documented with their own codes. Not to be reported for an edentulous space or an extraction site.

**D4264** Bone replacement graft - retained natural tooth - each additional site in quadrant Ⓑ  **S**

This procedure involves the use of grafts to stimulate periodontal regeneration when the disease process has led to a deformity of the bone. This procedure does not include flap entry and closure, wound debridement, osseous contouring, or the placement of biologic materials to aid in osseous tissue regeneration or barrier membranes. This procedure is performed concurrently with one or more bone replacement grafts to document the number of sites involved. Not to be reported for an edentulous space or an extraction site.

**D4265** Biologic materials to aid in soft and osseous tissue regeneration Ⓑ  **E1**

Biologic materials may be used alone or with other regenerative substrates such as bone and barrier membranes, depending upon their formulation and the presentation of the periodontal defect. This procedure does not include surgical entry and closure, wound debridement, osseous contouring, or the placement of graft materials and/or barrier membranes. Other separate procedures may be required concurrent to D4265 and should be reported using their own unique codes.

**D4266** Guided tissue regeneration - resorbable barrier, per site Ⓑ  **E1**

This procedure does not include flap entry and closure, or, when indicated, wound debridement, osseous contouring, bone replacement grafts, and placement of biologic materials to aid in osseous regeneration. This procedure can be used for periodontal and peri-implant defects.

**D4267** Guided tissue regeneration - nonresorbable barrier, per site, (includes membrane removal) Ⓑ  **E1**

This procedure does not include flap entry and closure, or, when indicated, wound debridement, osseous contouring, bone replacement grafts, and placement of biologic materials to aid in osseous regeneration. This procedure can be used for periodontal and peri-implant defects.

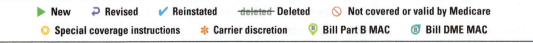

▶ New   ↺ Revised   ✔ Reinstated   ~~deleted~~ Deleted   ⊘ Not covered or valid by Medicare   ✱ Special coverage instructions   ✳ Carrier discretion   Ⓑ Bill Part B MAC   Ⓑ Bill DME MAC

**D4268** Surgical revision procedure, per tooth Ⓑ S

This procedure is to refine the results of a previously provided surgical procedure. This may require a surgical procedure to modify the irregular contours of hard or soft tissue. A mucoperiosteal flap may be elevated to allow access to reshape alveolar bone. The flaps are replaced or repositioned and sutured.

**D4270** Pedicle soft tissue graft procedure Ⓑ S

A pedicle flap of gingiva can be raised from an edentulous ridge, adjacent teeth, or from the existing gingiva on the tooth and moved laterally or coronally to replace alveolar mucosa as marginal tissue. The procedure can be used to cover an exposed root or to eliminate a gingival defect if the root is not too prominent in the arch.

**D4273** Autogenous connective tissue graft procedure (including donor and recipient surgical sites) first tooth, implant, or edentulous tooth position in graft Ⓑ S

There are two surgical sites. The recipient site utilizes a split thickness incision, retaining the overlapping flap of gingiva and/or mucosa. The connective tissue is dissected from a separate donor site leaving an epithelialized flap for closure.

**D4274** Mesial/distal wedge procedure, single tooth (when not performed in conjuction with surgical procedures in the same anatomical area) Ⓑ E1

This procedure is performed in an edentulous area adjacent to a tooth, allowing removal of a tissue wedge to gain access for debridement, permit close flap adaptation, and reduce pocket depths.

**D4275** Non-autogenous connective tissue graft (including recipient site and donor material) first tooth, implant, or edentulous tooth position in graft Ⓑ E1

There is only a recipient surgical site utilizing split thickness incision, retaining the overlaying flap of gingiva and/or mucosa. A donor surgical site is not present.

**D4276** Combined connective tissue and double pedicle graft, per tooth Ⓑ E1

Advanced gingival recession often cannot be corrected with a single procedure. Combined tissue grafting procedures are needed to achieve the desired outcome.

**D4277** Free soft tissue graft procedure (including recipient and donor surgical sites) first tooth, implant or edentulous tooth position in graft Ⓑ E1

**D4278** Free soft tissue graft procedure (including recipient and donor surgical sites) each additional contiguous tooth, implant or edentulous tooth position in same graft site Ⓑ E1

Used in conjunction with D4277.

**D4283** Autogenous connective tissue graft procedure (including donor and recipient surgical sites) - each additional contiguous tooth, implant or edentulous tooth position in same graft site Ⓑ E1

Used in conjunction with D4273.

**D4285** Non-autogenous connective tissue graft procedure (including recipient surgical site and donor material) - each additional contiguous tooth, implant or edentulous tooth position in same graft site Ⓑ E1

Used in conjunction with D4275.

## Non-Surgical Periodontal Services

**D4320** Provisional splinting - intracoronal Ⓑ E1

This is an interim stabilization of mobile teeth. A variety of methods and appliances may be employed for this purpose. Identify the teeth involved.

**D4321** Provisional splinting - extracoronal Ⓑ E1

This is an interim stabilization of mobile teeth. A variety of methods and appliances may be employed for this purpose. Identify the teeth involved.

---

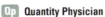 MIPS     Quantity Physician     Quantity Hospital    ♀ Female only

♂ Male only     Age     DMEPOS    A2-Z3 ASC Payment Indicator    A-Y ASC Status Indicator    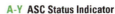 Coding Clinic

**D4341** Periodontal scaling and root planing - four or more teeth per quadrant ⑧ **E1**

This procedure involves instrumentation of the crown and root surfaces of the teeth to remove plaque and calculus from these surfaces. It is indicated for patients with periodontal disease and is therapeutic, not prophylactic, in nature. Root planing is the definitive procedure designed for the removal of cementum and dentin that is rough, and/or permeated by calculus or contaminated with toxins or microorganisms. Some soft tissue removal occurs. This procedure may be used as a definitive treatment in some stages of periodontal disease and/or as a part of pre-surgical procedures in others.

**D4342** Periodontal scaling and root planing - one to three teeth, per quadrant ⑧ **E1**

This procedure involves instrumentation of the crown and root surfaces of the teeth to remove plaque and calculus from these surfaces. It is indicated for patients with periodontal disease and is therapeutic, not prophylactic, in nature. Root planing is the definitive procedure designed for the removal of cementum and dentin that is rough, and/or permeated by calculus or contaminated with toxins or microorganisms. Some soft tissue removal occurs. This procedure may be used as a definitive treatment in some stages of periodontal disease and/or as a part of pre-surgical procedures in others.

**D4346** Scaling in presence of generalized moderate or severe gingival inflammation - full mouth, after oral evaluation ⑧ **E1**

The removal of plaque, calculus and stains from supra- and sub-gingival tooth surfaces when there is generalized moderate or severe gingival inflammation in the absence of periodontitis. It is indicated for patients who have swollen, inflamed gingiva, generalized suprabony pockets, and moderate to severe bleeding on probing. Should not be reported in conjunction with prophylaxis, scaling and root planing, or debridement procedures.

**D4355** Full mouth debridement to enable a comprehensive oral evaluation and diagnosis on a subsequent visit ⑧ **S**

Full mouth debridement involves the preliminary removal of plaque and calculus that interferes with the ability of the dentist to perform a comprehensive oral evaluation. Not to be completed on the same day as D0150, D0160, or D0180.

**D4381** Localized delivery of antimicrobial agents via a controlled release vehicle into diseased crevicular tissue, per tooth ⑧ **S**

FDA approved subgingival delivery devices containing antimicrobial medication(s) are inserted into periodontal pockets to suppress the pathogenic microbiota. These devices slowly release the pharmacological agents so they can remain at the intended site of action in a therapeutic concentration for a sufficient length of time.

## Other Periodontal Services

**D4910** Periodontal maintenance ⑧ **E1**

This procedure is instituted following periodontal therapy and continues at varying intervals, determined by the clinical evaluation of the dentist, for the life of the dentition or any implant replacements. It includes removal of the bacterial plaque and calculus from supragingival and subgingival regions, site specific scaling and root planing where indicated, and polishing the teeth. If new or recurring periodontal disease appears, additional diagnostic and treatment procedures must be considered.

**D4920** Unscheduled dressing change (by someone other than treating dentist or their staff) ⑧ **E1**

**D4921** Gingival irrigation - per quadrant ⑧ **E1**

Irrigation of gingival pockets with medicinal agent. Not to be used to report use of mouth rinses or non-invasive chemical debridement.

## None

**D4999** Unspecified periodontal procedure, by report ⑧ **E1**

Use for procedure that is not adequately described by a code. Describe procedure.

▶ New　↻ Revised　✔ Reinstated　~~deleted~~ Deleted　⊘ Not covered or valid by Medicare

⊙ Special coverage instructions　✱ Carrier discretion　⑧ Bill Part B MAC　Ⓓ Bill DME MAC

## Prosthodontics (removable)
### Complete Dentures (Including Routine Post-Delivery Care)

**D5110**  Complete denture - maxillary Ⓑ  E1

**D5120**  Complete denture - mandibular Ⓑ  E1

**D5130**  Immediate denture - maxillary Ⓑ  E1

Includes limited follow-up care only; does not include required future rebasing/relining procedure(s).

**D5140**  Immediate denture - mandibular Ⓑ  E1

Includes limited follow-up care only; does not include required future rebasing/relining procedure(s).

### Partial Dentures (Including Routine Post-Delivery Care)

**D5211**  Maxillary partial denture-resin base (including retentive/clasping materials, rests and teeth) Ⓑ  E1

Includes acrylic resin base denture with resin or wrought wire clasps.

**D5212**  Mandibular partial denture-resin base (including, retentive/clasping materials, rests and teeth) Ⓑ  E1

Includes acrylic resin base denture with resin or wrought wire clasps.

↻ **D5213**  Maxillary partial denture - cast metal framework with resin denture bases (including retentive/clasping materials, rests and teeth) Ⓑ  E1

↻ **D5214**  Mandibular partial denture - cast metal framework with resin denture bases (including retentive/clasping materials, rests and teeth) Ⓑ  E1

↻ **D5221**  Immediate maxillary partial denture - resin base (including retentive/clasping materials, rests and teeth) Ⓑ  E1

Includes limited follow-up care only; does not include future rebasing/relining procedure(s).

↻ **D5222**  Immediate mandibular partial denture - resin base (including retentive/clasping materials, rests and teeth) Ⓑ  E1

Includes limited follow-up care only; does not include future rebasing/relining procedure(s).

↻ **D5223**  Immediate maxillary partial denture - cast metal framework with resin denture bases (including retentive/clasping materials, rests and teeth) Ⓑ  E1

Includes limited follow-up care only; does not include future rebasing/relining procedure(s).

↻ **D5224**  Immediate mandibular partial denture - cast metal framework with resin denture bases (including retentive/clasping materials, rests and teeth) Ⓑ  E1

Includes limited follow-up care only; does not include future rebasing/relining procedure(s).

**D5225**  Maxillary partial denture - flexible base (including any clasps, rests and teeth) Ⓑ  E1

**D5226**  Mandibular partial denture - flexible base (including any clasps, rests and teeth) Ⓑ  E1

**D5282**  Removable unilateral partial denture - one piece cast metal (including clasps and teeth), maxillary Ⓑ  E1

**D5283**  Removable unilateral partial denture - one piece cast metal (including clasps and teeth), mandibular Ⓑ  E1

▶ **D5284**  Removable unilateral partial denture - one piece flexible base (including clasps and teeth) - per quadrant  E1

▶ **D5286**  Removable unilateral partial denture - one piece resin (including clasps and teeth) - per quadrant  E1

### Adjustment to Dentures

**D5410**  Adjust complete denture - maxillary Ⓑ  E1

**D5411**  Adjust complete denture - mandibular Ⓑ  E1

**D5421**  Adjust partial denture - maxillary Ⓑ  E1

**D5422**  Adjust partial denture - mandibular Ⓑ  E1

### Repairs to Complete Dentures

**D5511**  Repair broken complete denture base, mandibular Ⓑ  E1

**D5512**  Repair broken complete denture base, maxillary Ⓑ  E1

**D5520**  Replace missing or broken teeth-complete denture (each tooth) Ⓑ  E1

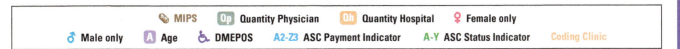

🐾 MIPS    Ⓞⓟ Quantity Physician    Ⓠⓗ Quantity Hospital    ♀ Female only
♂ Male only    Ⓐ Age    ♿ DMEPOS    A2-Z3 ASC Payment Indicator    A-Y ASC Status Indicator    Coding Clinic

DENTAL PROCEDURES   D5110 — D5520

## Repairs to Partial Dentures

**D5611** Repair resin partial denture base, mandibular Ⓑ **E1**

**D5612** Repair resin partial denture base, maxillary Ⓑ **E1**

**D5621** Repair cast partial framework, mandibular Ⓑ **E1**

**D5622** Repair cast partial framework, maxillary Ⓑ **E1**

**D5630** Repair or replace broken, retentive clasping materials - per tooth Ⓑ **E1**

**D5640** Replace broken teeth - per tooth Ⓑ **E1**

**D5650** Add tooth to existing partial denture Ⓑ **E1**

**D5660** Add clasp to existing partial denture - per tooth Ⓑ **E1**

**D5670** Replace all teeth and acrylic on cast metal framework (maxillary) Ⓑ **E1**

**D5671** Replace all teeth and acrylic on cast metal framework (mandibular) Ⓑ **E1**

## Denture Rebase Procedures

**D5710** Rebase complete maxillary denture Ⓑ**E1**

**D5711** Rebase complete mandibular denture Ⓑ **E1**

**D5720** Rebase maxillary partial denture Ⓑ **E1**

**D5721** Rebase mandibular partial denture Ⓑ **E1**

## Denture Reline Procedures

**D5730** Reline complete maxillary denture (chairside) Ⓑ **E1**

**D5731** Reline lower complete mandibular denture (chairside) Ⓑ **E1**

**D5740** Reline maxillary partial denture (chairside) Ⓑ **E1**

**D5741** Reline mandibular partial denture (chairside) Ⓑ **E1**

**D5750** Reline complete maxillary denture (laboratory) Ⓑ **E1**

**D5751** Reline complete mandibular denture (laboratory) Ⓑ **E1**

**D5760** Reline maxillary partial denture (laboratory) Ⓑ **E1**

**D5761** Reline mandibular partial denture (laboratory) Ⓑ **E1**

## Interim Prosthesis

**D5810** Interim complete denture (maxillary) Ⓑ **E1**

**D5811** Interim complete denture (mandibular) Ⓑ **E1**

**D5820** Interim partial denture (maxillary) Ⓑ **E1**

Includes any necessary clasps and rests.

**D5821** Interim partial denture (mandibular) Ⓑ **E1**

Includes any necessary clasps and rests.

## Other Removable Prosthetic Services

**D5850** Tissue conditioning, maxillary Ⓑ **E1**

Treatment reline using materials designed to heal unhealthy ridges prior to more definitive final restoration.

**D5851** Tissue conditioning, mandibular Ⓑ **E1**

Treatment reline using materials designed to heal unhealthy ridges prior to more definitive final restoration.

**D5862** Precision attachment, by report Ⓑ **E1**

Each set of male and female components should be reported as one precision attachment. Describe the type of attachment used.

**D5863** Overdenture - complete maxillary Ⓑ **E1**

**D5864** Overdenture - partial maxillary Ⓑ **E1**

**D5865** Overdenture - complete mandibular Ⓑ **E1**

**D5866** Overdenture - partial mandibular Ⓑ **E1**

**D5867** Replacement of replaceable part of semi-precision or precision attachment (male or female component) Ⓑ **E1**

**D5875** Modification of removable prosthesis following implant surgery Ⓑ **E1**

Attachment assemblies are reported using separate codes.

**D5876** Add metal substructure to acrylic full denture (per arch) Ⓑ **E1**

## None

**D5899** Unspecified removable prosthodontic procedure, by report Ⓑ **E1**

Use for a procedure that is not adequately described by a code. Describe procedure.

---

▶ New   ↩ Revised   ✔ Reinstated   ~~deleted~~ Deleted   ⊘ Not covered or valid by Medicare
⊙ Special coverage instructions   ✳ Carrier discretion   Ⓑ Bill Part B MAC   Ⓑ Bill DME MAC

## Maxillofacial Prosthetics

**D5911**  Facial moulage (sectional) Ⓑ  S

A sectional facial moulage impression is a procedure used to record the soft tissue contours of a portion of the face. Occasionally several separate sectional impressions are made, then reassembled to provide a full facial contour cast. The impression is utilized to create a partial facial moulage and generally is not reusable.

**D5912**  Facial moulage (complete) Ⓑ  S

Synonymous terminology: facial impression, face mask impression. A complete facial moulage impression is a procedure used to record the soft tissue contours of the whole face. The impression is utilized to create a facial moulage and generally is not reusable.

**D5913**  Nasal prosthesis Ⓑ  E1

Synonymous terminology: artificial nose. A removable prosthesis attached to the skin, which artificially restores part or all of the nose. Fabrication of a nasal prosthesis requires creation of an original mold. Additional prostheses usually can be made from the same mold, and assuming no further tissue changes occur, the same mold can be utilized for extended periods of time. When a new prosthesis is made from the existing mold, this procedure is termed a nasal prosthesis replacement.

*Cross Reference 21087*

**D5914**  Auricular prosthesis Ⓑ  E1

Synonymous terminology: artificial ear, ear prosthesis. A removable prosthesis, which artificially restores part or all of the natural ear. Usually, replacement prostheses can be made from the original mold if tissue bed changes have not occurred. Creation of an auricular prosthesis requires fabrication of a mold, from which additional prostheses usually can be made, as needed later (auricular prosthesis, replacement).

*Cross Reference 21086*

**D5915**  Orbital prosthesis Ⓑ  E1

A prosthesis, which artificially restores the eye, eyelids, and adjacent hard and soft tissue, lost as a result of trauma or surgery. Fabrication of an orbital prosthesis requires creation of an original mold. Additional prostheses usually can be made from the same mold, and assuming no further tissue changes occur, the same mold can be utilized for extended periods of time. When a new prosthesis is made from the existing mold, this procedure is termed an orbital prosthesis replacement.

*Cross Reference L8611*

**D5916**  Ocular prosthesis Ⓑ  E1

Synonymous terminology: artificial eye, glass eye. A prosthesis, which artificially replaces an eye missing as a result of trauma, surgery or congenital absence. The prosthesis does not replace missing eyelids or adjacent skin, mucosa or muscle. Ocular prostheses require semiannual or annual cleaning and polishing. Also, occasional revisions to re-adapt the prosthesis to the tissue bed may be necessary. Glass eyes are rarely made and cannot be re-adapted.

*Cross Reference V2623, V2629*

**D5919**  Facial prosthesis Ⓑ  E1

Synonymous terminology: prosthetic dressing. A removable prosthesis, which artificially replaces a portion of the face, lost due to surgery, trauma or congenital absence. Flexion of natural tissues may preclude adaptation and movement of the prosthesis to match the adjacent skin. Salivary leakage, when communicating with the oral cavity, adversely affects retention.

*Cross Reference 21088*

**D5922**  Nasal septal prosthesis Ⓑ  E1

Synonymous terminology: septal plug, septal button. Removable prosthesis to occlude (obturate) a hole within the nasal septal wall. Adverse chemical degradation in this moist environment may require frequent replacement. Silicone prostheses are occasionally subject to fungal invasion.

*Cross Reference 30220*

   MIPS  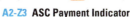 Quantity Physician  Quantity Hospital  ♀ Female only
♂ Male only  Ⓐ Age  DMEPOS  A2-Z3 ASC Payment Indicator  A-Y ASC Status Indicator  Coding Clinic
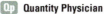  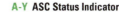

**173**

**D5923**    Ocular prosthesis, interim Ⓑ    E1

Synonymous terminology: eye shell, shell, ocular conformer, conformer. A temporary replacement generally made of clear acrylic resin for an eye lost due to surgery or trauma. No attempt is made to re-establish aesthetics. Fabrication of an interim ocular prosthesis generally implies subsequent fabrication of an aesthetic ocular prosthesis.

*Cross Reference 92330*

**D5924**    Cranial prosthesis Ⓑ    E1

Synonymous terminology: skull plate, cranioplasty prosthesis, cranial implant. A biocompatible, permanently implanted replacement of a portion of the skull bones; an artificial replacement for a portion of the skull bone.

*Cross Reference 62143*

**D5925**    Facial augmentation implant prosthesis Ⓑ    E1

Synonymous terminology: facial implant. An implantable biocompatible material generally onlayed upon an existing bony area beneath the skin tissue to fill in or collectively raise portions of the overlaying facial skin tissues to create acceptable contours. Although some forms of pre-made surgical implants are commercially available, the facial augmentation is usually custom made for surgical implantation for each individual patient due to the irregular or extensive nature of the facial deficit.

*Cross Reference 21208*

**D5926**    Nasal prosthesis, replacement Ⓑ    E1

Synonymous terminology: replacement nose. An artificial nose produced from a previously made mold. A replacement prosthesis does not require fabrication of a new mold. Generally, several prostheses can be made from the same mold assuming no changes occur in the tissue bed due to surgery or age related topographical variations.

*Cross Reference 21087*

**D5927**    Auricular prosthesis, replacement Ⓑ    E1

Synonymous terminology: replacement ear. An artificial ear produced from a previously made mold. A replacement prosthesis does not require fabrication of a new mold. Generally, several prostheses can be made from the same mold assuming no changes occur in the tissue bed due to surgery or age related topographical variations.

*Cross Reference 21086*

**D5928**    Orbital prosthesis, replacement Ⓑ    E1

A replacement for a previously made orbital prosthesis. A replacement prosthesis does not require fabrication of a new mold. Generally, several prostheses can be made from the same mold assuming no changes occur in the tissue bed due to surgery or age related topographical variations.

*Cross Reference 67550*

**D5929**    Facial prosthesis, replacement Ⓑ    E1

A replacement facial prosthesis made from the original mold. A replacement prosthesis does not require fabrication of a new mold. Generally, several prostheses can be made from the same mold assuming no changes occur in the tissue bed due to further surgery or age related topographical variations.

*Cross Reference 21088*

**D5931**    Obturator prosthesis, surgical Ⓑ    E1

Synonymous terminology: obturator, surgical stayplate, immediate temporary obturator. A temporary prosthesis inserted during or immediately following surgical or traumatic loss of a portion or all of one or both maxillary bones and contiguous alveolar structures (e.g., gingival tissue, teeth). Frequent revisions of surgical obturators are necessary during the ensuing healing phase (approximately six months). Some dentists prefer to replace many or all teeth removed by the surgical procedure in the surgical obturator, while others do not replace any teeth. Further surgical revisions may require fabrication of another surgical obturator (e.g., an initially planned small defect may be revised and greatly enlarged after the final pathology report indicates margins are not free of tumor).

*Cross Reference 21079*

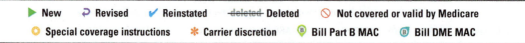

▶ New    ↻ Revised    ✔ Reinstated    ~~deleted~~ Deleted    ⊘ Not covered or valid by Medicare
✪ Special coverage instructions    ✳ Carrier discretion    Ⓑ Bill Part B MAC    Ⓓ Bill DME MAC

**D5932**  Obturator prosthesis, definitive Ⓑ  **E1**

Synonymous terminology: obturator. A prosthesis, which artificially replaces part or all of the maxilla and associated teeth, lost due to surgery, trauma or congenital defects. A definitive obturator is made when it is deemed that further tissue changes or recurrence of tumor are unlikely and a more permanent prosthetic rehabilitation can be achieved; it is intended for long-term use.

*Cross Reference 21080*

**D5933**  Obturator prosthesis, modification Ⓑ **E1**

Synonymous terminology: adjustment, denture adjustment, temporary or office reline. Revision or alteration of an existing obturator (surgical, interim, or definitive); possible modifications include relief of the denture base due to tissue compression, augmentation of the seal or peripheral areas to affect adequate sealing or separation between the nasal and oral cavities.

*Cross Reference 21080*

**D5934**  Mandibular resection prosthesis with guide flange Ⓑ  **E1**

Synonymous terminology: resection device, resection appliance. A prosthesis which guides the remaining portion of the mandible, left after a partial resection, into a more normal relationship with the maxilla. This allows for some tooth-to-tooth or an improved tooth contact. It may also artificially replace missing teeth and thereby increase masticatory efficiency.

*Cross Reference 21081*

**D5935**  Mandibular resection prosthesis without guide flange Ⓑ  **E1**

A prosthesis which helps guide the partially resected mandible to a more normal relation with the maxilla allowing for increased tooth contact. It does not have a flange or ramp, however, to assist in directional closure. It may replace missing teeth and thereby increase masticatory efficiency. Dentists who treat mandibulectomy patients may prefer to replace some, all or none of the teeth in the defect area. Frequently, the defect's margins preclude even partial replacement. Use of a guide (a mandibular resection prosthesis with a guide flange) may not be possible due to anatomical limitations or poor patient tolerance. Ramps, extended occlusal arrangements and irregular occlusal positioning relative to the denture foundation frequently preclude stability of the prostheses, and thus some prostheses are poorly tolerated under such adverse circumstances.

*Cross Reference 21081*

**D5936**  Obturator/prosthesis, interim Ⓑ  **E1**

Synonymous terminology: immediate postoperative obturator. A prosthesis which is made following completion of the initial healing after a surgical resection of a portion or all of one or both the maxillae; frequently many or all teeth in the defect area are replaced by this prosthesis. This prosthesis replaces the surgical obturator, which is usually inserted at, or immediately following the resection.

Generally, an interim obturator is made to facilitate closure of the resultant defect after initial healing has been completed. Unlike the surgical obturator, which usually is made prior to surgery and frequently revised in the operating room during surgery, the interim obturator is made when the defect margins are clearly defined and further surgical revisions are not planned. It is a provisional prosthesis, which may replace some or all lost teeth, and other lost bone and soft tissue structures. Also, it frequently must be revised (termed an obturator prosthesis modification) during subsequent dental procedures (e.g., restorations, gingival surgery) as well as to compensate for further tissue shrinkage before a definitive obturator prosthesis is made.

*Cross Reference 21079*

---

 **MIPS**      **Quantity Physician**      **Quantity Hospital**     ♀ **Female only**

♂ **Male only**      **Age**      **DMEPOS**     **A2-Z3 ASC Payment Indicator**     **A-Y ASC Status Indicator**     *Coding Clinic*

**D5937**   Trismus appliance (not for tm treatment) Ⓑ                              E1

Synonymous terminology: occlusal device for mandibular trismus, dynamic bite opener. A prosthesis, which assists the patient in increasing their oral aperture width in order to eat as well as maintain oral hygiene. Several versions and designs are possible, all intending to ease the severe lack of oral opening experienced by many patients immediately following extensive intraoral surgical procedures.

**D5951**   Feeding aid Ⓑ                                      E1

Synonymous terminology: feeding prosthesis. A prosthesis, which maintains the right and left maxillary segments of an infant cleft palate patient in their proper orientation until surgery is performed to repair the cleft. It closes the oral-nasal cavity defect, thus enhancing sucking and swallowing. Used on an interim basis, this prosthesis achieves separation of the oral and nasal cavities in infants born with wide clefts necessitating delayed closure. It is eliminated if surgical closure can be affected or, alternatively, with eruption of the deciduous dentition a pediatric speech aid may be made to facilitate closure of the defect.

**D5952**   Speech aid prosthesis, pediatric Ⓑ Ⓐ E1

Synonymous terminology: nasopharyngeal obturator, speech appliance, obturator, cleft palate appliance, prosthetic speech aid, speech bulb. A temporary or interim prosthesis used to close a defect in the hard and/or soft palate. It may replace tissue lost due to developmental or surgical alterations. It is necessary for the production of intelligible speech. Normal lateral growth of the palatal bones necessitates occasional replacement of this prosthesis. Intermittent revisions of the obturator section can assist in maintenance of palatalpharyngeal closure (termed a speech aid prosthesis modification). Frequently, such prostheses are not fabricated before the deciduous dentition is fully erupted since clasp retention is often essential.

*Cross Reference 21084*

**D5953**   Speech aid prosthesis, adult Ⓑ Ⓐ   E1

Synonymous terminology: prosthetic speech appliance, speech aid, speech bulb. A definitive prosthesis, which can improve speech in adult cleft palate patients either by obturating (sealing off) a palatal cleft or fistula, or occasionally by assisting an incompetent soft palate. Both mechanisms are necessary to achieve velopharyngeal competency. Generally, this prosthesis is fabricated when no further growth is anticipated and the objective is to achieve long-term use. Hence, more precise materials and techniques are utilized. Occasionally such procedures are accomplished in conjunction with precision attachments in crown work undertaken on some or all maxillary teeth to achieve improved aesthetics.

*Cross Reference 21084*

**D5954**   Palatal augmentation prosthesis Ⓑ   E1

Synonymous terminology: superimposed prosthesis, maxillary glossectomy prosthesis, maxillary speech prosthesis, palatal drop prosthesis. A removable prosthesis which alters the hard and/or soft palate's topographical form adjacent to the tongue.

*Cross Reference 21082*

**D5955**   Palatal lift prosthesis, definitive Ⓑ   E1

A prosthesis which elevates the soft palate superiorly and aids in restoration of soft palate functions which may be lost due to an acquired, congenital or developmental defect. A definitive palatal lift is usually made for patients whose experience with an interim palatal lift has been successful, especially if surgical alterations are deemed unwarranted.

*Cross Reference 21083*

---

▶ New   ↩ Revised   ✔ Reinstated   deleted Deleted   ⊘ Not covered or valid by Medicare
⊙ Special coverage instructions   ✳ Carrier discretion   Ⓑ Bill Part B MAC   Ⓑ Bill DME MAC

**D5958**  Palatal lift prosthesis, interim ⓑ **E1**

Synonymous terminology: diagnostic palatal lift. A prosthesis which elevates and assists in restoring soft palate function which may be lost due to clefting, surgery, trauma or unknown paralysis. It is intended for interim use to determine its usefulness in achieving palatalpharyngeal competency or enhance swallowing reflexes. This prosthesis is intended for interim use as a diagnostic aid to assess the level of possible improvement in speech intelligibility. Some clinicians believe use of a palatal lift on an interim basis may stimulate an otherwise flaccid soft palate to increase functional activity, subsequently lessening its need.

*Cross Reference 21083*

**D5959**  Palatal lift prosthesis, modification ⓑ **E1**

Synonymous terminology: revision of lift, adjustment. Alterations in the adaptation, contour, form or function of an existing palatal lift necessitated due to tissue impingement, lack of function, poor clasp adaptation or the like.

*Cross Reference 21083*

**D5960**  Speech aid prosthesis, modification ⓑ **E1**

Synonymous terminology: adjustment, repair, revision. Any revision of a pediatric or adult speech aid not necessitating its replacement. Frequently, revisions of the obturating section of any speech aid is required to facilitate enhanced speech intelligibility. Such revisions or repairs do not require complete remaking of the prosthesis, thus extending its longevity.

*Cross Reference 21084*

**D5982**  Surgical stent ⓑ **E1**

Synonymous terminology: periodontal stent, skin graft stent, columellar stent. Stents are utilized to apply pressure to soft tissues to facilitate healing and prevent cicatrization or collapse. A surgical stent may be required in surgical and post-surgical revisions to achieve close approximation of tissues. Usually such materials as temporary or interim soft denture liners, gutta percha, or dental modeling impression compound may be used.

*Cross Reference 21085*

**D5983**  Radiation carrier ⓑ **S**

Synonymous terminology: radiotherapy prosthesis, carrier prosthesis, radiation applicator, radium carrier, intracavity carrier, intracavity applicator. A device used to administer radiation to confined areas by means of capsules, beads or needles of radiation emitting materials such as radium or cesium. Its function is to hold the radiation source securely in the same location during the entire period of treatment. Radiation oncologists occasionally request these devices to achieve close approximation and controlled application of radiation to a tumor deemed amiable to eradication.

**D5984**  Radiation shield ⓑ **S**

Synonymous terminology: radiation stent, tongue protector, lead shield. An intraoral prosthesis designed to shield adjacent tissues from radiation during orthovoltage treatment of malignant lesions of the head and neck region.

**D5985**  Radiation cone locator ⓑ **S**

Synonymous terminology: docking device, cone locator. A prosthesis utilized to direct and reduplicate the path of radiation to an oral tumor during a split course of irradiation.

**D5986**  Fluoride gel carrier ⓑ **E1**

Synonymous terminology: fluoride applicator. A prosthesis, which covers the teeth in either dental arch and is used to apply topical fluoride in close proximity to tooth enamel and dentin for several minutes daily.

**D5987**  Commissure splint ⓑ **S**

Synonymous terminology: lip splint. A device placed between the lips, which assists in achieving increased opening between the lips. Use of such devices enhances opening where surgical, chemical or electrical alterations of the lips has resulted in severe restriction or contractures.

---

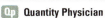 MIPS   Quantity Physician   Quantity Hospital  ♀ Female only

♂ Male only   Age  ♿ DMEPOS  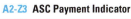 ASC Payment Indicator  A-Y ASC Status Indicator  Coding Clinic

**D5988** Surgical splint Ⓑ E1

Synonymous terminology: Gunning splint, modified Gunning splint, labiolingual splint, fenestrated splint, Kingsley splint, cast metal splint. Splints are designed to utilize existing teeth and/or alveolar processes as points of anchorage to assist in stabilization and immobilization of broken bones during healing. They are used to re-establish, as much as possible, normal occlusal relationships during the process of immobilization. Frequently, existing prostheses (e.g., a patient's complete dentures) can be modified to serve as surgical splints. Frequently, surgical splints have arch bars added to facilitate intermaxillary fixation. Rubber elastics may be used to assist in this process. Circummandibular eyelet hooks can be utilized for enhanced stabilization with wiring to adjacent bone.

**D5991** Vesicobullous disease medicament carrier Ⓑ E1

A custom fabricated carrier that covers the teeth and alveolar mucosa, or alveolar mucosa alone, and is used to deliver prescription medicaments for treatment of immunologically mediated vesiculobullous disease.

**D5992** Adjust maxillofacial prosthetic appliance, by report Ⓑ E1

**D5993** Maintenance and cleaning of a maxillofacial prosthesis (extra or intra-oral) other than required adjustments, by report Ⓑ E1

**D5994** Periodontal medicament carrier with peripheral seal - laboratory processed Ⓑ E1

A custom fabricated, laboratory processed carrier that covers the teeth and alveolar mucosa. Used as a vehicle to deliver prescribed medicaments for sustained contact with the gingiva, alveolar mucosa, and into the periodontal sulcus or pocket.

**D5999** Unspecified maxillofacial prosthesis, by report Ⓑ E1

Used for procedure that is not adequately described by a code. Describe procedure.

## Implant Services (D6010-D6199)

### D6010-D6199: FPD = fixed partial denture

### Surgical Services

**D6010** Surgical placement of implant body: endosteal implant Ⓑ E1

*Cross Reference 21248*

**D6011** Second stage implant surgery Ⓑ E1

Surgical access to an implant body for placement of a healing cap or to enable placement of an abutment.

**D6012** Surgical placement of interim implant body for transitional prosthesis: endosteal implant Ⓑ E1

Includes removal during later therapy to accommodate the definitive restoration, which may include placement of other implants.

**D6013** Surgical placement of mini implant Ⓑ E1

**D6040** Surgical placement: eposteal implant Ⓑ E1

An eposteal (subperiosteal) framework of a biocompatible material designed and fabricated to fit on the surface of the bone of the mandible or maxilla with permucosal extensions which provide support and attachment of a prosthesis. This may be a complete arch or unilateral appliance. Eposteal implants rest upon the bone and under the periosteum.

*Cross Reference 21245*

**D6050** Surgical placement: transosteal implant Ⓑ E1

A transosteal (transosseous) biocompatible device with threaded posts penetrating both the superior and inferior cortical bone plates of the mandibular symphysis and exiting through the permucosa providing support and attachment for a dental prosthesis. Transosteal implants are placed completely through the bone and into the oral cavity from extraoral or intraoral.

*Cross Reference 21244*

---

▶ New    ↩ Revised    ✔ Reinstated    ~~deleted~~ Deleted    ⊘ Not covered or valid by Medicare
✪ Special coverage instructions    ✳ Carrier discretion    Ⓑ Bill Part B MAC    Ⓓ Bill DME MAC

## Implant Supported Prosthetics

**D6051** Interim abutment - includes placement and removal ⓑ　　E1

　　*Includes placement and removal. A healing cap is not an interim abutment.*

**D6052** Semi-precision attachment abutment ⓑ　　E1

　　*Includes placement of keeper assembly.*

**D6055** Connecting bar — implant supported or abutment supported ⓑ　　E1

　　*Utilized to stabilize and anchor a prosthesis.*

**D6056** Prefabricated abutment - includes modification and placement ⓑ　　E1

　　*Modification of a prefabricated abutment may be necessary.*

**D6057** Custom fabricated abutment - includes placement ⓑ　　E1

　　*Created by a laboratory process, specific for an individual application.*

**D6058** Abutment supported porcelain/ceramic crown ⓑ　　E1

　　*A single crown restoration that is retained, supported and stabilized by an abutment on an implant.*

**D6059** Abutment supported porcelain fused to metal crown (high noble metal) ⓑ　　E1

　　*A single metal-ceramic crown restoration that is retained, supported and stabilized by an abutment on an implant.*

**D6060** Abutment supported porcelain fused to metal crown (predominantly base metal) ⓑ　　E1

　　*A single metal-ceramic crown restoration that is retained, supported and stabilized by an abutment on an implant.*

**D6061** Abutment supported porcelain fused to metal crown (noble metal) ⓑ　　E1

　　*A single metal-ceramic crown restoration that is retained, supported and stabilized by an abutment on an implant.*

**D6062** Abutment supported cast metal crown (high noble metal) ⓑ　　E1

　　*A single cast metal crown restoration that is retained, supported and stabilized by an abutment on an implant.*

**D6063** Abutment supported cast metal crown (predominantly base metal) ⓑ　　E1

　　*A single cast metal crown restoration that is retained, supported and stabilized by an abutment on an implant.*

**D6064** Abutment supported cast metal crown (noble metal) ⓑ　　E1

　　*A single cast metal crown restoration that is retained, supported and stabilized by an abutment on an implant.*

**D6065** Implant supported porcelain/ceramic crown ⓑ　　E1

　　*A single crown restoration that is retained, supported and stabilized by an implant.*

↩ **D6066** Implant supported crown - porcelain fused to high noble alloys ⓑ　　E1

　　*A single metal-ceramic crown restoration that is retained, supported and stabilized by an implant.*

↩ **D6067** Implant supported crown - high noble alloys ⓑ　　E1

　　*A single cast metal or milled crown restoration that is retained, supported and stabilized by an implant.*

**D6068** Abutment supported retainer for porcelain/ceramic FPD ⓑ　　E1

　　*A ceramic retainer for a fixed partial denture that gains retention, support and stability from an abutment on an implant.*

**D6069** Abutment supported retainer for porcelain fused to metal FPD (high noble metal) ⓑ　　E1

　　*A metal-ceramic retainer for a fixed partial denture that gains retention, support and stability from an abutment on an implant.*

**D6070** Abutment supported retainer for porcelain fused to metal FPD (predominantly base metal) ⓑ　　E1

　　*A metal-ceramic retainer for a fixed partial denture that gains retention, support and stability from an abutment on an implant.*

**D6071** Abutment supported retainer for porcelain fused to metal FPD (noble metal) ⓑ　　E1

　　*A metal-ceramic retainer for a fixed partial denture that gains retention, support and stability from an abutment on an implant.*

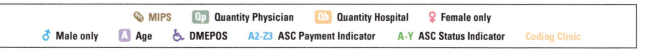

🐾 **MIPS**　　[Qp] **Quantity Physician**　　[Qh] **Quantity Hospital**　　♀ **Female only**
♂ **Male only**　　Ⓐ **Age**　　♿ **DMEPOS**　　A2-Z3 **ASC Payment Indicator**　　A-Y **ASC Status Indicator**　　**Coding Clinic**

**D6072** Abutment supported retainer for cast metal FPD (high noble metal) Ⓑ **E1**

A cast metal retainer for a fixed partial denture that gains retention, support and stability from an abutment on an implant.

**D6073** Abutment supported retainer for cast metal FPD (predominantly base metal) Ⓑ **E1**

A cast metal retainer for a fixed partial denture that gains retention, support and stability from an abutment on an implant.

**D6074** Abutment supported retainer for cast metal FPD (noble metal) Ⓑ **E1**

A cast metal retainer for a fixed partial denture that gains retention, support and stability from an abutment on an implant.

**D6075** Implant supported retainer for ceramic FPD Ⓑ **E1**

A ceramic retainer for a fixed partial denture that gains retention, support and stability from an implant.

↻ **D6076** Implant supported retainer for FPD - porcelain fused to high noble alloys Ⓑ **E1**

A metal-ceramic retainer for a fixed partial denture that gains retention, support and stability from an implant.

↻ **D6077** Implant supported retainer for metal FPD - high noble alloys Ⓑ **E1**

A cast metal retainer for a fixed partial denture that gains retention, support and stability from an implant.

## Other Implant Services

**D6080** Implant maintenance procedures when prostheses are removed and reinserted, including cleansing of prostheses and abutments Ⓑ **E1**

This procedure includes active debriding of the implant(s) and examination of all aspects of the implant system(s), including the occlusion and stability of the superstructure. The patient is also instructed in thorough daily cleansing of the implant(s). This is not a per implant code, and is indicated for implant supported fixed prostheses.

**D6081** Scaling and debridement in the presence of inflammation or mucositis of a single implant, including cleaning of the implant surfaces, without flap entry and closure Ⓑ **E1**

This procedure is not performed in conjunction with D1110, D4910, or D4346.

▶ **D6082** Implant supported crown - porcelain fused to predominantly base alloys **E1**

▶ **D6083** Implant supported crown - porcelain fused to noble alloys **E1**

▶ **D6084** Implant supported crown - porcelain fused to titanium and titanium alloys **E1**

**D6085** Provisional implant crown Ⓑ **E1**

Used when a period of healing is necessary prior to fabrication and placement of permanent prosthetic.

▶ **D6086** Implant supported crown - predominantly base alloys **E1**

▶ **D6087** Implant supported crown - noble alloys **E1**

▶ **D6088** Implant supported crown - titanium and titanium alloys **E1**

**D6090** Repair implant supported prosthesis by report Ⓑ **E1**

This procedure involves the repair or replacement of any part of the implant supported prosthesis.

*Cross Reference 21299*

**D6091** Replacement of semi-precision or precision attachment (male or female component) of implant/abutment supported prosthesis, per attachment Ⓑ **E1**

This procedure applies to the replaceable male or female component of the attachment.

**D6092** Re-cement or re-bond implant/abutment supported crown Ⓑ **E1**

**D6093** Re-cement or re-bond implant/abutment supported fixed partial denture Ⓑ **E1**

↻ **D6094** Abutment supported crown - titanium and titanium alloys Ⓑ **E1**

A single crown restoration that is retained, supported and stabilized by an abutment on an implant. May be cast or milled.

**D6095** Repair implant abutment, by report Ⓑ **E1**

This procedure involves the repair or replacement of any part of the implant abutment.

*Cross Reference 21299*

---

▶ New ↻ Revised ✔ Reinstated  ̶d̶e̶l̶e̶t̶e̶d̶ Deleted ⊘ Not covered or valid by Medicare
✪ Special coverage instructions ✳ Carrier discretion Ⓑ Bill Part B MAC Ⓑ Bill DME MAC

**D6096** Remove broken implant retaining screen ⓑ    E1

▶ **D6097** Abutment supported crown - porcelain fused to titanium and titanium alloys    E1

A single metal-ceramic crown restoration that is retained, supported, and stabilized by an abutment on an implant.

▶ **D6098** Implant supported retainer - porcelain fused to predominantly base alloys    E1

A metal-ceramic retainer for a fixed partial denture that gains retention, support, and stability from an abutment on an implant.

▶ **D6099** Implant supported retainer for FPD - porcelain fused to noble alloys    E1

A metal-ceramic retainer for a fixed partial denture that gains retention, support, and stability from an implant.

## Surgical Services

**D6100** Implant removal, by report ⓑ    E1

This procedure involves the surgical removal of an implant. Describe procedure.

*Cross Reference 21299*

**D6101** Debridement of a peri-implant defect or defects surrounding a single implant, and surface cleaning of exposed implant surfaces, including flap entry and closure ⓑ    E1

**D6102** Debridement and osseous contouring of a peri-implant defect or defects surrounding a single implant and includes surface cleaning of the exposed implant surfaces and flap entry and closure ⓑ    E1

**D6103** Bone graft for repair of peri-implant defect - does not include flap entry and closure ⓑ    E1

Placement of a barrier membrane or biologic materials to aid in osseous regeneration, are reported separately.

**D6104** Bone graft at time of implant placement ⓑ    E1

Placement of a barrier membrane, or biologic materials to aid in osseous regeneration are reported separately.

## Implant Supported Prosthetics

**D6110** Implant /abutment supported removable denture for edentulous arch - maxillary ⓑ    E1

**D6111** Implant /abutment supported removable denture for edentulous arch - mandibular ⓑ    E1

**D6112** Implant/abutment supported removable denture for partially edentulous arch - maxillary ⓑ    E1

**D6113** Implant/abutment supported removable denture for partially edentulous arch - mandibular ⓑ    E1

**D6114** Implant/abutment supported fixed denture for edentulous arch - maxillary ⓑ    E1

**D6115** Implant/abutment supported fixed denture for edentulous arch - mandibular ⓑ    E1

**D6116** Implant/abutment supported fixed denture for partially edentulous arch - maxillary ⓑ    E1

**D6117** Implant/abutment supported fixed denture for partially edentulous arch - mandibular ⓑ    E1

**D6118** Implant/abutment supported interim fixed denture for edentulous arch mandibular ⓑ    E1

Used when a period of healing is necessary prior to fabrication and placement of a permanent prosthetic.

**D6119** Implant/abutment supported interim fixed denture for edentulous arch maxillary ⓑ    E1

Used when a period of healing is necessary prior to fabrication and placement of a permanent prosthetic.

▶ **D6120** Implant supported retainer - porcelain fused to titanium and titanium alloys    E1

A metal-ceramic retainer for a fixed partial denture that gains retention, support, and stability from an implant.

▶ **D6121** Implant supported retainer for metal FPD - predominantly base alloys    E1

A metal-ceramic retainer for a fixed partial denture that gains retention, support, and stability from an implant.

▶ **D6122** Implant supported retainer for metal FPD - noble alloys    E1

A metal retainer for a fixed partial denture that gains retention, support, and stability from an implant.

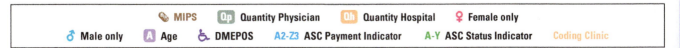

🐚 MIPS    📲 Quantity Physician    📲 Quantity Hospital    ♀ Female only
♂ Male only    🅐 Age    ♿ DMEPOS    A2-Z3 ASC Payment Indicator    A-Y ASC Status Indicator    Coding Clinic

▶ **D6123** Implant supported retainer for metal FPD - titanium and titanium alloys  E1

A metal retainer for a fixed partial denture that gains retention, support, and stability from an implant.

**D6190** Radiographic/surgical implant index, by report Ⓑ  E1

An appliance, designed to relate osteotomy or fixture position to existing anatomic structures, to be utilized during radiographic exposure for treatment planning and/or during osteotomy creation for fixture installation.

↻ **D6194** Abutment supported retainer crown for FPD – titanium and titanium alloys Ⓑ  E1

A retainer for a fixed partial denture that gains retention, support and stability from an abutment on an implant. May be cast or milled.

▶ **D6195** Abutment supported retainer - porcelain fused to titanium and titanium alloys  E1

A metal retainer for a fixed partial denture that gains retention, support, and stability from an implant.

**None**

**D6199** Unspecified implant procedure, by report Ⓑ  E1

Use for procedure that is not adequately described by a code. Describe procedure.

*Cross Reference 21299*

## Prosthodontics, fixed (D6205-D6999)
### Fixed Partial Denture Pontics

**D6205** Pontic - indirect resin based composite Ⓑ  E1

Not to be used as a temporary or provisional prosthesis.

**D6210** Pontic - cast high noble metal Ⓑ  E1

**D6211** Pontic - cast predominantly base metal Ⓑ  E1

**D6212** Pontic - cast noble metal Ⓑ  E1

↻ **D6214** Pontic - titanium and titanium alloys Ⓑ  E1

**D6240** Pontic - porcelain fused to high noble metal Ⓑ  E1

**D6241** Pontic - porcelain fused to predominantly base metal Ⓑ  E1

**D6242** Pontic - porcelain fused to noble metal Ⓑ  E1

*IOM: 100-02, 15, 150*

▶ **D6243** Pontic - porcelain fused to titanium and titanium alloys  E1

**D6245** Pontic - porcelain/ceramic Ⓑ  E1

**D6250** Pontic - resin with high noble metal Ⓑ  E1

**D6251** Pontic - resin with predominantly base metal Ⓑ  E1

**D6252** Pontic - resin with noble metal Ⓑ  E1

**D6253** Provisional pontic - further treatment or completion of diagnosis necessary prior to final impression Ⓑ  E1

Not to be used as a temporary pontic for routine prosthetic fixed partial dentures.

### Fixed Partial Denture Retainers – Inlays/Onlays

**D6545** Retainer - cast metal for resin bonded fixed prosthesis Ⓑ  E1

**D6548** Retainer - porcelain/ceramic for resin bonded fixed prosthesis Ⓑ  E1

**D6549** Retainer - for resin bonded fixed prosthesis Ⓑ  E1

**D6600** Retainer inlay - porcelain/ceramic, two surfaces Ⓑ  E1

**D6601** Retainer inlay - porcelain/ceramic, three or more surfaces Ⓑ  E1

**D6602** Retainer inlay - cast high noble metal, two surfaces Ⓑ  E1

**D6603** Retainer inlay - cast high noble metal, three or more surfaces Ⓑ  E1

**D6604** Retainer inlay - cast predominantly base metal, two surfaces Ⓑ  E1

**D6605** Retainer inlay - cast predominantly base metal, three or more surfaces Ⓞ Ⓑ E1

**D6606** Retainer inlay - cast noble metal, two surfaces Ⓑ  E1

**D6607** Retainer inlay - cast noble metal, three or more surfaces Ⓑ  E1

**D6608** Retainer onlay - porcelain/ceramic, two surfaces Ⓑ  E1

**D6609** Retainer onlay - porcelain/ceramic, three or more surfaces Ⓑ  E1

**D6610** Retainer onlay - cast high noble metal, two surfaces Ⓑ  E1

**D6611** Retainer onlay - cast high noble metal, three or more surfaces Ⓑ  E1

**D6612** Retainer onlay - cast predominantly base metal, two surfaces Ⓑ  E1

**D6613** Retainer onlay - cast predominantly base metal, three or more surfaces Ⓞ Ⓑ E1

---

| | | | | | |
|---|---|---|---|---|---|
| ▶ New | ↻ Revised | ✔ Reinstated | ~~deleted~~ Deleted | ⊘ Not covered or valid by Medicare | |
| ☼ Special coverage instructions | | ✳ Carrier discretion | | Ⓑ Bill Part B MAC | Ⓓ Bill DME MAC |

**D6614** Retainer onlay - cast noble metal, two surfaces Ⓑ E1

**D6615** Retainer onlay - cast noble metal, three or more surfaces Ⓑ E1

**D6624** Retainer inlay - titanium Ⓑ E1

**D6634** Retainer onlay - titanium Ⓑ E1

## Fixed Partial Denture Retainers – Crowns

**D6710** Retainer crown - indirect resin based composite Ⓑ E1

Not to be used as a temporary or provisional prosthesis.

**D6720** Retainer crown - resin with high noble metal Ⓑ E1

**D6721** Retainer crown - resin with predominantly base metal Ⓑ E1

**D6722** Retainer crown - resin with noble metal Ⓑ E1

**D6740** Retainer crown - porcelain/ceramic Ⓑ E1

**D6750** Retainer crown - porcelain fused to high noble metal Ⓑ E1

**D6751** Retainer crown - porcelain fused to predominantly base metal Ⓑ E1

**D6752** Retainer crown - porcelain fused to noble metal Ⓑ E1

▶ **D6753** Retainer crown - porcelain fused to titanium and titanium alloys E1

**D6780** Retainer crown - 3/4 cast high noble metal Ⓑ E1

**D6781** Retainer crown - 3/4 cast predominantly based metal Ⓑ E1

**D6782** Retainer crown - 3/4 cast noble metal Ⓑ E1

**D6783** Retainer crown - 3/4 porcelain/ceramic Ⓑ E1

▶ **D6784** Retainer crown 3/4 - titanium and titanium alloys E1

**D6790** Retainer crown - full cast high noble metal Ⓑ E1

**D6791** Retainer crown - full cast predominantly base metal Ⓑ E1

**D6792** Retainer crown - full cast noble metal Ⓑ E1

**D6793** Provisional retainer crown - further treatment or completion of diagnosis necessary prior to final impression Ⓑ E1

Not to be used as a temporary retainer crown for routine prosthetic fixed partial dentures.

↩ **D6794** Retainer crown - titanium and titanium alloys Ⓑ E1

## Other Fixed Partial Denture Services

**D6920** Connector bar Ⓑ S

A device attached to fixed partial denture retainer or coping which serves to stabilize and anchor a removable overdenture prosthesis.

**D6930** Re-cement or re-bond fixed partial denture Ⓑ E1

**D6940** Stress breaker Ⓑ E1

A non-rigid connector.

**D6950** Precision attachment Ⓑ E1

A male and female pair constitutes one precision attachment, and is separate from the prosthesis.

**D6980** Bridge repair necessitated by restorative material failure Ⓑ E1

**D6985** Pediatric partial denture, fixed Ⓑ Ⓐ E1

This prosthesis is used primarily for aesthetic purposes.

## None

**D6999** Unspecified fixed prosthodontic procedure, by report Ⓑ E1

Used for procedure that is not adequately described by a code. Describe procedure.

## Oral and Maxillofacial Surgery (D7111-D7999)
## Extractions (Includes Local Anesthesia, Suturing, If Needed, and Routine Postoperative Care)

**D7111** Extraction, coronal remnants - primary tooth Ⓑ S

Removal of soft tissue-retained coronal remnants.

**D7140** Extraction, erupted tooth or exposed root (elevation and/or forceps removal) Ⓑ S

Includes removal of tooth structure, minor smoothing of socket bone, and closure, as necessary.

**D7210** Extraction, erupted tooth requiring removal of bone and/or sectioning of tooth, and including elevation of mucoperiosteal flap if indicated Ⓑ S

Includes related cutting of gingiva and bone, removal of tooth structure, minor smoothing of socket bone and closure.

**D7220** Removal of impacted tooth - soft tissue Ⓑ S

Occlusal surface of tooth covered by soft tissue; requires mucoperiosteal flap elevation.

🐾 MIPS  Ⓠₚ Quantity Physician  Ⓠₕ Quantity Hospital  ♀ Female only
♂ Male only  Ⓐ Age  ♿ DMEPOS  A2-Z3 ASC Payment Indicator  A-Y ASC Status Indicator  Coding Clinic

DENTAL PROCEDURES  D6614 – D7220

183

**D7230**  Removal of impacted tooth - partially bony ⒷⒷ  **S**

Part of crown covered by bone; requires mucoperiosteal flap elevation and bone removal.

**D7240**  Removal of impacted tooth - completely bony Ⓑ  **S**

Most or all of crown covered by bone; requires mucoperiosteal flap elevation and bone removal.

**D7241**  Removal of impacted tooth - completely bony, with unusual surgical complications Ⓑ  **S**

Most or all of crown covered by bone; unusually difficult or complicated due to factors such as nerve dissection required, separate closure of maxillary sinus required or aberrant tooth position.

**D7250**  Removal of residual tooth roots (cutting procedure) Ⓑ  **S**

Includes cutting of soft tissue and bone, removal of tooth structure, and closure.

**D7251**  Coronectomy — intentional partial tooth removal Ⓑ  **E1**

Intentional partial tooth removal is performed when a neurovascular complication is likely if the entire impacted tooth is removed.

## Other Surgical Procedures

**D7260**  Oral antral fistula closure Ⓑ  **S**

Excision of fistulous tract between maxillary sinus and oral cavity and closure by advancement flap.

**D7261**  Primary closure of a sinus perforation Ⓑ  **S**

Subsequent to surgical removal of tooth, exposure of sinus requiring repair, or immediate closure of oroantral or oralnasal communication in absence of fistulous tract.

**D7270**  Tooth reimplantation and/or stabilization of accidentally evulsed or displaced tooth Ⓑ  **E1**

Includes splinting and/or stabilization.

**D7272**  Tooth transplantation (includes reimplantation from one site to another and splinting and/or stabilization) Ⓑ **E1**

**D7280**  Exposure of an unerupted tooth Ⓑ  **E1**

An incision is made and the tissue is reflected and bone removed as necessary to expose the crown of an impacted tooth not intended to be extracted.

**D7282**  Mobilization of erupted or malpositioned tooth to aid eruption Ⓑ  **E1**

To move/luxate teeth to eliminate ankylosis; not in conjunction with an extraction.

**D7283**  Placement of device to facilitate eruption of impacted tooth Ⓑ  **B**

Placement of an orthodontic bracket, band or other device on an unerupted tooth, after its exposure, to aid in its eruption. Report the surgical exposure separately using D7280.

**D7285**  Incisional biopsy of oral tissue - hard (bone, tooth) Ⓑ  **E1**

For partial removal of specimen only. This procedure involves biopsy of osseous lesions and is not used for apicoectomy/periradicular surgery. This procedure does not entail an excision.

*Cross Reference 20220, 20225, 20240, 20245*

**D7286**  Incisional biopsy of oral tissue - soft Ⓑ  **E1**

For partial removal of an architecturally intact specimen only. This procedure is not used at the same time as codes for apicoectomy/periradicular curettage. This procedure does not entail an excision.

*Cross Reference 40808*

**D7287**  Exfoliative cytological sample collection Ⓑ  **E1**

For collection of non-transepithelial cytology sample via mild scraping of the oral mucosa.

**D7288**  Brush biopsy - transepithelial sample collection Ⓑ  **B**

For collection of oral disaggregated transepithelial cells via rotational brushing of the oral mucosa.

**D7290**  Surgical repositioning of teeth Ⓑ  **E1**

Grafting procedure(s) is/are additional.

▶ **New**   ↩ **Revised**   ✔ **Reinstated**   ~~deleted~~ **Deleted**   ⃠ **Not covered or valid by Medicare**   ✪ **Special coverage instructions**   ✱ **Carrier discretion**   Ⓑ **Bill Part B MAC**   Ⓑ **Bill DME MAC**

DENTAL PROCEDURES

**D7291** Transseptal fiberotomy/supra crestal fiberotomy, by report Ⓑ    **S**

The supraosseous connective tissue attachment is surgically severed around the involved teeth. Where there are adjacent teeth, the transseptal fiberotomy of a single tooth will involve a minimum of three teeth. Since the incisions are within the gingival sulcus and tissue and the root surface is not instrumented, this procedure heals by the reunion of connective tissue with the root surface on which viable periodontal tissue is present (reattachment).

**D7292** Placement of temporary anchorage device [screw retained plate] requiring flap; includes device removal Ⓑ    **E1**

**D7293** Placement of temporary anchorage device requiring flap; includes device removal Ⓑ    **E1**

**D7294** Placement of temporary anchorage device without flap; includes device removal Ⓑ    **E1**

**D7295** Harvest of bone for use in autogenous grafting procedure Ⓑ    **E1**

Reported in addition to those autogenous graft placement procedures that do not include harvesting of bone.

**D7296** Corticotomy one to three teeth or tooth spaces, per quadrant Ⓑ    **E1**

This procedure involves creating multiple cuts, perforations, or removal of cortical, alveolar or basal bone of the jaw for the purpose of facilitating orthodontic repositioning of the dentition. This procedure includes flap entry and closure. Graft material and membrane, if used, should be reported separately.

**D7297** Corticotomy four or more teeth or tooth spaces, per quadrant Ⓑ    **E1**

This procedure involves creating multiple cuts, perforations, or removal of cortical, alveolar or basal bone of the jaw for the purpose of facilitating orthodontic repositioning of the dentition. This procedure includes flap entry and closure. Graft material and membrane, if used, should be reported separately.

## *Alveoloplasty – Preparation of Ridge*

**D7310** Alveoloplasty in conjunction with extractions - four or more teeth or tooth spaces, per quadrant Ⓑ    **E1**

The alveoloplasty is distinct (separate procedure) from extractions. Usually in preparation for a prosthesis or other treatments such as radiation therapy and transplant surgery.

*Cross Reference 41874*

**D7311** Alveoloplasty in conjunction with extractions - one to three teeth or tooth spaces, per quadrant Ⓑ    **E1**

The alveoloplasty is distinct (separate procedure) from extractions. Usually in preparation for a prosthesis or other treatments such as radiation therapy and transplant surgery.

**D7320** Alveoloplasty not in conjunction with extractions - four or more teeth or tooth spaces, per quadrant Ⓑ    **E1**

No extractions performed in an edentulous area. See D7310 if teeth are being extracted concurrently with the alveoloplasty. Usually in preparation for a prosthesis or other treatments such as radiation therapy and transplant surgery.

*Cross Reference 41870*

**D7321** Alveoloplasty not in conjunction with extractions - one to three teeth or tooth spaces, per quadrant Ⓑ    **B**

No extractions performed in an edentulous area. See D7311 if teeth are being extracted concurrently with the alveoloplasty. Usually in preparation for a prosthesis or other treatments such as radiation therapy and transplant surgery.

## *Vestibuloplasty*

**D7340** Vestibuloplasty - ridge extension (second epithelialization) Ⓑ    **E1**

*Cross Reference 40840, 40842, 40843, 40844*

**D7350** Vestibuloplasty - ridge extension (including soft tissue grafts, muscle reattachments, revision of soft tissue attachment, and management of hypertrophied and hyperplastic tissue) Ⓑ    **E1**

*Cross Reference 40845*

DENTAL PROCEDURES  D7291 – D7350

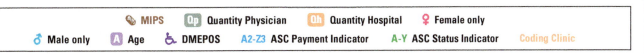

🐍 MIPS   Ⓠⓟ Quantity Physician   Ⓠⓗ Quantity Hospital   ♀ Female only   ♂ Male only   Ⓐ Age   ♿ DMEPOS   A2-Z3 ASC Payment Indicator   A-Y ASC Status Indicator   Coding Clinic

**185**

## Excision of Soft Tissue Lesions

**D7410** Excision of benign lesion up to 1.25 cm Ⓑ    E1

**D7411** Excision of benign lesion greater than 1.25 cm Ⓑ    E1

**D7412** Excision of benign lesion, complicated Ⓑ    E1

Requires extensive undermining with advancement or rotational flap closure.

**D7413** Excision of malignant lesion up to 1.25 cm Ⓑ    E1

**D7414** Excision of malignant lesion greater than 1.25 cm Ⓑ    E1

**D7415** Excision of malignant lesion, complicated Ⓑ    E1

Requires extensive undermining with advancement or rotational flap closure.

## Excision of Intra-Osseous Lesions

**D7440** Excision of malignant tumor - lesion diameter up to 1.25 cm Ⓑ    E1

**D7441** Excision of malignant tumor - lesion diameter greater than 1.25 cm Ⓑ    E1

**D7450** Removal of benign odontogenic cyst or tumor - lesion diameter up to 1.25 cm Ⓑ    E1

**D7451** Removal of benign odontogenic cyst or tumor - lesion diameter greater than 1.25 cm Ⓑ    E1

**D7460** Removal of benign nonodontogenic cyst or tumor - lesion diameter up to 1.25 cm Ⓑ    E1

**D7461** Removal of benign nonodontogenic cyst or tumor - lesion diameter greater than 1.25 cm Ⓑ    E1

## Excision of Soft Tissue Lesions

**D7465** Destruction of lesion(s) by physical or chemical methods, by report Ⓑ    E1

Examples include using cryo, laser or electro surgery.

Cross Reference 41850

## Excision of Bone Tissue

**D7471** Removal of lateral exostosis (maxilla or mandible) Ⓑ    E1

Cross Reference 21031, 21032

**D7472** Removal of torus palatinus Ⓑ    E1

**D7473** Removal of torus mandibularis Ⓑ    E1

**D7485** Reduction of osseous tuberosity Ⓑ    E1

**D7490** Radical resection of maxilla or mandible Ⓑ    E1

Partial resection of maxilla or mandible; removal of lesion and defect with margin of normal appearing bone. Reconstruction and bone grafts should be reported separately.

Cross Reference 21095

## Surgical Incision

**D7510** Incision and drainage of abscess - intraoral soft tissue Ⓑ    E1

Involves incision through mucosa, including periodontal origins.

Cross Reference 41800

**D7511** Incision and drainage of abscess - intraoral soft tissue - complicated (includes drainage of multiple fascial spaces) Ⓑ    B

Incision is made intraorally and dissection is extended into adjacent fascial space(s) to provide adequate drainage of abscess/cellulitis.

**D7520** Incision and drainage of abscess - extraoral soft tissue Ⓑ    E1

Involves incision through skin.

Cross Reference 41800

**D7521** Incision and drainage of abscess - extraoral soft tissue - complicated (includes drainage of multiple fascial spaces) Ⓑ    B

Incision is made extraorally and dissection is extended into adjacent fascial space(s) to provide adequate drainage of abscess/cellulitis.

**D7530** Removal of foreign body from mucosa, skin, or subcutaneous alveolar tissue Ⓑ    E1

Cross Reference 41805, 41828

**D7540** Removal of reaction-producing foreign bodies, musculoskeletal system Ⓑ    E1

May include, but is not limited to, removal of splinters, pieces of wire, etc., from muscle and/or bone.

Cross Reference 20520, 41800, 41806

**D7550** Partial ostectomy/sequestrectomy for removal of non-vital bone Ⓑ    E1

Removal of loose or sloughed-off dead bone caused by infection or reduced blood supply.

Cross Reference 20999

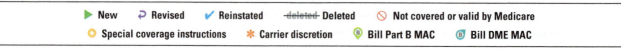

▶ New    ↻ Revised    ✔ Reinstated    ~~deleted~~ Deleted    ⊘ Not covered or valid by Medicare

✿ Special coverage instructions    ✱ Carrier discretion    Ⓑ Bill Part B MAC    Ⓓ Bill DME MAC

**D7560** Maxillary sinusotomy for removal of tooth fragment or foreign body Ⓑ  E1

*Cross Reference 31020*

## Treatment of Closed Fractures

**D7610** Maxilla - open reduction (teeth immobilized, if present) Ⓑ  E1

Teeth may be wired, banded or splinted together to prevent movement. Incision required for interosseous fixation.

**D7620** Maxilla - closed reduction (teeth immobilized if present) Ⓑ  E1

No incision required to reduce fracture. See D7610 if interosseous fixation is applied.

**D7630** Mandible - open reduction (teeth immobilized, if present) Ⓑ  E1

Teeth may be wired, banded or splinted together to prevent movement. Incision required to reduce fracture.

**D7640** Mandible - closed reduction (teeth immobilized if present) Ⓑ  E1

No incision required to reduce fracture. See D7630 if interosseous fixation is applied.

**D7650** Malar and/or zygomatic arch - open reduction Ⓑ  E1

**D7660** Malar and/or zygomatic arch - closed reduction Ⓑ  E1

**D7670** Alveolus - closed reduction, may include stabilization of teeth Ⓑ  E1

Teeth may be wired, banded or splinted together to prevent movement.

**D7671** Alveolus - open reduction, may include stabilization of teeth Ⓑ  E1

Teeth may be wired, banded or splinted together to prevent movement.

**D7680** Facial bones - complicated reduction with fixation and multiple surgical approaches Ⓑ  E1

Facial bones include upper and lower jaw, cheek, and bones around eyes, nose, and ears.

## Treatment of Open Fractures

**D7710** Maxilla - open reduction Ⓑ  E1

Incision required to reduce fracture.

*Cross Reference 21346*

**D7720** Maxilla - closed reduction Ⓑ  E1

*Cross Reference 21345*

**D7730** Mandible - open reduction Ⓑ  E1

Incision required to reduce fracture.

*Cross Reference 21461, 21462*

**D7740** Mandible - closed reduction Ⓑ  E1

*Cross Reference 21455*

**D7750** Malar and/or zygomatic arch - open reduction Ⓑ  E1

Incision required to reduce fracture.

*Cross Reference 21360, 21365*

**D7760** Malar and/or zygomatic arch - closed reduction Ⓑ  E1

*Cross Reference 21355*

**D7770** Alveolus - open reduction stabilization of teeth Ⓑ  E1

Fractured bone(s) are exposed to mouth or outside the face. Incision required to reduce fracture.

*Cross Reference 21422*

**D7771** Alveolus, closed reduction stabilization of teeth Ⓑ  E1

Fractured bone(s) are exposed to mouth or outside the face.

**D7780** Facial bones - complicated reduction with fixation and multiple approaches Ⓑ  E1

Incision required to reduce fracture. Facial bones include upper and lower jaw, cheek, and bones around eyes, nose, and ears.

*Cross Reference 21433, 21435*

## Reduction of Dislocation and Management of Other Temporomandibular Joint Dysfunction

**D7810** Open reduction of dislocation Ⓑ  E1

Access to TMJ via surgical opening.

*Cross Reference 21490*

**D7820** Closed reduction of dislocation Ⓑ  E1

Joint manipulated into place; no surgical exposure.

*Cross Reference 21480*

**D7830** Manipulation under anesthesia Ⓑ  E1

Usually done under general anesthesia or intravenous sedation.

*Cross Reference 00190*

**D7840** Condylectomy Ⓑ  E1

Removal of all or portion of the mandibular condyle (separate procedure).

*Cross Reference 21050*

| | | | |
|---|---|---|---|
| 🦤 MIPS | Qp Quantity Physician | Qh Quantity Hospital | ♀ Female only |
| ♂ Male only | A Age | ♿ DMEPOS | A2-Z3 ASC Payment Indicator | A-Y ASC Status Indicator | Coding Clinic |

**D7850** Surgical discectomy, with/without implant Ⓑ      E1

Excision of the intra-articular disc of a joint.

*Cross Reference 21060*

**D7852** Disc repair Ⓑ      E1

Repositioning and/or sculpting of disc; repair of perforated posterior attachment.

*Cross Reference 21299*

**D7854** Synovectomy Ⓑ      E1

Excision of a portion or all of the synovial membrane of a joint.

*Cross Reference 21299*

**D7856** Myotomy Ⓑ      E1

Cutting of muscle for therapeutic purposes (separate procedure).

*Cross Reference 21299*

**D7858** Joint reconstruction Ⓑ      E1

Reconstruction of osseous components including or excluding soft tissues of the joint with autogenous, homologous, or alloplastic materials.

*Cross Reference 21242, 21243*

**D7860** Arthrotomy Ⓑ      E1

Cutting into joint (separate procedure).

**D7865** Arthroplasty Ⓑ      E1

Reduction of osseous components of the joint to create a pseudoarthrosis or eliminate an irregular remodeling pattern (osteophytes).

*Cross Reference 21240*

**D7870** Arthrocentesis Ⓑ      E1

Withdrawal of fluid from a joint space by aspiration.

*Cross Reference 21060*

**D7871** Non-arthroscopic lysis and lavage Ⓑ E1

Inflow and outflow catheters are placed into the joint space. The joint is lavaged and manipulated as indicated in an effort to release minor adhesions and synovial vacuum phenomenon as well as to remove inflammation products from the joint space.

**D7872** Arthroscopy - diagnosis, with or without biopsy Ⓑ      E1

*Cross Reference 29800*

**D7873** Arthroscopy: lavage and lysis of adhesions Ⓑ      E1

Removal of adhesions using the arthroscope and lavage of the joint cavities.

*Cross Reference 29804*

**D7874** Arthroscopy: disc repositioning and stabilization Ⓑ      E1

Repositioning and stabilization of disc using arthroscopic techniques.

*Cross Reference 29804*

**D7875** Arthroscopy: synovectomy Ⓑ      E1

Removal of inflamed and hyperplastic synovium (partial/complete) via an arthroscopic technique.

*Cross Reference 29804*

**D7876** Arthroscopy: discectomy Ⓑ      E1

Removal of disc and remodeled posterior attachment via the arthroscope.

*Cross Reference 29804*

**D7877** Arthroscopy: debridement Ⓑ      E1

Removal of pathologic hard and/or soft tissue using the arthroscope.

*Cross Reference 29804*

**D7880** Occlusal orthotic device, by report Ⓑ E1

Presently includes splints provided for treatment of temporomandibular joint dysfunction.

*Cross Reference 21499*

**D7881** Occlusal orthotic device adjustment Ⓑ      E1

**D7899** Unspecified TMD therapy, by report Ⓑ      E1

Used for procedure that is not adequately described by a code. Describe procedure.

*Cross Reference 21499*

## *Repair of Traumatic Wounds*

**D7910** Suture of recent small wounds up to 5 cm Ⓑ      E1

*Cross Reference 12011, 12013*

---

▶ New    ↻ Revised    ✔ Reinstated    ~~deleted~~ Deleted    ⃠ Not covered or valid by Medicare

✲ Special coverage instructions    ✳ Carrier discretion    Ⓑ Bill Part B MAC    Ⓑ Bill DME MAC

## Complicated Suturing (Reconstruction Requiring Delicate Handling of Tissue and Wide Undermining for Meticulous Closure)

**D7911** Complicated suture - up to 5 cm ⒷE1

*Cross Reference 12051, 12052*

**D7912** Complicated suture - greater than 5 cm ⒷE1

*Cross Reference 13132*

## Other Repair Procedures

**D7920** Skin graft (identify defect covered, location, and type of graft) ⒷE1

**D7921** Collection and application of autologous blood concentrate product ⒷE1

▶ **D7922** Placement of intra-socket biological dressing to aid in hemostasis or clot stabilization, per site E1

This procedure can be performed at time and/or after extraction to aid in hemostasis. The socket is packed with a hemostatic agent to aid in hemostasis and or clot stabilization.

**D7940** Osteoplasty - for orthognathic deformities ⒷS

Reconstruction of jaws for correction of congenital, developmental or acquired traumatic or surgical deformity.

**D7941** Osteotomy - mandibular rami ⒷE1

*Cross Reference 21193, 21195, 21196*

**D7943** Osteotomy - mandibular rami with bone graft; includes obtaining the graft ⒷE1

*Cross Reference 21194*

**D7944** Osteotomy - segmented or subapical ⒷE1

Report by range of tooth numbers within segment.

*Cross Reference 21198, 21206*

**D7945** Osteotomy - body of mandible ⒷE1

Sectioning of lower jaw. This includes exposure, bone cut, fixation, routine wound closure and normal post-operative follow-up care.

*Cross Reference 21193, 21194, 21195, 21196*

**D7946** LeFort I (maxilla - total) ⒷE1

Sectioning of the upper jaw. This includes exposure, bone cuts, downfracture, repositioning, fixation, routine wound closure and normal post-operative follow-up care.

*Cross Reference 21147*

**D7947** LeFort I (maxilla - segmented) ⒷE1

When reporting a surgically assisted palatal expansion without downfracture, this code would entail a reduced service and should be "by report."

*Cross Reference 21145, 21146*

**D7948** LeFort II or LeFort III (osteoplasty of facial bones for midface hypoplasia or retrusion) - without bone graft ⒷE1

Sectioning of upper jaw. This includes exposure, bone cuts, downfracture, segmentation of maxilla, repositioning, fixation, routine wound closure and normal post-operative follow-up care.

*Cross Reference 21150*

**D7949** LeFort II or LeFort III - with bone graft ⒷE1

Includes obtaining autografts.

**D7950** Osseous, osteoperiosteal, or cartilage graft of the mandible or maxilla - autogenous or nonautogenous, by report ⒷE1

This procedure is for ridge augmentation or reconstruction to increase height, width and/or volume of residual alveolar ridge. It includes obtaining graft material. Placement of a barrier membrane, if used, should be reported separately.

*Cross Reference 21247*

**D7951** Sinus augmentation with bone or bone substitutes ⒷE1

The augmentation of the sinus cavity to increase alveolar height for reconstruction of edentulous portions of the maxilla. This procedure is performed via a lateral open approach. This includes obtaining the bone or bone substitutes. Placement of a barrier membrane if used should be reported separately.

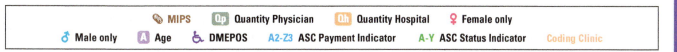

🔖 MIPS    Ⓠp Quantity Physician    Ⓠh Quantity Hospital    ♀ Female only    ♂ Male only    Ⓐ Age    ♿ DMEPOS    A2-Z3 ASC Payment Indicator    A-Y ASC Status Indicator    Coding Clinic

**D7952** Sinus augmentation via a vertical approach Ⓑ    E1

The augmentation of the sinus to increase alveolar height by vertical access through the ridge crest by raising the floor of the sinus and grafting as necessary. This includes obtaining the bone or bone substitutes.

**D7953** Bone replacement graft for ridge preservation - per site Ⓑ    E1

Graft is placed in an extraction or implant removal site at the time of the extraction or removal to preserve ridge integrity (e.g., clinically indicated in preparation for implant reconstruction or where alveolar contour is critical to planned prosthetic reconstruction). Does not include obtaining graft material. Membrane, if used should be reported separately.

**D7955** Repair of maxillofacial soft and/or hard tissue defect Ⓑ    E1

Reconstruction of surgical, traumatic, or congenital defects of the facial bones, including the mandible, may utilize graft materials in conjunction with soft tissue procedures to repair and restore the facial bones to form and function. This does not include obtaining the graft and these procedures may require multiple surgical approaches. This procedure does not include edentulous maxilla and mandibular reconstruction for prosthetic considerations.

*Cross Reference 21299*

**D7960** Frenulectomy - also known as frenectomy or frenotomy - separate procedure not incidental to another procedure Ⓑ    E1

Removal or release of mucosal and muscle elements of a buccal, labial or lingual frenum that is associated with a pathological condition, or interferes with proper oral development or treatment.

*Cross Reference 40819, 41010, 41115*

**D7963** Frenuloplasty Ⓑ    E1

Excision of frenum with accompanying excision or repositioning of aberrant muscle and z-plasty or other local flap closure.

**D7970** Excision of hyperplastic tissue - per arch Ⓑ    E1

**D7971** Excision of pericoronal gingival Ⓑ    E1

Removal of inflammatory or hypertrophied tissues surrounding partially erupted/impacted teeth.

*Cross Reference 41821*

**D7972** Surgical reduction of fibrous tuberosity Ⓑ    E1

**D7979** Non surgical sialolithotomy Ⓑ    E1

A sialolith is removed from the gland or ductal portion of the gland without surgical incision into the gland or the duct of the gland; for example via manual manipulation, ductal dilation, or any other non-surgical method.

**D7980** Surgical sialolithotomy Ⓑ    E1

Procedure by which a stone within a salivary gland or its duct is removed, either intraorally or extraorally.

*Cross Reference 42330, 42335, 42340*

**D7981** Excision of salivary gland, by report Ⓑ    E1

*Cross Reference 42408*

**D7982** Sialodochoplasty Ⓑ    E1

Procedure for the repair of a defect and/or restoration of a portion of a salivary gland duct.

*Cross Reference 42500*

**D7983** Closure of salivary fistula Ⓑ    E1

Closure of an opening between a salivary duct and/or gland and the cutaneous surface, or an opening into the oral cavity through other than the normal anatomic pathway.

*Cross Reference 42600*

**D7990** Emergency tracheotomy Ⓑ    E1

Formation of a tracheal opening usually below the cricoid cartilage to allow for respiratory exchange.

*Cross Reference 21070*

**D7991** Coronoidectomy Ⓑ    E1

Removal of the coronoid process of the mandible.

*Cross Reference 21070*

**D7995** Synthetic graft - mandible or facial bones, by report Ⓑ    E1

Includes allogenic material.

*Cross Reference 21299*

**D7996** Implant-mandible for augmentation purposes (excluding alveolar ridge), by report Ⓑ    E1

*Cross Reference 21299*

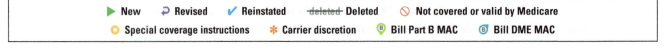

▶ New    ↵ Revised    ✔ Reinstated    ~~deleted~~ Deleted    ⊘ Not covered or valid by Medicare
   ✿ Special coverage instructions    ✳ Carrier discretion    Ⓑ Bill Part B MAC    Ⓓ Bill DME MAC

**D7997** Appliance removal (not by dentist who placed appliance), includes removal of archbar Ⓑ E1

**D7998** Intraoral placement of a fixation device not in conjunction with a fracture Ⓑ E1

The placement of intermaxillary fixation appliance for documented medically accepted treatments not in association with fractures.

## None

**D7999** Unspecified oral surgery procedure, by report Ⓑ E1

Used for procedure that is not adequately described by a code. Describe procedure.

*Cross Reference 21299*

## Orthodontics (D8010-D8999)
### Limited Orthodontic Treatment

**D8010** Limited orthodontic treatment of the primary dentition Ⓑ E1

**D8020** Limited orthodontic treatment of the transitional dentition Ⓑ E1

**D8030** Limited orthodontic treatment of the adolescent dentition Ⓑ Ⓐ E1

**D8040** Limited orthodontic treatment of the adult dentition Ⓑ Ⓐ E1

### Interceptive Orthodontic Treatment

**D8050** Interceptive orthodontic treatment of the primary dentition Ⓑ E1

**D8060** Interceptive orthodontic treatment of the transitional dentition Ⓑ E1

### Comprehensive Orthodontic Treatment

**D8070** Comprehensive orthodontic treatment of the transitional dentition Ⓑ E1

**D8080** Comprehensive orthodontic treatment of the adolescent dentition Ⓑ Ⓐ E1

**D8090** Comprehensive orthodontic treatment of the adult dentition Ⓑ Ⓐ E1

### Minor Treatment to Control Harmful Habits

**D8210** Removable appliance therapy Ⓑ E1

Removable indicates patient can remove; includes appliances for thumb sucking and tongue thrusting.

**D8220** Fixed appliance therapy Ⓑ E1

Fixed indicates patient cannot remove appliance; includes appliances for thumb sucking and tongue thrusting.

### Other Orthodontic Services

**D8660** Pre-orthodontic treatment examination to monitor growth and development Ⓑ E1

Periodic observation of patient dentition, at intervals established by the dentist, to determine when orthodontic treatment should begin. Diagnostic procedures are documented separately.

**D8670** Periodic orthodontic treatment visit Ⓑ E1

**D8680** Orthodontic retention (removal of appliances, construction and placement of retainer(s)) Ⓑ E1

**D8681** Removable orthodontic retainer adjustment Ⓑ E1

**D8690** Orthodontic treatment (alternative billing to a contract fee) Ⓑ E1

Services provided by dentist other than original treating dentist. A method of payment between the provider and responsible party for services that reflect an open-ended fee arrangement.

~~D8691 Repair of orthodontic appliance~~ ✖

~~D8692 Replacement of lost or broken retainer~~ ✖

~~D8693 Re-cement or re-bond of fixed retainer~~ ✖

~~D8694 Repair of fixed retainers, includes reattachment~~ ✖

**D8695** Removal of fixed orthodontic appliances for reasons other than completion of treatment Ⓑ E1

▶ **D8696** Repair of orthodontic appliance - maxillary E1

Does not include bracket and standard fixed orthodontic appliances. It does include functional appliances and palatal expanders.

▶ **D8697** Repair of orthodontic appliance - mandibular E1

Does not include bracket and standard fixed orthodontic appliances. It does include functional appliances and palatal expanders.

▶ **D8698** Re-cement or re-bond fixed retainer - maxillary E1

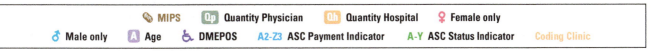

MIPS   Ⓠⓟ Quantity Physician   Ⓠⓗ Quantity Hospital   ♀ Female only
♂ Male only   Ⓐ Age   DMEPOS   A2-Z3 ASC Payment Indicator   A-Y ASC Status Indicator   Coding Clinic

▶ **D8699** Re-cement or re-bond fixed retainer - mandibular **E1**

▶ **D8701** Repair of fixed retainer, includes reattachment - maxillary **E1**

▶ **D8702** Repair of fixed retainer, includes reattachment - mandibular **E1**

▶ **D8703** Replacement of lost or broken retainer - maxillary **E1**

▶ **D8704** Replacement of lost or broken retainer - mandibular **E1**

## None

**D8999** Unspecified orthodontic procedure, by report Ⓑ **E1**

Used for procedure that is not adequately described by a code. Describe procedure.

## Adjunctive General Services (D9110-D9999)
### Unclassified Treatment

**D9110** Palliative (emergency) treatment of dental pain - minor procedures Ⓑ **N**

This is typically reported on a "per visit" basis for emergency treatment of dental pain.

**D9120** Fixed partial denture sectioning Ⓑ **E1**

Separation of one or more connections between abutments and/or pontics when some portion of a fixed prosthesis is to remain intact and serviceable following sectioning and extraction or other treatment. Includes all recontouring and polishing of retained portions.

**D9130** Temporomandibular joint dysfunction - non-invasive physical therapies Ⓑ **E1**

### Anesthesia

**D9210** Local anesthesia not in conjunction with operative or surgical procedures Ⓑ **E1**

Cross Reference 90784

**D9211** Regional block anesthesia Ⓑ **E1**

Cross Reference 01995

**D9212** Trigeminal division block anesthesia Ⓑ **E1**

Cross Reference 64400

**D9215** Local anesthesia in conjunction with operative or surgical procedures Ⓑ **E1**

Cross Reference 90784

**D9219** Evaluation for moderate sedation or general anesthesia Ⓑ Ⓐ **E1**

**D9222** Deep sedation/general anesthesia first 15 minutes Ⓑ **E1**

Anesthesia time begins when the doctor administering the anesthetic agent initiates the appropriate anesthesia and non-invasive monitoring protocol and remains in continuous attendance of the patient. Anesthesia services are considered completed when the patient may be safely left under the observation of trained personnel and the doctor may safely leave the room to attend to other patients or duties.

The level of anesthesia is determined by the anesthesia provider's documentation of the anesthetic effects upon the central nervous system and not dependent upon the route of administration.

**D9223** Deep sedation/general anesthesia - each subsequent 15 minute increment Ⓑ **E1**

**D9230** Inhalation of nitrous oxide/analgesia, anxiolysis Ⓑ **N**

**D9239** Intravenous moderate (conscious) sedation/analgesia - first 15 minutes Ⓑ **E1**

Anesthesia time begins when the doctor administering the anesthetic agent initiates the appropriate anesthesia and non-invasive monitoring protocol and remains in continuous attendance of the patient. Anesthesia services are considered completed when the patient may be safely left under the observation of trained personnel and the doctor may safely leave the room to attend to other patients or duties.

The level of anesthesia is determined by the anesthesia provider's documentation of the anesthetic effects upon the central nervous system and not dependent upon the route of administration.

**D9243** Intravenous moderate (conscious) sedation/analgesia - each subsequent 15 minute increment Ⓑ **E1**

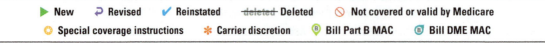

▶ New  ↻ Revised  ✔ Reinstated  ~~deleted~~ Deleted  ⊘ Not covered or valid by Medicare  ✿ Special coverage instructions  ✱ Carrier discretion  Ⓑ Bill Part B MAC  Ⓑ Bill DME MAC

**D9248** Non-intravenous conscious sedation Ⓑ      **N**

This includes non-IV minimal and moderate sedation. A medically controlled state of depressed consciousness while maintaining the patient's airway, protective reflexes and the ability to respond to stimulation or verbal commands. It includes non-intravenous administration of sedative and/or analgesic agent(s) and appropriate monitoring.

The level of anesthesia is determined by the anesthesia provider's documentation of the anesthetic's effects upon the central nervous system and not dependent upon the route of administration.

## Professional Consultation

**D9310** Consultation - diagnostic service provided by dentist or physician other than requesting dentist or physician Ⓑ      **E1**

A patient encounter with a practitioner whose opinion or advice regarding evaluation and/or management of a specific problem; may be requested by another practitioner or appropriate source. The consultation includes an oral evaluation. The consulted practitioner may initiate diagnostic and/or therapeutic services.

**D9311** Consultation with a medical health care professional Ⓑ      **E1**

Treating dentist consults with a medical health care professional concerning medical issues that may affect patient's planned dental treatment.

## Professional Visits

**D9410** House/extended care facility call Ⓑ      **E1**

Includes visits to nursing homes, long-term care facilities, hospice sites, institutions, etc. Report in addition to reporting appropriate code numbers for actual services performed.

**D9420** Hospital or ambulatory surgical center call Ⓑ      **E1**

Care provided outside the dentist's office to a patient who is in a hospital or ambulatory surgical center. Services delivered to the patient on the date of service are documented separately using the applicable procedure codes.

**D9430** Office visit for observation (during regularly scheduled hours) - no other services performed Ⓑ      **E1**

**D9440** Office visit-after regularly scheduled hours Ⓑ      **E1**

*Cross Reference 99050*

**D9450** Case presentation, detailed and extensive treatment planning Ⓑ      **E1**

Established patient. Not performed on same day as evaluation.

## Drugs

**D9610** Therapeutic parenteral drug, single administration Ⓑ      **E1**

Includes single administration of antibiotics, steroids, anti-inflammatory drugs, or other therapeutic medications. This code should not be used to report administration of sedative, anesthetic or reversal agents.

**D9612** Therapeutic parenteral drugs, two or more administrations, different medications Ⓑ      **E1**

Includes multiple administrations of antibiotics, steroids, anti-inflammatory drugs or other therapeutic medications. This code should not be used to report administration of sedatives, anesthetic or reversal agents. This code should be reported when two or more different medications are necessary and should not be reported in addition to code D9610 on the same date.

**D9613** Infiltration of sustained release therapeutic drug - single or multiple sites      **E1**

**D9630** Drugs or medicaments dispensed in the office for home use Ⓑ      **B**

Includes, but is not limited to oral antibiotics, oral analgesics, and topical fluoride; does not include writing prescriptions.

## Miscellaneous Services

**D9910** Application of desensitizing medicament Ⓑ      **E1**

Includes in-office treatment for root sensitivity. Typically reported on a "per visit" basis for application of topical fluoride. This code is not to be used for bases, liners or adhesives used under restorations.

---

 MIPS    **Qp** Quantity Physician   **Qh** Quantity Hospital   ♀ Female only

♂ Male only    **A** Age    DMEPOS   **A2-Z3** ASC Payment Indicator   **A-Y** ASC Status Indicator   Coding Clinic

**D9911** Application of desensitizing resin for cervical and/or root surface, per tooth Ⓑ    E1

Typically reported on a "per tooth" basis for application of adhesive resins. This code is not to be used for bases, liners, or adhesives used under restorations.

**D9920** Behavior management, by report Ⓑ    E1

May be reported in addition to treatment provided. Should be reported in 15-minute increments.

**D9930** Treatment of complications (postsurgical) - unusual circumstances, by report Ⓑ    S

For example, treatment of a dry socket following extraction or removal of bony sequestrum.

**D9932** Cleaning and inspection of removable complete denture, maxillary Ⓑ    E1

This procedure does not include any adjustments.

**D9933** Cleaning and inspection of removable complete denture, mandibular Ⓑ    E1

This procedure does not include any adjustments.

**D9934** Cleaning and inspection of removable partial denture, maxillary Ⓑ    E1

This procedure does not include any adjustments.

**D9935** Cleaning and inspection of removable partial denture, mandibular Ⓑ    E1

This procedure does not include any adjustments.

**D9941** Fabrication of athletic mouthguard Ⓞ E1

*Cross Reference 21089*

**D9942** Repair and/or reline of occlusal guard Ⓑ    E1

**D9943** Occlusal guard adjustment Ⓑ    E1

**D9944** Occlusal guard - hard appliance, full arch    E1

**D9945** Occlusal guard - soft appliance, full arch    E1

**D9946** Occlusal guard - hard appliance, partial arch Ⓞ    E1

**D9950** Occlusion analysis - mounted case Ⓞ    S

Includes, but is not limited to, facebow, interocclusal records tracings, and diagnostic wax-up; for diagnostic casts, see D0470.

**D9951** Occlusal adjustment - limited Ⓑ    S

May also be known as equilibration; reshaping the occlusal surfaces of teeth to create harmonious contact relationships between the maxillary and mandibular teeth. Presently includes discing/odontoplasty/enamoplasty. Typically reported on a "per visit" basis. This should not be reported when the procedure only involves bite adjustment in the routine post-delivery care for a direct/indirect restoration or fixed/removable prosthodontics.

**D9952** Occlusal adjustment - complete Ⓑ    S

Occlusal adjustment may require several appointments of varying length, and sedation may be necessary to attain adequate relaxation of the musculature. Study casts mounted on an articulating instrument may be utilized for analysis of occlusal disharmony. It is designed to achieve functional relationships and masticatory efficiency in conjunction with restorative treatment, orthodontics, orthognathic surgery, or jaw trauma when indicated. Occlusal adjustment enhances the healing potential of tissues affected by the lesions of occlusal trauma.

**D9961** Duplicate/copy of patient's records Ⓞ E1

**D9970** Enamel microabrasion Ⓑ    E1

The removal of discolored surface enamel defects resulting from altered mineralization or decalcification of the superficial enamel layer. Submit per treatment visit.

**D9971** Odontoplasty 1 - 2 teeth; includes removal of enamel projections Ⓑ    E1

**D9972** External bleaching - per arch - performed in office Ⓑ    E1

**D9973** External bleaching - per tooth Ⓑ    E1

**D9974** Internal bleaching - per tooth Ⓑ    E1

**D9975** External bleaching for home application, per arch; includes materials and fabrication of custom trays Ⓑ    E1

## Non-Clinical Procedures

**D9985** Sales tax Ⓑ    E1

**D9986** Missed appointment Ⓞ    E1

**D9987** Cancelled appointment Ⓑ    E1

**D9990** Certified translation or sign-language services - per visit Ⓞ    E1

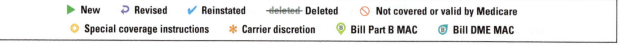

▶ New    ↻ Revised    ✔ Reinstated    ~~deleted~~ Deleted    ⊘ Not covered or valid by Medicare    Ⓞ Special coverage instructions    ✳ Carrier discretion    Ⓑ Bill Part B MAC    Ⓓ Bill DME MAC

**D9991** Dental case management - addressing appointment compliance barriers ⑧ E1

Individualized efforts to assist a patient to maintain scheduled appointments by solving transportation challenges or other barriers.

**D9992** Dental case management - care coordination ⑧ E1

Assisting in a patient's decisions regarding the coordination of oral health care services across multiple providers, provider types, specialty areas of treatment, health care settings, health care organizations and payment systems. This is the additional time and resources expended to provide experience or expertise beyond that possessed by the patient.

**D9993** Dental case management - motivational interviewing ⑧ E1

Patient-centered, personalized counseling using methods such as Motivational Interviewing (MI) to identify and modify behaviors interfering with positive oral health outcomes. This is a separate service from traditional nutritional or tobacco counseling.

**D9994** Dental case management - patient education to improve oral health literacy ⑧ E1

Individual, customized communication of information to assist the patient in making appropriate health decisions designed to improve oral health literacy, explained in a manner acknowledging economic circumstances and different cultural beliefs, values, attitudes, traditions and language preferences, and adopting information and services to these differences, which requires the expenditure of time and resources beyond that of an oral evaluation or case presentation.

**D9995** Teledentistry synchronous; real-time encounter ⑧ E1

Reported in addition to other procedures (e.g., diagnostic) delivered to the patient on the date of service.

**D9996** Teledentistry asynchronous; information stored and forwarded to dentist for subsequent review ⑧ E1

Reported in addition to other procedures (e.g., diagnostic) delivered to the patient on the date of service.

▶ **D9997** Dental case management - patients with special health care needs E1

Special treatment considerations for patients/individuals with physical, medical, developmental or cognitive conditions resulting in substantial functional limitations, which require that modifications be made to delivery of treatment to provide comprehensive oral health care services.

*None*

**D9999** Unspecified adjunctive procedure, by report ⑧ E1

Used for procedure that is not adequately described by a code. Describe procedure.

*Cross Reference 21499*

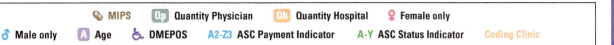

🖐 MIPS    Qp Quantity Physician    Qh Quantity Hospital    ♀ Female only

♂ Male only    A Age    ♿ DMEPOS    A2-Z3 ASC Payment Indicator    A-Y ASC Status Indicator    Coding Clinic

## DURABLE MEDICAL EQUIPMENT (E0100-E8002)

### Canes

⚙ **E0100**  Cane, includes canes of all materials, adjustable or fixed, with tip Ⓑ Qp Qh ♿  Y

*IOM: 100-02, 15, 110.1; 100-03, 4, 280.1; 100-03, 4, 280.2*

⚙ **E0105**  Cane, quad or three prong, includes canes of all materials, adjustable or fixed, with tips Ⓑ Qp Qh ♿  Y

*IOM: 100-02, 15, 110.1; 100-03, 4, 280.1; 100-03, 4, 280.2*

**Coding Clinic: 2016, Q3, P3**

### Crutches

⚙ **E0110**  Crutches, forearm, includes crutches of various materials, adjustable or fixed, pair, complete with tips and handgrips Ⓑ Qp Qh ♿  Y

Crutches are covered when prescribed for a patient who is normally ambulatory but suffers from a condition that impairs ambulation. Provides minimal to moderate weight support while ambulating.

*IOM: 100-02, 15, 110.1; 100-03, 4, 280.1*

⚙ **E0111**  Crutch forearm, includes crutches of various materials, adjustable or fixed, each, with tips and handgrips Ⓑ Qp Qh ♿  Y

*IOM: 100-02, 15, 110.1; 100-03, 4, 280.1*

⚙ **E0112**  Crutches, underarm, wood, adjustable or fixed, pair, with pads, tips, and handgrips Ⓑ Qp Qh ♿  Y

*IOM: 100-02, 15, 110.1; 100-03, 4, 280.1*

⚙ **E0113**  Crutch underarm, wood, adjustable or fixed, each, with pad, tip, and handgrip Ⓑ Qp Qh ♿  Y

*IOM: 100-02, 15, 110.1; 100-03, 4, 280.1*

⚙ **E0114**  Crutches, underarm, other than wood, adjustable or fixed, pair, with pads, tips and handgrips Ⓑ Qp Qh ♿  Y

*IOM: 100-02, 15, 110.1; 100-03, 4, 280.1*

⚙ **E0116**  Crutch, underarm, other than wood, adjustable or fixed, with pad, tip, handgrip, with or without shock absorber, each Ⓑ Qp Qh ♿  Y

*IOM: 100-02, 15, 110.1; 100-03, 4, 280.1*

⚙ **E0117**  Crutch, underarm, articulating, spring assisted, each Ⓑ Qp Qh ♿  Y

*IOM: 100-02, 15, 110.1*

✳ **E0118**  Crutch substitute, lower leg platform, with or without wheels, each Ⓑ Qp Qh  E1

### Walkers

⚙ **E0130**  Walker, rigid (pickup), adjustable or fixed height Ⓑ Qp Qh ♿  Y

Standard walker criteria for payment: Individual has a mobility limitation that significantly impairs ability to participate in mobility-related activities of daily living that cannot be adequately or safely addressed by a cane. The patient is able to use the walker safely; the functional mobility deficit can be resolved with use of a standard walker.

*IOM: 100-02, 15, 110.1; 100-03, 4, 280.1*

⚙ **E0135**  Walker, folding (pickup), adjustable or fixed height Ⓑ Qp Qh ♿  Y

*IOM: 100-02, 15, 110.1; 100-03, 4, 280.1*

⚙ **E0140**  Walker, with trunk support, adjustable or fixed height, any type Ⓑ Qp Qh ♿  Y

*IOM: 100-02, 15, 110.1; 100-03, 4, 280.1*

⚙ **E0141**  Walker, rigid, wheeled, adjustable or fixed height Ⓑ Qp Qh ♿  Y

*IOM: 100-02, 15, 110.1; 100-03, 4, 280.1*

⚙ **E0143**  Walker, folding, wheeled, adjustable or fixed height Ⓑ Qp Qh ♿  Y

*IOM: 100-02, 15, 110.1; 100-03, 4, 280.1*

⚙ **E0144**  Walker, enclosed, four sided framed, rigid or folding, wheeled, with posterior seat Ⓑ Qp Qh ♿  Y

*IOM: 100-02, 15, 110.1; 100-03, 4, 280.1*

⚙ **E0147**  Walker, heavy duty, multiple braking system, variable wheel resistance Ⓑ Qp Qh ♿  Y

Heavy-duty walker is labeled as capable of supporting more than 300 pounds

*IOM: 100-02, 15, 110.1; 100-03, 4, 280.1*

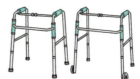

**Figure 11**  Walkers.

---

▶ New  ↻ Revised  ✔ Reinstated  ~~deleted~~ Deleted  ⃠ Not covered or valid by Medicare
⚙ Special coverage instructions  ✳ Carrier discretion  Ⓑ Bill Part B MAC  Ⓑ Bill DME MAC

* **E0148** Walker, heavy duty, without wheels, rigid or folding, any type, each 🅑 Qp Qh ♿ Y

  *Heavy-duty walker is labeled as capable of supporting more than 300 pounds*

* **E0149** Walker, heavy duty, wheeled, rigid or folding, any type 🅑 Qp Qh ♿ Y

  *Heavy-duty walker is labeled as capable of supporting more than 300 pounds*

* **E0153** Platform attachment, forearm crutch, each 🅑 Qp Qh ♿ Y

* **E0154** Platform attachment, walker, each 🅑 Qp Qh ♿ Y

* **E0155** Wheel attachment, rigid pick-up walker, per pair 🅑 Qp Qh ♿ Y

## Attachments

* **E0156** Seat attachment, walker 🅑 Qp Qh ♿ Y

* **E0157** Crutch attachment, walker, each 🅑 Qp Qh ♿ Y

* **E0158** Leg extensions for walker, per set of four (4) 🅑 Qp Qh ♿ Y

  *Leg extensions are considered medically necessary DME for patients 6 feet tall or more.*

* **E0159** Brake attachment for wheeled walker, replacement, each 🅑 Qp Qh ♿ Y

## Sitz Bath/Equipment

⚙ **E0160** Sitz type bath or equipment, portable, used with or without commode 🅑 Qp Qh ♿ Y

  *IOM: 100-03, 4, 280.1*

⚙ **E0161** Sitz type bath or equipment, portable, used with or without commode, with faucet attachment/s 🅑 Qp Qh ♿ Y

  *IOM: 100-03, 4, 280.1*

⚙ **E0162** Sitz bath chair 🅑 Qp Qh ♿ Y

  *IOM: 100-03, 4, 280.1*

## Commodes

⚙ **E0163** Commode chair, mobile or stationary, with fixed arms 🅑 Qp Qh ♿ Y

  *IOM: 100-02, 15, 110.1; 100-03, 4, 280.1*

⚙ **E0165** Commode chair, mobile or stationary, with detachable arms 🅑 Qp Qh ♿ Y

  *IOM: 100-02, 15, 110.1; 100-03, 4, 280.1*

⚙ **E0167** Pail or pan for use with commode chair, replacement only 🅑 Qp Qh ♿ Y

  *IOM: 100-03, 4, 280.1*

* **E0168** Commode chair, extra wide and/or heavy duty, stationary or mobile, with or without arms, any type, each 🅑 Qp Qh ♿ Y

  *Extra-wide or heavy duty commode chair is labeled as capable of supporting more than 300 pounds*

* **E0170** Commode chair with integrated seat lift mechanism, electric, any type 🅑 Qp Qh ♿ Y

* **E0171** Commode chair with integrated seat lift mechanism, non-electric, any type 🅑 Qp Qh ♿ Y

⊘ **E0172** Seat lift mechanism placed over or on top of toilet, any type 🅑 Qp Qh E1

  *Medicare Statute 1861 SSA*

* **E0175** Foot rest, for use with commode chair, each 🅑 Qp Qh ♿ Y

## Decubitus Care Equipment

⚙ **E0181** Powered pressure reducing mattress overlay/pad, alternating, with pump, includes heavy duty 🅑 Qp Qh ♿ Y

  *Requires the provider to determine medical necessity compliance. To demonstrate the requirements in the medical policy were met, attach KX.*

  *IOM: 100-03, 4, 280.1; 100-08, 5, 5.2.3*

⚙ **E0182** Pump for alternating pressure pad, for replacement only 🅑 Qp Qh ♿ Y

  *IOM: 100-03, 4, 280.1; 100-08, 5, 5.2.3*

⚙ **E0184** Dry pressure mattress 🅑 Qp Qh ♿ Y

  *IOM: 100-03, 4, 280.1; 100-08, 5, 5.2.3*

⚙ **E0185** Gel or gel-like pressure pad for mattress, standard mattress length and width 🅑 Qp Qh ♿ Y

  *IOM: 100-03, 4, 280.1; 100-08, 5, 5.2.3*

⚙ **E0186** Air pressure mattress 🅑 Qp Qh ♿ Y

  *IOM: 100-03, 4, 280.1*

⚙ **E0187** Water pressure mattress 🅑 Qp Qh ♿ Y

  *IOM: 100-03, 4, 280.1*

⚙ **E0188** Synthetic sheepskin pad 🅑 Qp Qh ♿ Y

  *IOM: 100-03, 4, 280.1; 100-08, 5, 5.2.3*

⚙ **E0189** Lambswool sheepskin pad, any size 🅑 Qp Qh ♿ Y

  *IOM: 100-03, 4, 280.1; 100-08, 5, 5.2.3*

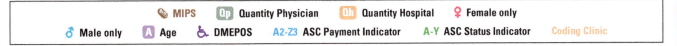

MIPS   Qp Quantity Physician   Qh Quantity Hospital   ♀ Female only   ♂ Male only   A Age   ♿ DMEPOS   A2-Z3 ASC Payment Indicator   A-Y ASC Status Indicator   Coding Clinic

⊛ **E0190** Positioning cushion/pillow/wedge, any shape or size, includes all components and accessories ⑬ Qp Qh     E1

*IOM: 100-02, 15, 110.1*

✳ **E0191** Heel or elbow protector, each ⑬ Qp Qh ♿     Y

✳ **E0193** Powered air flotation bed (low air loss therapy) ⑬ Qp Qh ♿     Y

⊛ **E0194** Air fluidized bed ⑬ Qp Qh ♿     Y

*IOM: 100-03, 4, 280.1*

⊛ **E0196** Gel pressure mattress ⑬ Qp Qh ♿     Y

*IOM: 100-03, 4, 280.1*

⊛ **E0197** Air pressure pad for mattress, standard mattress length and width ⑬ Qp Qh ♿     Y

*IOM: 100-03, 4, 280.1*

⊛ **E0198** Water pressure pad for mattress, standard mattress length and width ⑬ Qp Qh ♿     Y

*IOM: 100-03, 4, 280.1*

⊛ **E0199** Dry pressure pad for mattress, standard mattress length and width ⑬ Qp Qh ♿     Y

*IOM: 100-03, 4, 280.1*

## Heat/Cold Application

⊛ **E0200** Heat lamp, without stand (table model), includes bulb, or infrared element ⑬ Qp Qh ♿     Y

Covered when medical review determines patient's medical condition is one for which application of heat by heat lamp is therapeutically effective

*IOM: 100-02, 15, 110.1; 100-03, 4, 280.1*

✳ **E0202** Phototherapy (bilirubin) light with photometer ⑬ Qp Qh ♿     Y

⊘ **E0203** Therapeutic lightbox, minimum 10,000 lux, table top model ⑬ Qp Qh     E1

*IOM: 100-03, 4, 280.1*

⊛ **E0205** Heat lamp, with stand, includes bulb, or infrared element ⑬ Qp Qh ♿     Y

*IOM: 100-02, 15, 110.1; 100-03, 4, 280.1*

⊛ **E0210** Electric heat pad, standard ⑬ Qp Qh ♿     Y

Flexible device containing electric resistive elements producing heat; has fabric cover to prevent burns; with or without timing devices for automatic shut-off

*IOM: 100-03, 4, 280.1*

⊛ **E0215** Electric heat pad, moist ⑬ Qp Qh ♿     Y

Flexible device containing electric resistive elements producing heat. Must have component that will absorb and retain liquid (water).

*IOM: 100-03, 4, 280.1*

⊛ **E0217** Water circulating heat pad with pump ⑬ Qp Qh ♿     Y

Consists of flexible pad containing series of channels through which water is circulated by means of electrical pumping mechanism and heated in external reservoir

*IOM: 100-03, 4, 280.1*

⊛ **E0218** Fluid circulating cold pad with pump, any type ⑬ Qp Qh     Y

*IOM: 100-03, 4, 280.1*

✳ **E0221** Infrared heating pad system ⑬ Qp Qh     Y

⊛ **E0225** Hydrocollator unit, includes pads ⑬ Qp Qh ♿     Y

*IOM: 100-02, 15, 230; 100-03, 4, 280.1*

⊘ **E0231** Non-contact wound warming device (temperature control unit, AC adapter and power cord) for use with warming card and wound cover ⑬ Qp Qh     E1

*IOM: 100-02, 16, 20*

⊘ **E0232** Warming card for use with the non-contact wound warming device and non-contact wound warming wound cover ⑬ Qp Qh     E1

*IOM: 100-02, 16, 20*

⊛ **E0235** Paraffin bath unit, portable, (see medical supply code A4265 for paraffin) ⑬ Qp Qh ♿     Y

Ordered by physician and patient's condition expected to be relieved by long-term use of modality

*IOM: 100-02, 15, 230; 100-03, 4, 280.1*

⊛ **E0236** Pump for water circulating pad ⑬ Qp Qh ♿     Y

*IOM: 100-03, 4, 280.1*

⊛ **E0239** Hydrocollator unit, portable ⑬ Qp Qh ♿     Y

*IOM: 100-02, 15, 230; 100-03, 4, 280.1*

## Bath and Toilet Aids

⊘ **E0240** Bath/shower chair, with or without wheels, any size ⑬ Qp Qh     E1

*IOM: 100-03, 4, 280.1*

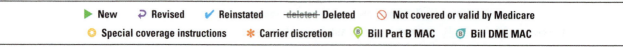

▶ New    ↻ Revised    ✔ Reinstated    ~~deleted~~ Deleted    ⊘ Not covered or valid by Medicare
⊛ Special coverage instructions    ✳ Carrier discretion    ⑬ Bill Part B MAC    ⑬ Bill DME MAC

⊘ **E0241**  Bath tub wall rail, each Ⓑ Qp Qh    E1
*IOM: 100-02, 15, 110.1; 100-03, 4, 280.1*

⊘ **E0242**  Bath tub rail, floor base Ⓑ Qp Qh    E1
*IOM: 100-02, 15, 110.1; 100-03, 4, 280.1*

⊘ **E0243**  Toilet rail, each Ⓑ Qp Qh    E1
*IOM: 100-02, 15, 110.1; 100-03, 4, 280.1*

⊘ **E0244**  Raised toilet seat Ⓑ Qp Qh    E1
*IOM: 100-03, 4, 280.1*

⊘ **E0245**  Tub stool or bench Ⓑ Qp Qh    E1
*IOM: 100-03, 4, 280.1*

✳ **E0246**  Transfer tub rail
attachment Ⓑ Qp Qh    E1

✿ **E0247**  Transfer bench for tub or toilet
with or without commode
opening Ⓑ Qp Qh    E1
*IOM: 100-03, 4, 280.1*

✿ **E0248**  Transfer bench, heavy duty, for tub
or toilet with or without commode
opening Ⓑ Qp Qh    E1

Heavy duty transfer bench is labeled
as capable of supporting more than
300 pounds
*IOM: 100-03, 4, 280.1*

## Pad for Heating Unit

✿ **E0249**  Pad for water circulating heat unit, for
replacement only Ⓑ Qp Qh &    Y

Describes durable replacement pad
used with water circulating heat pump
system
*IOM: 100-03, 4, 280.1*

## Hospital Beds and Accessories

✿ **E0250**  Hospital bed, fixed height, with any
type side rails, with
mattress Ⓑ Qp Qh ♿    Y
*IOM: 100-02, 15, 110.1; 100-03, 4, 280.7*

✿ **E0251**  Hospital bed, fixed height, with any
type side rails, without
mattress Ⓑ Qp Qh ♿    Y
*IOM: 100-02, 15, 110.1; 100-03, 4, 280.7*

✿ **E0255**  Hospital bed, variable height, hi-lo,
with any type side rails, with
mattress Ⓑ Qp Qh ♿    Y
*IOM: 100-02, 15, 110.1; 100-03, 4, 280.7*

✿ **E0256**  Hospital bed, variable height, hi-lo,
with any type side rails, without
mattress Ⓑ Qp Qh &    Y
*IOM: 100-02, 15, 110.1; 100-03, 4, 280.7*

✿ **E0260**  Hospital bed, semi-electric (head and
foot adjustment), with any type side
rails, with mattress Ⓑ Qp Qh &    Y
*IOM: 100-02, 15, 110.1; 100-03, 4, 280.7*

✿ **E0261**  Hospital bed, semi-electric (head and
foot adjustment), with any type side
rails, without mattress Ⓑ Qp Qh &    Y
*IOM: 100-02, 15, 110.1; 100-03, 4, 280.7*

✿ **E0265**  Hospital bed, total electric (head, foot
and height adjustments), with any type
side rails, with mattress Ⓑ Qp Qh & Y
*IOM: 100-02, 15, 110.1; 100-03, 4, 280.7*

✿ **E0266**  Hospital bed, total electric (head, foot
and height adjustments), with any type
side rails, without
mattress Ⓑ Qp Qh &    Y
*IOM: 100-02, 15, 110.1; 100-03, 4, 280.7*

⊘ **E0270**  Hospital bed, institutional type
includes: oscillating, circulating
and Stryker frame, with
mattress Ⓑ Qp Qh    E1
*IOM: 100-03, 4, 280.1*

✿ **E0271**  Mattress, innerspring Ⓑ Qp Qh &    Y
*IOM: 100-03, 4, 280.1; 100-03, 4, 280.7*

✿ **E0272**  Mattress, foam rubber Ⓑ Qp Qh & Y
*IOM: 100-03, 4, 280.1; 100-03, 4, 280.7*

⊘ **E0273**  Bed board Ⓑ Qp Qh    E1
*IOM: 100-03, 4, 280.1*

⊘ **E0274**  Over-bed table Ⓑ Qp Qh    E1
*IOM: 100-03, 4, 280.1*

✿ **E0275**  Bed pan, standard, metal or
plastic Ⓑ Qp Qh &    Y
*IOM: 100-03, 4, 280.1*

✿ **E0276**  Bed pan, fracture, metal or
plastic Ⓑ Qp Qh &    Y
*IOM: 100-03, 4, 280.1*

✿ **E0277**  Powered pressure-reducing air
mattress Ⓑ Qp Qh &    Y
*IOM: 100-03, 4, 280.1*

✳ **E0280**  Bed cradle, any type Ⓑ Qp Qh &    Y

✿ **E0290**  Hospital bed, fixed height,
without side rails, with
mattress Ⓑ Qp Qh ♿    Y
*IOM: 100-02, 15, 110.1; 100-03, 4, 280.7*

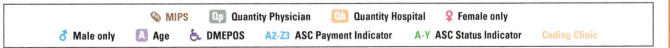

🐾 MIPS    Qp Quantity Physician    Qh Quantity Hospital    ♀ Female only
♂ Male only    Ⓐ Age    & DMEPOS    A2-Z3 ASC Payment Indicator    A-Y ASC Status Indicator    Coding Clinic

⚙ **E0291** Hospital bed, fixed height, without side rails, without mattress Ⓑ Qp Qh ♿    Y

*IOM: 100-02, 15, 110.1; 100-03, 4, 280.7*

⚙ **E0292** Hospital bed, variable height, hi-lo, without side rails, with mattress Ⓑ Qp Qh ♿    Y

*IOM: 100-02, 15, 110.1; 100-03, 4, 280.7*

⚙ **E0293** Hospital bed, variable height, hi-lo, without side rails, without mattress Ⓑ Qp Qh ♿    Y

*IOM: 100-02, 15, 110.1; 100-03, 4, 280.7*

⚙ **E0294** Hospital bed, semi-electric (head and foot adjustment), without side rails, with mattress Ⓑ Qp Qh ♿    Y

*IOM: 100-02, 15, 110.1; 100-03, 4, 280.7*

⚙ **E0295** Hospital bed, semi-electric (head and foot adjustment), without side rails, without mattress Ⓑ Qp Qh ♿    Y

*IOM: 100-02, 15, 110.1; 100-03, 4, 280.7*

⚙ **E0296** Hospital bed, total electric (head, foot and height adjustments), without side rails, with mattress Ⓑ Qp Qh ♿    Y

*IOM: 100-02, 15, 110.1; 100-03, 4, 280.7*

⚙ **E0297** Hospital bed, total electric (head, foot and height adjustments), without side rails, without mattress Ⓑ Qp Qh ♿    Y

*IOM: 100-02, 15, 110.1; 100-03, 4, 280.7*

✳ **E0300** Pediatric crib, hospital grade, fully enclosed, with or without top enclosure Ⓑ Qp Qh Ⓐ ♿    Y

⚙ **E0301** Hospital bed, heavy duty, extra wide, with weight capacity greater than 350 pounds, but less than or equal to 600 pounds, with any type side rails, without mattress Ⓑ Qp Qh ♿    Y

*IOM: 100-03, 4, 280.7*

⚙ **E0302** Hospital bed, extra heavy duty, extra wide, with weight capacity greater than 600 pounds, with any type side rails, without mattress Ⓑ Qp Qh ♿    Y

*IOM: 100-03, 4, 280.7*

⚙ **E0303** Hospital bed, heavy duty, extra wide, with weight capacity greater than 350 pounds, but less than or equal to 600 pounds, with any type side rails, with mattress Ⓑ Qp Qh ♿    Y

*IOM: 100-03, 4, 280.7*

⚙ **E0304** Hospital bed, extra heavy duty, extra wide, with weight capacity greater than 600 pounds, with any type side rails, with mattress Ⓑ Qp Qh ♿    Y

*IOM: 100-03, 4, 280.7*

⚙ **E0305** Bed side rails, half length Ⓑ Qp Qh ♿    Y

*IOM: 100-03, 4, 280.7*

⚙ **E0310** Bed side rails, full length Ⓑ Qp Qh ♿    Y

*IOM: 100-03, 4, 280.7*

⊘ **E0315** Bed accessory: board, table, or support device, any type Ⓑ Qp Qh    E1

*IOM: 100-03, 4, 280.1*

✳ **E0316** Safety enclosure frame/canopy for use with hospital bed, any type Ⓑ Qp Qh ♿    Y

⚙ **E0325** Urinal; male, jug-type, any material Ⓑ Qp Qh ♂ ♿    Y

*IOM: 100-03, 4, 280.1*

⚙ **E0326** Urinal; female, jug-type, any material Ⓑ Qp Qh ♀ ♿    Y

*IOM: 100-03, 4, 280.1*

✳ **E0328** Hospital bed, pediatric, manual, 360 degree side enclosures, top of headboard, footboard and side rails up to 24 inches above the spring, includes mattress Ⓑ Qp Qh Ⓐ    Y

✳ **E0329** Hospital bed, pediatric, electric or semi-electric, 360 degree side enclosures, top of headboard, footboard and side rails up to 24 inches above the spring, includes mattress Ⓑ Qp Qh Ⓐ    Y

✳ **E0350** Control unit for electronic bowel irrigation/evacuation system Ⓑ Qp Qh    E1

Pulsed Irrigation Enhanced Evacuation (PIEE) is pulsed irrigation of severely impacted fecal material and may be necessary for patients who have not responded to traditional bowel program.

✳ **E0352** Disposable pack (water reservoir bag, speculum, valving mechanism and collection bag/box) for use with the electronic bowel irrigation/evacuation system Ⓑ Qp Qh    E1

Therapy kit includes 1 B-Valve circuit, 2 containment bags, 1 lubricating jelly, 1 bed pad, 1 tray liner-waste disposable bag, and 2 hose clamps

✳ **E0370** Air pressure elevator for heel Ⓑ Qp Qh    E1

---

| ▶ New | ↺ Revised | ✔ Reinstated | ~~deleted~~ Deleted | ⊘ Not covered or valid by Medicare |
|---|---|---|---|---|
| ⚙ Special coverage instructions | ✳ Carrier discretion | Ⓑ Bill Part B MAC | Ⓑ Bill DME MAC | |

✳ **E0371** Non powered advanced pressure reducing overlay for mattress, standard mattress length and width Ⓑ Qp Qh ♿    Y

*Patient has at least one large Stage III or Stage IV pressure sore (greater than 2 × 2 cm.) on trunk, with only two turning surfaces on which to lie*

✳ **E0372** Powered air overlay for mattress, standard mattress length and width Ⓑ Qp Qh ♿    Y

✳ **E0373** Non powered advanced pressure reducing mattress Ⓑ Qp Qh ♿    Y

## Oxygen and Related Respiratory Equipment

✪ **E0424** Stationary compressed gaseous oxygen system, rental; includes container, contents, regulator, flowmeter, humidifier, nebulizer, cannula or mask, and tubing Ⓑ Qp Qh ♿    Y

*IOM: 100-03, 4, 280.1; 100-04, 20, 30.6*

✪ **E0425** Stationary compressed gas system, purchase; includes regulator, flowmeter, humidifier, nebulizer, cannula or mask, and tubing Ⓑ Qp Qh    E1

*IOM: 100-03, 4, 280.1; 100-04, 20, 30.6*

✪ **E0430** Portable gaseous oxygen system, purchase; includes regulator, flowmeter, humidifier, cannula or mask, and tubing Ⓑ Qp Qh    E1

*IOM: 100-03, 4, 280.1; 100-04, 20, 30.6*

✪ **E0431** Portable gaseous oxygen system, rental; includes portable container, regulator, flowmeter, humidifier, cannula or mask, and tubing Ⓑ Qp Qh ♿    Y

*IOM: 100-03, 4, 280.1; 100-04, 20, 30.6*

✳ **E0433** Portable liquid oxygen system, rental; home liquefier used to fill portable liquid oxygen containers, includes portable containers, regulator, flowmeter, humidifier, cannula or mask and tubing, with or without supply reservoir and contents gauge Ⓑ Qh ♿    Y

✪ **E0434** Portable liquid oxygen system, rental; includes portable container, supply reservoir, humidifier, flowmeter, refill adaptor, contents gauge, cannula or mask, and tubing Ⓑ Qp Qh ♿    Y

*Fee schedule payments for stationary oxygen system rentals are all-inclusive and represent monthly allowance for beneficiary. Non-Medicare payers may rent device to beneficiaries, or arrange for purchase of device.*

*IOM: 100-03, 4, 280.1; 100-04, 20, 30.6*

✪ **E0435** Portable liquid oxygen system, purchase; includes portable container, supply reservoir, flowmeter, humidifier, contents gauge, cannula or mask, tubing and refill adaptor Ⓑ Qp Qh    E1

*IOM: 100-03, 4, 280.1; 100-04, 20, 30.6*

✪ **E0439** Stationary liquid oxygen system, rental; includes container, contents, regulator, flowmeter, humidifier, nebulizer, cannula or mask, and tubing Ⓑ Qp Qh ♿    Y

*This allowance includes payment for equipment, contents, and accessories furnished during rental month*

*IOM: 100-03, 4, 280.1; 100-04, 20, 30.6*

✪ **E0440** Stationary liquid oxygen system, purchase; includes use of reservoir, contents indicator, regulator, flowmeter, humidifier, nebulizer, cannula or mask, and tubing Ⓑ Qp Qh    E1

*IOM: 100-03, 4, 280.1; 100-04, 20, 30.6*

✪ **E0441** Stationary oxygen contents, gaseous, 1 month's supply = 1 unit Ⓑ Qp Qh ♿ Y

*IOM: 100-03, 4, 280.1; 100-04, 20, 30.6*

✪ **E0442** Stationary oxygen contents, liquid, 1 month's supply = 1 unit Ⓑ Qp Qh ♿ Y

*IOM: 100-03, 4, 280.1; 100-04, 20, 30.6*

✪ **E0443** Portable oxygen contents, gaseous, 1 month's supply = 1 unit Ⓑ Qp Qh ♿ Y

*IOM: 100-03, 4, 280.1; 100-04, 20, 30.6*

✪ **E0444** Portable oxygen contents, liquid, 1 month's supply = 1 unit Ⓑ Qp Qh ♿ Y

*IOM: 100-03, 4, 280.1; 100-04, 20, 30.6*

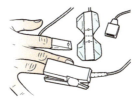

**Figure 12** Oximeter device.

---

🐾 **MIPS**    Qp **Quantity Physician**    Qh **Quantity Hospital**    ♀ **Female only**

♂ **Male only**    Ⓐ **Age**    ♿ **DMEPOS**    A2-Z3 **ASC Payment Indicator**    A-Y **ASC Status Indicator**    *Coding Clinic*

✳ **E0445** Oximeter device for measuring blood oxygen levels non-invasively ⑧ Qp Qh **N**

✳ **E0446** Topical oxygen delivery system, not otherwise specified, includes all supplies and accessories ⑧ Qp Qh **A**

✿ **E0447** Portable oxygen contents, liquid, 1 month's supply = 1 unit, prescribed amount at rest or nighttime exceeds 4 liters per minute (lpm) **Y**

✿ **E0455** Oxygen tent, excluding croup or pediatric tents ⑧ Qp Qh **Y**

*IOM: 100-03, 4, 280.1; 100-04, 20, 30.6*

⊘ **E0457** Chest shell (cuirass) ⑧ Qp Qh **E1**

⊘ **E0459** Chest wrap ⑧ Qp Qh **E1**

✳ **E0462** Rocking bed with or without side rails ⑧ Qp Qh ♿ **Y**

✿ **E0465** Home ventilator, any type, used with invasive interface (e.g., tracheostomy tube) ⑧ Qp Qh ♿ **Y**

*IOM: 100-03, 4, 280.1*

✿ **E0466** Home ventilator, any type, used with non-invasive interface (e.g., mask, chest shell) ⑧ Qp Qh ♿ **Y**

*IOM: 100-03, 4, 280.1*

✿ **E0467** Home ventilator, multi-function respiratory device, also performs any or all of the additional functions of oxygen concentration, drug nebulization, aspiration, and cough stimulation, includes all accessories, components and supplies for all functions **Y**

✿ **E0470** Respiratory assist device, bi-level pressure capability, without backup rate feature, used with noninvasive interface, e.g., nasal or facial mask (intermittent assist device with continuous positive airway pressure device) ⑧ Qp Qh ♿ **Y**

*IOM: 100-03, 4, 240.2*

✿ **E0471** Respiratory assist device, bi-level pressure capability, with back-up rate feature, used with noninvasive interface, e.g., nasal or facial mask (intermittent assist device with continuous positive airway pressure device) ⑧ Qp Qh ♿ **Y**

*IOM: 100-03, 4, 240.2*

✿ **E0472** Respiratory assist device, bi-level pressure capability, with backup rate feature, used with invasive interface, e.g., tracheostomy tube (intermittent assist device with continuous positive airway pressure device) ⑧ Qp Qh ♿ **Y**

*IOM: 100-03, 4, 240.2*

✿ **E0480** Percussor, electric or pneumatic, home model ⑧ Qp Qh ♿ **Y**

*IOM: 100-03, 4, 240.2*

⊘ **E0481** Intrapulmonary percussive ventilation system and related accessories ⑧ Qp Qh **E1**

*IOM: 100-03, 4, 240.2*

✳ **E0482** Cough stimulating device, alternating positive and negative airway pressure ⑧ Qp Qh **Y**

✳ **E0483** High frequency chest wall oscillation system, includes all accessories and supplies, each ⑧ Qp Qh ♿ **Y**

✳ **E0484** Oscillatory positive expiratory pressure device, non-electric, any type, each ⑧ Qp Qh **Y**

✳ **E0485** Oral device/appliance used to reduce upper airway collapsibility, adjustable or non-adjustable, prefabricated, includes fitting and adjustment ⑧ Qp Qh ♿ **Y**

✳ **E0486** Oral device/appliance used to reduce upper airway collapsibility, adjustable or non-adjustable, custom fabricated, includes fitting and adjustment ⑧ Qp Qh ♿ **Y**

✿ **E0487** Spirometer, electronic, includes all accessories ⑧ Qp Qh **N**

## IPPB Machines

✿ **E0500** IPPB machine, all types, with built-in nebulization; manual or automatic valves; internal or external power source ⑧ Qp Qh ♿ **Y**

*IOM: 100-03, 4, 240.2*

## Humidifiers/Nebulizers/Compressors for Use with Oxygen IPPB Equipment

✿ **E0550** Humidifier, durable for extensive supplemental humidification during IPPB treatments or oxygen delivery ⑧ Qp Qh ♿ **Y**

*IOM: 100-03, 4, 240.2*

✿ **E0555** Humidifier, durable, glass or autoclavable plastic bottle type, for use with regulator or flowmeter ⑧ Qp Qh **Y**

*IOM: 100-03, 4, 280.1; 100-04, 20, 30.6*

✿ **E0560** Humidifier, durable for supplemental humidification during IPPB treatment or oxygen delivery ⑧ Qp Qh ♿ **Y**

*IOM: 100-03, 4, 280.1*

▶ New   ↻ Revised   ✔ Reinstated   ~~deleted~~ Deleted   ⊘ Not covered or valid by Medicare
✿ Special coverage instructions   ✳ Carrier discretion   Ⓑ Bill Part B MAC   ⑧ Bill DME MAC

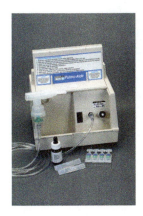

**Figure 13**   Nebulizer

* **E0561**   Humidifier, non-heated, used with positive airway pressure device Ⓑ Qp Qh 👤   Y

* **E0562**   Humidifier, heated, used with positive airway pressure device Ⓑ Qp Qh 👤   Y

* **E0565**   Compressor, air power source for equipment which is not self-contained or cylinder driven Ⓑ Qp Qh 👤   Y

⚙ **E0570**   Nebulizer, with compressor Ⓑ Qp Qh 👤   Y

*IOM: 100-03, 4, 240.2; 100-03, 4, 280.1*

* **E0572**   Aerosol compressor, adjustable pressure, light duty for intermittent use Ⓑ Qp Qh 👤   Y

* **E0574**   Ultrasonic/electronic aerosol generator with small volume nebulizer Ⓑ Qp Qh 👤   Y

⚙ **E0575**   Nebulizer, ultrasonic, large volume Ⓑ Qp Qh 👤   Y

*IOM: 100-03, 4, 240.2*

⚙ **E0580**   Nebulizer, durable, glass or autoclavable plastic, bottle type, for use with regulator or flowmeter Ⓑ Qp Qh 👤   Y

*IOM: 100-03, 4, 240.2; 100-03, 4, 280.1*

⚙ **E0585**   Nebulizer, with compressor and heater Ⓑ Qp Qh 👤   Y

*IOM: 100-03, 4, 240.2; 100-03, 4, 280.1*

## Suction Pump/CPAP

⚙ **E0600**   Respiratory suction pump, home model, portable or stationary, electric Ⓑ Qp Qh 👤   Y

*IOM: 100-03, 4, 240.2*

⚙ **E0601**   Continuous positive airway pressure (CPAP) device Ⓑ Qp Qh 👤   Y

*IOM: 100-03, 4, 240.4*

## Breast Pump

* **E0602**   Breast pump, manual, any type Ⓑ Qp Qh ♀ 👤   Y

Bill either manual breast pump or breast pump kit

* **E0603**   Breast pump, electric (AC and/or DC), any type Ⓑ Qp Qh ♀   N

* **E0604**   Breast pump, hospital grade, electric (AC and/or DC), any type Ⓑ Qp Qh ♀   A

## Other Breathing Aids

⚙ **E0605**   Vaporizer, room type Ⓑ Qp Qh 👤   Y

*IOM: 100-03, 4, 240.2*

⚙ **E0606**   Postural drainage board Ⓑ Qp Qh 👤 Y

*IOM: 100-03, 4, 240.2*

## Monitoring Equipment

⚙ **E0607**   Home blood glucose monitor Ⓑ Qp Qh 👤   Y

Document recipient or caregiver is competent to monitor equipment and that device is designed for home rather than clinical use

*IOM: 100-03, 4, 280.1; 100-03, 1, 40.2*

⚙ **E0610**   Pacemaker monitor, self-contained, (checks battery depletion, includes audible and visible check systems) Ⓑ Qp Qh 👤   Y

*IOM: 100-03, 1, 20.8*

⚙ **E0615**   Pacemaker monitor, self-contained, checks battery depletion and other pacemaker components, includes digital/visible check systems Ⓑ Qp Qh 👤   Y

*IOM: 100-03, 1, 20.8*

* **E0616**   Implantable cardiac event recorder with memory, activator and programmer Ⓑ Qp Qh   N

Assign when two 30-day pre-symptom external loop recordings fail to establish a definitive diagnosis

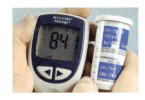

**Figure 14**   Glucose monitor.

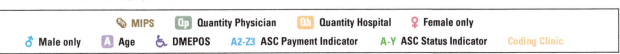

🔖 **MIPS**     Qp **Quantity Physician**     Qh **Quantity Hospital**     ♀ **Female only**

♂ **Male only**     Ⓐ **Age**     👤 **DMEPOS**     A2-Z3 **ASC Payment Indicator**     A-Y **ASC Status Indicator**     Coding Clinic

* **E0617** External defibrillator with integrated electrocardiogram analysis ⑧ Qp Qh ♿ Y

* **E0618** Apnea monitor, without recording feature ⑧ Qp Qh ♿ Y

* **E0619** Apnea monitor, with recording feature ⑧ Qp Qh ♿ Y

* **E0620** Skin piercing device for collection of capillary blood, laser, each ⑧ Qp Qh ♿ Y

## Patient Lifts

⊛ **E0621** Sling or seat, patient lift, canvas or nylon ⑧ Qp Qh ♿ Y
*IOM: 100-03, 4, 240.2, 280.4*

⊘ **E0625** Patient lift, bathroom or toilet, not otherwise classified ⑧ Qp Qh E1
*IOM: 100-03, 4, 240.2*

⊛ **E0627** Seat lift mechanism, electric, any type ⑧ Qp Qh ♿ Y
*IOM: 100-03, 4, 280.4; 100-04, 4, 20*

⊛ **E0629** Seat lift mechanism, non-electric, any type ⑧ Qp Qh ♿ Y
*IOM: 100-04, 4, 20*

⊛ **E0630** Patient lift, hydraulic or mechanical, includes any seat, sling, strap(s) or pad(s) ⑧ Qp Qh ♿ Y
*IOM: 100-03, 4, 240.2*

⊛ **E0635** Patient lift, electric, with seat or sling ⑧ Qp Qh ♿ Y
*IOM: 100-03, 4, 240.2*

* **E0636** Multipositional patient support system, with integrated lift, patient accessible controls ⑧ Qp Qh ♿ Y

⊘ **E0637** Combination sit to stand frame/table system, any size including pediatric, with seat lift feature, with or without wheels ⑧ Qp Qh E1
*IOM: 100-03, 4, 240.2*

⊘ **E0638** Standing frame/table system, one position (e.g., upright, supine or prone stander), any size including pediatric, with or without wheels ⑧ Qp Qh E1
*IOM: 100-03, 4, 240.2*

* **E0639** Patient lift, moveable from room to room with disassembly and reassembly, includes all components/accessories ⑧ Qp Qh ♿ E1

* **E0640** Patient lift, fixed system, includes all components/accessories ⑧ Qp Qh ♿ E1

⊘ **E0641** Standing frame/table system, multi-position (e.g., three-way stander), any size including pediatric, with or without wheels ⑧ Qp Qh E1
*IOM: 100-03, 4, 240.2*

⊘ **E0642** Standing frame/table system, mobile (dynamic stander), any size including pediatric ⑧ Qp Qh E1
*IOM: 100-03, 4, 240.2*

## Pneumatic Compressor and Appliances

⊛ **E0650** Pneumatic compressor, non-segmental home model ⑧ Qp Qh ♿ Y

Lymphedema pumps are classified as segmented or nonsegmented, depending on whether distinct segments of devices can be inflated sequentially.
*IOM: 100-03, 4, 280.6*

⊛ **E0651** Pneumatic compressor, segmental home model without calibrated gradient pressure ⑧ Qp Qh ♿ Y
*IOM: 100-03, 4, 280.6*

⊛ **E0652** Pneumatic compressor, segmental home model with calibrated gradient pressure ⑧ Qp Qh ♿ Y
*IOM: 100-03, 4, 280.6*

⊛ **E0655** Non-segmental pneumatic appliance for use with pneumatic compressor, half arm ⑧ Qp Qh ♿ Y
*IOM: 100-03, 4, 280.6*

⊛ **E0656** Segmental pneumatic appliance for use with pneumatic compressor, trunk ⑧ Qp Qh ♿ Y

⊛ **E0657** Segmental pneumatic appliance for use with pneumatic compressor, chest ⑧ Qp Qh ♿ Y

⊛ **E0660** Non-segmental pneumatic appliance for use with pneumatic compressor, full leg ⑧ Qp Qh ♿ Y
*IOM: 100-03, 4, 280.6*

⊛ **E0665** Non-segmental pneumatic appliance for use with pneumatic compressor, full arm ⑧ Qp Qh ♿ Y
*IOM: 100-03, 4, 280.6*

⊛ **E0666** Non-segmental pneumatic appliance for use with pneumatic compressor, half leg ⑧ Qp Qh ♿ Y
*IOM: 100-03, 4, 280.6*

---

▶ New ↩ Revised ✔ Reinstated ~~deleted~~ Deleted ⊘ Not covered or valid by Medicare
⊛ Special coverage instructions * Carrier discretion ⑧ Bill Part B MAC ⑧ Bill DME MAC

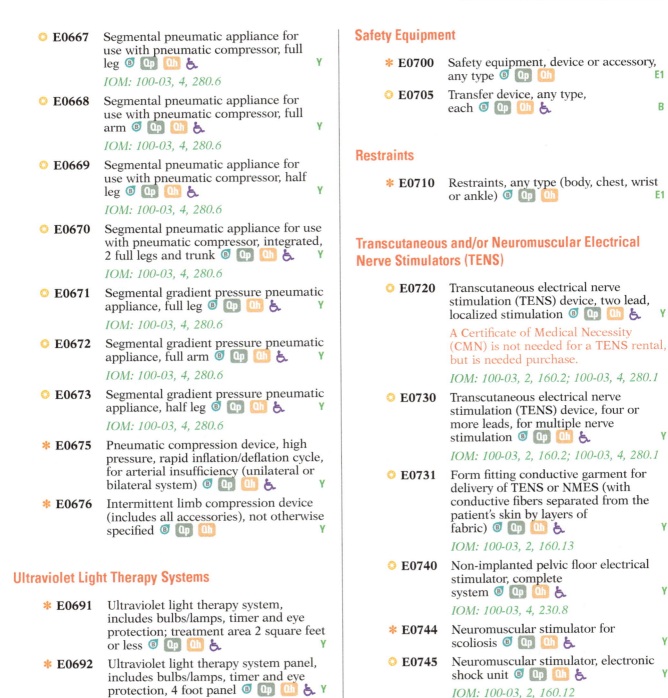

⚙ **E0667** Segmental pneumatic appliance for use with pneumatic compressor, full leg Ⓑ Qp Qh ♿     Y

*IOM: 100-03, 4, 280.6*

⚙ **E0668** Segmental pneumatic appliance for use with pneumatic compressor, full arm Ⓑ Qp Qh ♿     Y

*IOM: 100-03, 4, 280.6*

⚙ **E0669** Segmental pneumatic appliance for use with pneumatic compressor, half leg Ⓑ Qp Qh ♿     Y

*IOM: 100-03, 4, 280.6*

⚙ **E0670** Segmental pneumatic appliance for use with pneumatic compressor, integrated, 2 full legs and trunk Ⓑ Qp Qh ♿     Y

*IOM: 100-03, 4, 280.6*

⚙ **E0671** Segmental gradient pressure pneumatic appliance, full leg Ⓑ Qp Qh ♿     Y

*IOM: 100-03, 4, 280.6*

⚙ **E0672** Segmental gradient pressure pneumatic appliance, full arm Ⓑ Qp Qh ♿     Y

*IOM: 100-03, 4, 280.6*

⚙ **E0673** Segmental gradient pressure pneumatic appliance, half leg Ⓑ Qp Qh ♿     Y

*IOM: 100-03, 4, 280.6*

✳ **E0675** Pneumatic compression device, high pressure, rapid inflation/deflation cycle, for arterial insufficiency (unilateral or bilateral system) Ⓑ Qp Qh ♿     Y

✳ **E0676** Intermittent limb compression device (includes all accessories), not otherwise specified Ⓑ Qp Qh     Y

## Ultraviolet Light Therapy Systems

✳ **E0691** Ultraviolet light therapy system, includes bulbs/lamps, timer and eye protection; treatment area 2 square feet or less Ⓑ Qp Qh ♿     Y

✳ **E0692** Ultraviolet light therapy system panel, includes bulbs/lamps, timer and eye protection, 4 foot panel Ⓑ Qp Qh ♿    Y

✳ **E0693** Ultraviolet light therapy system panel, includes bulbs/lamps, timer and eye protection, 6 foot panel Ⓑ Qp Qh ♿    Y

✳ **E0694** Ultraviolet multidirectional light therapy system in 6 foot cabinet, includes bulbs/lamps, timer and eye protection Ⓑ Qp Qh ♿     Y

## Safety Equipment

✳ **E0700** Safety equipment, device or accessory, any type Ⓑ Qp Qh     E1

⚙ **E0705** Transfer device, any type, each Ⓑ Qp Qh ♿     B

## Restraints

✳ **E0710** Restraints, any type (body, chest, wrist or ankle) Ⓑ Qp Qh     E1

## Transcutaneous and/or Neuromuscular Electrical Nerve Stimulators (TENS)

⚙ **E0720** Transcutaneous electrical nerve stimulation (TENS) device, two lead, localized stimulation Ⓑ Qp Qh ♿     Y

A Certificate of Medical Necessity (CMN) is not needed for a TENS rental, but is needed purchase.

*IOM: 100-03, 2, 160.2; 100-03, 4, 280.1*

⚙ **E0730** Transcutaneous electrical nerve stimulation (TENS) device, four or more leads, for multiple nerve stimulation Ⓑ Qp Qh ♿     Y

*IOM: 100-03, 2, 160.2; 100-03, 4, 280.1*

⚙ **E0731** Form fitting conductive garment for delivery of TENS or NMES (with conductive fibers separated from the patient's skin by layers of fabric) Ⓑ Qp Qh ♿     Y

*IOM: 100-03, 2, 160.13*

⚙ **E0740** Non-implanted pelvic floor electrical stimulator, complete system Ⓑ Qp Qh ♿     Y

*IOM: 100-03, 4, 230.8*

✳ **E0744** Neuromuscular stimulator for scoliosis Ⓑ Qp Qh ♿     Y

⚙ **E0745** Neuromuscular stimulator, electronic shock unit Ⓑ Qp Qh ♿     Y

*IOM: 100-03, 2, 160.12*

⚙ **E0746** Electromyography (EMG), biofeedback device Ⓑ Qp Qh     N

*IOM: 100-03, 1, 30.1*

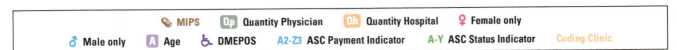

🐾 MIPS    Qp **Quantity Physician**    Qh **Quantity Hospital**    ♀ **Female only**

♂ **Male only**    Ⓐ **Age**    ♿ **DMEPOS**    A2-Z3 **ASC Payment Indicator**    A-Y **ASC Status Indicator**    Coding Clinic

⚙ **E0747** Osteogenesis stimulator, electrical, non-invasive, other than spinal applications Ⓑ ⓆⓅ Ⓠⓗ ♿ Y

*Devices are composed of two basic parts: Coils that wrap around cast and pulse generator that produces electric current*

⚙ **E0748** Osteogenesis stimulator, electrical, non-invasive, spinal applications Ⓑ ⓆⓅ Ⓠⓗ ♿ Y

*Device should be applied within 30 days as adjunct to spinal fusion surgery*

⚙ **E0749** Osteogenesis stimulator, electrical, surgically implanted Ⓑ ⓆⓅ Ⓠⓗ ♿ N

✳ **E0755** Electronic salivary reflex stimulator (intra-oral/non-invasive) Ⓑ ⓆⓅ Ⓠⓗ E1

✳ **E0760** Osteogenesis stimulator, low intensity ultrasound, non-invasive Ⓑ ⓆⓅ Ⓠⓗ ♿ Y

*Ultrasonic osteogenesis stimulator may not be used concurrently with other noninvasive stimulators*

⚙ **E0761** Non-thermal pulsed high frequency radiowaves, high peak power electromagnetic energy treatment device Ⓑ ⓆⓅ Ⓠⓗ E1

✳ **E0762** Transcutaneous electrical joint stimulation device system, includes all accessories Ⓑ ⓆⓅ Ⓠⓗ ♿ B

⚙ **E0764** Functional neuromuscular stimulator, transcutaneous stimulation of sequential muscle groups of ambulation with computer control, used for walking by spinal cord injured, entire system, after completion of training program Ⓑ ⓆⓅ Ⓠⓗ ♿ Y

*IOM: 100-03, 2, 160.12*

✳ **E0765** FDA approved nerve stimulator, with replaceable batteries, for treatment of nausea and vomiting Ⓑ ⓆⓅ Ⓠⓗ ♿ Y

✳ **E0766** Electrical stimulation device used for cancer treatment, includes all accessories, any type Ⓑ ⓆⓅ Ⓠⓗ Y

⚙ **E0769** Electrical stimulation or electromagnetic wound treatment device, not otherwise classified Ⓑ ⓆⓅ Ⓠⓗ B

*IOM: 100-04, 32, 11.1*

⚙ **E0770** Functional electrical stimulator, transcutaneous stimulation of nerve and/or muscle groups, any type, complete system, not otherwise specified Ⓑ ⓆⓅ Ⓠⓗ Y

## Infusion Supplies

✳ **E0776** IV pole Ⓑ ⓆⓅ Ⓠⓗ ♿ Y

*PEN: On Fee Schedule*

✳ **E0779** Ambulatory infusion pump, mechanical, reusable, for infusion 8 hours or greater Ⓑ ⓆⓅ Ⓠⓗ ♿ Y

*Requires prior authorization and copy of invoice*

*This is a capped rental infusion pump modifier. The correct monthly modifier (KH, KI, KJ) is used to indicate which month the rental is for (i.e., KH, month 1; KI, months 2 and 3; KJ, months 4 through 13).*

✳ **E0780** Ambulatory infusion pump, mechanical, reusable, for infusion less than 8 hours Ⓑ ⓆⓅ Ⓠⓗ Y

*Requires prior authorization and copy of invoice*

⚙ **E0781** Ambulatory infusion pump, single or multiple channels, electric or battery operated with administrative equipment, worn by patient Ⓑ ⓆⓅ Ⓠⓗ ♿ Y

*IOM: 100-03, 1, 50.3*

⚙ **E0782** Infusion pump, implantable, non-programmable (includes all components, e.g., pump, cathether, connectors, etc.) Ⓑ ⓆⓅ Ⓠⓗ ♿ N

*IOM: 100-03, 1, 50.3*

⚙ **E0783** Infusion pump system, implantable, programmable (includes all components, e.g., pump, catheter, connectors, etc.) Ⓑ ⓆⓅ Ⓠⓗ ♿ N

*IOM: 100-03, 1, 50.3*

⚙ **E0784** External ambulatory infusion pump, insulin Ⓑ ⓆⓅ Ⓠⓗ ♿ Y

*IOM: 100-03, 4, 280.14*

⚙ **E0785** Implantable intraspinal (epidural/intrathecal) catheter used with implantable infusion pump, replacement Ⓑ ⓆⓅ Ⓠⓗ ♿ N

*IOM: 100-03, 1, 50.3*

⚙ **E0786** Implantable programmable infusion pump, replacement (excludes implantable intraspinal catheter) Ⓑ ⓆⓅ Ⓠⓗ ♿ N

*IOM: 100-03, 1, 50.3*

▶ ✳ **E0787** External ambulatory infusion pump, insulin, dosage rate adjustment using therapeutic continuous glucose sensing Y

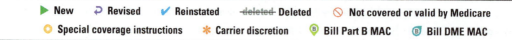

▶ New  ↻ Revised  ✔ Reinstated  ~~deleted~~ Deleted  ⊘ Not covered or valid by Medicare
⚙ Special coverage instructions  ✳ Carrier discretion  Ⓑ Bill Part B MAC  Ⓑ Bill DME MAC

⊛ **E0791** Parenteral infusion pump, stationary, single or multi-channel Ⓑ Qp Qh ♿ Y

*IOM: 100-02, 15, 120; 100-03, 3, 180.2; 100-04, 20, 100.2.2*

## Traction Equipment and Orthopedic Devices

⊛ **E0830** Ambulatory traction device, all types, each Ⓑ Qp Qh N

*IOM: 100-03, 4, 280.1*

⊛ **E0840** Traction frame, attached to headboard, cervical traction Ⓑ Qp Qh ♿ Y

*IOM: 100-03, 4, 280.1*

✳ **E0849** Traction equipment, cervical, free-standing stand/frame, pneumatic, applying traction force to other than mandible Ⓑ Qp Qh ♿ Y

⊛ **E0850** Traction stand, free standing, cervical traction Ⓑ Qp Qh ♿ Y

*IOM: 100-03, 4, 280.1*

✳ **E0855** Cervical traction equipment not requiring additional stand or frame Ⓑ Qp Qh ♿ Y

✳ **E0856** Cervical traction device, with inflatable air bladder(s) Ⓑ Qp Qh ♿ Y

⊛ **E0860** Traction equipment, overdoor, cervical Ⓑ Qp Qh ♿ Y

*IOM: 100-03, 4, 280.1*

⊛ **E0870** Traction frame, attached to footboard, extremity traction, (e.g., Buck's) Ⓑ Qp Qh ♿ Y

*IOM: 100-03, 4, 280.1*

⊛ **E0880** Traction stand, free standing, extremity traction (e.g., Buck's) Ⓑ Qp Qh ♿ Y

*IOM: 100-03, 4, 280.1*

⊛ **E0890** Traction frame, attached to footboard, pelvic traction Ⓑ Qp Qh ♿ Y

*IOM: 100-03, 4, 280.1*

⊛ **E0900** Traction stand, free standing, pelvic traction (e.g., Buck's) Ⓑ Qp Qh ♿ Y

*IOM: 100-03, 4, 280.1*

⊛ **E0910** Trapeze bars, A/K/A patient helper, attached to bed, with grab bar Ⓑ Qp Qh ♿ Y

*IOM: 100-03, 4, 280.1*

⊛ **E0911** Trapeze bar, heavy duty, for patient weight capacity greater than 250 pounds, attached to bed, with grab bar Ⓑ Qp Qh ♿ Y

*IOM: 100-03, 4, 280.1*

⊛ **E0912** Trapeze bar, heavy duty, for patient weight capacity greater than 250 pounds, free standing, complete with grab bar Ⓑ Qp Qh ♿ Y

*IOM: 100-03, 4, 280.1*

⊛ **E0920** Fracture frame, attached to bed, includes weights Ⓑ Qp Qh ♿ Y

*IOM: 100-03, 4, 280.1*

⊛ **E0930** Fracture frame, free standing, includes weights Ⓑ Qp Qh ♿ Y

*IOM: 100-03, 4, 280.1*

⊛ **E0935** Continuous passive motion exercise device for use on knee only Ⓑ Qp Qh ♿ Y

To qualify for coverage, use of device must commence within two days following surgery

*IOM: 100-03, 4, 280.1*

⊘ **E0936** Continuous passive motion exercise device for use other than knee Ⓑ Qp Qh E1

⊛ **E0940** Trapeze bar, free standing, complete with grab bar Ⓑ Qp Qh ♿ Y

*IOM: 100-03, 4, 280.1*

⊛ **E0941** Gravity assisted traction device, any type Ⓑ Qp Qh ♿ Y

*IOM: 100-03, 4, 280.1*

✳ **E0942** Cervical head harness/halter Ⓑ Qp Qh ♿ Y

✳ **E0944** Pelvic belt/harness/boot Ⓑ Qp Qh ♿ Y

✳ **E0945** Extremity belt/harness Ⓑ Qp Qh ♿ Y

⊛ **E0946** Fracture, frame, dual with cross bars, attached to bed (e.g., Balken, 4 poster) Ⓑ Qp Qh ♿ Y

*IOM: 100-03, 4, 280.1*

⊛ **E0947** Fracture frame, attachments for complex pelvic traction Ⓑ Qp Qh ♿ Y

*IOM: 100-03, 4, 280.1*

⊛ **E0948** Fracture frame, attachments for complex cervical traction Ⓑ Qp Qh ♿ Y

*IOM: 100-03, 4, 280.1*

## Wheelchair Accessories

⊛ **E0950** Wheelchair accessory, tray, each Ⓑ Qp Qh ♿ Y

*IOM: 100-03, 4, 280.1*

---

| 🖾 MIPS | Qp Quantity Physician | Qh Quantity Hospital | ♀ Female only | |
|---|---|---|---|---|
| ♂ Male only | Ⓐ Age | ♿ DMEPOS | A2-Z3 ASC Payment Indicator | A-Y ASC Status Indicator | Coding Clinic |

✳ **E0951** Heel loop/holder, any type, with or without ankle strap, each Ⓑ Qp Qh ♿     Y

⚙ **E0952** Toe loop/holder, any type, each Ⓑ Qp Qh ♿     Y

    *IOM: 100-03, 4, 280.1*

✳ **E0953** Wheelchair accessory, lateral thigh or knee support, any type, including fixed mounting hardware, each     Y

✳ **E0954** Wheelchair accessory, foot box, any type, includes attachment and mounting hardware, each foot     Y

✳ **E0955** Wheelchair accessory, headrest, cushioned, any type, including fixed mounting hardware, each Ⓑ Qp Qh ♿     Y

✳ **E0956** Wheelchair accessory, lateral trunk or hip support, any type, including fixed mounting hardware, each Ⓑ Qp Qh ♿     Y

✳ **E0957** Wheelchair accessory, medial thigh support, any type, including fixed mounting hardware, each Ⓑ Qp Qh ♿     Y

⚙ **E0958** Manual wheelchair accessory, one-arm drive attachment, each Ⓑ Qp Qh ♿     Y

    *IOM: 100-03, 4, 280.1*

✳ **E0959** Manual wheelchair accessory, adapter for amputee, each Ⓑ Qp Qh ♿     B

    *IOM: 100-03, 4, 280.1*

✳ **E0960** Wheelchair accessory, shoulder harness/straps or chest strap, including any type mounting hardware Ⓑ Qp Qh ♿     Y

✳ **E0961** Manual wheelchair accessory, wheel lock brake extension (handle), each Ⓑ Qp Qh ♿     B

    *IOM: 100-03, 4, 280.1*

✳ **E0966** Manual wheelchair accessory, headrest extension, each Ⓑ Qp Qh ♿     B

    *IOM: 100-03, 4, 280.1*

⚙ **E0967** Manual wheelchair accessory, hand rim with projections, any type, replacement only, each Ⓑ Qp Qh ♿     Y

    *IOM: 100-03, 4, 280.1*

⚙ **E0968** Commode seat, wheelchair Ⓑ Qp Qh ♿     Y

    *IOM: 100-03, 4, 280.1*

⚙ **E0969** Narrowing device, wheelchair Ⓑ ♿     Y

    *IOM: 100-03, 4, 280.1*

🚫 **E0970** No. 2 footplates, except for elevating leg rest Ⓑ Qp Qh     E1

    *IOM: 100-03, 4, 280.1*

    *Cross Reference K0037, K0042*

✳ **E0971** Manual wheelchair accessory, anti-tipping device, each Ⓑ Qp Qh ♿     B

    *IOM: 100-03, 4, 280.1*

    *Cross Reference K0021*

⚙ **E0973** Wheelchair accessory, adjustable height, detachable armrest, complete assembly, each Ⓑ Qp Qh ♿     B

    *IOM: 100-03, 4, 280.1*

⚙ **E0974** Manual wheelchair accessory, anti-rollback device, each Ⓑ Qp Qh ♿     B

    *IOM: 100-03, 4, 280.1*

✳ **E0978** Wheelchair accessory, positioning belt/safety belt/pelvic strap, each Ⓑ Qp Qh ♿     B

✳ **E0980** Safety vest, wheelchair Ⓑ ♿     Y

✳ **E0981** Wheelchair accessory, seat upholstery, replacement only, each Ⓑ Qp Qh ♿     Y

✳ **E0982** Wheelchair accessory, back upholstery, replacement only, each Ⓑ Qp Qh ♿     Y

✳ **E0983** Manual wheelchair accessory, power add-on to convert manual wheelchair to motorized wheelchair, joystick control Ⓑ Qp Qh ♿     Y

✳ **E0984** Manual wheelchair accessory, power add-on to convert manual wheelchair to motorized wheelchair, tiller control Ⓑ Qp Qh ♿     Y

✳ **E0985** Wheelchair accessory, seat lift mechanism Ⓑ Qp Qh ♿     Y

✳ **E0986** Manual wheelchair accessory, push-rim activated power assist system Ⓑ Qp Qh ♿     Y

✳ **E0988** Manual wheelchair accessory, lever-activated, wheel drive, pair Ⓑ Qp Qh ♿     Y

✳ **E0990** Wheelchair accessory, elevating leg rest, complete assembly, each Ⓑ Qp Qh ♿     B

    *IOM: 100-03, 4, 280.1*

✳ **E0992** Manual wheelchair accessory, solid seat insert Ⓑ Qp Qh ♿     B

⚙ **E0994** Arm rest, each Ⓑ Qp Qh ♿     Y

    *IOM: 100-03, 4, 280.1*

✳ **E0995** Wheelchair accessory, calf rest/pad, replacement only, each Ⓑ Qp Qh ♿     B

    *IOM: 100-03, 4, 280.1*

---

▶ New    ↩ Revised    ✔ Reinstated    ~~deleted~~ Deleted    🚫 Not covered or valid by Medicare

⚙ Special coverage instructions    ✳ Carrier discretion    Ⓑ Bill Part B MAC    Ⓑ Bill DME MAC

✳ **E1002** Wheelchair accessory, power seating system, tilt only Ⓑ Qp Qh ♿     Y

✳ **E1003** Wheelchair accessory, power seating system, recline only, without shear reduction Ⓑ Qp Qh ♿     Y

✳ **E1004** Wheelchair accessory, power seating system, recline only, with mechanical shear reduction Ⓑ Qp Qh ♿     Y

✳ **E1005** Wheelchair accessory, power seating system, recline only, with power shear reduction Ⓑ Qp Qh ♿     Y

✳ **E1006** Wheelchair accessory, power seating system, combination tilt and recline, without shear reduction Ⓑ Qp Qh ♿     Y

✳ **E1007** Wheelchair accessory, power seating system, combination tilt and recline, with mechanical shear reduction Ⓑ Qp Qh ♿     Y

✳ **E1008** Wheelchair accessory, power seating system, combination tilt and recline, with power shear reduction Ⓑ Qp Qh ♿     Y

✳ **E1009** Wheelchair accessory, addition to power seating system, mechanically linked leg elevation system, including pushrod and leg rest, each Ⓑ Qp Qh ♿     Y

✳ **E1010** Wheelchair accessory, addition to power seating system, power leg elevation system, including leg rest, pair Ⓑ Qp Qh ♿     Y

✿ **E1011** Modification to pediatric size wheelchair, width adjustment package (not to be dispensed with initial chair) Ⓑ Qp Qh Ⓐ ♿     Y

        *IOM: 100-03, 4, 280.1*

✳ **E1012** Wheelchair accessory, addition to power seating system, center mount power elevating leg rest/platform, complete system, any type, each Qp Qh ♿     Y

✿ **E1014** Reclining back, addition to pediatric size wheelchair Ⓑ Qp Qh Ⓐ ♿     Y

        *IOM: 100-03, 4, 280.1*

✿ **E1015** Shock absorber for manual wheelchair, each Ⓑ Qp Qh ♿     Y

        *IOM: 100-03, 4, 280.1*

✿ **E1016** Shock absorber for power wheelchair, each Ⓑ Qp Qh ♿     Y

        *IOM: 100-03, 4, 280.1*

✿ **E1017** Heavy duty shock absorber for heavy duty or extra heavy duty manual wheelchair, each Ⓑ Qp Qh ♿     Y

        *IOM: 100-03, 4, 280.1*

✿ **E1018** Heavy duty shock absorber for heavy duty or extra heavy duty power wheelchair, each Ⓑ Qp Qh ♿     Y

        *IOM: 100-03, 4, 280.1*

✿ **E1020** Residual limb support system for wheelchair, any type Ⓑ Qp Qh ♿     Y

        *IOM: 100-03, 3, 280.3*

✳ **E1028** Wheelchair accessory, manual swing-away, retractable or removable mounting hardware for joystick, other control interface or positioning accessory Ⓑ Qp Qh ♿     Y

✳ **E1029** Wheelchair accessory, ventilator tray, fixed Ⓑ Qp Qh ♿     Y

✳ **E1030** Wheelchair accessory, ventilator tray, gimbaled Ⓑ Qp Qh ♿     Y

## Rollabout Chair, Transfer System, Transport Chair

✿ **E1031** Rollabout chair, any and all types with casters 5" or greater Ⓑ Qp Qh ♿     Y

        *IOM: 100- 03, 4, 280.1*

✿ **E1035** Multi-positional patient transfer system, with integrated seat, operated by care giver, patient weight capacity up to and including 300 lbs Ⓑ Qp Qh ♿     Y

        *IOM: 100-02, 15, 110*

✳ **E1036** Multi-positional patient transfer system, extra-wide, with integrated seat, operated by caregiver, patient weight capacity greater than 300 lbs Ⓑ Qh ♿     Y

✿ **E1037** Transport chair, pediatric size Ⓑ Qp Qh Ⓐ ♿     Y

        *IOM: 100-03, 4, 280.1*

✿ **E1038** Transport chair, adult size, patient weight capacity up to and including 300 pounds Ⓑ Qp Qh Ⓐ ♿     Y

        *IOM: 100-03, 4, 280.1*

✳ **E1039** Transport chair, adult size, heavy duty, patient weight capacity greater than 300 pounds Ⓑ Qp Qh Ⓐ ♿     Y

## Wheelchair: Fully Reclining

✿ **E1050** Fully-reclining wheelchair, fixed full length arms, swing away detachable elevating leg rests Ⓑ Qp Qh ♿     Y

        *IOM: 100-03, 4, 280.1*

---

🔬 MIPS    Qp Quantity Physician    Qh Quantity Hospital    ♀ Female only
♂ Male only    Ⓐ Age    ♿ DMEPOS    A2-Z3 ASC Payment Indicator    A-Y ASC Status Indicator    Coding Clinic

⚙ **E1060** Fully-reclining wheelchair, detachable arms, desk or full length, swing away detachable elevating legrests Ⓑ Qp Qh ♿     Y

*IOM: 100-03, 4, 280.1*

⚙ **E1070** Fully-reclining wheelchair, detachable arms (desk or full length) swing away detachable footrests Ⓑ Qp Qh ♿    Y

*IOM: 100-03, 4, 280.1*

### Wheelchair: Hemi

⚙ **E1083** Hemi-wheelchair, fixed full length arms, swing away detachable elevating leg rest Ⓑ Qp Qh ♿     Y

*IOM: 100-03, 4, 280.1*

⚙ **E1084** Hemi-wheelchair, detachable arms desk or full length arms, swing away detachable elevating leg rests Ⓑ Qp Qh ♿     Y

*IOM: 100-03, 4, 280.1*

⊘ **E1085** Hemi-wheelchair, fixed full length arms, swing away detachable foot rests Ⓑ Qp Qh     E1

*IOM: 100-03, 4, 280.1*

*Cross Reference K0002*

⊘ **E1086** Hemi-wheelchair, detachable arms desk or full length, swing away detachable footrests Ⓑ Qp Qh     E1

*IOM: 100-03, 4, 280.1*

*Cross Reference K0002*

### Wheelchair: High-strength Lightweight

⚙ **E1087** High strength lightweight wheelchair, fixed full length arms, swing away detachable elevating leg rests Ⓑ Qp Qh ♿     Y

*IOM: 100-03, 4, 280.1*

⚙ **E1088** High strength lightweight wheelchair, detachable arms desk or full length, swing away detachable elevating leg rests Ⓑ Qp Qh ♿     Y

*IOM: 100-03, 4, 280.1*

⊘ **E1089** High strength lightweight wheelchair, fixed length arms, swing away detachable footrest Ⓑ Qp Qh     E1

*IOM: 100-03, 4, 280.1*

*Cross Reference K0004*

⊘ **E1090** High strength lightweight wheelchair, detachable arms desk or full length, swing away detachable foot rests Ⓑ Qp Qh     E1

*IOM: 100-03, 4, 280.1*

*Cross Reference K0004*

### Wheelchair: Wide Heavy Duty

⚙ **E1092** Wide heavy duty wheelchair, detachable arms (desk or full length) swing away detachable elevating leg rests Ⓑ Qp Qh ♿     Y

*IOM: 100-03, 4, 280.1*

⚙ **E1093** Wide heavy duty wheelchair, detachable arms (desk or full length arms), swing away detachable foot rests Ⓑ Qp Qh ♿     Y

*IOM: 100-03, 4, 280.1*

### Wheelchair: Semi-reclining

⚙ **E1100** Semi-reclining wheelchair, fixed full length arms, swing away detachable elevating leg rests Ⓑ Qp Qh ♿     Y

*IOM: 100-03, 4, 280.1*

⚙ **E1110** Semi-reclining wheelchair, detachable arms (desk or full length), elevating leg rest Ⓑ Qp Qh ♿     Y

*IOM: 100-03, 4, 280.1*

### Wheelchair: Standard

⊘ **E1130** Standard wheelchair, fixed full length arms, fixed or swing away detachable footrests Ⓑ Qp Qh     E1

*IOM: 100-03, 4, 280.1*

*Cross Reference K0001*

⊘ **E1140** Wheelchair, detachable arms, desk or full length, swing away detachable footrests Ⓑ Qp Qh     E1

*IOM: 100-03, 4, 280.1*

*Cross Reference K0001*

⚙ **E1150** Wheelchair, detachable arms, desk or full length, swing away detachable elevating legrests Ⓑ Qp Qh ♿     Y

*IOM: 100-03, 4, 280.1*

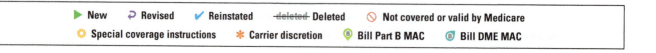

▶ New    ↻ Revised    ✔ Reinstated    ~~deleted~~ Deleted    ⊘ Not covered or valid by Medicare

⚙ Special coverage instructions    ✳ Carrier discretion    Ⓑ Bill Part B MAC    Ⓑ Bill DME MAC

⚙ **E1160** Wheelchair, fixed full length arms, swing away detachable elevating legrests Ⓑ Qp Qh ♿ Y
*IOM: 100-03, 4, 280.1*

✳ **E1161** Manual adult size wheelchair, includes tilt in space Ⓑ Qp Qh A ♿ Y

## Wheelchair: Amputee

⚙ **E1170** Amputee wheelchair, fixed full length arms, swing away detachable elevating legrests Ⓑ Qp Qh ♿ Y
*IOM: 100-03, 4, 280.1*

⚙ **E1171** Amputee wheelchair, fixed full length arms, without footrests or legrest Ⓑ Qp Qh ♿ Y
*IOM: 100-03, 4, 280.1*

⚙ **E1172** Amputee wheelchair, detachable arms (desk or full length) without footrests or legrest Ⓑ Qp Qh ♿ Y
*IOM: 100-03, 4, 280.1*

⚙ **E1180** Amputee wheelchair, detachable arms (desk or full length) swing away detachable footrests Ⓑ Qp Qh ♿ Y
*IOM: 100-03, 4, 280.1*

⚙ **E1190** Amputee wheelchair, detachable arms (desk or full length), swing away detachable elevating legrests Ⓑ Qp Qh ♿ Y
*IOM: 100-03, 4, 280.1*

⚙ **E1195** Heavy duty wheelchair, fixed full length arms, swing away detachable elevating legrests Ⓑ Qp Qh ♿ Y
*IOM: 100-03, 4, 280.1*

⚙ **E1200** Amputee wheelchair, fixed full length arms, swing away detachable footrest Ⓑ Qp Qh ♿ Y
*IOM: 100-03, 4, 280.1*

## Wheelchair: Other and Accessories

⚙ **E1220** Wheelchair; specially sized or constructed (indicate brand name, model number, if any) and justification Ⓑ Qp Qh Y
*IOM: 100-03, 4, 280.3*

⚙ **E1221** Wheelchair with fixed arm, footrests Ⓑ Qp Qh ♿ Y
*IOM: 100-03, 4, 280.3*

⚙ **E1222** Wheelchair with fixed arm, elevating legrests Ⓑ Qp Qh ♿ Y
*IOM: 100-03, 4, 280.3*

⚙ **E1223** Wheelchair with detachable arms, footrests Ⓑ Qp Qh ♿ Y
*IOM: 100-03, 4, 280.3*

⚙ **E1224** Wheelchair with detachable arms, elevating legrests Ⓑ Qp Qh ♿ Y
*IOM: 100-03, 4, 280.3*

⚙ **E1225** Wheelchair accessory, manual semi-reclining back, (recline greater than 15 degrees, but less than 80 degrees), each Ⓑ Qp Qh ♿ Y
*IOM: 100-03, 4, 280.3*

⚙ **E1226** Wheelchair accessory, manual fully reclining back, (recline greater than 80 degrees), each Ⓑ Qp Qh ♿ B
*IOM: 100-03, 4, 280.1*

⚙ **E1227** Special height arms for wheelchair Ⓑ ♿ Y
*IOM: 100-03, 4, 280.3*

⚙ **E1228** Special back height for wheelchair Ⓑ Qp Qh ♿ Y
*IOM: 100-03, 4, 280.3*

## Wheelchair: Pediatric

✳ **E1229** Wheelchair, pediatric size, not otherwise specified Ⓑ Qp Qh A Y

⚙ **E1230** Power operated vehicle (three or four wheel non-highway), specify brand name and model number Ⓑ Qp Qh ♿ Y

*Patient is unable to operate manual wheelchair; patient capable of safely operating controls for scooter; patient can transfer safely in and out of scooter*

*IOM: 100-08, 5, 5.2.3*

⚙ **E1231** Wheelchair, pediatric size, tilt-in-space, rigid, adjustable, with seating system Ⓑ Qp Qh A ♿ Y
*IOM: 100-03, 4, 280.1*

⚙ **E1232** Wheelchair, pediatric size, tilt-in-space, folding, adjustable, with seating system Ⓑ Qp Qh A ♿ Y
*IOM: 100-03, 4, 280.1*

⚙ **E1233** Wheelchair, pediatric size, tilt-in-space, rigid, adjustable, without seating system Ⓑ Qp Qh A ♿ Y
*IOM: 100-03, 4, 280.1*

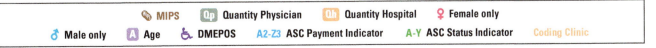

🖐 **MIPS**   Qp **Quantity Physician**   Qh **Quantity Hospital**   ♀ **Female only**
♂ **Male only**   A **Age**   ♿ **DMEPOS**   A2-Z3 **ASC Payment Indicator**   A-Y **ASC Status Indicator**   **Coding Clinic**

⚙ **E1234** Wheelchair, pediatric size, tilt-in-space, folding, adjustable, without seating system Ⓑ Qp Qh Ⓐ ♿     Y
*IOM: 100-03, 4, 280.1*

⚙ **E1235** Wheelchair, pediatric size, rigid, adjustable, with seating system Ⓑ Qp Qh A ♿     Y
*IOM: 100-03, 4, 280.1*

⚙ **E1236** Wheelchair, pediatric size, folding, adjustable, with seating system Ⓑ Qp Qh Ⓐ ♿     Y
*IOM: 100-03, 4, 280.1*

⚙ **E1237** Wheelchair, pediatric size, rigid, adjustable, without seating system Ⓑ Qp Qh A ♿     Y
*IOM: 100-03, 4, 280.1*

⚙ **E1238** Wheelchair, pediatric size, folding, adjustable, without seating system Ⓑ Qp Qh Ⓐ ♿     Y
*IOM: 100-03, 4, 280.1*

✳ **E1239** Power wheelchair, pediatric size, not otherwise specified Ⓑ Qh Ⓐ     Y

## Wheelchair: Lightweight

⚙ **E1240** Lightweight wheelchair, detachable arms (desk or full length) swing away detachable, elevating leg rests Ⓑ Qp Qh ♿     Y
*IOM: 100-03, 4, 280.1*

🚫 **E1250** Lightweight wheelchair, fixed full length arms, swing away detachable footrest Ⓑ Qp Qh     E1
*IOM: 100-03, 4, 280.1*
*Cross Reference K0003*

🚫 **E1260** Lightweight wheelchair, detachable arms (desk or full length) swing away detachable footrest Ⓑ Qp Qh     E1
*IOM: 100-03, 4, 280.1*
*Cross Reference K0003*

⚙ **E1270** Lightweight wheelchair, fixed full length arms, swing away detachable elevating legrests Ⓑ Qp Qh ♿     Y
*IOM: 100-03, 4, 280.1*

## Wheelchair: Heavy Duty

⚙ **E1280** Heavy duty wheelchair, detachable arms (desk or full length), elevating legrests Ⓑ Qp Qh ♿     Y
*IOM: 100-03, 4, 280.1*

🚫 **E1285** Heavy duty wheelchair, fixed full length arms, swing away detachable footrest Ⓑ Qp Qh     E1
*IOM: 100-03, 4, 280.1*
*Cross Reference K0006*

🚫 **E1290** Heavy duty wheelchair, detachable arms (desk or full length) swing away detachable footrest Ⓑ Qp Qh     E1
*IOM: 100-03, 4, 280.1*
*Cross Reference K0006*

⚙ **E1295** Heavy duty wheelchair, fixed full length arms, elevating legrest Ⓑ Qp Qh ♿   Y
*IOM: 100-03, 4, 280.1*

⚙ **E1296** Special wheelchair seat height from floor Ⓑ ♿     Y
*IOM: 100-03, 4, 280.3*

⚙ **E1297** Special wheelchair seat depth, by upholstery Ⓑ ♿     Y
*IOM: 100-03, 4, 280.3*

⚙ **E1298** Special wheelchair seat depth and/or width, by construction Ⓑ ♿     Y
*IOM: 100-03, 4, 280.3*

## Whirlpool Equipment

🚫 **E1300** Whirlpool, portable (overtub type) Ⓑ Qp Qh     E1
*IOM: 100-03, 4, 280.1*

⚙ **E1310** Whirlpool, non-portable (built-in type) Ⓑ Qp Qh ♿     Y
*IOM: 100-03, 4, 280.1*

## Additional Oxygen Related Equipment

✳ **E1352** Oxygen accessory, flow regulator capable of positive inspiratory pressure Ⓑ Qp Qh     Y

⚙ **E1353** Regulator Ⓑ Qp Qh &     Y
*IOM: 100-03, 4, 240.2*

✳ **E1354** Oxygen accessory, wheeled cart for portable cylinder or portable concentrator, any type, replacement only, each Ⓑ Qp Qh     Y

⚙ **E1355** Stand/rack Ⓑ Qp Qh &     Y
*IOM: 100-03, 4, 240.2*

✳ **E1356** Oxygen accessory, battery pack/cartridge for portable concentrator, any type, replacement only, each Ⓑ Qp Qh     Y

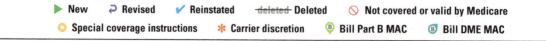

▶ New    ⤶ Revised    ✔ Reinstated    ~~deleted~~ Deleted    🚫 Not covered or valid by Medicare
⚙ Special coverage instructions    ✳ Carrier discretion    Ⓑ Bill Part B MAC    Ⓑ Bill DME MAC

**E1357** Oxygen accessory, battery charger for portable concentrator, any type, replacement only, each Ⓑ Qp Qh   Y

**E1358** Oxygen accessory, DC power adapter for portable concentrator, any type, replacement only, each Ⓑ Qp Qh   Y

**E1372** Immersion external heater for nebulizer Ⓑ Qp Qh ♿   Y

*IOM: 100-03, 4, 240.2*

**E1390** Oxygen concentrator, single delivery port, capable of delivering 85 percent or greater oxygen concentration at the prescribed flow rate Qp Qh ♿   Y

*IOM: 100-03, 4, 240.2*

**E1391** Oxygen concentrator, dual delivery port, capable of delivering 85 percent or greater oxygen concentration at the prescribed flow rate, each Ⓑ Qp Qh ♿   Y

*IOM: 100-03, 4, 240.2*

**E1392** Portable oxygen concentrator, rental Ⓑ Qp Qh ♿   Y

*IOM: 100-03, 4, 240.2*

**E1399** Durable medical equipment, miscellaneous Ⓑ Ⓑ   Y

Example: Therapeutic exercise putty; rubber exercise tubing; anti-vibration gloves

On DMEPOS fee schedule as a payable replacement for miscellaneous implanted or non-implanted items

**E1405** Oxygen and water vapor enriching system with heated delivery Ⓑ Qp Qh ♿   Y

*IOM: 100-03, 4, 240.2*

**E1406** Oxygen and water vapor enriching system without heated delivery Ⓑ Qp Qh ♿   Y

*IOM: 100-03, 4, 240.2*

## Artificial Kidney Machines and Accessories

**E1500** Centrifuge, for dialysis Ⓑ Qp Qh   A

**E1510** Kidney, dialysate delivery syst kidney machine, pump recirculating, air removal syst. flowrate meter, power off, heater and temperature control with alarm, I.V. poles, pressure gauge, concentrate container Ⓑ Qp Qh   A

**E1520** Heparin infusion pump for hemodialysis Ⓑ Qp Qh   A

**E1530** Air bubble detector for hemodialysis, each, replacement Ⓑ Qp Qh   A

**E1540** Pressure alarm for hemodialysis, each, replacement Ⓑ Qp Qh   A

**E1550** Bath conductivity meter for hemodialysis, each Ⓑ Qp Qh   A

**E1560** Blood leak detector for hemodialysis, each, replacement Ⓑ Qp Qh   A

**E1570** Adjustable chair, for ESRD patients Ⓑ Qp Qh   A

**E1575** Transducer protectors/fluid barriers for hemodialysis, any size, per 10 Ⓑ Qp Qh   A

**E1580** Unipuncture control system for hemodialysis Ⓑ Qp Qh   A

**E1590** Hemodialysis machine Ⓑ Qp Qh   A

**E1592** Automatic intermittent peritoneal dialysis system Ⓑ Qp Qh   A

**E1594** Cycler dialysis machine for peritoneal dialysis Ⓑ Qp Qh   A

**E1600** Delivery and/or installation charges for hemodialysis equipment Ⓑ Qp Qh   A

**E1610** Reverse osmosis water purification system, for hemodialysis Ⓑ Qp Qh   A

*IOM: 100-03, 4, 230.7*

**E1615** Deionizer water purification system, for hemodialysis Ⓑ Qp Qh   A

*IOM: 100-03, 4, 230.7*

**E1620** Blood pump for hemodialysis replacement Ⓑ Qp Qh   A

**E1625** Water softening system, for hemodialysis Ⓑ Qp Qh   A

*IOM: 100-03, 4, 230.7*

**E1630** Reciprocating peritoneal dialysis system Ⓑ Qp Qh   A

**E1632** Wearable artificial kidney, each Ⓑ Qp Qh   A

**E1634** Peritoneal dialysis clamps, each Ⓑ Qp Qh   B

*IOM: 100-04, 8, 60.4.2; 100-04, 8, 90.1; 100-04, 18, 80; 100-04, 18, 90*

**E1635** Compact (portable) travel hemodialyzer system Ⓑ Qp Qh   A

**E1636** Sorbent cartridges, for hemodialysis, per 10 Ⓑ Qp Qh   A

**E1637** Hemostats, each Ⓑ Qp Qh   A

**E1639** Scale, each Ⓑ Qp Qh   A

**E1699** Dialysis equipment, not otherwise specified Ⓑ   A

## Jaw Motion Rehabilitation System

* **E1700** Jaw motion rehabilitation system Ⓑ Qp Qh ♿     Y

     Must be prescribed by physician

* **E1701** Replacement cushions for jaw motion rehabilitation system, pkg. of 6 Ⓑ Qp Qh ♿     Y

* **E1702** Replacement measuring scales for jaw motion rehabilitation system, pkg. of 200 Ⓑ Qp Qh ♿     Y

## Other Orthopedic Devices

* **E1800** Dynamic adjustable elbow extension/flexion device, includes soft interface material Ⓑ Qp Qh ♿     Y

* **E1801** Static progressive stretch elbow device, extension and/or flexion, with or without range of motion adjustment, includes all components and accessories Ⓑ Qp Qh ♿     Y

* **E1802** Dynamic adjustable forearm pronation/supination device, includes soft interface material Ⓑ Qp Qh ♿     Y

* **E1805** Dynamic adjustable wrist extension/flexion device, includes soft interface material Ⓑ Qp Qh ♿     Y

* **E1806** Static progressive stretch wrist device, flexion and/or extension, with or without range of motion adjustment, includes all components and accessories Ⓑ Qp Qh ♿     Y

* **E1810** Dynamic adjustable knee extension/flexion device, includes soft interface material Ⓑ Qp Qh ♿     Y

* **E1811** Static progressive stretch knee device, extension and/or flexion, with or without range of motion adjustment, includes all components and accessories Ⓑ Qp Qh ♿     Y

* **E1812** Dynamic knee, extension/flexion device with active resistance control Ⓑ Qp Qh ♿     Y

* **E1815** Dynamic adjustable ankle extension/flexion device, includes soft interface material Ⓑ Qp Qh ♿     Y

* **E1816** Static progressive stretch ankle device, flexion and/or extension, with or without range of motion adjustment, includes all components and accessories Ⓑ Qp Qh ♿     Y

* **E1818** Static progressive stretch forearm pronation/supination device with or without range of motion adjustment, includes all components and accessories Ⓑ Qp Qh ♿     Y

* **E1820** Replacement soft interface material, dynamic adjustable extension/flexion device Ⓑ Qp Qh ♿     Y

* **E1821** Replacement soft interface material/cuffs for bi-directional static progressive stretch device Ⓑ Qp Qh ♿     Y

* **E1825** Dynamic adjustable finger extension/flexion device, includes soft interface material Ⓑ Qp Qh ♿     Y

* **E1830** Dynamic adjustable toe extension/flexion device, includes soft interface material Ⓑ Qp Qh ♿     Y

* **E1831** Static progressive stretch toe device, extension and/or flexion, with or without range of motion adjustment, includes all components and accessories Ⓑ Qp Qh ♿     Y

* **E1840** Dynamic adjustable shoulder flexion/abduction/rotation device, includes soft interface material Ⓑ Qp Qh ♿     Y

* **E1841** Static progressive stretch shoulder device, with or without range of motion adjustment, includes all components and accessories Ⓑ Qp Qh ♿     Y

## Miscellaneous

* **E1902** Communication board, non-electronic augmentative or alternative communication device Ⓑ Qp Qh     Y

* **E2000** Gastric suction pump, home model, portable or stationary, electric Ⓑ Qp Qh ♿     Y

⚙ **E2100** Blood glucose monitor with integrated voice synthesizer Ⓑ Qp Qh ♿     Y

     *IOM: 100-03, 4, 230.16*

⚙ **E2101** Blood glucose monitor with integrated lancing/blood sample Ⓑ Qp Qh ♿     Y

     *IOM: 100-03, 4, 230.16*

* **E2120** Pulse generator system for tympanic treatment of inner ear endolymphatic fluid Ⓑ Qp Qh ♿     Y

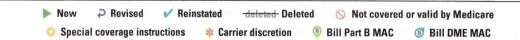

▶ New    ↻ Revised    ✔ Reinstated    ~~deleted~~ Deleted    ⊘ Not covered or valid by Medicare
⚙ Special coverage instructions    ✱ Carrier discretion    Ⓑ Bill Part B MAC    Ⓑ Bill DME MAC

## Wheelchair Assessories: Manual and Power

* **E2201** Manual wheelchair accessory, nonstandard seat frame, width greater than or equal to 20 inches and less than 24 inches Ⓑ Qp Qh ♿ Y

* **E2202** Manual wheelchair accessory, nonstandard seat frame width, 24-27 inches Ⓑ Qp Qh ♿ Y

* **E2203** Manual wheelchair accessory, nonstandard seat frame depth, 20 to less than 22 inches Ⓑ Qp Qh ♿ Y

* **E2204** Manual wheelchair accessory, nonstandard seat frame depth, 22 to 25 inches Ⓑ Qp Qh ♿ Y

* **E2205** Manual wheelchair accessory, handrim without projections (includes ergonomic or contoured), any type, replacement only, each Ⓑ Qp Qh ♿ Y

* **E2206** Manual wheelchair accessory, wheel lock assembly, complete, replacement only, each Ⓑ Qp Qh ♿ Y

* **E2207** Wheelchair accessory, crutch and cane holder, each Ⓑ Qp Qh ♿ Y

* **E2208** Wheelchair accessory, cylinder tank carrier, each Ⓑ Qp Qh ♿ Y

* **E2209** Accessory arm trough, with or without hand support, each Ⓑ Qp Qh ♿ Y

* **E2210** Wheelchair accessory, bearings, any type, replacement only, each Ⓑ Qp Qh ♿ Y

* **E2211** Manual wheelchair accessory, pneumatic propulsion tire, any size, each Ⓑ Qp Qh ♿ Y

* **E2212** Manual wheelchair accessory, tube for pneumatic propulsion tire, any size, each Ⓑ Qp Qh ♿ Y

* **E2213** Manual wheelchair accessory, insert for pneumatic propulsion tire (removable), any type, any size, each Ⓑ Qp Qh ♿ Y

* **E2214** Manual wheelchair accessory, pneumatic caster tire, any size, each Ⓑ Qp Qh ♿ Y

* **E2215** Manual wheelchair accessory, tube for pneumatic caster tire, any size, each Ⓑ Qp Qh ♿ Y

* **E2216** Manual wheelchair accessory, foam filled propulsion tire, any size, each Ⓑ Qp Qh ♿ Y

* **E2217** Manual wheelchair accessory, foam filled caster tire, any size, each Ⓑ Qp Qh ♿ Y

* **E2218** Manual wheelchair accessory, foam propulsion tire, any size, each Ⓑ Qp Qh ♿ Y

* **E2219** Manual wheelchair accessory, foam caster tire, any size, each Ⓑ Qp Qh ♿ Y

* **E2220** Manual wheelchair accessory, solid (rubber/plastic) propulsion tire, any size, replacement only, each Ⓑ Qp Qh ♿ Y

* **E2221** Manual wheelchair accessory, solid (rubber/plastic) caster tire (removable), any size, replacement only, each Ⓑ Qp Qh ♿ Y

* **E2222** Manual wheelchair accessory, solid (rubber/plastic) caster tire with integrated wheel, any size, replacement only, each Ⓑ Qp Qh ♿ Y

* **E2224** Manual wheelchair accessory, propulsion wheel excludes tire, any size, replacement only, each Ⓑ Qp Qh ♿ Y

* **E2225** Manual wheelchair accessory, caster wheel excludes tire, any size, replacement only, each Ⓑ Qp Qh ♿ Y

* **E2226** Manual wheelchair accessory, caster fork, any size, replacement only, each Ⓑ Qp Qh ♿ Y

* **E2227** Manual wheelchair accessory, gear reduction drive wheel, each Ⓑ Qp Qh ♿ Y

* **E2228** Manual wheelchair accessory, wheel braking system and lock, complete, each Ⓑ Qp Qh ♿ Y

* **E2230** Manual wheelchair accessory, manual standing system Ⓑ Qp Qh Y

* **E2231** Manual wheelchair accessory, solid seat support base (replaces sling seat), includes any type mounting hardware Ⓑ Qp Qh ♿ Y

* **E2291** Back, planar, for pediatric size wheelchair including fixed attaching hardware Ⓑ Qp Qh Ⓐ Y

* **E2292** Seat, planar, for pediatric size wheelchair including fixed attaching hardware Ⓑ Qp Qh Ⓐ Y

* **E2293** Back, contoured, for pediatric size wheelchair including fixed attaching hardware Ⓑ Qp Qh Ⓐ Y

* **E2294** Seat, contoured, for pediatric size wheelchair including fixed attaching hardware Ⓑ Qp Qh Ⓐ Y

* **E2295** Manual wheelchair accessory, for pediatric size wheelchair, dynamic seating frame, allows coordinated movement of multiple positioning features Ⓑ Qp Qh Ⓐ Y

* **E2300** Wheelchair accessory, power seat elevation system, any type Ⓑ Qp Qh Y

🪙 **MIPS**   Qp **Quantity Physician**   Qh **Quantity Hospital**   ♀ **Female only**
♂ **Male only**   Ⓐ **Age**   ♿ **DMEPOS**   A2-Z3 **ASC Payment Indicator**   A-Y **ASC Status Indicator**   **Coding Clinic**

DURABLE MEDICAL EQUIPMENT  E2201 — E2300

215

✳ **E2301** Wheelchair accessory, power standing system, any type Ⓑ Qp Qh Y

✳ **E2310** Power wheelchair accessory, electronic connection between wheelchair controller and one power seating system motor, including all related electronics, indicator feature, mechanical function selection switch, and fixed mounting hardware Ⓑ Qp Qh ♿ Y

✳ **E2311** Power wheelchair accessory, electronic connection between wheelchair controller and two or more power seating system motors, including all related electronics, indicator feature, mechanical function selection switch, and fixed mounting hardware Ⓑ Qp Qh ♿ Y

✳ **E2312** Power wheelchair accessory, hand or chin control interface, mini-proportional remote joystick, proportional, including fixed mounting hardware Ⓑ Qp Qh ♿ Y

✳ **E2313** Power wheelchair accessory, harness for upgrade to expandable controller, including all fasteners, connectors and mounting hardware, each Ⓑ Qp Qh ♿ Y

✳ **E2321** Power wheelchair accessory, hand control interface, remote joystick, nonproportional, including all related electronics, mechanical stop switch, and fixed mounting hardware Ⓑ Qp Qh ♿ Y

✳ **E2322** Power wheelchair accessory, hand control interface, multiple mechanical switches, nonproportional, including all related electronics, mechanical stop switch, and fixed mounting hardware Ⓑ Qp Qh ♿ Y

✳ **E2323** Power wheelchair accessory, specialty joystick handle for hand control interface, prefabricated Ⓑ Qp Qh ♿ Y

✳ **E2324** Power wheelchair accessory, chin cup for chin control interface Ⓑ Qp Qh ♿ Y

✳ **E2325** Power wheelchair accessory, sip and puff interface, nonproportional, including all related electronics, mechanical stop switch, and manual swingaway mounting hardware Ⓑ Qp Qh ♿ Y

✳ **E2326** Power wheelchair accessory, breath tube kit for sip and puff interface Ⓑ Qp Qh ♿ Y

✳ **E2327** Power wheelchair accessory, head control interface, mechanical, proportional, including all related electronics, mechanical direction change switch, and fixed mounting hardware Ⓑ Qp Qh ♿ Y

✳ **E2328** Power wheelchair accessory, head control or extremity control interface, electronic, proportional, including all related electronics and fixed mounting hardware Ⓑ Qp Qh ♿ Y

✳ **E2329** Power wheelchair accessory, head control interface, contact switch mechanism, nonproportional, including all related electronics, mechanical stop switch, mechanical direction change switch, head array, and fixed mounting hardware Ⓑ Qp Qh ♿ Y

✳ **E2330** Power wheelchair accessory, head control interface, proximity switch mechanism, nonproportional, including all related electronics, mechanical stop switch, mechanical direction change switch, head array, and fixed mounting hardware Ⓑ Qp Qh ♿ Y

✳ **E2331** Power wheelchair accessory, attendant control, proportional, including all related electronics and fixed mounting hardware Ⓑ Qp Qh Y

✳ **E2340** Power wheelchair accessory, nonstandard seat frame width, 20-23 inches Qp Qh ♿ Y

✳ **E2341** Power wheelchair accessory, nonstandard seat frame width, 24-27 inches Ⓑ Qp Qh ♿ Y

✳ **E2342** Power wheelchair accessory, nonstandard seat frame depth, 20 or 21 inches Ⓑ Qp Qh ♿ Y

✳ **E2343** Power wheelchair accessory, nonstandard seat frame depth, 22-25 inches Ⓑ Qp Qh ♿ Y

✳ **E2351** Power wheelchair accessory, electronic interface to operate speech generating device using power wheelchair control interface Ⓑ Qp Qh ♿ Y

✳ **E2358** Power wheelchair accessory, Group 34 non-sealed lead acid battery, each Ⓑ Qp Qh Y

✳ **E2359** Power wheelchair accessory, Group 34 sealed lead acid battery, each (e.g., gel cell, absorbed glassmat) Ⓑ Qp Qh ♿ Y

✳ **E2360** Power wheelchair accessory, 22 NF non-sealed lead acid battery, each Ⓑ ♿ Y

---

▶ New   ↻ Revised   ✔ Reinstated   ~~deleted~~ Deleted   ⊘ Not covered or valid by Medicare
⬡ Special coverage instructions   ✳ Carrier discretion   Ⓑ Bill Part B MAC   Ⓓ Bill DME MAC

* **E2361** Power wheelchair accessory, 22NF sealed lead acid battery, each (e.g., gel cell, absorbed glassmat) Ⓑ Qp Qh ♿      Y

* **E2362** Power wheelchair accessory, group 24 non-sealed lead acid battery, each Ⓑ ♿      Y

* **E2363** Power wheelchair accessory, group 24 sealed lead acid battery, each (e.g., gel cell, absorbed glassmat) Ⓑ Qp Qh ♿      Y

* **E2364** Power wheelchair accessory, U-1 non-sealed lead acid battery, each Ⓑ ♿      Y

* **E2365** Power wheelchair accessory, U-1 sealed lead acid battery, each (e.g., gel cell, absorbed glassmat) Ⓑ Qp Qh ♿      Y

* **E2366** Power wheelchair accessory, battery charger, single mode, for use with only one battery type, sealed or non-sealed, each Ⓑ Qp Qh ♿      Y

* **E2367** Power wheelchair accessory, battery charger, dual mode, for use with either battery type, sealed or non-sealed, each Ⓑ Qp Qh ♿      Y

* **E2368** Power wheelchair component, drive wheel motor, replacement only Ⓑ Qp Qh ♿      Y

* **E2369** Power wheelchair component, drive wheel gear box, replacement only Ⓑ Qp Qh ♿      Y

* **E2370** Power wheelchair component, integrated drive wheel motor and gear box combination, replacement only Ⓑ Qp Qh ♿      Y

* **E2371** Power wheelchair accessory, group 27 sealed lead acid battery, (e.g., gel cell, absorbed glass mat), each Ⓑ Qp Qh ♿      Y

* **E2372** Power wheelchair accessory, group 27 non-sealed lead acid battery, each Ⓑ ♿      Y

* **E2373** Power wheelchair accessory, hand or chin control interface, compact remote joystick, proportional, including fixed mounting hardware Ⓑ Qp Qh ♿      Y

✿ **E2374** Power wheelchair accessory, hand or chin control interface, standard remote joystick (not including controller), proportional, including all related electronics and fixed mounting hardware, replacement only Ⓑ Qp Qh ♿      Y

✿ **E2375** Power wheelchair accessory, non-expandable controller, including all related electronics and mounting hardware, replacement only Ⓑ Qp Qh ♿      Y

✿ **E2376** Power wheelchair accessory, expandable controller, including all related electronics and mounting hardware, replacement only Ⓑ Qp Qh ♿      Y

✿ **E2377** Power wheelchair accessory, expandable controller, including all related electronics and mounting hardware, upgrade provided at initial issue Ⓑ Qp Qh ♿      Y

* **E2378** Power wheelchair component, actuator, replacement only Ⓑ Qp Qh ♿      Y

✿ **E2381** Power wheelchair accessory, pneumatic drive wheel tire, any size, replacement only, each Ⓑ Qp Qh ♿      Y

✿ **E2382** Power wheelchair accessory, tube for pneumatic drive wheel tire, any size, replacement only, each Ⓑ Qp Qh ♿      Y

✿ **E2383** Power wheelchair accessory, insert for pneumatic drive wheel tire (removable), any type, any size, replacement only, each Ⓑ Qp Qh ♿      Y

✿ **E2384** Power wheelchair accessory, pneumatic caster tire, any size, replacement only, each Ⓑ Qp Qh ♿      Y

✿ **E2385** Power wheelchair accessory, tube for pneumatic caster tire, any size, replacement only, each Ⓑ Qp Qh ♿ Y

✿ **E2386** Power wheelchair accessory, foam filled drive wheel tire, any size, replacement only, each Ⓑ Qp Qh ♿      Y

✿ **E2387** Power wheelchair accessory, foam filled caster tire, any size, replacement only, each Ⓑ Qp Qh ♿      Y

✿ **E2388** Power wheelchair accessory, foam drive wheel tire, any size, replacement only, each Ⓑ Qp Qh ♿      Y

✿ **E2389** Power wheelchair accessory, foam caster tire, any size, replacement only, each Ⓑ Qp Qh ♿      Y

✿ **E2390** Power wheelchair accessory, solid (rubber/plastic) drive wheel tire, any size, replacement only, each Ⓑ Qp Qh ♿      Y

✿ **E2391** Power wheelchair accessory, solid (rubber/plastic) caster tire (removable), any size, replacement only, each Ⓑ Qp Qh ♿      Y

✿ **E2392** Power wheelchair accessory, solid (rubber/plastic) caster tire with integrated wheel, any size, replacement only, each Ⓑ Qp Qh ♿      Y

---

| 🖎 MIPS | Qp Quantity Physician | Qh Quantity Hospital | ♀ Female only |
|---|---|---|---|
| ♂ Male only | Ⓐ Age | ♿ DMEPOS | A2-Z3 ASC Payment Indicator | A-Y ASC Status Indicator | Coding Clinic |

⊛ **E2394**   Power wheelchair accessory, drive wheel excludes tire, any size, replacement only, each Ⓑ Qp Qh ♿ Y

⊛ **E2395**   Power wheelchair accessory, caster wheel excludes tire, any size, replacement only, each Ⓑ Qp Qh ♿ Y

⊛ **E2396**   Power wheelchair accessory, caster fork, any size, replacement only, each Ⓑ Qp Qh ♿ Y

✱ **E2397**   Power wheelchair accessory, lithium-based battery, each Ⓑ Qp Qh ♿ Y

▶ ✱ **E2398**   Wheelchair accessory, dynamic positioning hardware for back Y

## Negative Pressure

✱ **E2402**   Negative pressure wound therapy electrical pump, stationary or portable Ⓑ Qp Qh ♿ Y

Document at least every 30 calendar days the quantitative wound characteristics, including wound surface area (length, width and depth).

Medicare coverage up to a maximum of 15 dressing kits (A6550) per wound per month unless documentation states that the wound size requires more than one dressing kit for each dressing change.

## Speech Device

⊛ **E2500**   Speech generating device, digitized speech, using pre-recorded messages, less than or equal to 8 minutes recording time Ⓑ Qp Qh ♿ Y

*IOM: 100-03, 1, 50.1*

⊛ **E2502**   Speech generating device, digitized speech, using pre-recorded messages, greater than 8 minutes but less than or equal to 20 minutes recording time Ⓑ Qp Qh ♿ Y

*IOM: 100-03, 1, 50.1*

⊛ **E2504**   Speech generating device, digitized speech, using pre-recorded messages, greater than 20 minutes but less than or equal to 40 minutes recording time Ⓑ Qp Qh ♿ Y

*IOM: 100-03, 1, 50.1*

⊛ **E2506**   Speech generating device, digitized speech, using pre-recorded messages, greater than 40 minutes recording time Ⓑ Qp Qh ♿ Y

*IOM: 100-03, 1, 50.1*

⊛ **E2508**   Speech generating device, synthesized speech, requiring message formulation by spelling and access by physical contact with the device Ⓑ Qp Qh ♿ Y

*IOM: 100-03, 1, 50.1*

⊛ **E2510**   Speech generating device, synthesized speech, permitting multiple methods of message formulation and multiple methods of device access Ⓑ Qp Qh ♿ Y

*IOM: 100-03, 1, 50.1*

⊛ **E2511**   Speech generating software program, for personal computer or personal digital assistant Ⓑ Qp Qh ♿ Y

*IOM: 100-03, 1, 50.1*

⊛ **E2512**   Accessory for speech generating device, mounting system Ⓑ Qp Qh ♿ Y

*IOM: 100-03, 1, 50.1*

⊛ **E2599**   Accessory for speech generating device, not otherwise classified Ⓑ Y

*IOM: 100-03, 1, 50.1*

## Wheelchair: Cushion

✱ **E2601**   General use wheelchair seat cushion, width less than 22 inches, any depth Ⓑ Qp Qh ♿ Y

✱ **E2602**   General use wheelchair seat cushion, width 22 inches or greater, any depth Ⓑ Qp Qh ♿ Y

✱ **E2603**   Skin protection wheelchair seat cushion, width less than 22 inches, any depth Ⓑ Qp Qh ♿ Y

✱ **E2604**   Skin protection wheelchair seat cushion, width 22 inches or greater, any depth Ⓑ Qp Qh ♿ Y

✱ **E2605**   Positioning wheelchair seat cushion, width less than 22 inches, any depth Ⓑ Qp Qh ♿ Y

✱ **E2606**   Positioning wheelchair seat cushion, width 22 inches or greater, any depth Ⓑ Qp Qh ♿ Y

✱ **E2607**   Skin protection and positioning wheelchair seat cushion, width less than 22 inches, any depth Ⓑ Qp Qh ♿ Y

✱ **E2608**   Skin protection and positioning wheelchair seat cushion, width 22 inches or greater, any depth Ⓑ Qp Qh ♿ Y

✱ **E2609**   Custom fabricated wheelchair seat cushion, any size Ⓑ Qp Qh Y

✱ **E2610**   Wheelchair seat cushion, powered Ⓑ B

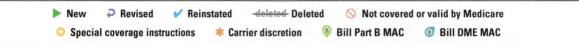

▶ New   ↻ Revised   ✔ Reinstated   ~~deleted~~ Deleted   ⊘ Not covered or valid by Medicare
⊛ Special coverage instructions   ✱ Carrier discretion   Ⓑ Bill Part B MAC   Ⓑ Bill DME MAC

* **E2611** General use wheelchair back cushion, width less than 22 inches, any height, including any type mounting hardware Ⓑ Qp Qh ♿    Y

* **E2612** General use wheelchair back cushion, width 22 inches or greater, any height, including any type mounting hardware Ⓑ Qp Qh ♿    Y

* **E2613** Positioning wheelchair back cushion, posterior, width less than 22 inches, any height, including any type mounting hardware Ⓑ Qp Qh ♿    Y

* **E2614** Positioning wheelchair back cushion, posterior, width 22 inches or greater, any height, including any type mounting hardware Ⓑ Qp Qh ♿    Y

* **E2615** Positioning wheelchair back cushion, posterior-lateral, width less than 22 inches, any height, including any type mounting hardware Ⓑ Qp Qh ♿    Y

* **E2616** Positioning wheelchair back cushion, posterior-lateral, width 22 inches or greater, any height, including any type mounting hardware Ⓑ Qp Qh ♿    Y

* **E2617** Custom fabricated wheelchair back cushion, any size, including any type mounting hardware Ⓑ Qp Qh    Y

* **E2619** Replacement cover for wheelchair seat cushion or back cushion, each Ⓑ Qp Qh ♿    Y

* **E2620** Positioning wheelchair back cushion, planar back with lateral supports, width less than 22 inches, any height, including any type mounting hardware Ⓑ Qp Qh ♿    Y

* **E2621** Positioning wheelchair back cushion, planar back with lateral supports, width 22 inches or greater, any height, including any type mounting hardware Ⓑ Qp Qh ♿    Y

## Wheelchair: Skin Protection

* **E2622** Skin protection wheelchair seat cushion, adjustable, width less than 22 inches, any depth Ⓑ Qp Qh ♿    Y

* **E2623** Skin protection wheelchair seat cushion, adjustable, width 22 inches or greater, any depth Ⓑ Qp Qh ♿    Y

* **E2624** Skin protection and positioning wheelchair seat cushion, adjustable, width less than 22 inches, any depth Ⓑ Qp Qh ♿    Y

* **E2625** Skin protection and positioning wheelchair seat cushion, adjustable, width 22 inches or greater, any depth Ⓑ Qp Qh ♿    Y

## Wheelchair: Arm Support

* **E2626** Wheelchair accessory, shoulder elbow, mobile arm support attached to wheelchair, balanced, adjustable Ⓑ Qp Qh ♿    Y

* **E2627** Wheelchair accessory, shoulder elbow, mobile arm support attached to wheelchair, balanced, adjustable rancho type Ⓑ Qp Qh ♿    Y

* **E2628** Wheelchair accessory, shoulder elbow, mobile arm support attached to wheelchair, balanced, reclining Ⓑ Qp Qh ♿    Y

* **E2629** Wheelchair accessory, shoulder elbow, mobile arm support attached to wheelchair, balanced, friction arm support (friction dampening to proximal and distal joints) Ⓑ Qp Qh ♿    Y

* **E2630** Wheelchair accessory, shoulder elbow, mobile arm support, monosuspension arm and hand support, overhead elbow forearm hand sling support, yoke type suspension support Ⓑ Qp Qh ♿    Y

* **E2631** Wheelchair accessory, addition to mobile arm support, elevating proximal arm Ⓑ Qp Qh ♿    Y

* **E2632** Wheelchair accessory, addition to mobile arm support, offset or lateral rocker arm with elastic balance control Ⓑ Qp Qh ♿    Y

* **E2633** Wheelchair accessory, addition to mobile arm support, supinator Ⓑ Qp Qh ♿    Y

## Pediatric Gait Trainer

⊘ **E8000** Gait trainer, pediatric size, posterior support, includes all accessories and components Ⓑ Ⓐ    E1

⊘ **E8001** Gait trainer, pediatric size, upright support, includes all accessories and components Ⓑ Ⓐ    E1

⊘ **E8002** Gait trainer, pediatric size, anterior support, includes all accessories and components Ⓑ Ⓐ    E1

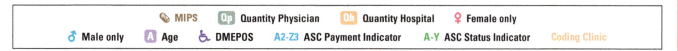

## TEMPORARY PROCEDURES/ PROFESSIONAL SERVICES (G0000-G9999)

**NOTE:** Series "G", "K", and "Q" in the Level II coding are reserved for CMS assignment. "G", "K", and "Q" codes are temporary national codes for items or services requiring uniform national coding between one year's update and the next. Sometimes "temporary" codes remain for more than one update. If "G", "K", and "Q" codes are not converted to permanent codes in Level I or Level II series in the following update, they will remain active until converted in following years or until CMS notifies contractors to delete them. All active "G", "K", and "Q" codes at the time of update will be included on the update file for contractors. In addition, deleted codes are retained on the file for informational purposes, with a deleted indicator, for four years.

### Vaccine Administration

✳ **G0008** Administration of influenza virus vaccine ⑧ Qp Qh                    S

Coinsurance and deductible do not apply. If provided, report significant, separately identifiable E/M for medically necessary services (Z23).

*Coding Clinic: 2016, Q4, P3*

✳ **G0009** Administration of pneumococcal vaccine ⑧ Qp Qh                    S

Reported once in a lifetime based on risk; Medicare covers cost of vaccine and administration (Z23)

Copayment, coinsurance, and deductible waived. (https://www.cms. gov/MLNProducts/downloads/MPS_ QuickReferenceChart_1.pdf)

*Coding Clinic: 2016, Q4, P3*

✳ **G0010** Administration of hepatitis B vaccine ⑧ Qp Qh                    S

Report for other than OPPs. Coinsurance and deductible apply; Medicare covers both cost of vaccine and administration (Z23)

Copayment/coinsurance and deductible are waived. (https://www.cms.gov/ MLNProducts/downloads/MPS_ QuickReferenceChart_1.pdf)

*Coding Clinic: 2016, Q4, P3*

### Semen Analysis

✳ **G0027** Semen analysis; presence and/or motility of sperm excluding Huhner ⑨ Qp Qh ♂                    Q4

*Laboratory Certification: Hematology*

### Administration, Payment and Care Management Services

✳ **G0068** Professional services for the administration of anti-infective, pain management, chelation, pulmonary hypertension, and/or inotropic infusion drug(s) for each infusion drug administration calendar day in the individual's home, each 15 minutes ⑧ A

✳ **G0069** Professional services for the administration of subcutaneous immunotherapy for each infusion drug administration calendar day in the individual's home, each 15 minutes ⑧ A

✳ **G0070** Professional services for the administration of chemotherapy for each infusion drug administration calendar day in the individual's home, each 15 minutes ⑧ A

✳ **G0071** Payment for communication technology-based services for 5 minutes or more of a virtual (non-face-to-face) communication between an rural health clinic (RHC) or federally qualified health center (FQHC) practitioner and RHC or FQHC patient, or 5 minutes or more of remote evaluation of recorded video and/or images by an RHC or FQHC practitioner, occurring in lieu of an office visit; RHC or FQHC only ⑧ A

✳ **G0076** Brief (20 minutes) care management home visit for a new patient. For use only in a Medicare-approved CMMI model. (Services must be furnished within a beneficiary's home, domiciliary, rest home, assisted living and/or nursing facility.) ⑧ B

✳ **G0077** Limited (30 minutes) care management home visit for a new patient. For use only in a Medicare-approved CMMI model. (Services must be furnished within a beneficiary's home, domiciliary, rest home, assisted living and/or nursing facility.) ⑧ B

✳ **G0078** Moderate (45 minutes) care management home visit for a new patient. For use only in a Medicare-approved CMMI model. (Services must be furnished within a beneficiary's home, domiciliary, rest home, assisted living and/or nursing facility.) ⑧ B

| ▶ New | ↻ Revised | ✔ Reinstated | deleted Deleted | ⊘ Not covered or valid by Medicare |
|---|---|---|---|---|
| ⊕ Special coverage instructions | | ✳ Carrier discretion | ⑧ Bill Part B MAC | ⑧ Bill DME MAC |

* **G0079** Comprehensive (60 minutes) care management home visit for a new patient. For use only in a Medicare-approved CMMI model. (Services must be furnished within a beneficiary's home, domiciliary, rest home, assisted living and/or nursing facility.) Ⓑ **B**

* **G0080** Extensive (75 minutes) care management home visit for a new patient. For use only in a Medicare-approved CMMI model. (Services must be furnished within a beneficiary's home, domiciliary, rest home, assisted living and/or nursing facility.) Ⓑ **B**

* **G0081** Brief (20 minutes) care management home visit for an existing patient. For use only in a Medicare-approved CMMI model. (Services must be furnished within a beneficiary's home, domiciliary, rest home, assisted living and/or nursing facility.) Ⓑ **B**

* **G0082** Limited (30 minutes) care management home visit for an existing patient. For use only in a Medicare-approved CMMI model. (Services must be furnished within a beneficiary's home, domiciliary, rest home, assisted living and/or nursing facility.) Ⓑ **B**

* **G0083** Moderate (45 minutes) care management home visit for an existing patient. For use only in a Medicare-approved CMMI model. (Services must be furnished within a beneficiary's home, domiciliary, rest home, assisted living and/or nursing facility.) Ⓑ **B**

* **G0084** Comprehensive (60 minutes) care management home visit for an existing patient. For use only in a Medicare-approved CMMI model. (Services must be furnished within a beneficiary's home, domiciliary, rest home, assisted living and/or nursing facility.) Ⓑ **B**

* **G0085** Extensive (75 minutes) care management home visit for an existing patient. For use only in a Medicare-approved CMMI model. (Services must be furnished within a beneficiary's home, domiciliary, rest home, assisted living and/or nursing facility.) Ⓑ **B**

* **G0086** Limited (30 minutes) care management home care plan oversight. For use only in a Medicare-approved CMMI model. (Services must be furnished within a beneficiary's home, domiciliary, rest home, assisted living and/or nursing facility.) Ⓑ **B**

* **G0087** Comprehensive (60 minutes) care management home care plan oversight. For use only in a Medicare-approved CMMI model. (Services must be furnished within a beneficiary's home, domiciliary, rest home, assisted living and/or nursing facility.) Ⓑ **B**

## Screening Services

○ **G0101** Cervical or vaginal cancer screening; pelvic and clinical breast examination Ⓑ Qp Qh **S**

Covered once every two years and annually if high risk for cervical/vaginal cancer, or if childbearing age patient has had an abnormal Pap smear in preceding three years. High risk diagnosis, Z77.9

Coding Clinic: 2002, Q4, P8

○ **G0102** Prostate cancer screening; digital rectal examination Ⓑ Qp Qh **N**

Covered annually by Medicare (Z12.5). Not separately payable with an E/M code (99201-99499).

IOM: 100-02, 6, 10; 100-04, 4, 240; 100-04, 18, 50.1

○ **G0103** Prostate cancer screening; prostate specific antigen test (PSA) Ⓑ Qp Qh **A**

Covered annually by Medicare (Z12.5)

IOM: 100-02, 6, 10; 100-04, 4, 240; 100-04, 18, 50

Laboratory Certification: Routine chemistry

○ **G0104** Colorectal cancer screening; flexible sigmoidoscopy Ⓑ Qp Qh **T**

Covered once every 48 months for beneficiaries age 50+

Co-insurance waived under Section 4104.

Coding Clinic: 2011, Q2, P4

○ **G0105** Colorectal cancer screening; colonoscopy on individual at high risk Ⓑ Qp Qh **T**

Screening colonoscopy covered once every 24 months for high risk for developing colorectal cancer. May use modifier 53 if appropriate (physician fee schedule).

Co-insurance waived under Section 4104.

Coding Clinic: 2018, Q2, P4; 2011, Q2, P4

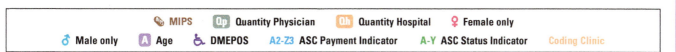

🐾 MIPS   Qp Quantity Physician   Qh Quantity Hospital   ♀ Female only
♂ Male only   A Age   DMEPOS   A2-Z3 ASC Payment Indicator   A-Y ASC Status Indicator   Coding Clinic

TEMPORARY PROCEDURES/PROFESSIONAL SERVICES   G0079 — G0105

◎ ○ **G0106** Colorectal cancer screening; alternative to G0104, screening sigmoidoscopy, barium enema ◉ Qp Qh                    S

Barium enema (not high risk) (alternative to G0104). Covered once every 4 years for beneficiaries age 50+. Use modifier 26 for professional component only.

*Coding Clinic: 2011, Q2, P4*

## Diabetes Management Training Services

◎ ✳ **G0108** Diabetes outpatient self-management training services, individual, per 30 minutes ⑧ Qp Qh                    A

Report for beneficiaries diagnosed with diabetes.

Effective January 2011, DSMT will be included in the list of reimbursable Medicare telehealth services.

◎ ✳ **G0109** Diabetes outpatient self-management training services, group session (2 or more) per 30 minutes ⑧ Qp Qh          A

Report for beneficiaries diagnosed with diabetes.

Effective January 2011, DSMT will be included in the list of reimbursable Medicare telehealth services.

## Screening Services

◎ ✳ **G0117** Glaucoma screening for high risk patients furnished by an optometrist or ophthalmologist ⑧ Qp Qh          S

Covered once per year (full 11 months between screenings). Bundled with all other ophthalmic services provided on same day. Diagnosis code Z13.5.

◎ ✳ **G0118** Glaucoma screening for high risk patient furnished under the direct supervision of an optometrist or ophthalmologist ⑧ Qp Qh          S

Covered once per year (full 11 months between screenings). Diagnosis code Z13.5.

◎ ○ **G0120** Colorectal cancer screening; alternative to G0105, screening colonoscopy, barium enema. ⑧ Qp Qh          S

Barium enema for patients with a high risk of developing colorectal. Covered once every 2 years. Used as an alternative to G0105. Use modifier 26 for professional component only.

◎ ○ **G0121** Colorectal cancer screening; colonoscopy on individual not meeting criteria for high risk ⑧ Qp Qh          T

Screening colonoscopy for patients that are not high risk. Covered once every 10 years, but not within 48 months of a G0104. For non-Medicare patients report 45378.

Co-insurance waived under Section 4104.

*Coding Clinic: 2018, Q2, P4*

◎ ⊘ **G0122** Colorectal cancer screening; barium enema ⑧          E1

Medicare: this service is denied as noncovered, because it fails to meet the requirements of the benefit. The beneficiary is liable for payment.

○ **G0123** Screening cytopathology, cervical or vaginal (any reporting system), collected in preservative fluid, automated thin layer preparation, screening by cytotechnologist under physician supervision ⑧ Qp Qh ♀          A

Use G0123 or G0143 or G0144 or G0145 or G0147 or G0148 or P3000 for Pap smears NOT requiring physician interpretation (technical component).

*IOM: 100-03, 3, 190.2; 100-04, 18, 30*

*Laboratory Certification: Cytology*

○ **G0124** Screening cytopathology, cervical or vaginal (any reporting system), collected in preservative fluid, automated thin layer preparation, requiring interpretation by physician ⑧ Qp Qh ♀          B

Report professional component for Pap smears requiring physician interpretation.

*IOM: 100-03, 3, 190.2; 100-04, 18, 30*

*Laboratory Certification: Cytology*

## Miscellaneous Services, Diagnostic and Therapeutic

○ **G0127** Trimming of dystrophic nails, any number ⑧ Qp Qh          Q1

Must be used with a modifier (Q7, Q8, or Q9) to show that the foot care service is needed because the beneficiary has a systemic disease. Limit 1 unit of service.

*IOM: 100-02, 15, 290*

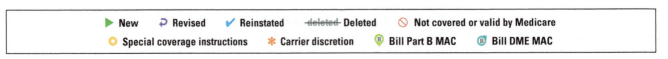

▶ New   ↻ Revised   ✔ Reinstated   ~~deleted~~ Deleted   ⊘ Not covered or valid by Medicare
○ Special coverage instructions   ✳ Carrier discretion   ⑧ Bill Part B MAC   ⑧ Bill DME MAC

⊕ **G0128** Direct (face-to-face with patient) skilled nursing services of a registered nurse provided in a comprehensive outpatient rehabilitation facility, each 10 minutes beyond the first 5 minutes ⑧ Qp Qh **B**

A separate nursing service that is clearly identifiable in the Plan of Treatment and not part of other services. Documentation must support this service. Examples include: Insertion of a urinary catheter, intramuscular injections, bowel disimpaction, nursing assessment, and education. Restricted coverage by Medicare.

*Medicare Statute 1833(a)*

✳ **G0129** Occupational therapy services requiring the skills of a qualified occupational therapist, furnished as a component of a partial hospitalization treatment program, per session (45 minutes or more) ⑧ Qh **P**

⊕ **G0130** Single energy x-ray absorptiometry (SEXA) bone density study, one or more sites; appendicular skeleton (peripheral) (e.g., radius, wrist, heel) ⑧ Qp Qh **Z3 S**

Covered every 24 months (more frequently if medically necessary). Use modifier 26 for professional component only.

Preventive service; no deductible

*IOM: 100-03, 2, 150.3; 100-04, 13, 140.1*

✳ **G0141** Screening cytopathology smears, cervical or vaginal, performed by automated system, with manual rescreening, requiring interpretation by physician ⑧ Qp Qh ♀ **B**

Co-insurance, copay, and deductible waived

Report professional component for Pap smears requiring physician interpretation. Refer to diagnosis of Z92.89, Z12.4, Z12.72, or Z12.89 to report appropriate risk level.

*Laboratory Certification: Cytology*

✳ **G0143** Screening cytopathology, cervical or vaginal (any reporting system), collected in preservative fluid, automated thin layer preparation, with manual screening and rescreening by cytotechnologist under physician supervision ⑧ Qp Qh ♀ **A**

Co-insurance, copay, and deductible waived

*Laboratory Certification: Cytology*

✳ **G0144** Screening cytopathology, cervical or vaginal (any reporting system), collected in preservative fluid, automated thin layer preparation, with screening by automated system, under physician supervision ⑧ Qp Qh ♀ **A**

Co-insurance, copay, and deductible waived

*Laboratory Certification: Cytology*

✳ **G0145** Screening cytopathology, cervical or vaginal (any reporting system), collected in preservative fluid, automated thin layer preparation, with screening by automated system and manual rescreening under physician supervision ⑧ Qp Qh ♀ **A**

Co-insurance, copay, and deductible waived

*Laboratory Certification: Cytology*

✳ **G0147** Screening cytopathology smears, cervical or vaginal; performed by automated system under physician supervision ⑧ Qp Qh ♀ **A**

Co-insurance, copay, and deductible waived

*Laboratory Certification: Cytology*

✳ **G0148** Screening cytopathology smears, cervical or vaginal; performed by automated system with manual rescreening ⑧ Qp Qh ♀ **A**

Co-insurance, copay, and deductible waived

*Laboratory Certification: Cytology*

✳ **G0151** Services performed by a qualified physical therapist in the home health or hospice setting, each 15 minutes ⑧ **B**

✳ **G0152** Services performed by a qualified occupational therapist in the home health or hospice setting, each 15 minutes ⑧ **B**

✳ **G0153** Services performed by a qualified speech-language pathologist in the home health or hospice setting, each 15 minutes ⑧ **B**

⊘ ✳ **G0155** Services of clinical social worker in home health or hospice settings, each 15 minutes ⑧ **B**

✳ **G0156** Services of home health/health aide in home health or hospice settings, each 15 minutes ⑧ **B**

✳ **G0157** Services performed by a qualified physical therapist assistant in the home health or hospice setting, each 15 minutes ⑧ **B**

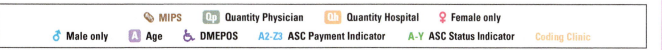

| 🏷 MIPS | Qp Quantity Physician | Qh Quantity Hospital | ♀ Female only |
| --- | --- | --- | --- |
| ♂ Male only | A Age | ♿ DMEPOS | A2-Z3 ASC Payment Indicator | A-Y ASC Status Indicator | Coding Clinic |

✳ **G0158** Services performed by a qualified occupational therapist assistant in the home health or hospice setting, each 15 minutes ⑧                B

✳ **G0159** Services performed by a qualified physical therapist, in the home health setting, in the establishment or delivery of a safe and effective physical therapy maintenance program, each 15 minutes ⑧                B

✳ **G0160** Services performed by a qualified occupational therapist, in the home health setting, in the establishment or delivery of a safe and effective occupational therapy maintenance program, each 15 minutes ⑧                B

✳ **G0161** Services performed by a qualified speech-language pathologist, in the home health setting, in the establishment or delivery of a safe and effective speech-language pathology maintenance program, each 15 minutes ⑧                B

✳ **G0162** Skilled services by a registered nurse (RN) for management and evaluation of the plan of care; each 15 minutes (the patient's underlying condition or complication requires an RN to ensure that essential non-skilled care achieves its purpose in the home health or hospice setting) ⑧                B

*Transmittal No. 824 (CR7182)*

⊛ **G0166** External counterpulsation, per treatment session ⑧ Qp Qh                Q1

*IOM: 100-03, 1, 20.20*

✳ **G0168** Wound closure utilizing tissue adhesive(s) only ⑧ Qp Qh                B

Report for wound closure with only tissue adhesive. If a practitioner utilizes tissue adhesive in addition to staples or sutures to close a wound, HCPCS code G0168 is not separately reportable, but is included in the tissue repair.

The only closure material used for a simple repair, coverage based on payer.

Coding Clinic: 2005, Q1, P5; 2001, Q4, P12; Q3, P13

✳ **G0175** Scheduled interdisciplinary team conference (minimum of three exclusive of patient care nursing staff) with patient present ⑧ Qp Qh                V

⊛ **G0176** Activity therapy, such as music, dance, art or play therapies not for recreation, related to the care and treatment of patient's disabling mental health problems, per session (45 minutes or more) ⑧ Qh                P

*Paid in partial hospitalization*

⊛ **G0177** Training and educational services related to the care and treatment of patient's disabling mental health problems per session (45 minutes or more) ⑧ Qp Qh                N

*Paid in partial hospitalization*

✳ **G0179** Physician recertification for Medicare-covered home health services under a home health plan of care (patient not present), including contacts with home health agency and review of reports of patient status required by physicians to affirm the initial implementation of the plan of care that meets patient's needs, per recertification period ⑧ Qp Qh                M

The recertification code is used after a patient has received services for at least 60 days (or one certification period) when the physician signs the certification after the initial certification period.

✳ **G0180** Physician certification for Medicare-covered home health services under a home health plan of care (patient not present), including contacts with home health agency and review of reports of patient status required by physicians to affirm the initial implementation of the plan of care that meets patient's needs, per certification period ⑧ Qp Qh                M

This code can be billed only when the patient has not received Medicare covered home health services for at least 60 days.

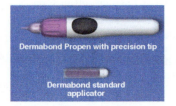

Dermabond Propen with precision tip

Dermabond standard applicator

**Figure 15**  Tissue adhesive.

▶ New    ↻ Revised    ✔ Reinstated    ~~deleted~~ Deleted    ⊘ Not covered or valid by Medicare
⊛ Special coverage instructions    ✳ Carrier discretion    ⑧ Bill Part B MAC    ⑧ Bill DME MAC

224

\* **G0181** Physician supervision of a patient receiving Medicare-covered services provided by a participating home health agency (patient not present) requiring complex and multidisciplinary care modalities involving regular physician development and/or revision of care plans, review of subsequent reports of patient status, review of laboratory and other studies, communication (including telephone calls) with other health care professionals involved in the patient's care, integration of new information into the medical treatment plan and/or adjustment of medical therapy, within a calendar month, 30 minutes or more ⑧ Qp Qh    M

*Coding Clinic: 2015, Q2, P10*

\* **G0182** Physician supervision of a patient under a Medicare-approved hospice (patient not present) requiring complex and multidisciplinary care modalities involving regular physician development and/or revision of care plans, review of subsequent reports of patient status, review of laboratory and other studies, communication (including telephone calls) with other health care professionals involved in the patient's care, integration of new information into the medical treatment plan and/or adjustment of medical therapy, within a calendar month, 30 minutes or more ⑧ Qp Qh    M

*Coding Clinic: 2015, Q2, P10*

\* **G0186** Destruction of localized lesion of choroid (for example, choroidal neovascularization); photocoagulation, feeder vessel technique (one or more sessions) ⑧ Qp Qh    T

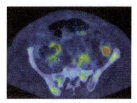

**Figure 16**  PET scan.

🚫 **G0219** PET imaging whole body; melanoma for non-covered indications ⑧    E1

Example: Assessing regional lymph nodes in melanoma.

*IOM: 100-03, 4, 220.6*

*Coding Clinic: 2007, Q1, P6*

🚫 **G0235** PET imaging, any site, not otherwise specified ⑧ Qp Qh    E1

Example: Prostate cancer diagnosis and initial staging.

*IOM: 100-03, 4, 220.6*

*Coding Clinic: 2007, Q1, P6*

\* **G0237** Therapeutic procedures to increase strength or endurance of respiratory muscles, face to face, one on one, each 15 minutes (includes monitoring) ⑧ Qp Qh    S

\* **G0238** Therapeutic procedures to improve respiratory function, other than described by G0237, one on one, face to face, per 15 minutes (includes monitoring) ⑧ Qp Qh    S

\* **G0239** Therapeutic procedures to improve respiratory function or increase strength or endurance of respiratory muscles, two or more individuals (includes monitoring) ⑧ Qp Qh    S

🔧 ⚙ **G0245** Initial physician evaluation and management of a diabetic patient with diabetic sensory neuropathy resulting in a loss of protective sensation (LOPS) which must include (1) the diagnosis of LOPS, (2) a patient history, (3) a physical examination that consist of at least the following elements: (A) visual inspection of the forefoot, hindfoot and toe web spaces, (B) evaluation of a protective sensation, (C) evaluation of foot structure and biomechanics, (D) evaluation of vascular status and skin integrity, and (E) evaluation and recommendation of footwear, and (4) patient education ⑧ Qp Qh    V

*IOM: 100-03, 1, 70.2.1*

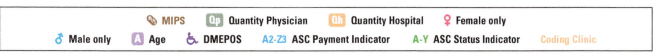

🔧 **MIPS**    Qp **Quantity Physician**    Qh **Quantity Hospital**    ♀ **Female only**    ♂ **Male only**    Ⓐ **Age**    ♿ **DMEPOS**    A2-Z3 **ASC Payment Indicator**    A-Y **ASC Status Indicator**    **Coding Clinic**

**G0246** Follow-up physician evaluation and management of a diabetic patient with diabetic sensory neuropathy resulting in a loss of protective sensation (LOPS) to include at least the following: (1) a patient history, (2) a physical examination that includes: (A) visual inspection of the forefoot, hindfoot and toe web spaces, (B) evaluation of protective sensation, (C) evaluation of foot structure and biomechanics, (D) evaluation of vascular status and skin integrity, and (E) evaluation and recommendation of footwear, and (3) patient education ⑧ Qp Qh     V

*IOM: 100-03, 1, 70.2.1; 100-02, 15, 290*

**G0247** Routine foot care by a physician of a diabetic patient with diabetic sensory neuropathy resulting in a loss of protective sensation (LOPS) to include, the local care of superficial wounds (i.e., superficial to muscle and fascia) and at least the following if present: (1) local care of superficial wounds, (2) debridement of corns and calluses, and (3) trimming and debridement of nails ⑧ Qp Qh     Q1

*IOM: 100-03, 1, 70.2.1*

**G0248** Demonstration, prior to initiation, of home INR monitoring for patient with either mechanical heart valve(s), chronic atrial fibrillation, or venous thromboembolism who meets Medicare coverage criteria, under the direction of a physician; includes: face-to-face demonstration of use and care of the INR monitor, obtaining at least one blood sample, provision of instructions for reporting home INR test results, and documentation of patient's ability to perform testing and report results ⑧ Qp Qh     V

**G0249** Provision of test materials and equipment for home INR monitoring of patient with either mechanical heart valve(s), chronic atrial fibrillation, or venous thromboembolism who meets Medicare coverage criteria; includes provision of materials for use in the home and reporting of test results to physician; testing not occurring more frequently than once a week; testing materials, billing units of service include 4 tests ⑧ Qp Qh     V

**G0250** Physician review, interpretation, and patient management of home INR testing for patient with either mechanical heart valve(s), chronic atrial fibrillation, or venous thromboembolism who meets Medicare coverage criteria; testing not occurring more frequently than once a week; billing units of service include 4 tests ⑧ Qp Qh     M

**G0252** PET imaging, full and partial-ring PET scanners only, for initial diagnosis of breast cancer and/or surgical planning for breast cancer (e.g., initial staging of axillary lymph nodes) ⑧     E1

*IOM: 100-03, 4, 220.6*

Coding Clinic: 2007, Q1, P6

**G0255** Current perception threshold/sensory nerve conduction test (SNCT), per limb, any nerve ⑧     E1

*IOM: 100-03, 2, 160.23*

**G0257** Unscheduled or emergency dialysis treatment for an ESRD patient in a hospital outpatient department that is not certified as an ESRD facility ⑧ Qp Qh     S

Coding Clinic: 2003, Q1, P9

**G0259** Injection procedure for sacroiliac joint; arthrography ⑧ Qp Qh     N

Replaces 27096 for reporting injections for Medicare beneficiaries

Used by Part A only (facility), not priced by Part B Medicare.

**G0260** Injection procedure for sacroiliac joint; provision of anesthetic, steroid and/or other therapeutic agent, with or without arthrography ⑧ Qp Qh     T

ASCs report when a therapeutic sacroiliac joint injection is administered in ASC

**G0268** Removal of impacted cerumen (one or both ears) by physician on same date of service as audiologic function testing ⑧ Qp Qh     N

Report only when a physician, not an audiologist, performs the procedure.

Use with DX H61.2- when performed by physician.

Coding Clinic: 2016, Q2, P2-3; 2003, Q1, P12

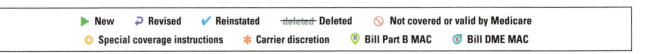

▶ New    ↻ Revised    ✔ Reinstated    ~~deleted~~ Deleted    ⊘ Not covered or valid by Medicare
⚙ Special coverage instructions    ✳ Carrier discretion    ⑧ Bill Part B MAC    ⑧ Bill DME MAC

⚙ **G0269** Placement of occlusive device into either a venous or arterial access site, post surgical or interventional procedure (e.g., angioseal plug, vascular plug) ⑧ Qh　　　　N

*Report for replacement of vasoseal. Hospitals may report the closure device as a supply with C1760. Bundled status on Physician Fee Schedule.*

*Coding Clinic: 2011, Q3, P4; 2010, Q4, P6*

✱ **G0270** Medical nutrition therapy; reassessment and subsequent intervention(s) following second referral in same year for change in diagnosis, medical condition or treatment regimen (including additional hours needed for renal disease), individual, face to face with the patient, each 15 minutes ⑧ Qp Qh　　A

*Requires physician referral for beneficiaries with diabetes or renal disease. Services must be provided by dietitian/nutritionist. Co-insurance and deductible waived.*

✱ **G0271** Medical nutrition therapy, reassessment and subsequent intervention(s) following second referral in same year for change in diagnosis, medical condition, or treatment regimen (including additional hours needed for renal disease), group (2 or more individuals), each 30 minutes ⑧ Qp Qh　　A

*Requires physician referral for beneficiaries with diabetes or renal disease. Services must be provided by dietitian/nutritionist. Co-insurance and deductible waived.*

⚙ **G0276** Blinded procedure for lumbar stenosis, percutaneous image-guided lumbar decompression (PILD) or placebo-control, performed in an approved coverage with evidence development (CED) clinical trial ⑧ Qp Qh　　J1

⚙ **G0277** Hyperbaric oxygen under pressure, full body chamber, per 30 minute interval ⑧ Qp Qh　　S

*IOM: 100-03, 1, 20.29*

*Coding Clinic: 2015, Q3, P7*

✱ **G0278** Iliac and/or femoral artery angiography, non-selective, bilateral or ipsilateral to catheter insertion, performed at the same time as cardiac catheterization and/or coronary angiography, includes positioning or placement of the catheter in the distal aorta or ipsilateral femoral or iliac artery, injection of dye, production of permanent images, and radiologic supervision and interpretation (list separately in addition to primary procedure) ⑧ Qp Qh　　N

*Medicare specific code not reported for iliac injection used as a guiding shot for a closure device*

*Coding Clinic: 2011, Q3, P4; 2006, Q4, P7*

✱ **G0279** Diagnostic digital breast tomosynthesis, unilateral or bilateral (list separately in addition to G0204 or G0206) ⑧　　A

✱ **G0281** Electrical stimulation, (unattended), to one or more areas, for chronic stage III and stage IV pressure ulcers, arterial ulcers, diabetic ulcers, and venous stasis ulcers not demonstrating measurable signs of healing after 30 days of conventional care, as part of a therapy plan of care ⑧ Qp Qh　　A

*Reported by encounter/areas and not by site. Therapists report G0281 and G0283 rather than 97014.*

⊘ **G0282** Electrical stimulation, (unattended), to one or more areas, for wound care other than described in G0281 ⑧　　E1

*IOM: 100-03, 4, 270.1*

✱ **G0283** Electrical stimulation (unattended), to one or more areas for indication(s) other than wound care, as part of a therapy plan of care ⑧ Qp Qh　　A

*Reported by encounter/areas and not by site. Therapists report G0281 and G0283 rather than 97014.*

✱ **G0288** Reconstruction, computed tomographic angiography of aorta for surgical planning for vascular surgery ⑨ Qp Qh　　N

* **G0289** Arthroscopy, knee, surgical, for removal of loose body, foreign body, debridement/shaving of articular cartilage (chondroplasty) at the time of other surgical knee arthroscopy in a different compartment of the same knee Ⓑ Qp Qh       N

Add-on code reported with knee arthroscopy code for major procedure performed-reported once per extra compartment

"The code may be reported twice (or with a unit of two) if the physician performs these procedures in two compartments, in addition to the compartment where the main procedure was performed." (http://www.ama-assn.org/resources/doc/cpt/orthopaedics.pdf)

○ **G0293** Noncovered surgical procedure(s) using conscious sedation, regional, general or spinal anesthesia in a Medicare qualifying clinical trial, per day Ⓑ Qp Qh       Q1

○ **G0294** Noncovered procedure(s) using either no anesthesia or local anesthesia only, in a Medicare qualifying clinical trial, per day Ⓑ Qp Qh       Q1

⊘ **G0295** Electromagnetic therapy, to one or more areas, for wound care other than described in G0329 or for other uses Ⓑ       E1

*IOM: 100-03, 4, 270.1*

* **G0296** Counseling visit to discuss need for lung cancer screening (LDCT) using low dose CT scan (service is for eligibility determination and shared decision making) ⊙ Qp Qh       S

* **G0297** Low dose CT scan (LDCT) for lung cancer screening Ⓑ Qp Qh       S

* **G0299** Direct skilled nursing services of a registered nurse (RN) in the home health or hospice setting, each 15 minutes Ⓑ       B

* **G0300** Direct skilled nursing services of a licensed practical nurse (LPN) in the home health or hospice setting, each 15 minutes Ⓑ       B

* **G0302** Pre-operative pulmonary surgery services for preparation for LVRS, complete course of services, to include a minimum of 16 days of services Ⓑ Qp Qh       S

* **G0303** Pre-operative pulmonary surgery services for preparation for LVRS, 10 to 15 days of services Ⓑ Qp Qh       S

* **G0304** Pre-operative pulmonary surgery services for preparation for LVRS, 1 to 9 days of services Qp Qh       S

* **G0305** Post-discharge pulmonary surgery services after LVRS, minimum of 6 days of services Ⓑ Qp Qh       S

* **G0306** Complete CBC, automated (HgB, HCT, RBC, WBC, without platelet count) and automated WBC differential count Ⓑ Qp Qh       Q4

*Laboratory Certification: Hematology*

* **G0307** Complete CBC, automated (HgB, HCT, RBC, WBC; without platelet count) Ⓑ Qp Qh       Q4

*Laboratory Certification: Hematology*

○ **G0328** Colorectal cancer screening; fecal occult blood test, immunoassay, 1-3 simultaneous Ⓑ Qp Qh       A

Co-insurance and deductible waived

Reported for Medicare patients 501; one FOBT per year, with either G0107 (guaiac-based) or G0328 (immunoassay-based)

*Laboratory Certification: Routine chemistry,Hematology*

Coding Clinic: 2012, Q2, P9

* **G0329** Electromagnetic therapy, to one or more areas for chronic stage III and stage IV pressure ulcers, arterial ulcers, and diabetic ulcers and venous stasis ulcers not demonstrating measurable signs of healing after 30 days of conventional care as part of a therapy plan of care Ⓑ Qp Qh       A

○ **G0333** Pharmacy dispensing fee for inhalation drug(s); initial 30-day supply as a beneficiary Ⓑ Qp Qh       M

Medicare will reimburse an initial dispensing fee to a pharmacy for initial 30-day period of inhalation drugs furnished through DME.

US machine

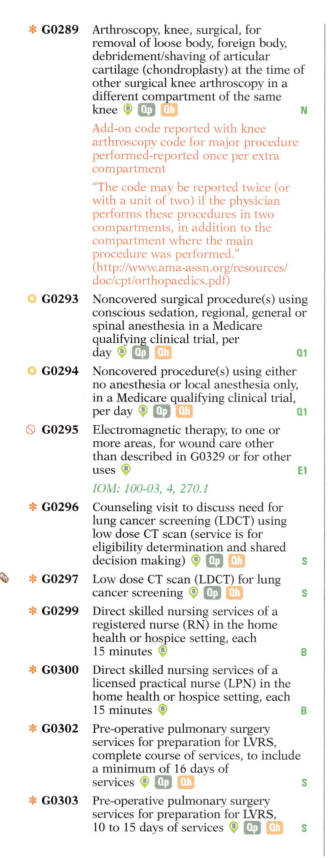

Electromagnetic device

**Figure 17**   Electromagnetic device.

▶ New       ↻ Revised       ✔ Reinstated       ~~deleted~~ Deleted       ⊘ Not covered or valid by Medicare

○ Special coverage instructions       * Carrier discretion       Ⓑ Bill Part B MAC       Ⓓ Bill DME MAC

\* **G0337** Hospice evaluation and counseling services, pre-election Ⓑ Qp Qh **B**

\* **G0339** Image-guided robotic linear accelerator-based stereotactic radiosurgery, complete course of therapy in one session or first session of fractionated treatment ♥ Qp Qh **B**

\* **G0340** Image-guided robotic linear accelerator-based stereotactic radiosurgery, delivery including collimator changes and custom plugging, fractionated treatment, all lesions, per session, second through fifth sessions, maximum five sessions per course of treatment ♥ Qp Qh **B**

✿ **G0341** Percutaneous islet cell transplant, includes portal vein catheterization and infusion Ⓑ Qp Qh **C**

*IOM: 100-03, 4, 260.3; 100-04, 32, 70*

✿ **G0342** Laparoscopy for islet cell transplant, includes portal vein catheterization and infusion ♥ Qp Qh **C**

*IOM: 100-03, 4, 260.3*

✿ **G0343** Laparotomy for islet cell transplant, includes portal vein catheterization and infusion Ⓑ Qp Qh **C**

*IOM: 100-03, 4, 260.3*

~~G0365~~ ~~Vessel mapping of vessels for hemodialysis access (services for preoperative vessel mapping prior to creation of hemodialysis access using an autogenous hemodialysis conduit, including arterial inflow and venous outflow)~~ ✖

✿ **G0372** Physician service required to establish and document the need for a power mobility device ♥ Qp Qh **M**

Providers should bill the E/M code and G0372 on the same claim.

## Hospital Services: Observation and Emergency Department

✿ **G0378** Hospital observation service, per hour Ⓑ Qh **N**

Report all related services in addition to G0378. Report units of hours spent in observation (rounded to the nearest hour). Hospitals report the ED or clinic visit with a CPT code or, if applicable, G0379 (direct admit to observation) and G0378 (hospital observation services, per hour).

Coding Clinic: 2007, Q1, P10; 2006, Q3, P7-8

✿ **G0379** Direct admission of patient for hospital observation care Ⓑ Qp Qh **J2**

Report all related services in addition to G0379. Report units of hours spent in observation (rounded to the nearest hour). Hospitals report the ED or clinic visit with a CPT code or, if applicable, G0379 (direct admit to observation) and G0378 (hospital observation services, per hour).

Coding Clinic: 2007, Q1, P7

\* **G0380** Level 1 hospital emergency department visit provided in a type B emergency department; (the ED must meet at least one of the following requirements: (1) it is licensed by the state in which it is located under applicable state law as an emergency room or emergency department; (2) it is held out to the public (by name, posted signs, advertising, or other means) as a place that provides care for emergency medical conditions on an urgent basis without requiring a previously scheduled appointment; or (3) during the calendar year immediately preceding the calendar year in which a determination under 42 CFR 489.24 is being made, based on a representative sample of patient visits that occurred during that calendar year, it provides at least one-third of all of its outpatient visits for the treatment of emergency medical conditions on an urgent basis without requiring a previously scheduled appointment) Ⓑ Qh **J2**

Coding Clinic: 2009, Q1, P4; 2007, Q2, P1

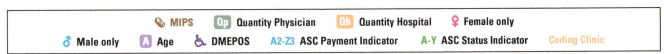

🖐 MIPS    Qp Quantity Physician    Qh Quantity Hospital    ♀ Female only
♂ Male only    Ⓐ Age    ♿ DMEPOS    A2-Z3 ASC Payment Indicator    A-Y ASC Status Indicator    Coding Clinic

* **G0381** Level 2 hospital emergency department visit provided in a type B emergency department; (the ED must meet at least one of the following requirements: (1) it is licensed by the state in which it is located under applicable state law as an emergency room or emergency department; (2) it is held out to the public (by name, posted signs, advertising, or other means) as a place that provides care for emergency medical conditions on an urgent basis without requiring a previously scheduled appointment; or (3) during the calendar year immediately preceding the calendar year in which a determination under 42 CFR 489.24 is being made, based on a representative sample of patient visits that occurred during that calendar year, it provides at least one-third of all of its outpatient visits for the treatment of emergency medical conditions on an urgent basis without requiring a previously scheduled appointment) Ⓑ Qh J2

*Coding Clinic: 2009, Q1, P4; 2007, Q2, P1*

* **G0382** Level 3 hospital emergency department visit provided in a type B emergency department; (the ED must meet at least one of the following requirements: (1) it is licensed by the state in which it is located under applicable state law as an emergency room or emergency department; (2) it is held out to the public (by name, posted signs, advertising, or other means) as a place that provides care for emergency medical conditions on an urgent basis without requiring a previously scheduled appointment; or (3) during the calendar year immediately preceding the calendar year in which a determination under 42 CFR 489.24 is being made, based on a representative sample of patient visits that occurred during that calendar year, it provides at least one-third of all of its outpatient visits for the treatment of emergency medical conditions on an urgent basis without requiring a previously scheduled appointment) Ⓑ Qh J2

*Coding Clinic: 2009, Q1, P4; 2007, Q2, P1*

* **G0383** Level 4 hospital emergency department visit provided in a type B emergency department; (the ED must meet at least one of the following requirements: (1) it is licensed by the state in which it is located under applicable state law as an emergency room or emergency department; (2) it is held out to the public (by name, posted signs, advertising, or other means) as a place that provides care for emergency medical conditions on an urgent basis without requiring a previously scheduled appointment; or (3) during the calendar year immediately preceding the calendar year in which a determination under 42 CFR 489.24 is being made, based on a representative sample of patient visits that occurred during that calendar year, it provides at least one-third of all of its outpatient visits for the treatment of emergency medical conditions on an urgent basis without requiring a previously scheduled appointment) Ⓑ Qh J2

*Coding Clinic: 2009, Q1, P4; 2007, Q2, P1*

* **G0384** Level 5 hospital emergency department visit provided in a type B emergency department; (the ED must meet at least one of the following requirements: (1) it is licensed by the state in which it is located under applicable state law as an emergency room or emergency department; (2) it is held out to the public (by name, posted signs, advertising, or other means) as a place that provides care for emergency medical conditions on an urgent basis without requiring a previously scheduled appointment; or (3) during the calendar year immediately preceding the calendar year in which a determination under 42 CFR 489.24 is being made, based on a representative sample of patient visits that occurred during that calendar year, it provides at least one-third of all of its outpatient visits for the treatment of emergency medical conditions on an urgent basis without requiring a previously scheduled appointment) Ⓑ Qh J2

*Coding Clinic: 2009, Q1, P4; 2007, Q2, P1*

### Trauma Response Team

⊕ **G0390** Trauma response team associated with hospital critical care service Ⓑ Qh S

*Coding Clinic: 2007, Q2, P5*

---

▶ New   ↻ Revised   ✔ Reinstated   ~~deleted~~ Deleted   ⊘ Not covered or valid by Medicare
⊕ Special coverage instructions   * Carrier discretion   Ⓑ Bill Part B MAC   Ⓑ Bill DME MAC

## Alcohol Substance Abuse Assessment and Intervention

**\* G0396** Alcohol and/or substance (other than tobacco) abuse structured assessment (e.g., audit, DAST), and brief intervention 15 to 30 minutes ⓥ **Qp** **Qh**     S

Bill instead of 99408 and 99409

**\* G0397** Alcohol and/or substance (other than tobacco) abuse structured assessment (e.g., audit, DAST), and intervention, greater than 30 minutes ⓑ **Qp** **Qh**     S

Bill instead of 99408 and 99409

## Home Sleep Study Test

**\* G0398** Home sleep study test (HST) with type II portable monitor, unattended; minimum of 7 channels: EEG, EOG, EMG, ECG/heart rate, airflow, respiratory effort and oxygen saturation ⓥ **Qp** **Qh**     S

**\* G0399** Home sleep test (HST) with type III portable monitor, unattended; minimum of 4 channels: 2 respiratory movement/airflow, 1 ECG/heart rate and 1 oxygen saturation ⓥ **Qp** **Qh**     S

**\* G0400** Home sleep test (HST) with type IV portable monitor, unattended; minimum of 3 channels ⓑ **Qp** **Qh**     S

## Initial Examination for Medicare Enrollment

**\* G0402** Initial preventive physical examination; face-to-face visit, services limited to new beneficiary during the first 12 months of Medicare enrollment ⓑ **Qp** **Qh**     V

Depending on circumstances, 99201-99215 may be assigned with modifier 25 to report an E/M service as a significant, separately identifiable service in addition to the Initial Preventive Physical Examination (IPPE), G0402.

Copayment and coinsurance waived, deductible waived.

Coding Clinic: 2009, Q4, P8

## Electrocardiogram

**\* G0403** Electrocardiogram, routine ECG with 12 leads; performed as a screening for the initial preventive physical examination with interpretation and report ⓑ **Qp** **Qh**     M

Optional service may be ordered or performed at discretion of physician. Once in a life-time screening, stemming from a referral from Initial Preventive Physical Examination (IPPE). Both deductible and co-payment apply.

**\* G0404** Electrocardiogram, routine ECG with 12 leads; tracing only, without interpretation and report, performed as a screening for the initial preventive physical examination ⓥ **Qp** **Qh**     S

**\* G0405** Electrocardiogram, routine ECG with 12 leads; interpretation and report only, performed as a screening for the initial preventive physical examination ⓥ **Qp** **Qh**     B

## Follow-up Telehealth Consultation

**\* G0406** Follow-up inpatient consultation, limited, physicians typically spend 15 minutes communicating with the patient via telehealth ⓑ **Qp** **Qh**     B

These telehealth modifers are required when billing for telehealth services with codes G0406-G0408 and G0425-G0427:

• GT, via interactive audio and video telecommunications system

• GQ, via asynchronous telecommunications system

**\* G0407** Follow-up inpatient consultation, intermediate, physicians typically spend 25 minutes communicating with the patient via telehealth ⓑ **Qp** **Qh**     B

**\* G0408** Follow-up inpatient consultation, complex, physicians typically spend 35 minutes communicating with the patient via telehealth ⓑ **Qp** **Qh**     B

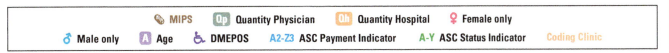

MIPS   **Qp** Quantity Physician   **Qh** Quantity Hospital   ♀ Female only
♂ Male only   Ⓐ Age   DMEPOS   A2-Z3 ASC Payment Indicator   A-Y ASC Status Indicator   Coding Clinic

TEMPORARY PROCEDURES/PROFESSIONAL SERVICES

G0396 — G0408

**231**

## Psychological Services

✳ **G0409**  Social work and psychological services, directly relating to and/or furthering the patient's rehabilitation goals, each 15 minutes, face-to-face; individual (services provided by a CORF-qualified social worker or psychologist in a CORF) Ⓑ  **B**

✳ **G0410**  Group psychotherapy other than of a multiple-family group, in a partial hospitalization setting, approximately 45 to 50 minutes Ⓑ Qp Qh  **P**

*Coding Clinic: 2009, Q4, P9, 10*

✳ **G0411**  Interactive group psychotherapy, in a partial hospitalization setting, approximately 45 to 50 minutes Ⓑ Qp Qh  **P**

*Coding Clinic: 2009, Q4, P9, 10*

## Fracture Treatment

✳ **G0412**  Open treatment of iliac spine(s), tuberosity avulsion, or iliac wing fracture(s), unilateral or bilateral for pelvic bone fracture patterns which do not disrupt the pelvic ring includes internal fixation, when performed Ⓑ Qp Qh  **C**

✳ **G0413**  Percutaneous skeletal fixation of posterior pelvic bone fracture and/or dislocation, for fracture patterns which disrupt the pelvic ring, unilateral or bilateral, (includes ilium, sacroiliac joint and/or sacrum) Ⓑ Qp Qh  **J1**

✳ **G0414**  Open treatment of anterior pelvic bone fracture and/or dislocation for fracture patterns which disrupt the pelvic ring, unilateral or bilateral, includes internal fixation when performed (includes pubic symphysis and/or superior/inferior rami) Ⓑ Qp Qh  **C**

✳ **G0415**  Open treatment of posterior pelvic bone fracture and/or dislocation, for fracture patterns which disrupt the pelvic ring, unilateral or bilateral, includes internal fixation, when performed (includes ilium, sacroiliac joint and/or sacrum) Ⓑ Qp Qh  **C**

## Surgical Pathology: Prostate Biopsy

✳ **G0416**  Surgical pathology, gross and microscopic examinations for prostate needle biopsy, any method Ⓑ Qp Qh ♂  **Q2**

This testing requires a facility to have either a CLIA certificate of registration (certificate type code 9), a CLIA certificate of compliance (certificate type code 1), or a CLIA certificate of accreditation (certificate type code 3). A facility without a valid, current, CLIA certificate, with a current CLIA certificate of waiver (certificate type code 2) or with a current CLIA certificate for provider-performed microscopy procedures (certificate type code 4), must not be permitted to be paid for these tests. This code has a TC, 26 (physician), or gobal component.

*Laboratory Certification: Histopathology*

*Coding Clinic: 2013, Q2, P6*

## Educational Services

✳ **G0420**  Face-to-face educational services related to the care of chronic kidney disease; individual, per session, per one hour Ⓑ Qp Qh  **A**

CKD is kidney damage of 3 months or longer, regardless of the cause of kidney damage. Sessions billed in increments of one hour (if session is less than one hour, it must last at least 31 minutes to be billable. Sessions less than one hour and longer than 31 minutes is billable as one session. No more than 6 sessions of KDE services in a beneficiary's lifetime.

✳ **G0421**  Face-to-face educational services related to the care of chronic kidney disease; group, per session, per one hour Ⓑ Qp Qh  **A**

Group setting: 2 to 20, report codes G0420 and G0421 with diagnosis code N18.4.

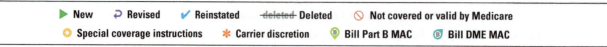

▶ New  ↻ Revised  ✔ Reinstated  ~~deleted~~ Deleted  ⊘ Not covered or valid by Medicare
⊕ Special coverage instructions  ✳ Carrier discretion  Ⓑ Bill Part B MAC  Ⓒ Bill DME MAC

## Cardiac and Pulmonary Rehabilitation

\* **G0422** Intensive cardiac rehabilitation; with or without continuous ECG monitoring with exercise, per session Ⓑ Qp Qh    S

Includes the same service as 93798 but at a greater frequency; may be reported with as many as six hourly sessions on a single date of service. Includes medical nutrition services to reduce cardiac disease risk factors.

\* **G0423** Intensive cardiac rehabilitation; with or without continuous ECG monitoring; without exercise, per session Ⓑ Qp Qh    S

Includes the same service as 93797 but at a greater frequency; may be reported with as many as six hourly sessions on a single date of service. Includes medical nutrition services to reduce cardiac disease risk factors.

\* **G0424** Pulmonary rehabilitation, including exercise (includes monitoring), one hour, per session, up to two sessions per day Ⓑ Qp Qh    S

Includes therapeutic services and all related monitoring services to improve respiratory function. Do not report with G0237, G0238, or G0239.

## Initial Telehealth Consultation

\* **G0425** Telehealth consultation, emergency department or initial inpatient, typically 30 minutes communicating with the patient via telehealth Ⓑ Qp Qh    B

Problem Focused: Problem focused history and examination, with straightforward medical decision making complexity. Typically 30 minutes communicating with patient via telehealth.

\* **G0426** Initial inpatient telehealth consultation, emergency department or initial inpatient, typically 50 minutes communicating with the patient via telehealth Ⓑ Qp Qh    B

Detailed: Detailed history and examination, with moderate medical decision making complexity. Typically 50 minutes communicating with patient via telehealth.

\* **G0427** Initial inpatient telehealth consultation, emergency department or initial inpatient, typically 70 minutes or more communicating with the patient via telehealth Ⓑ Qp Qh    B

Comprehensive: Comprehensive history and examination, with high medical decision making complexity. Typically 70 minutes or more communicating with patient via telehealth.

## Fillers

⊘ **G0428** Collagen meniscus implant procedure for filling meniscal defects (e.g., cmi, collagen scaffold, menaflex) Ⓑ    E1

\* **G0429** Dermal filler injection(s) for the treatment of facial lipodystrophy syndrome (LDS) (e.g., as a result of highly active antiretroviral therapy) Ⓑ Qp Qh    T

Designated for dermal fillers Sculptra&reg; and Radiesse (Medicare). (https://www.cms.gov/ContractorLearningResources/downloads/JA6953.pdf)

Coding Clinic: 2010, Q3, P8

## Laboratory Screening

\* **G0432** Infectious agent antibody detection by enzyme immunoassay (EIA) technique, HIV-1 and/or HIV-2, screening Ⓑ Qp Qh    A

*Laboratory Certification: Virology, General immunology*

Coding Clinic: 2010, Q2, P10

\* **G0433** Infectious agent antibody detection by enzyme-linked immunosorbent assay (ELISA) technique, HIV-1 and/or HIV-2, screening Ⓑ Qp Qh    A

*Laboratory Certification: Virology, General immunology*

Coding Clinic: 2010, Q2, P10

\* **G0435** Infectious agent antibody detection by rapid antibody test, HIV-1 and/or HIV-2, screening Ⓑ Qp Qh    A

Coding Clinic: 2010, Q2, P10

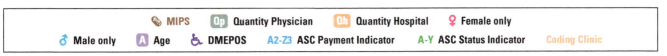

🔖 MIPS    Qp Quantity Physician    Qh Quantity Hospital    ♀ Female only    ♂ Male only    Ⓐ Age    ♿ DMEPOS    A2-Z3 ASC Payment Indicator    A-Y ASC Status Indicator    Coding Clinic

TEMPORARY PROCEDURES/PROFESSIONAL SERVICES    G0422 — G0435

## Counselling, Wellness, and Screening Services

✳ **G0438** Annual wellness visit; includes a personalized prevention plan of service (pps), initial visit Ⓑ Qp Qh      A

✳ **G0439** Annual wellness visit, includes a personalized prevention plan of service (pps), subsequent visit Ⓑ Qp Qh      A

✳ **G0442** Annual alcohol misuse screening, 15 minutes Ⓑ Qp Qh      S

*Coding Clinic: 2012, Q1, P7*

✳ **G0443** Brief face-to-face behavioral counseling for alcohol misuse, 15 minutes Ⓑ Qp Qh      S

*Coding Clinic: 2012, Q1, P7*

✳ **G0444** Annual depression screening, 15 minutes Ⓑ Qp Qh      S

✳ **G0445** High intensity behavioral counseling to prevent sexually transmitted infection; face-to-face, individual, includes: education, skills training and guidance on how to change sexual behavior; performed semi-annually, 30 minutes Ⓑ Qp Qh      S

✳ **G0446** Annual, face-to-face intensive behavioral therapy for cardiovascular disease, individual, 15 minutes Ⓑ Qp Qh      S

*Coding Clinic: 2012, Q2, P8*

✳ **G0447** Face-to-face behavioral counseling for obesity, 15 minutes Ⓑ Qp Qh      S

*Coding Clinic: 2012, Q1, P8*

✳ **G0448** Insertion or replacement of a permanent pacing cardioverter-defibrillator system with transvenous lead(s), single or dual chamber with insertion of pacing electrode, cardiac venous system, for left ventricular pacing Ⓑ Qp Qh      B

✳ **G0451** Development testing, with interpretation and report, per standardized instrument form Ⓑ Qp Qh      Q3

## Miscellaneous Services

✳ **G0452** Molecular pathology procedure; physician interpretation and report Ⓑ Qp Qh      B

✳ **G0453** Continuous intraoperative neurophysiology monitoring, from outside the operating room (remote or nearby), per patient, (attention directed exclusively to one patient) each 15 minutes (list in addition to primary procedure) Ⓑ Qp Qh      N

✳ **G0454** Physician documentation of face-to-face visit for durable medical equipment determination performed by nurse practitioner, physician assistant or clinical nurse specialist Ⓑ Qp Qh      B

✳ **G0455** Preparation with instillation of fecal microbiota by any method, including assessment of donor specimen Ⓑ Qp Qh      Q1

*Coding Clinic: 2013, Q3, P8*

✳ **G0458** Low dose rate (LDR) prostate brachytherapy services, composite rate Ⓑ Qp Qh      B

✳ **G0459** Inpatient telehealth pharmacologic management, including prescription, use, and review of medication with no more than minimal medical psychotherapy Ⓑ Qp Qh      B

✳ **G0460** Autologous platelet rich plasma for chronic wounds/ulcers, including phlebotomy, centrifugation, and all other preparatory procedures, administration and dressings, per treatment Ⓑ Qp Qh      T

✳ **G0463** Hospital outpatient clinic visit for assessment and management of a patient Ⓑ Qp Qh      J2

✳ **G0464** Colorectal cancer screening; stool-based DNA and fecal occult hemoglobin (e.g., KRAS, NDRG4 and BMP3) Ⓑ

*Cross Reference 81528*

*Laboratory Certification: General immunology, Routine chemistry, Clinical cytogenetics*

## Federally Qualified Health Center Visits

✳ **G0466** Federally qualified health center (FQHC) visit, new patient; a medically-necessary, face-to-face encounter (one-on-one) between a new patient and a FQHC practitioner during which time one or more FQHC services are rendered and includes a typical bundle of Medicare-covered services that would be furnished per diem to a patient receiving a FQHC visit Ⓑ Qp Qh      A

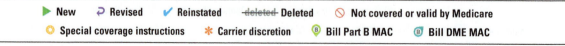

▶ New    ↻ Revised    ✔ Reinstated    ~~deleted~~ Deleted    ⊘ Not covered or valid by Medicare
⊛ Special coverage instructions    ✳ Carrier discretion    Ⓑ Bill Part B MAC    Ⓓ Bill DME MAC

* **G0467** Federally qualified health center (FQHC) visit, established patient; a medically-necessary, face-to-face encounter (one-on-one) between an established patient and a FQHC practitioner during which time one or more FQHC services are rendered and includes a typical bundle of Medicare-covered services that would be furnished per diem to a patient receiving a FQHC visit Ⓑ Qp Qh    A

* **G0468** Federally qualified health center (FQHC) visit, IPPE or AWV; a FQHC visit that includes an initial preventive physical examination (IPPE) or annual wellness visit (AWV) and includes a typical bundle of Medicare-covered services that would be furnished per diem to a patient receiving an IPPE or AWV Ⓑ Qp Qh    A

* **G0469** Federally qualified health center (FQHC) visit, mental health, new patient; a medically-necessary, face-to-face mental health encounter (one-on-one) between a new patient and a FQHC practitioner during which time one or more FQHC services are rendered and includes a typical bundle of Medicare-covered services that would be furnished per diem to a patient receiving a mental health visit Ⓑ Qp Qh    A

* **G0470** Federally qualified health center (FQHC) visit, mental health, established patient; a medically-necessary, face-to-face mental health encounter (one-on-one) between an established patient and a FQHC practitioner during which time one or more FQHC services are rendered and includes a typical bundle of Medicare-covered services that would be furnished per diem to a patient receiving a mental health visit Ⓑ Qp Qh    A

## Other Miscellaneous Services

* **G0471** Collection of venous blood by venipuncture or urine sample by catheterization from an individual in a skilled nursing facility (SNF) or by a laboratory on behalf of a home health agency (HHA) Ⓑ Qp Qh    A

* **G0472** Hepatitis C antibody screening, for individual at high risk and other covered indication(s) Ⓑ Qp Qh    A

*Medicare Statute 1861SSA*

*Laboratory Certification: General immunology*

* **G0473** Face-to-face behavioral counseling for obesity, group (2-10), 30 minutes Ⓑ Qp Qh    S

* **G0475** HIV antigen/antibody, combination assay, screening Ⓑ Qp Qh    A

*Laboratory Certification: Virology, General immunology*

* **G0476** Infectious agent detection by nucleic acid (DNA or RNA); human papillomavirus (HPV), high-risk types (e.g., 16, 18, 31, 33, 35, 39, 45, 51, 52, 56, 58, 59, 68) for cervical cancer screening, must be performed in addition to pap test Ⓑ Qp Qh    A

*Laboratory Certification: Virology*

## Drug Tests

* **G0480** Drug test(s), definitive, utilizing drug identification methods able to identify individual drugs and distinguish between structural isomers (but not necessarily stereoisomers), including, but not limited to GC/MS (any type, single or tandem) and LC/MS (any type, single or tandem and excluding immunoassays (e.g., IA, EIA, ELISA, EMIT, FPIA) and enzymatic methods (e.g., alcohol dehydrogenase)); qualitative or quantitative, all sources(s), includes specimen validity testing, per day, 1-7 drug class(es), including metabolite(s) if performed Ⓑ Qp Qh    Q4

*Coding Clinic: 2018, Q1, P5*

* **G0481** Drug test(s), definitive, utilizing drug identification methods able to identify individual drugs and distinguish between structural isomers (but not necessarily stereoisomers), including, but not limited to GC/MS (any type, single or tandem) and LC/MS (any type, single or tandem and excluding immunoassays (e.g., IA, EIA, ELISA, EMIT, FPIA) and enzymatic methods (e.g., alcohol dehydrogenase)); qualitative or quantitative, all sources(s), includes specimen validity testing, per day, 8-14 drug class(es), including metabolite(s) if performed Ⓑ Qp Qh    Q4

*Coding Clinic: 2018, Q1, P5*

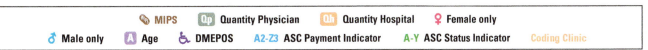

**TEMPORARY PROCEDURES/PROFESSIONAL SERVICES  G0467 — G0481**

**235**

✳ **G0482** Drug test(s), definitive, utilizing drug identification methods able to identify individual drugs and distinguish between structural isomers (but not necessarily stereoisomers), including, but not limited to GC/MS (any type, single or tandem) and LC/MS (any type, single or tandem and excluding immunoassays (e.g., IA, EIA, ELISA, EMIT, FPIA) and enzymatic methods (e.g., alcohol dehydrogenase)); qualitative or quantitative, all sources(s), includes specimen validity testing, per day, 15-21 drug class(es), including metabolite(s) if performed Ⓑ Qp Qh     Q4

*Coding Clinic: 2018, Q1, P5*

✳ **G0483** Drug test(s), definitive, utilizing drug identification methods able to identify individual drugs and distinguish between structural isomers (but not necessarily stereoisomers), including, but not limited to GC/MS (any type, single or tandem) and LC/MS (any type, single or tandem and excluding immunoassays (e.g., IA, EIA, ELISA, EMIT, FPIA) and enzymatic methods (e.g., alcohol dehydrogenase)); qualitative or quantitative, all sources(s), includes specimen validity testing, per day, 22 or more drug class(es), including metabolite(s) if performed Ⓑ Qp Qh     Q4

*Coding Clinic: 2018, Q1, P5*

## Home Health Nursing Visit: Area of Shortage

✳ **G0490** Face-to-face home health nursing visit by a rural health clinic (RHC) or federally qualified health center (FQHC) in an area with a shortage of home health agencies (services limited to RN or LPN only) Ⓑ     A

## Dialysis Procedure

✳ **G0491** Dialysis procedure at a Medicare certified esrd facility for acute kidney injury without ESRD Ⓑ Qp Qh     B

✳ **G0492** Dialysis procedure with single evaluation by a physician or other qualified health care professional for acute kidney injury without ESRD Ⓑ Qp Qh     B

## Home Health or Hospice: Skilled Services

✳ **G0493** Skilled services of a registered nurse (RN) for the observation and assessment of the patient's condition, each 15 minutes (the change in the patient's condition requires skilled nursing personnel to identify and evaluate the patient's need for possible modification of treatment in the home health or hospice setting) Ⓑ     B

✳ **G0494** Skilled services of a licensed practical nurse (LPN) for the observation and assessment of the patient's condition, each 15 minutes (the change in the patient's condition requires skilled nursing personnel to identify and evaluate the patient's need for possible modification of treatment in the home health or hospice setting) Ⓑ     B

✳ **G0495** Skilled services of a registered nurse (RN), in the training and/or education of a patient or family member, in the home health or hospice setting, each 15 minutes Ⓑ     B

✳ **G0496** Skilled services of a licensed practical nurse (LPN), in the training and/or education of a patient or family member, in the home health or hospice setting, each 15 minutes Ⓑ     B

## Chemotherapy Administration

✳ **G0498** Chemotherapy administration, intravenous infusion technique; initiation of infusion in the office/clinic setting using office/clinic pump/supplies, with continuation of the infusion in the community setting (e.g., home, domiciliary, rest home or assisted living) using a portable pump provided by the office/clinic, includes follow up office/clinic visit at the conclusion of the infusion Ⓑ Qp Qh     S

## Hepatitis B Screening

✳ **G0499** Hepatitis B screening in non-pregnant, high risk individual includes hepatitis B surface antigen (HBsAG), antibodies to HBsAG (anti-HBs) and antibodies to hepatitis B core antigen (anti-hbc), and is followed by a neutralizing confirmatory test, when performed, only for an initially reactive HBsAG result Ⓑ Qp Qh     A

*Laboratory Certification: Virology*

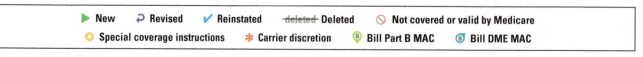

▶ New    ⮂ Revised    ✔ Reinstated    ~~deleted~~ Deleted    ⊘ Not covered or valid by Medicare
⟳ Special coverage instructions    ✳ Carrier discretion    Ⓑ Bill Part B MAC    Ⓓ Bill DME MAC

## Moderate Sedation Services

\* **G0500** Moderate sedation services provided by the same physician or other qualified health care professional performing a gastrointestinal endoscopic service that sedation supports, requiring the presence of an independent trained observer to assist in the monitoring of the patient's level of consciousness and physiological status; initial 15 minutes of intra-service time; patient age 5 years or older (additional time may be reported with 99153, as appropriate) ⓑ **Qp** **Qh** **N**

## Resource-Intensive Service

\* **G0501** Resource-intensive services for patients for whom the use of specialized mobility-assistive technology (such as adjustable height chairs or tables, patient lift, and adjustable padded leg supports) is medically necessary and used during the provision of an office/outpatient, evaluation and management visit (list separately in addition to primary service) ⓑ **N**

## Psychiatric Care Management

\* **G0506** Comprehensive assessment of and care planning for patients requiring chronic care management services (list separately in addition to primary monthly care management service) ⓑ **Qp** **Qh** **N**

## Critical Care Telehealth Consultation

\* **G0508** Telehealth consultation, critical care, initial , physicians typically spend 60 minutes communicating with the patient and providers via telehealth ⓑ **Qp** **Qh** **B**

\* **G0509** Telehealth consultation, critical care, subsequent, physicians typically spend 50 minutes communicating with the patient and providers via telehealth ⓑ **Qp** **Qh** **B**

## Rural Health Clinic: Management and Care

⊙ **G0511** Rural health clinic or federally qualified health center (RHC or FQHC) only, general care management, 20 minutes or more of clinical staff time for chronic care management services or behavioral health integration services directed by an RHC or FQHC practitioner (physician, NP, PA, or CNM), per calendar month **A**

⊙ **G0512** Rural health clinic or federally qualified health center (RHC/FQHC) only, psychiatric collaborative care model (psychiatric CoCM), 60 minutes or more of clinical staff time for psychiatric CoCM services directed by an RHC or FQHC practitioner (physician, NP, PA, or CNM) and including services furnished by a behavioral health care manager and consultation with a psychiatric consultant, per calendar month **A**

## Prolonged Preventive Services

\* **G0513** Prolonged preventive service(s) (beyond the typical service time of the primary procedure), in the office or other outpatient setting requiring direct patient contact beyond the usual service; first 30 minutes (list separately in addition to code for preventive service) **N**

\* **G0514** Prolonged preventive service(s) (beyond the typical service time of the primary procedure), in the office or other outpatient setting requiring direct patient contact beyond the usual service; each additional 30 minutes (list separately in addition to code G0513 for additional 30 minutes of preventive service) **N**

## Cognitive Development

~~G0515 Development of cognitive skills to improve attention, memory, problem-solving (includes compensatory training), direct (one-on-one) patient contact, each 15 minutes~~ ✖

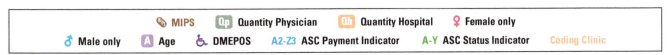

## Non-biodegradable Drug Delivery Implants: Removal and Insertion

＊ **G0516** Insertion of non-biodegradable drug delivery implants, 4 or more (services for subdermal rod implant) Q1

＊ **G0517** Removal of non-biodegradable drug delivery implants, 4 or more (services for subdermal implants) Q1

＊ **G0518** Removal with reinsertion, non-biodegradable drug delivery implants, 4 or more (services for subdermal implants) Q1

## Drug Test

＊ **G0659** Drug test(s), definitive, utilizing drug identification methods able to identify individual drugs and distinguish between structural isomers (but not necessarily stereoisomers), including but not limited to GC/MS (any type, single or tandem) and LC/MS (any type, single or tandem), excluding immunoassays (e.g., IA, EIA, ELISA, EMIT, FPIA) and enzymatic methods (e.g., alcohol dehydrogenase), performed without method or drug-specific calibration, without matrix-matched quality control material, or without use of stable isotope or other universally recognized internal standard(s) for each drug, drug metabolite or drug class per specimen; qualitative or quantitative, all sources, includes specimen validity testing, per day, any number of drug classes Q4

## Quality Care Measures: Cataract Surgery

＊ **G0913** Improvement in visual function achieved within 90 days following cataract surgery Ⓑ M

＊ **G0914** Patient care survey was not completed by patient Ⓑ M

＊ **G0915** Improvement in visual function not achieved within 90 days following cataract surgery Ⓑ M

＊ **G0916** Satisfaction with care achieved within 90 days following cataract surgery Ⓑ M

＊ **G0917** Patient satisfaction survey was not completed by patient Ⓑ M

＊ **G0918** Satisfaction with care not achieved within 90 days following cataract surgery Ⓑ M

## Clinical Decision Support Mechanism

▶ ＊ **G1000** Clinical decision support mechanism applied pathways, as defined by the Medicare Appropriate Use Criteria Program E1

▶ ＊ **G1001** Clinical decision support mechanism evicore, as defined by the Medicare Appropriate Use Criteria Program E1

▶ ＊ **G1002** Clinical decision support mechanism medcurrent, as defined by the Medicare Appropriate Use Criteria Program E1

▶ ＊ **G1003** Clinical decision support mechanism medicalis, as defined by the Medicare Appropriate Use Criteria Program E1

▶ ＊ **G1004** Clinical decision support mechanism national decision support company, as defined by the Medicare Appropriate Use Criteria Program E1

▶ ＊ **G1005** Clinical decision support mechanism national imaging associates, as defined by the Medicare Appropriate Use Criteria Program E1

▶ ＊ **G1006** Clinical decision support mechanism test appropriate, as defined by the Medicare Appropriate Use Criteria Program E1

▶ ＊ **G1007** Clinical decision support mechanism aim specialty health, as defined by the Medicare Appropriate Use Criteria Program E1

▶ ＊ **G1008** Clinical decision support mechanism cranberry peak, as defined by the Medicare Appropriate Use Criteria Program E1

▶ ＊ **G1009** Clinical decision support mechanism sage health management solutions, as defined by the Medicare Appropriate Use Criteria Program E1

▶ ＊ **G1010** Clinical decision support mechanism stanson, as defined by the Medicare Appropriate Use Criteria Program E1

▶ ＊ **G1011** Clinical decision support mechanism, qualified tool not otherwise specified, as defined by the Medicare Appropriate Use Criteria Program E1

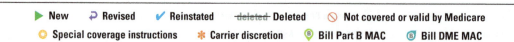

▶ New  ↻ Revised  ✔ Reinstated  ~~deleted~~ Deleted  ⊘ Not covered or valid by Medicare  ⊙ Special coverage instructions  ＊ Carrier discretion  Ⓑ Bill Part B MAC  Ⓑ Bill DME MAC

## Therapy, Evaluation and Assessment

✳ **G2000** Blinded administration of convulsive therapy procedure, either electroconvulsive therapy (ECT, current covered gold standard) or magnetic seizure therapy (MST, non-covered experimental therapy), performed in an approved IDE-based clinical trial, per treatment session **S**

✳ **G2010** Remote evaluation of recorded video and/or images submitted by an established patient (e.g., store and forward), including interpretation with follow-up with the patient within 24 business hours, not originating from a related E/M service provided within the previous 7 days nor leading to an E/M service or procedure within the next 24 hours or soonest available appointment **M**

✳ **G2011** Alcohol and/or substance (other than tobacco) abuse structured assessment (e.g., AUDIT, DAST), and brief intervention, 5-14 minutes **S**

✳ **G2012** Brief communication technology-based service, e.g., virtual check-in, by a physician or other qualified health care professional who can report evaluation and management services, provided to an established patient, not originating from a related E/M service provided within the previous 7 days nor leading to an E/M service or procedure within the next 24 hours or soonest available appointment; 5-10 minutes of medical discussion **M**

▶ ✳ **G2021** Health care practitioners rendering treatment in place (TIP) **E1**

▶ ✳ **G2022** A model participant (ambulance supplier/provider), the beneficiary refuses services covered under the model (transport to an alternate destination/treatment in place) **E1**

▶ ✳ **G2058** Chronic care management services, each additional 20 minutes of clinical staff time directed by a physician or other qualified health care professional, per calendar month (list separately in addition to code for primary procedure). (Do not report G2058 for care management services of less than 20 minutes additional to the first 20 minutes of chronic care management services during a calendar month.) (Use G2058 in conjunction with 99490.) (Do not report 99490, G2058 in the same calendar month as 99487, 99489, 99491.) **N**

▶ ✳ **G2061** Qualified nonphysician healthcare professional online assessment, for an established patient, for up to seven days, cumulative time during the 7 days; 5-10 minutes **M**

▶ ✳ **G2062** Qualified nonphysician healthcare professional online assessment service, for an established patient, for up to seven days, cumulative time during the 7 days; 11-20 minutes **M**

▶ ✳ **G2063** Qualified nonphysician qualified healthcare professional assessment service, for an established patient, for up to seven days, cumulative time during the 7 days; 21 or more minutes **M**

▶ ✳ **G2064** Comprehensive care management services for a single high-risk disease, e.g., principal care management, at least 30 minutes of physician or other qualified health care professional time per calendar month with the following elements: one complex chronic condition lasting at least 3 months, which is the focus of the care plan, the condition is of sufficient severity to place patient at risk of hospitalization or have been the cause of a recent hospitalization, the condition requires development or revision of disease-specific care plan, the condition requires frequent adjustments in the medication regimen, and/or the management of the condition is unusually complex due to comorbidities **M**

▶ ✳ **G2065** Comprehensive care management for a single high-risk disease services, e.g. principal care management, at least 30 minutes of clinical staff time directed by a physician or other qualified health care professional, per calendar month with the following elements: one complex chronic condition lasting at least 3 months, which is the focus of the care plan, the condition is of sufficient severity to place patient at risk of hospitalization or have been cause of a recent hospitalization, the condition requires development or revision of disease-specific care plan, the condition requires frequent adjustments in the medication regimen, and/or the management of the condition is unusually complex due to comorbidities **S**

---

🏷 **MIPS**   **Qp** Quantity Physician   **Qh** Quantity Hospital   ♀ **Female only**
♂ **Male only**   **A** Age   ♿ **DMEPOS**   **A2-Z3** ASC Payment Indicator   **A-Y** ASC Status Indicator   Coding Clinic

▶ ＊ **G2066** Interrogation device evaluation(s), (remote) up to 30 days; implantable cardiovascular physiologic monitor system, implantable loop recorder system, or subcutaneous cardiac rhythm monitor system, remote data acquisition(s), receipt of transmissions and technician review, technical support and distribution of results **Q1**

▶ ＊ **G2067** Medication assisted treatment, methadone; weekly bundle including dispensing and/or administration, substance use counseling, individual and group therapy, and toxicology testing, if performed (provision of the services by a Medicare-enrolled opioid treatment program) **E1**

▶ ＊ **G2068** Medication assisted treatment, buprenorphine (oral); weekly bundle including dispensing and/or administration, substance use counseling, individual and group therapy, and toxicology testing if performed (provision of the services by a Medicare-enrolled opioid treatment program) **E1**

▶ ＊ **G2069** Medication assisted treatment, buprenorphine (injectable); weekly bundle including dispensing and/or administration, substance use counseling, individual and group therapy, and toxicology testing if performed (provision of the services by a Medicare-enrolled opioid treatment program) **E1**

▶ ＊ **G2070** Medication assisted treatment, buprenorphine (implant insertion); weekly bundle including dispensing and/or administration, substance use counseling, individual and group therapy, and toxicology testing if performed (provision of the services by a Medicare-enrolled opioid treatment program) **E1**

▶ ＊ **G2071** Medication assisted treatment, buprenorphine (implant removal); weekly bundle including dispensing and/or administration, substance use counseling, individual and group therapy, and toxicology testing if performed (provision of the services by a Medicare-enrolled opioid treatment program) **E1**

▶ ＊ **G2072** Medication assisted treatment, buprenorphine (implant insertion and removal); weekly bundle including dispensing and/or administration, substance use counseling, individual and group therapy, and toxicology testing if performed (provision of the services by a Medicare-enrolled opioid treatment program) **E1**

▶ ＊ **G2073** Medication assisted treatment, naltrexone; weekly bundle including dispensing and/or administration, substance use counseling, individual and group therapy, and toxicology testing if performed (provision of the services by a Medicare-enrolled opioid treatment program) **E1**

▶ ＊ **G2074** Medication assisted treatment, weekly bundle not including the drug, including substance use counseling, individual and group therapy, and toxicology testing if performed (provision of the services by a Medicare-enrolled opioid treatment program) **E1**

▶ ＊ **G2075** Medication assisted treatment, medication not otherwise specified; weekly bundle including dispensing and/or administration, substance use counseling, individual and group therapy, and toxicology testing, if performed (provision of the services by a Medicare-enrolled opioid treatment program) **E1**

▶ ＊ **G2076** Intake activities, including initial medical examination that is a complete, fully documented physical evaluation and initial assessment by a program physician or a primary care physician, or an authorized healthcare professional under the supervision of a program physician qualified personnel that includes preparation of a treatment plan that includes the patient's short-term goals and the tasks the patient must perform to complete the short-term goals; the patient's requirements for education, vocational rehabilitation, and employment; and the medical, psycho-social, economic, legal, or other supportive services that a patient needs, conducted by qualified personnel (provision of the services by a Medicare-enrolled opioid treatment program); list separately in addition to code for primary procedure **E1**

▶ New  ↻ Revised  ✓ Reinstated  ~~deleted~~ Deleted  ⊘ Not covered or valid by Medicare
⬡ Special coverage instructions  ＊ Carrier discretion  Ⓑ Bill Part B MAC  Ⓑ Bill DME MAC

▶ ✳ **G2077** Periodic assessment; assessing periodically by qualified personnel to determine the most appropriate combination of services and treatment (provision of the services by a Medicare-enrolled opioid treatment program); list separately in addition to code for primary procedure  **E1**

▶ ✳ **G2078** Take-home supply of methadone; up to 7 additional day supply (provision of the services by a Medicare-enrolled opioid treatment program); list separately in addition to code for primary procedure  **E1**

▶ ✳ **G2079** Take-home supply of buprenorphine (oral); up to 7 additional day supply (provision of the services by a Medicare-enrolled opioid treatment program); list separately in addition to code for primary procedure  **E1**

▶ ✳ **G2080** Each additional 30 minutes of counseling in a week of medication assisted treatment, (provision of the services by a Medicare-enrolled opioid treatment program); list separately in addition to code for primary procedure  **E1**

▶ ✳ **G2081** Patients age 66 and older in institutional special needs plans (SNP) or residing in long-term care with a POS code 32, 33, 34, 54 or 56 for more than 90 days during the measurement period  **M**

▶ ✳ **G2082** Office or other outpatient visit for the evaluation and management of an established patient that requires the supervision of a physician or other qualified health care professional and provision of up to 56 mg of esketamine nasal self-administration, includes 2 hours post-administration observation  **S**

▶ ✳ **G2083** Office or other outpatient visit for the evaluation and management of an established patient that requires the supervision of a physician or other qualified health care professional and provision of greater than 56 mg esketamine nasal self-administration, includes 2 hours post-administration observation  **S**

▶ ✳ **G2086** Office-based treatment for opioid use disorder, including development of the treatment plan, care coordination, individual therapy and group therapy and counseling; at least 70 minutes in the first calendar month  **S**

▶ ✳ **G2087** Office-based treatment for opioid use disorder, including care coordination, individual therapy and group therapy and counseling; at least 60 minutes in a subsequent calendar month  **S**

▶ ✳ **G2088** Office-based treatment for opioid use disorder, including care coordination, individual therapy and group therapy and counseling; each additional 30 minutes beyond the first 120 minutes (list separately in addition to code for primary procedure)  **N**

▶ ✳ **G2089** Most recent hemoglobin A1c (HbA1c) level 7.0 to 9.0%  **N1 M**

▶ ✳ **G2090** Patients 66 years of age and older with at least one claim/encounter for frailty during the measurement period and a dispensed medication for dementia during the measurement period or the year prior to the measurement period  **N1 M**

▶ ✳ **G2091** Patients 66 years of age and older with at least one claim/encounter for frailty during the measurement period and either one acute inpatient encounter with a diagnosis of advanced illness or two outpatient, observation, ED or nonacute inpatient encounters on different dates of service with an advanced illness diagnosis during the measurement period or the year prior to the measurement period  **N1 M**

▶ ✳ **G2092** Angiotensin converting enzyme (ACE) inhibitor or angiotensin receptor blocker (ARB) or angiotensin receptor-neprilysin inhibitor (AMI) therapy prescribed or currently being taken  **N1 M**

▶ ✳ **G2093** Documentation of medical reason(s) for not prescribing ACE inhibitor or ARB or AMI therapy (e.g., hypotensive patients who are at immediate risk of cardiogenic shock, hospitalized patients who have experienced marked azotemia, allergy, intolerance, other medical reasons)  **N1 M**

▶ ✳ **G2094** Documentation of patient reason(s) for not prescribing ACE inhibitor or ARB or AMI therapy (e.g., patient declined, other patient reasons)  **N1 M**

▶ ✳ **G2095** Documentation of system reason(s) for not prescribing ACE inhibitor or ARB or AMI therapy (e.g., other system reasons)  **N1 M**

▶ ✳ **G2096** Angiotensin converting enzyme (ACE) inhibitor or angiotensin receptor blocker (ARB) or angiotensin receptor-neprilysin inhibitor (AMI) therapy was not prescribed, reason not given  **N1 M**

| 🖱 MIPS | 〔Qp〕 Quantity Physician | 〔Qh〕 Quantity Hospital | ♀ Female only |
|---|---|---|---|
| ♂ Male only | 〔A〕 Age | ♿ DMEPOS | A2-Z3 ASC Payment Indicator | A-Y ASC Status Indicator | Coding Clinic |

▶ ＊ **G2097** Children with a competing diagnosis for upper respiratory infection within three days of diagnosis of pharyngitis (e.g., intestinal infection, pertussis, bacterial infection, lyme disease, otitis media, acute sinusitis, acute pharyngitis, acute tonsillitis, chronic sinusitis, infection of the pharynx/larynx/tonsils/adenoids, prostatitis, cellulitis, mastoiditis, or bone infections, acute lymphadenitis, impetigo, skin staph infections, pneumonia/gonococcal infections, venereal disease (syphilis, chlamydia, inflammatory diseases [female reproductive organs]), infections of the kidney, cystitis or UTI   N1 M

▶ ＊ **G2098** Patients 66 years of age and older with at least one claim/encounter for frailty during the measurement period and a dispensed medication for dementia during the measurement period or the year prior to the measurement period   N1 M

▶ ＊ **G2099** Patients 66 years of age and older with at least one claim/encounter for frailty during the measurement period and either one acute inpatient encounter with a diagnosis of advanced illness or two outpatient, observation, ED or nonacute inpatient encounters on different dates of service with an advanced illness diagnosis during the measurement period or the year prior to the measurement period   N1 M

▶ ＊ **G2100** Patients 66 years of age and older with at least one claim/encounter for frailty during the measurement period and a dispensed medication for dementia during the measurement period or the year prior to the measurement period   N1 M

▶ ＊ **G2101** Patients 66 years of age and older with at least one claim/encounter for frailty during the measurement period and either one acute inpatient encounter with a diagnosis of advanced illness or two outpatient, observation, ED or nonacute inpatient encounters on different dates of service with an advanced illness diagnosis during the measurement period or the year prior to the measurement period   N1 M

▶ ＊ **G2102** Dilated retinal eye exam with interpretation by an ophthalmologist or optometrist documented and reviewed   N1 M

▶ ＊ **G2103** Seven standard field stereoscopic photos with interpretation by an ophthalmologist or optometrist documented and reviewed   N1 M

▶ ＊ **G2104** Eye imaging validated to match diagnosis from seven standard field stereoscopic photos results documented and reviewed   N1 M

▶ ＊ **G2105** Patients age 66 or older in institutional special needs plans (SNP) or residing in long-term care with POS code 32, 33, 34, 54 or 56 for more than 90 days during the measurement period   N1 M

▶ ＊ **G2106** Patients 66 years of age and older with at least one claim/encounter for frailty during the measurement period and a dispensed medication for dementia during the measurement period or the year prior to the measurement period   N1 M

▶ ＊ **G2107** Patients 66 years of age and older with at least one claim/encounter for frailty during the measurement period and either one acute inpatient encounter with a diagnosis of advanced illness or two outpatient, observation, ED or nonacute inpatient encounters on different dates of service with an advanced illness diagnosis during the measurement period or the year prior to the measurement period   N1 M

▶ ＊ **G2108** Patients age 66 or older in institutional special needs plans (SNP) or residing in long-term care with POS code 32, 33, 34, 54 or 56 for more than 90 days during the measurement period   N1 M

▶ ＊ **G2109** Patients 66 years of age and older with at least one claim/encounter for frailty during the measurement period and a dispensed medication for dementia during the measurement period or the year prior to the measurement period   N1 M

▶ ＊ **G2110** Patients 66 years of age and older with at least one claim/encounter for frailty during the measurement period and either one acute inpatient encounter with a diagnosis of advanced illness or two outpatient, observation, ED or nonacute inpatient encounters on different dates of service with an advanced illness diagnosis during the measurement period or the year prior to the measurement period   N1 M

▶ ＊ **G2112** Patient receiving <=5 mg daily prednisone (or equivalent), or RA activity is worsening, or glucocorticoid use is for less than 6 months   N1 M

---

▶ New   ↻ Revised   ✔ Reinstated   deleted Deleted   ⊘ Not covered or valid by Medicare   ⊙ Special coverage instructions   ＊ Carrier discretion   Ⓑ Bill Part B MAC   Ⓓ Bill DME MAC

▶ ✳ **G2113** Patient receiving >5 mg daily prednisone (or equivalent) for longer than 6 months, and improvement or no change in disease activity **N1 M**

▶ ✳ **G2114** Patients 66-80 years of age with at least one claim/encounter for frailty during the measurement period and a dispensed medication for dementia during the measurement period or the year prior to the measurement period **N1 M**

▶ ✳ **G2115** Patients 66 years of age and older with at least one claim/encounter for frailty during the measurement period and a dispensed medication for dementia during the measurement period or the year prior to the measurement period **N1 M**

▶ ✳ **G2116** Patients 66 years of age and older with at least one claim/encounter for frailty during the measurement period and either one acute inpatient encounter with a diagnosis of advanced illness or two outpatient, observation, ED or nonacute inpatient encounters on different dates of service with an advanced illness diagnosis during the measurement period or the year prior to the measurement period **N1 M**

▶ ✳ **G2117** Patients 66-80 years of age with at least one claim/encounter for frailty during the measurement period and either one acute inpatient encounter with a diagnosis of advanced illness or two outpatient, observation, ED or nonacute inpatient encounters on different dates of service with an advanced illness diagnosis during the measurement period or the year prior to the measurement period **N1 M**

▶ ✳ **G2118** Patients 81 years of age and older with a evidence of frailty during the measurement period **N1 M**

▶ ✳ **G2119** Within the past 2 years, calcium and/or vitamin D optimization has been ordered or performed **N1 M**

▶ ✳ **G2120** Within the past 2 years, calcium and/or vitamin D optimization has not been ordered or performed **N1 M**

▶ ✳ **G2121** Psychosis, depression, anxiety, apathy, and impulse control disorder assessed **N1 M**

▶ ✳ **G2122** Psychosis, depression, anxiety, apathy, and impulse control disorder not assessed **N1 M**

▶ ✳ **G2123** Patients 66-80 years of age and had at least one claim/encounter for frailty during the measurement period and either one acute inpatient encounter with a diagnosis of advanced illness or two outpatient, observation, ED or nonacute inpatient encounters on different dates of service with an advanced illness diagnosis during the measurement period or the year prior to the measurement period **N1 M**

▶ ✳ **G2124** Patients 66-80 years of age and had at least one claim/encounter for frailty during the measurement period and a dispensed dementia medication **N1 M**

▶ ✳ **G2125** Patients 81 years of age and older with evidence of frailty during the measurement period **N1 M**

▶ ✳ **G2126** Patients 66 years of age or older and had at least one claim/encounter for frailty during the measurement period and either one acute inpatient encounter with a diagnosis of advanced illness or two outpatient, observation, ED or nonacute inpatient encounters on different dates of service with an advanced illness diagnosis during the measurement period or the year prior to the measurement period **N1 M**

▶ ✳ **G2127** Patients 66 years of age or older and had at least one claim/encounter for frailty during the measurement period and a dispensed dementia medication **N1 M**

▶ ✳ **G2128** Documentation of medical reason(s) for not on a daily aspirin or other antiplatelet (e.g. history of gastrointestinal bleed, intra-cranial bleed, blood disorders, idiopathic thrombocytopenic purpura [ITP], gastric bypass or documentation of active anticoagulant use during the measurement period) **N1 M**

▶ ✳ **G2129** Procedure-related BP's not taken during an outpatient visit. Examples include same day surgery, ambulatory service center, G.I. lab, dialysis, infusion center, chemotherapy **N1 M**

▶ ✳ **G2130** Patients age 66 or older in institutional special needs plans (SNP) or residing in long-term care with POS code 32, 33, 34, 54 or 56 for more than 90 days during the measurement period **N1 M**

▶ ✳ **G2131** Patients 81 years and older with a diagnosis of frailty **N1 M**

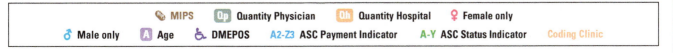

🐌 MIPS  💠 Quantity Physician  💠 Quantity Hospital  ♀ Female only
♂ Male only  🅐 Age  ♿ DMEPOS  A2-Z3 ASC Payment Indicator  A-Y ASC Status Indicator  Coding Clinic

▶ ✳ **G2132** Patients 66-80 years of age with at least one claim/encounter for frailty during the measurement period and a dispensed medication for dementia during the measurement period or the year prior to the measurement period     **N1 M**

▶ ✳ **G2133** Patients 66-80 years of age with at least one claim/encounter for frailty during the measurement period and either one acute inpatient encounter with a diagnosis of advanced illness or two outpatient, observation, ED or nonacute inpatient encounters on different dates of service with an advanced illness diagnosis during the measurement period or the year prior to the measurement period     **N1 M**

▶ ✳ **G2134** Patients 66 years of age or older with at least one claim/encounter for frailty during the measurement period and a dispensed medication for dementia during the measurement period or the year prior to the measurement period     **N1 M**

▶ ✳ **G2135** Patients 66 years of age or older with at least one claim/encounter for frailty during the measurement period and either one acute inpatient encounter with a diagnosis of advanced illness or two outpatient, observation, ED or nonacute inpatient encounters on different dates of service with an advanced illness diagnosis during the measurement period or the year prior to the measurement period     **N1 M**

▶ ✳ **G2136** Back pain measured by the Visual Analog Scale (VAS) at three months (6 - 20 weeks) postoperatively was less than or equal to 3.0 or back pain measured by the Visual Analog Scale (VAS) within three months preoperatively and at three months (6 - 20 weeks) postoperatively demonstrated an improvement of 5.0 points or greater     **N1 M**

▶ ✳ **G2137** Back pain measured by the Visual Analog Scale (VAS) at three months (6 - 20 weeks) postoperatively was greater than 3.0 and back pain measured by the Visual Analog Scale (VAS) within three months preoperatively and at three months (6 - 20 weeks) postoperatively demonstrated a change of less than an improvement of 5.0 points     **N1 M**

▶ ✳ **G2138** Back pain as measured by the Visual Analog Scale (VAS) at one year (9 to 15 months) postoperatively was less than or equal to 3.0 or back pain measured by the Visual Analog Scale (VAS) within three months preoperatively and at one year (9 to 15 months) postoperatively demonstrated a change of 5.0 points or greater     **N1 M**

▶ ✳ **G2139** Back pain measured by the Visual Analog Scale (VAS) pain at one year (9 to 15 months) postoperatively was greater than 3.0 and back pain measured by the Visual Analog Scale (VAS) within three months preoperatively and at one year (9 to 15 months) postoperatively demonstrated a change of less than 5.0     **N1 M**

▶ ✳ **G2140** Leg pain measured by the Visual Analog Scale (VAS) at three months (6 - 20 weeks) postoperatively was less than or equal to 3.0 or leg pain measured by the Visual Analog Scale (VAS) within three months preoperatively and at three months (6 - 20 weeks) postoperatively demonstrated an improvement of 5.0 points or greater     **N1 M**

▶ ✳ **G2141** Leg pain measured by the Visual Analog Scale (VAS) at three months (6 - 20 weeks) postoperatively was greater than 3.0 and leg pain measured by the Visual Analog Scale (VAS) within three months preoperatively and at three months (6 - 20 weeks) postoperatively demonstrated less than an improvement of 5.0 points     **N1 M**

▶ ✳ **G2142** Functional status measured by the Oswestry Disability Index (ODI version 2.1a) at one year (9 to 15 months) postoperatively was less than or equal to 22 or functional status measured by the ODI version 2.1a within three months preoperatively and at one year (9 to 15 months) postoperatively demonstrated a change of 30 points or greater     **N1 M**

▶ ✳ **G2143** Functional status measured by the Oswestry Disability Index (ODI version 2.1a) at one year (9 to 15 months) postoperatively was greater than 22 and functional status measured by the ODI version 2.1a within three months preoperatively and at one year (9 to 15 months) postoperatively demonstrated a change of less than 30 points     **N1 M**

---

▶ New    ↻ Revised    ✔ Reinstated    ~~deleted~~ Deleted    ⊘ Not covered or valid by Medicare

⊙ Special coverage instructions    ✳ Carrier discretion    Ⓑ Bill Part B MAC    Ⓑ Bill DME MAC

▶ ✳ **G2144** Functional status measured by the Oswestry Disability Index (ODI version 2.1a) at three months (6 - 20 weeks) postoperatively was less than or equal to 22 or functional status measured by the ODI version 2.1a within three months preoperatively and at three months (6 - 20 weeks) postoperatively demonstrated a change of 30 points or greater

▶ ✳ **G2145** Functional status measured by the Oswestry Disability Index (ODI version 2.1a) at three months (6 - 20 weeks) postoperatively was greater than 22 and functional status measured by the ODI version 2.1a within three months preoperatively and at three months (6 - 20 weeks) postoperatively demonstrated a change of less than 30 points   N1 M

▶ ✳ **G2146** Leg pain as measured by the Visual Analog Scale (VAS) at one year (9 to 15 months) postoperatively was less than or equal to 3.0 or leg pain measured by the Visual Analog Scale (VAS) within three months preoperatively and at one year (9 to 15 months) postoperatively demonstrated an improvement of 5.0 points or greater   N1 M

▶ ✳ **G2147** Leg pain measured by the Visual Analog Scale (VAS) at one year (9 to 15 months) postoperatively was greater than 3.0 and leg pain measured by the Visual Analog Scale (VAS) within three months preoperatively and at one year (9 to 15 months) postoperatively demonstrated less than an improvement of 5.0 points   N1 M

▶ ✳ **G2148** Performance met: multimodal pain management was used   N1 M

▶ ✳ **G2149** Documentation of medical reason(s) for not using multimodal pain management (e.g., allergy to multiple classes of analgesics, intubated patient, hepatic failure, patient reports no pain during pacu stay, other medical reason(s))   N1 M

▶ ✳ **G2150** Performance not met: multimodal pain management was not used   N1 M

▶ ✳ **G2151** Patients with diagnosis of a degenerative neurological condition such as ALS, MS, Parkinson's diagnosed at any time before or during the episode of care   N1 M

▶ ✳ **G2152** Performance met: the residual change score is equal to or greater than 0   N1 M

▶ ✳ **G2153** In hospice or using hospice services during the measurement period   N1 M

▶ ✳ **G2154** Patient received at least one Td vaccine or one Tdap vaccine between nine years prior to the start of the measurement period and the end of the measurement period   N1 M

▶ ✳ **G2155** Patient had history of at least one of the following contraindications any time during or before the measurement period: anaphylaxis due to Tdap vaccine, anaphylaxis due to Td vaccine or its components; encephalopathy due to Tdap or Td vaccination (post tetanus vaccination encephalitis, post diphtheria vaccination encephalitis or post pertussis vaccination encephalitis)   N1 M

▶ ✳ **G2156** Patient did not receive at least one Td vaccine or one Tdap vaccine between nine years prior to the start of the measurement period and the end of the measurement period; or have history of at least one of the following contraindications any time during or before the measurement period: anaphylaxis due to Tdap vaccine, anaphylaxis due to Td vaccine or its components; encephalopathy due to Tdap or Td vaccination (post tetanus vaccination encephalitis, post diphtheria vaccination encephalitis or post pertussis vaccination encephalitis)   N1 M

▶ ✳ **G2157** Patients received both the 13-valent pneumococcal conjugate vaccine and the 23-valent pneumococcal polysaccharide vaccine at least 12 months apart, with the first occurrence after the age of 60 before or during the measurement period

▶ ✳ **G2158** Patient had prior pneumococcal vaccine adverse reaction any time during or before the measurement period   N1 M

▶ ✳ **G2159** Patient did not receive both the 13-valent pneumococcal conjugate vaccine and the 23-valent pneumococcal polysaccharide vaccine at least 12 months apart, with the first occurrence after the age of 60 before or during measurement period; or have prior pneumococcal vaccine adverse reaction any time during or before the measurement period   N1 M

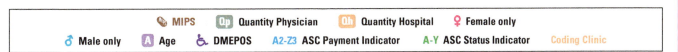

🐾 MIPS     Qp Quantity Physician     Qh Quantity Hospital     ♀ Female only
♂ Male only     A Age     ♿ DMEPOS     A2-Z3 ASC Payment Indicator     A-Y ASC Status Indicator     Coding Clinic

▶ ✳ **G2160** Patient received at least one dose of the herpes zoster live vaccine or two doses of the herpes zoster recombinant vaccine (at least 28 days apart) anytime on or after the patient's 50th birthday before or during the measurement period    N1 M

▶ ✳ **G2161** Patient had prior adverse reaction caused by zoster vaccine or its components any time during or before the measurement period    N1 M

▶ ✳ **G2162** Patient did not receive at least one dose of the herpes zoster live vaccine or two doses of the herpes zoster recombinant vaccine (at least 28 days apart) anytime on or after the patient's 50th birthday before or during the measurement period; or have prior adverse reaction caused by zoster vaccine or its components any time during or before the measurement period    N1 M

▶ ✳ **G2163** Patient received an influenza vaccine on or between July 1 of the year prior to the measurement period and June 30 of the measurement period    N1 M

▶ ✳ **G2164** Patient had a prior influenza virus vaccine adverse reaction any time before or during the measurement period    N1 M

▶ ✳ **G2165** Patient did not receive an influenza vaccine on or between July 1 of the year prior to the measurement period and June 30 of the measurement period; or did not have a prior influenza virus vaccine adverse reaction any time before or during the measurement period    N1 M

▶ ✳ **G2166** Patient refused to participate at admission and/or discharge; patient unable to complete the neck FS prom at admission or discharge due to cognitive deficit, visual deficit, motor deficit, language barrier, or low reading level, and a suitable proxy/recorder is not available; patient self-discharged early; medical reason    N1 M

▶ ✳ **G2167** Performance not met: the residual change score is less than 0    N1 M

## Guidance

⊙ **G6001** Ultrasonic guidance for placement of radiation therapy fields  Ⓑ Qp Qh    B

✳ **G6002** Stereoscopic x-ray guidance for localization of target volume for the delivery of radiation therapy  Ⓑ Qp Qh    B

## Radiation Treatment

✳ **G6003** Radiation treatment delivery, single treatment area, single port or parallel opposed ports, simple blocks or no blocks: up to 5 mev  Ⓑ Qp Qh    B

✳ **G6004** Radiation treatment delivery, single treatment area, single port or parallel opposed ports, simple blocks or no blocks: 6-10 mev  Ⓑ Qp Qh    B

✳ **G6005** Radiation treatment delivery, single treatment area, single port or parallel opposed ports, simple blocks or no blocks: 11-19 mev  Ⓑ Qp Qh    B

✳ **G6006** Radiation treatment delivery, single treatment area, single port or parallel opposed ports, simple blocks or no blocks: 20 mev or greater  Ⓑ Qp Qh    B

✳ **G6007** Radiation treatment delivery, 2 separate treatment areas, 3 or more ports on a single treatment area, use of multiple blocks: up to 5 mev  Ⓑ Qp Qh    B

✳ **G6008** Radiation treatment delivery, 2 separate treatment areas, 3 or more ports on a single treatment area, use of multiple blocks: 6-10 mev  Qp Qh    B

✳ **G6009** Radiation treatment delivery, 2 separate treatment areas, 3 or more ports on a single treatment area, use of multiple blocks: 11-19 mev  Ⓑ Qp Qh    B

✳ **G6010** Radiation treatment delivery, 2 separate treatment areas, 3 or more ports on a single treatment area, use of multiple blocks: 20 mev or greater  Ⓑ Qp Qh    B

✳ **G6011** Radiation treatment delivery, 3 or more separate treatment areas, custom blocking, tangential ports, wedges, rotational beam, compensators, electron beam; up to 5 mev  Ⓑ Qp Qh    B

✳ **G6012** Radiation treatment delivery, 3 or more separate treatment areas, custom blocking, tangential ports, wedges, rotational beam, compensators, electron beam; 6-10 mev  Ⓑ Qp Qh    B

✳ **G6013** Radiation treatment delivery, 3 or more separate treatment areas, custom blocking, tangential ports, wedges, rotational beam, compensators, electron beam; 11-19 mev  Ⓑ Qp Qh    B

✳ **G6014** Radiation treatment delivery, 3 or more separate treatment areas, custom blocking, tangential ports, wedges, rotational beam, compensators, electron beam; 20 mev or greater  Ⓑ Qp Qh    B

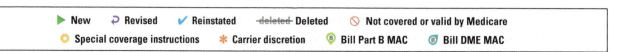

▶ New   ↻ Revised   ✔ Reinstated   ~~deleted~~ Deleted   ⊘ Not covered or valid by Medicare
⊙ Special coverage instructions   ✳ Carrier discretion   Ⓑ Bill Part B MAC   Ⓓ Bill DME MAC

* **G6015** Intensity modulated treatment delivery, single or multiple fields/arcs, via narrow spatially and temporally modulated beams, binary, dynamic MLC, per treatment session ⑧ Qp Qh  B

* **G6016** Compensator-based beam modulation treatment delivery of inverse planned treatment using 3 or more high resolution (milled or cast) compensator, convergent beam modulated fields, per treatment session ⑧ Qp Qh  B

* **G6017** Intra-fraction localization and tracking of target or patient motion during delivery of radiation therapy (e.g., 3D positional tracking, gating, 3D surface tracking), each fraction of treatment ⑧ Qp Qh  B

## Quality Measures

* **G8395** Left ventricular ejection fraction (LVEF) >=40% or documentation as normal or mildly depressed left ventricular systolic function ⑧  M

* **G8396** Left ventricular ejection fraction (LVEF) not performed or documented ⑧  M

* **G8397** Dilated macular or fundus exam performed, including documentation of the presence or absence of macular edema and level of severity of retinopathy ⑧  M

* **G8398** Dilated macular or fundus exam not performed ⑧  M

* **G8399** Patient with documented results of a central dual-energy x-ray absorptiometry (DXA) ever being performed ⑧  M

* **G8400** Patient with central dual-energy x-ray absorptiometry (DXA) results not documented ⑧  M

* **G8404** Lower extremity neurological exam performed and documented ⑧  M

* **G8405** Lower extremity neurological exam not performed ⑧  M

* **G8410** Footwear evaluation performed and documented ⑧  M

* **G8415** Footwear evaluation was not performed ⑧  M

* **G8416** Clinician documented that patient was not an eligible candidate for footwear evaluation measure ⑧  M

* **G8417** BMI is documented above normal parameters and a follow-up plan is documented ⑧  M

* **G8418** BMI is documented below normal parameters and a follow-up plan is documented ⑧  M

* **G8419** BMI is documented outside normal parameters, no follow-up plan documented, no reason given ⑧  M

* **G8420** BMI is documented within normal parameters and no follow-up plan is required ⑧  M

* **G8421** BMI not documented and no reason is given ⑧  M

* **G8422** BMI not documented, documentation the patient is not eligible for BMI calculation ⑧  M

* **G8427** Eligible clinician attests to documenting in the medical record they obtained, updated, or reviewed the patient's current medications ⑧  M

* **G8428** Current list of medications not documented as obtained, updated, or reviewed by the eligible clinician, reason not given ⑧  M

* **G8430** Eligible clinician attests to documenting in the medical record the patient is not eligible for a current list of medications being obtained, updated, or reviewed by the eligible clinician ⑧  M

* **G8431** Screening for depression is documented as being positive and a follow-up plan is documented ⑧  M

* **G8432** Depression screening not documented, reason not given ⑧  M

* **G8433** Screening for depression not completed, documented reason ⑧  M

* **G8442** Pain assessment not documented as being performed, documentation the patient is not eligible for a pain assessment using a standardized tool at the time of the encounter ⑧  M

* **G8450** Beta-blocker therapy prescribed ⑧  M

* **G8451** beta therapy for LVEF <40% not prescribed for reasons documented by the clinician (e.g., low blood pressure, fluid overload, asthma, patients recently treated with an intravenous positive inotropic agent, allergy, intolerance, other medical reasons, patient declined, other patient reasons or other reasons attributable to the healthcare system) ⑧  M

* **G8452** Beta-blocker therapy not prescribed ⑧  M

* **G8465** High or very high risk of recurrence of prostate cancer ⑧ ♂  M

---

🔁 MIPS   Qp Quantity Physician   Qh Quantity Hospital   ♀ Female only
♂ Male only   Ⓐ Age   ♿ DMEPOS   A2-Z3 ASC Payment Indicator   A-Y ASC Status Indicator   Coding Clinic

* **G8473** Angiotensin converting enzyme (ACE) inhibitor or angiotensin receptor blocker (ARB) therapy prescribed ⑬ M

* **G8474** Angiotensin converting enzyme (ACE) inhibitor or angiotensin receptor blocker (ARB) therapy not prescribed for reasons documented by the clinician (e.g., allergy, intolerance, pregnancy, renal failure due to ACE inhibitor, diseases of the aortic or mitral valve, other medical reasons) or (e.g., patient declined, other patient reasons) or (e.g., lack of drug availability, other reasons attributable to the health care system) ⑬ M

* **G8475** Angiotensin converting enzyme (ACE) inhibitor or angiotensin receptor blocker (ARB) therapy not prescribed, reason not given ⑬ M

* **G8476** Most recent blood pressure has a systolic measurement of <140 mmHg and a diastolic measurement of <90 mmHg ⑬ M

* **G8477** Most recent blood pressure has a systolic measurement of >=140 mmHg and/or a diastolic measurement of >=90 mmHg ⑬ M

* **G8478** Blood pressure measurement not performed or documented, reason not given ⑬ M

* **G8482** Influenza immunization administered or previously received ⑬ M

* **G8483** Influenza immunization was not administered for reasons documented by clinician (e.g., patient allergy or other medical reasons, patient declined or other patient reasons, vacine not available or other system reasons) ⑬ M

* **G8484** Influenza immunization was not administered, reason not given ⑬ M

* **G8506** Patient receiving angiotensin converting enzyme (ACE) inhibitor or angiotensin receptor blocker (ARB) therapy ⑬ M

* **G8509** Pain assessment documented as positive using a standardized tool, follow-up plan not documented, reason not given ⑬ M

* **G8510** Screening for depression is documented as negative, a follow-up plan is not required ⑬ M

* **G8511** Screening for depression documented as positive, follow up plan not documented, reason not given ⑬ M

* **G8535** Elder maltreatment screen not documented; documentation that patient is not eligible for the elder maltreatment screen at the time of the encounter ⑬ Ⓐ M

* **G8536** No documentation of an elder maltreatment screen, reason not given ⑬ Ⓐ M

* **G8539** Functional outcome assessment documented as positive using a standardized tool and a care plan based on identified deficiencies on the date of functional outcome assessment is documented ⑬ M

* **G8540** Functional outcome assessment not documented as being performed, documentation the patient is not eligible for a functional outcome assessment using a standardized tool at the time of the encounter ⑬ M

* **G8541** Functional outcome assessment using a standardized tool not documented, reason not given ⑬ M

* **G8542** Functional outcome assessment using a standardized tool is documented; no functional deficiencies identified, care plan not required ⑬ M

* **G8543** Documentation of a positive functional outcome assessment using a standardized tool; care plan not documented, reason not given ⑬ M

* **G8559** Patient referred to a physician (preferably a physician with training in disorders of the ear) for an otologic evaluation ⑬ M

* **G8560** Patient has a history of active drainage from the ear within the previous 90 days ⑬ M

* **G8561** Patient is not eligible for the referral for otologic evaluation for patients with a history of active drainage measure ⑬ M

* **G8562** Patient does not have a history of active drainage from the ear within the previous 90 days ⑬ M

* **G8563** Patient not referred to a physician (preferably a physician with training in disorders of the ear) for an otologic evaluation, reason not given ⑬ M

* **G8564** Patient was referred to a physician (preferably a physician with training in disorders of the ear) for an otologic evaluation, reason not specified ⑬ M

* **G8565** Verification and documentation of sudden or rapidly progressive hearing loss ⑬ M

---

▶ New  ↩ Revised  ✔ Reinstated  ~~deleted~~ Deleted  ⊘ Not covered or valid by Medicare
⊛ Special coverage instructions  * Carrier discretion  ⑬ Bill Part B MAC  Ⓑ Bill DME MAC

**G8566** Patient is not eligible for the "referral for otologic evaluation for sudden or rapidly progressive hearing loss" measure Ⓑ M

**G8567** Patient does not have verification and documentation of sudden or rapidly progressive hearing loss Ⓑ M

**G8568** Patient was not referred to a physician (preferably a physician with training in disorders of the ear) for an otologic evaluation, reason not given Ⓑ M

**G8569** Prolonged postoperative intubation (>24 hrs) required Ⓑ M

**G8570** Prolonged postoperative intubation (>24 hrs) not required Ⓑ M

**G8571** Development of deep sternal wound infection/mediastinitis within 30 days postoperatively Ⓑ M

**G8572** No deep sternal wound infection/mediastinitis Ⓑ M

**G8573** Stroke following isolated CABG surgery Ⓑ M

**G8574** No stroke following isolated CABG surgery Ⓑ M

**G8575** Developed postoperative renal failure or required dialysis Ⓑ M

**G8576** No postoperative renal failure/dialysis not required Ⓑ M

**G8577** Re-exploration required due to mediastinal bleeding with or without tamponade, graft occlusion, valve disfunction, or other cardiac reason Ⓑ M

**G8578** Re-exploration not required due to mediastinal bleeding with or without tamponade, graft occlusion, valve dysfunction, or other cardiac reason Ⓑ M

**G8598** Aspirin or another antiplatelet therapy used Ⓑ M

**G8599** Aspirin or another antiplatelet therapy not used, reason not given Ⓑ M

**G8600** IV T-PA initiated within three hours (<=180 minutes) of time last known well Ⓑ M

**G8601** IV T-PA not initiated within three hours (<=180 minutes) of time last known well for reasons documented by clinician Ⓑ M

**G8602** IV T-PA not initiated within three hours (<=180 minutes) of time last known well, reason not given Ⓑ M

**G8627** Surgical procedure performed within 30 days following cataract surgery for major complications (e.g., retained nuclear fragments, endophthalmitis, dislocated or wrong power IOL, retinal detachment, or wound dehiscence) Ⓑ M

**G8628** Surgical procedure not performed within 30 days following cataract surgery for major complications (e.g., retained nuclear fragments, endophthalmitis, dislocated or wrong power IOL, retinal detachment, or wound dehiscence) Ⓑ M

**G8633** Pharmacologic therapy (other than minierals/vitamins) for osteoporosis prescribed ⑤ M

**G8635** Pharmacologic therapy for osteoporosis was not prescribed, reason not given ⑤ M

**G8647** Risk-adjusted functional status change residual score for the knee impairment successfully calculated and the score was equal to zero (0) or greater than zero (>0) ⑤ M

**G8648** Risk-adjusted functional status change residual score for the knee impairment successfully calculated and the score was less than zero (<0) Ⓑ M

G8649 Risk-adjusted functional status change residual scores for the knee impairment not measured because the patient did not complete FOTO'S status survey near discharge, not appropriate ✖

**G8650** Risk-adjusted functional status change residual scores for the knee impairment not measured because the patient did not complete the knee FS prom at initial evaluation and/or near discharge, reason not given Ⓑ M

**G8651** Risk-adjusted functional status change residual score for the hip impairment successfully calculated and the score was equal to zero (0) or greater than zero (>0) ⑤ M

**G8652** Risk-adjusted functional status change residual score for the hip impairment successfully calculated and the score was less than zero (<0) Ⓑ M

G8653 Risk-adjusted functional status change residual scores for the hip impairment not measured because the patient did not complete follow up status survey near discharge, patient not appropriate ✖

MIPS    Qp Quantity Physician    Qh Quantity Hospital    ♀ Female only

♂ Male only    A Age    ♿ DMEPOS    A2-Z3 ASC Payment Indicator    A-Y ASC Status Indicator    Coding Clinic

* **G8654** Risk-adjusted functional status change residual scores for the hip impairment not measured because the patient did not complete FOTO'S functional intake on admission and/or follow up status survey near discharge, reason not given Ⓑ M

* **G8655** Risk-adjusted functional status change residual score for the foot or ankle impairment successfully calculated and the score was equal to zero (0) or greater than zero (>0) Ⓑ M

* **G8656** Risk-adjusted functional status change residual score for the foot or ankle impairment successfully calculated and the score was less than zero (<0) Ⓑ M

~~G8657~~ ~~Risk-adjusted functional status change residual scores for the foot or ankle impairment not measured because the patient did not complete FOTO'S status survey near discharge, patient not appropriate~~ ✖

* **G8658** Risk-adjusted functional status change residual scores for the foot or ankle impairment not measured because the patient did not complete FOTO'S functional intake on admission and/or follow up status survey near discharge, reason not given Ⓑ M

* **G8659** Risk-adjusted functional status change residual score for the low back impairment successfully calculated and the score was equal to zero (0) or greater than zero (>0) Ⓑ M

* **G8660** Risk-adjusted functional status change residual score for the low back impairment successfully calculated and the score was less than zero (<0) Ⓑ M

* **G8661** Risk-adjusted functional status change residual scores for the low back impairment not measured because the patient did not complete FOTO'S status survey near discharge, patient not appropriate Ⓑ M

↺ * **G8662** Risk-adjusted functional status change residual scores for the low back impairment not measured because the patient did not complete the low back FS prom at initial evaluation and/or near discharge, reason not given Ⓑ M

* **G8663** Risk-adjusted functional status change residual score for the shoulder impairment successfully calculated and the score was equal to zero (0) or greater than zero (>0) Ⓑ M

* **G8664** Risk-adjusted functional status change residual score for the shoulder impairment successfully calculated and the score was less than zero (<0) Ⓑ M

~~G8665~~ ~~Risk-adjusted functional status change residual scores for the shoulder impairment not measured because the patient did not complete FOTO'S functional status survey near discharge, patient not appropriate~~ ✖

↺ * **G8666** Risk-adjusted functional status change residual scores for the shoulder impairment not measured because the patient did not complete the shoulder FS prom at initial evaluation and/or near discharge, reason not given Ⓑ M

* **G8667** Risk-adjusted functional status change residual score for the elbow, wrist or hand impairment successfully calculated and the score was equal to zero (0) or greater than zero (>0) Ⓑ M

* **G8668** Risk-adjusted functional status change residual score for the elbow, wrist or hand impairment successfully calculated and the score was less than zero (<0) Ⓑ M

~~G8669~~ ~~Risk-adjusted functional status change residual scores for the elbow, wrist or hand impairment not measured because the patient did not complete the FS status survey near discharge, patient not appropriate~~ ✖

↺ * **G8670** Risk-adjusted functional status change residual scores for the elbow, wrist or hand impairment not measured because the patient did not complete the the elbow/wrist/hand FS prom at initial evaluation near discharge, reason not given Ⓑ M

* **G8671** Risk-adjusted functional status change residual score for the neck, cranium, mandible, thoracic spine, ribs, or other general orthopaedic impairment successfully calculated and the score was equal to zero (0) or greater than zero (>0) Ⓑ M

* **G8672** Risk-adjusted functional status change residual score for the neck, cranium, mandible, thoracic spine, ribs, or other general orthopaedic impairment successfully calculated and the score was less than zero (<0) Ⓑ M

~~G8673~~ ~~Risk-adjusted functional status change residual scores for the neck, cranium, mandible, thoracic spine, ribs, or other general orthopaedic impairment not measured because the patient did not complete the FS status survey near discharge, patient not appropriate~~ ✖

▶ New    ↺ Revised    ✔ Reinstated    ~~deleted~~ Deleted    ⊘ Not covered or valid by Medicare
⊛ Special coverage instructions    * Carrier discretion    Ⓑ Bill Part B MAC    Ⓓ Bill DME MAC

⬥ ↩ ✴ **G8674** Risk-adjusted functional status change residual scores for the neck, cranium, mandible, thoracic spine, ribs, or other general orthopaedic impairment not measured because the patient did not complete the general orthopedic FS prom at initial evaluation near discharge, reason not given Ⓑ    M

⬥ ✴ **G8694** Left ventriucular ejection fraction (LVEF) <40% Ⓑ    M

⬥ ✴ **G8708** Patient not prescribed or dispensed antibiotic Ⓑ    M

⬥ ✴ **G8709** Patient prescribed or dispensed antibiotic for documented medical reason(s) within three days after the initial diagnosis of URI (e.g., intestinal infection, pertussis, bacterial infection, Lyme disease, otitis media, acute sinusitis, acute pharyngitis, acute tonsillitis, chronic sinusitis, infection of the pharynx/larynx/tonsils/adenoids, prostatitis, cellulitis, mastoiditis, or bone infections, acute lymphadenitis, impetigo, skin staph infections, pneumonia/gonococcal infections, venereal disease [syphilis, chlamydia, inflammatory diseases (female reproductive organs)], infections of the kidney, cystitis or UTI, and acne) Ⓑ    M

⬥ ✴ **G8710** Patient prescribed or dispensed antibiotic Ⓑ    M

⬥ ✴ **G8711** Prescribed or dispensed antibiotic Ⓑ   M

✴ **G8712** Antibiotic not prescribed or dispensed Ⓑ    M

⬥ ✴ **G8721** PT category (primary tumor), PN category (regional lymph nodes), and histologic grade were documented in pathology report Ⓑ    M

⬥ ✴ **G8722** Documentation of medical reason(s) for not including the PT category, the PN category or the histologic grade in the pathology report (e.g., re-excision without residual tumor; non-carcinomasanal canal) Ⓑ    M

⬥ ✴ **G8723** Specimen site is other than anatomic location of primary tumor Ⓑ    M

⬥ ✴ **G8724** PT category, PN category and histologic grade were not documented in the pathology report, reason not given Ⓑ   M

⬥ ✴ **G8730** Pain assessment documented as positive using a standardized tool and a follow-up plan is documented Ⓖ    M

⬥ ✴ **G8731** Pain assessment using a standardized tool is documented as negative, no follow-up plan required Ⓖ    M

⬥ ✴ **G8732** No documentation of pain assessment, reason not given Ⓑ    M

⬥ ✴ **G8733** Elder maltreatment screen documented as positive and a follow-up plan is documented Ⓑ Ⓐ    M

⬥ ✴ **G8734** Elder maltreatment screen documented as negative, no follow-up required Ⓑ Ⓐ    M

⬥ ✴ **G8735** Elder maltreatment screen documented as positive, follow-up plan not documented, reason not given Ⓑ Ⓐ   M

⬥ ✴ **G8749** Absence of signs of melanoma (tenderness, jaundice, localized neurologic signs such as weakness, or any other sign suggesting systemic spread) or absence of symptoms of melanoma (cough, dyspnea, pain, paresthesia, or any other symptom suggesting the possibility of systemic spread of melanoma) Ⓑ    M

⬥ ✴ **G8752** Most recent systolic blood pressure <140 mmhg Ⓑ    M

⬥ ✴ **G8753** Most recent systolic blood pressure >=140 mmhg Ⓑ    M

⬥ ✴ **G8754** Most recent diastolic blood pressure <90 mmhg Ⓑ    M

⬥ ✴ **G8755** Most recent diastolic blood pressure >=90 mmhg Ⓑ    M

⬥ ✴ **G8756** No documentation of blood pressure measurement, reason not given Ⓑ    M

⬥ ✴ **G8783** Normal blood pressure reading documented, follow-up not required Ⓑ    M

⬥ ✴ **G8785** Blood pressure reading not documented, reason not given Ⓑ    M

⬥ ✴ **G8797** Specimen site other than anatomic location of esophagus Ⓑ    M

⬥ ✴ **G8798** Specimen site other than anatomic location of prostate Ⓑ    M

⬥ ✴ **G8806** Performance of trans-abdominal or trans-vaginal ultrasound and pregnancy location documented Ⓑ    M

⬥ ✴ **G8807** Trans-abdominal or trans-vaginal ultrasound not performed for reasons documented by clinician (e.g., patient has visited the ED multiple times within 72 hours, patient has a documented intrauterine pregnancy [IUP]) Ⓑ    M

⬥ ✴ **G8808** Trans-abdominal or trans-vaginal ultrasound not performed, reason not given Ⓑ    M

⬥ ✴ **G8809** Rh-immunoglobulin (RhoGAM) ordered Ⓑ    M

---

⬥ MIPS    Ⓠⓟ Quantity Physician    Ⓠⓗ Quantity Hospital    ♀ Female only

♂ Male only    Ⓐ Age    & DMEPOS    A2-Z3 ASC Payment Indicator    A-Y ASC Status Indicator    Coding Clinic

* **G8810** Rh-immunoglobulin (RhoGAM) not ordered for reasons documented by clinician (e.g., patient had prior documented report of RhoGAM within 12 weeks, patient refusal) Ⓑ   M

* **G8811** Documentation RH-immunoglobulin (RhoGAM) was not ordered, reason not given Ⓑ   M

* **G8815** Documented reason in the medical records for why the statin therapy was not prescribed (i.e., lower extremity bypass was for a patient with non-artherosclerotic disease) Ⓑ   M

* **G8816** Statin medication prescribed at discharge Ⓑ   M

* **G8817** Statin therapy not prescribed at discharge, reason not given Ⓑ   M

* **G8818** Patient discharge to home no later than post-operative day #7 Ⓑ   M

* **G8825** Patient not discharged to home by post-operative day #7 Ⓑ   M

* **G8826** Patient discharge to home no later than post-operative day #2 following EVAR Ⓑ   M

* **G8833** Patient not discharged to home by post-operative day #2 following EVAR Ⓑ   M

* **G8834** Patient discharged to home no later than post-operative day #2 following CEA Ⓑ   M

* **G8838** Patient not discharged to home by post-operative day #2 following CEA Ⓑ   M

* **G8839** Sleep apnea symptoms assessed, including presence or absence of snoring and daytime sleepiness Ⓑ   M

* **G8840** Documentation of reason(s) for not documenting an assessment of sleep symptoms (e.g., patient didn't have initial daytime sleepiness, patient visited between initial testing and initiation of therapy) Ⓑ   M

* **G8841** Sleep apnea symptoms not assessed, reason not given Ⓑ   M

* **G8842** Apnea Hypopnea Index (AHI) or Respiratory Disturbance Index (RDI) measured at the time of initial diagnosis Ⓑ   M

* **G8843** Documentation of reason(s) for not measuring an Apnea Hypopnea Index (AHI) or a Respiratory Disturbance Index (RDI) at the time of initial diagnosis (e.g., psychiatric disease, dementia, patient declined, financial, insurance coverage, test ordered but not yet completed) Ⓑ   M

* **G8844** Apnea Hypopnea Index (AHI) or Respiratory Disturbance Index (RDI) not measured at the time of initial diagnosis, reason not given Ⓑ   M

* **G8845** Positive airway pressure therapy prescribed Ⓑ   M

* **G8846** Moderate or severe obstructive sleep apnea (Apnea Hypopnea Index (AHI) or Respiratory Disturbance Index (RDI) of 15 or greater) Ⓑ   M

* **G8849** Documentation of reason(s) for not prescribing positive airway pressure therapy (e.g., patient unable to tolerate, alternative therapies use, patient declined, financial, insurance coverage) Ⓑ   M

* **G8850** Positive airway pressure therapy not prescribed, reason not given Ⓑ   M

* **G8851** Objective measurement of adherence to positive airway pressure therapy, documented Ⓑ   M

* **G8852** Positive airway pressure therapy prescribed Ⓑ   M

* **G8854** Documentation of reason(s) for not objectively measuring adherence to positive airway pressure therapy (e.g., patient didn't bring data from continuous positive airway pressure [CPAP], therapy was not yet initiated, not available on machine) Ⓑ   M

* **G8855** Objective measurement of adherence to positive airway pressure therapy not performed, reason not given Ⓑ   M

* **G8856** Referral to a physician for an otologic evaluation performed Ⓑ   M

* **G8857** Patient is not eligible for the referral for otologic evaluation measure (e.g., patients who are already under the care of a physician for acute or chronic dizziness) Ⓑ   M

* **G8858** Referral to a physician for an otologic evaluation not performed, reason not given Ⓑ   M

~~G8861~~ ~~Within the past 2 years, central dual-energy x-ray absorptiometry (DXA) ordered and documented, review of systems and medication history or pharmacologic therapy (other than minerals/vitamins) for osteoporosis prescribed~~ ✖

* **G8863** Patients not assessed for risk of bone loss, reason not given Ⓑ   M

* **G8864** Pneumococcal vaccine administered or previously received Ⓑ   M

---

\* **G8865** Documentation of medical reason(s) for not administering or previously receiving pneumococcal vaccine (e.g., patient allergic reaction, potential adverse drug reaction) Ⓑ M

\* **G8866** Documentation of patient reason(s) for not administering or previously receiving pneumococcal vaccine (e.g., patient refusal) Ⓑ M

\* **G8867** Pneumococcal vaccine not administered or previously received, reason not given Ⓑ M

\* **G8869** Patient has documented immunity to hepatitis B and initiating anti-TNF therapy Ⓑ M

\* **G8872** Excised tissue evaluated by imaging intraoperatively to confirm successful inclusion of targeted lesion Ⓑ M

\* **G8873** Patients with needle localization specimens which are not amenable to intraoperative imaging such as MRI needle wire localization, or targets which are tentatively identified on mammogram or ultrasound which do not contain a biopsy marker but which can be verified on intraoperative inspection or pathology (e.g., needle biopsy site where the biopsy marker is remote from the actual biopsy site) Ⓑ M

\* **G8874** Excised tissue not evaluated by imaging intraoperatively to confirm successful inclusion of targeted lesion Ⓑ M

\* **G8875** Clinician diagnosed breast cancer preoperatively by a minimally invasive biopsy method Ⓑ M

\* **G8876** Documentation of reason(s) for not performing minimally invasive biopsy to diagnose breast cancer preoperatively (e.g., lesion too close to skin, implant, chest wall, etc., lesion could not be adequately visualized for needle biopsy, patient condition prevents needle biopsy [weight, breast thickness, etc.], duct excision without imaging abnormality, prophylactic mastectomy, reduction mammoplasty, excisional biopsy performed by another physician) Ⓑ M

\* **G8877** Clinician did not attempt to achieve the diagnosis of breast cancer preoperatively by a minimally invasive biopsy method, reason not given Ⓑ M

\* **G8878** Sentinel lymph node biopsy procedure performed Ⓑ M

\* **G8880** Documentation of reason(s) sentinel lymph node biopsy not performed (e.g., reasons could include but not limited to; non-invasive cancer, incidental discovery of breast cancer on prophylactic mastectomy, incidental discovery of breast cancer on reduction mammoplasty, pre-operative biopsy proven lymph node (LN) metastases, inflammatory carcinoma, stage 3 locally advanced cancer, recurrent invasive breast cancer, clinically node positive after neoadjuvant systemic therapy, patient refusal after informed consent; patient with significant age, comorbidities, or limited life expectancy and favorable tumor; adjuvant systemic therapy unlikely to change) Ⓑ M

\* **G8881** Stage of breast cancer is greater than T1N0M0 or T2N0M0 Ⓑ M

\* **G8882** Sentinel lymph node biopsy procedure not performed, reason not given Ⓑ M

\* **G8883** Biopsy results reviewed, communicated, tracked and documented Ⓑ M

\* **G8884** Clinician documented reason that patient's biopsy results were not reviewed Ⓑ M

\* **G8885** Biopsy results not reviewed, communicated, tracked or documented Ⓑ M

\* **G8907** Patient documented not to have experienced any of the following events: a burn prior to discharge; a fall within the facility; wrong site/side/patient/procedure/implant event; or a hospital transfer or hospital admission upon discharge from the facility Ⓑ M

\* **G8908** Patient documented to have received a burn prior to discharge Ⓑ M

\* **G8909** Patient documented not to have received a burn prior to discharge Ⓑ M

\* **G8910** Patient documented to have experienced a fall within ASC Ⓑ M

\* **G8911** Patient documented not to have experienced a fall within ambulatory surgical center Ⓑ M

\* **G8912** Patient documented to have experienced a wrong site, wrong side, wrong patient, wrong procedure or wrong implant event Ⓑ M

\* **G8913** Patient documented not to have experienced a wrong site, wrong side, wrong patient, wrong procedure or wrong implant event Ⓑ M

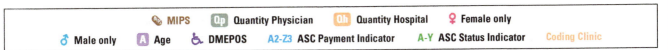

🦪 MIPS    Ⓠp Quantity Physician    Ⓠh Quantity Hospital    ♀ Female only

♂ Male only    Ⓐ Age    ♿ DMEPOS    A2-Z3 ASC Payment Indicator    A-Y ASC Status Indicator    Coding Clinic

* **G8914** Patient documented to have experienced a hospital transfer or hospital admission upon discharge from ASC ⑧     M

* **G8915** Patient documented not to have experienced a hospital transfer or hospital admission upon discharge from ASC ⑧     M

* **G8916** Patient with preoperative order for IV antibiotic surgical site infection (SSI) prophylaxis, antibiotic initiated on time ⑧     M

* **G8917** Patient with preoperative order for IV antibiotic surgical site infection (SSI) prophylaxis, antibiotic not initiated on time ⑧     M

* **G8918** Patient without preoperative order for IV antibiotic surgical site infection(SSI) prophylaxis ⑧     M

* **G8923** Left ventricular ejection fraction (LVEF) <40% or documentation of moderately or severely depressed left ventricular systolic function ⑧     M

* **G8924** Spirometry test results demonstrate FEV1/FVC <70%, FEV <60% predicted and patient has COPD symptoms (e.g., dyspnea, cough/sputum, wheezing) ⑧     M

* **G8925** Spirometry test results demonstrate FEV1 >=60% FEV1/FVC >=70%, predicted or patient does not have COPD symptoms ⑧     M

* **G8926** Spirometry test not performed or documented, reason not given ⑧     M

* **G8934** Left ventricular ejection fraction (LVEF) <40% or documentation of moderately or severely depressed left ventricular systolic function ⑧     M

* **G8935** Clinician prescribed angiotensin converting enzyme (ACE) inhibitor or angiotensin receptor blocker (ARB) therapy ⑧     M

* **G8936** Clinician documented that patient was not an eligible candidate for angiotensin converting enzyme (ACE) inhibitor or angiotensin receptor blocker (ARB) therapy (e.g., allergy, intolerance, pregnancy, renal failure due to ace inhibitor, diseases of the aortic or mitral valve, other medical reasons) or (e.g., patient declined, other patient reasons) or (e.g., lack of drug availability, other reasons attributable to the health care system) ⑧     M

* **G8937** Clinician did not prescribe angiotensin converting enzyme (ACE) inhibitor or angiotensin receptor blocker (ARB) therapy, reason not given ⑧     M

* **G8938** BMI is documented as being outside of normal limits, follow-up plan is not documented, documentation the patient is not eligible ⑧     M

* **G8939** Pain assessment documented as positive, follow-up plan not documented, documentation the patient is not eligible at the time of the encounter at the time of the encounter ⑧     M

* **G8941** Elder maltreatment screen documented as positive, follow-up plan not documented, documentation the patient is not eligible for follow-up plan at the time of the encounter ⑧ Ⓐ     M

* **G8942** Functional outcomes assessment using a standardized tool is documented within the previous 30 days and care plan, based on identified deficiencies on the date of the functional outcome assessment, is documented ⑧     M

* **G8944** AJCC melanoma cancer stage 0 through IIC melanoma ⑧     M

* **G8946** Minimally invasive biopsy method attempted but not diagnostic of breast cancer (e.g., high risk lesion of breast such as atypical ductal hyperplasia, lobular neoplasia, atypical lobular hyperplasia, lobular carcinoma in situ, atypical columnar hyperplasia, flat epithelial atypia, radial scar, complex sclerosing lesion, papillary lesion, or any lesion with spindle cells) ⑧     M

* **G8950** Pre-hypertensive or hypertensive blood pressure reading documented, and the indicated follow-up documented ⑧     M

* **G8952** Pre-hypertensive or hypertensive blood pressure reading documented, indicated follow-up not documented, reason not given ⑧     M

* **G8955** Most recent assessment of adequacy of volume management documented ⑧ M

* **G8956** Patient receiving maintenance hemodialysis in an outpatient dialysis facility ⑧     M

* **G8958** Assessment of adequacy of volume management not documented, reason not given ⑧     M

* **G8959** Clinician treating major depressive disorder communicates to clinician treating comorbid condition ⑧     M

---

▶ New    ↻ Revised    ✔ Reinstated    ~~deleted~~ Deleted    ⊘ Not covered or valid by Medicare

⊕ Special coverage instructions    * Carrier discretion    ⑧ Bill Part B MAC    ⑬ Bill DME MAC

* **G8960** Clinician treating major depressive disorder did not communicate to clinician treating comorbid condition, reason not given Ⓑ   M

* **G8961** Cardiac stress imaging test primarily performed on low-risk surgery patient for preoperative evaluation within 30 days preceding this surgery Ⓑ   M

* **G8962** Cardiac stress imaging test performed on patient for any reason including those who did not have low risk surgery or test that was performed more than 30 days preceding low risk surgery Ⓑ M

* **G8963** Cardiac stress imaging performed primarily for monitoring of asymptomatic patient who had PCI within 2 years Ⓑ   M

* **G8964** Cardiac stress imaging test performed primarily for any other reason than monitoring of asymptomatic patient who had PCI within 2 years (e.g., symptomatic patient, patient greater than 2 years since PCI, initial evaluation, etc.) Ⓑ   M

* **G8965** Cardiac stress imaging test primarily performed on low CHD risk patient for initial detection and risk assessment Ⓑ   M

* **G8966** Cardiac stress imaging test performed on symptomatic or higher than low CHD risk patient or for any reason other than initial detection and risk assessment Ⓑ   M

* **G8967** Warfarin or another FDA-approved oral anticoagulant is prescribed Ⓑ   M

* **G8968** Documentation of medical reason(s) for not prescribing warfarin or another FDA-approved anticoagulant (e.g., atrial appendage device in place) Ⓑ   M

* **G8969** Documentation of patient reason(s) for not prescribing warfarin or another FDA-approved oral anticoagulant that is FDA approved for the prevention of thromboembolism (e.g., patient choice of having atrial appendage device placed) Ⓑ   M

* **G8970** No risk factors or one moderate risk factor for thromboembolism Ⓑ   M

* **G8973** Most recent hemoglobin (Hgb) level <10 g/dl Ⓑ   M

* **G8974** Hemoglobin level measurement not documented, reason not given Ⓑ   M

* **G8975** Documentation of medical reason(s) for patient having a hemoglobin level <10 g/dl (e.g., patients who have non-renal etiologies of anemia [e.g., sickle cell anemia or other hemoglobinopathies, hypersplenism, primary bone marrow disease, anemia related to chemotherapy for diagnosis of malignancy, postoperative bleeding, active bloodstream or peritoneal infection], other medical reasons) Ⓠ   M

* **G8976** Most recent hemoglobin (Hgb) level >=10 g/dl Ⓑ   M

## Functional Limitation

G8978   Mobility: walking & moving around functional limitation, current status, at therapy episode outset and at reporting intervals ✖

G8979   Mobility: walking & moving around functional limitation, projected goal status, at therapy episode outset, at reporting intervals, and at discharge or to end reporting ✖

G8980   Mobility: walking & moving around functional limitation, discharge status, at discharge from therapy or to end reporting ✖

G8981   Changing and maintaining body position functional limitation, current status, at therapy episode outset and at reporting intervals ✖

G8982   Changing and maintaining body position functional limitation, projected goal status, at therapy episode outset, at reporting intervals, and at discharge or to end reporting ✖

G8983   Changing and maintaining body position functional limitation, discharge status, at discharge from therapy or to end reporting ✖

G8984   Carrying, moving and handling objects functional limitation, current status, at therapy episode outset and at reporting intervals ✖

G8985   Carrying, moving and handling objects, projected goal status, at therapy episode outset, at reporting intervals, and at discharge or to end reporting ✖

G8986   Carrying, moving & handling objects functional limitation, discharge status, at discharge from therapy or to end reporting ✖

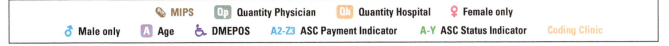

🐚 MIPS   Ⓠᵖ Quantity Physician   Ⓠₕ Quantity Hospital   ♀ Female only

♂ Male only   Ⓐ Age   ♿ DMEPOS   A2-Z3 ASC Payment Indicator   A-Y ASC Status Indicator   Coding Clinic

G8987   Self-care functional limitation, current status, at therapy episode outset and at reporting intervals   ✖

G8988   Self-care functional limitation, projected goal status, at therapy episode outset, at reporting intervals, and at discharge or to end reporting   ✖

G8989   Self-care functional limitation, discharge status, at discharge from therapy or to end reporting   ✖

G8990   Other physical or occupational therapy primary functional limitation, current status, at therapy episode outset and at reporting intervals   ✖

G8991   Other physical or occupational therapy primary functional limitation, projected goal status, at therapy episode outset, at reporting intervals, and at discharge or to end reporting   ✖

G8992   Other physical or occupational therapy primary functional limitation, discharge status, at discharge from therapy or to end reporting   ✖

G8993   Other physical or occupational therapy subsequent functional limitation, current status, at therapy episode outset and at reporting intervals   ✖

G8994   Other physical or occupational therapy subsequent functional limitation, projected goal status, at therapy episode outset, at reporting intervals, and at discharge or to end reporting   ✖

G8995   Other physical or occupational therapy subsequent functional limitation, discharge status, at discharge from therapy or to end reporting   ✖

G8996   Swallowing functional limitation, current status at therapy episode outset and at reporting intervals   ✖

G8997   Swallowing functional limitation, projected goal status, at therapy episode outset, at reporting intervals, and at discharge or to end reporting   ✖

G8998   Swallowing functional limitation, discharge status, at discharge from therapy or to end reporting   ✖

G8999   Motor speech functional limitation, current status at therapy episode outset and at reporting intervals   ✖

## Coordinated Care

✪ **G9001** Coordinated care fee, initial rate Ⓑ   B

✪ **G9002** Coordinated care fee, maintenance rate Ⓑ   B

✪ **G9003** Coordinated care fee, risk adjusted high, initial Ⓑ   B

✪ **G9004** Coordinated care fee, risk adjusted low, initial Ⓑ   B

✪ **G9005** Coordinated care fee, risk adjusted maintenance Ⓑ   B

✪ **G9006** Coordinated care fee, home monitoring Ⓑ   B

✪ **G9007** Coordinated care fee, scheduled team conference Ⓑ   B

✪ **G9008** Coordinated care fee, physician coordinated care oversight services Ⓑ   B

✪ **G9009** Coordinated care fee, risk adjusted maintenance, level 3 Ⓑ   B

✪ **G9010** Coordinated care fee, risk adjusted maintenance, level 4 Ⓑ   B

✪ **G9011** Coordinated care fee, risk adjusted maintenance, level 5 Ⓑ   B

✪ **G9012** Other specified case management services not elsewhere classified Ⓑ   B

## Demonstration Project

⊘ **G9013** ESRD demo basic bundle Level I Ⓑ   E1

⊘ **G9014** ESRD demo expanded bundle including venous access and related services Ⓑ   E1

⊘ **G9016** Smoking cessation counseling, individual, in the absence of or in addition to any other evaluation and management service, per session (6-10 minutes) [demo project code only] Ⓑ   E1

G9017   Amantadine hydrochloride, oral, per 100 mg (for use in a Medicare-approved demonstration project)   ✖

G9018   Zanamivir, inhalation powder, administered through inhaler, per 10 mg (for use in a Medicare-approved demonstration project)   ✖

G9019   Oseltamivir phosphate, oral, per 75 mg (for use in a Medicare-approved demonstration project)   ✖

G9020   Rimantadine hydrochloride, oral, per 100 mg (for use in a Medicare-approved demonstration project)   ✖

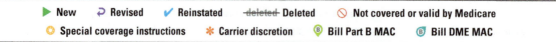

▶ New    ↻ Revised    ✔ Reinstated    ~~deleted~~ Deleted    ⊘ Not covered or valid by Medicare
✪ Special coverage instructions    ✶ Carrier discretion    Ⓑ Bill Part B MAC    Ⓑ Bill DME MAC

~~G9033~~ ~~Amantadine hydrochloride, oral,~~ ✖
~~brand, per 100 mg (for use in a~~
~~Medicare-approved demonstration~~
~~project)~~

~~G9034~~ ~~Zanamivir, inhalation powder,~~ ✖
~~administered through inhaler, brand,~~
~~per 10 mg (for use in a Medicare-~~
~~approved demonstration project)~~

~~G9035~~ ~~Oseltamivir phosphate, oral, brand, per~~ ✖
~~75 mg (for use in a Medicare-approved~~
~~demonstration project)~~

~~G9036~~ ~~Rimantadine hydrochloride, oral,~~ ✖
~~brand, per 100 mg (for use in a~~
~~Medicare-approved demonstration~~
~~project)~~

⊘ **G9050** Oncology; primary focus of visit; work-up, evaluation, or staging at the time of cancer diagnosis or recurrence (for use in a Medicare-approved demonstration project) Ⓑ  E1

⊘ **G9051** Oncology; primary focus of visit; treatment decision-making after disease is staged or restaged, discussion of treatment options, supervising/coordinating active cancer directed therapy or managing consequences of cancer directed therapy (for use in a Medicare-approved demonstration project) Ⓑ  E1

⊘ **G9052** Oncology; primary focus of visit; surveillance for disease recurrence for patient who has completed definitive cancer-directed therapy and currently lacks evidence of recurrent disease; cancer directed therapy might be considered in the future (for use in a Medicare-approved demonstration project) Ⓑ  E1

⊘ **G9053** Oncology; primary focus of visit; expectant management of patient with evidence of cancer for whom no cancer directed therapy is being administered or arranged at present; cancer directed therapy might be considered in the future (for use in a Medicare-approved demonstration project) Ⓑ  E1

⊘ **G9054** Oncology; primary focus of visit; supervising, coordinating or managing care of patient with terminal cancer or for whom other medical illness prevents further cancer treatment; includes symptom management, end-of-life care planning, management of palliative therapies (for use in a Medicare-approved demonstration project) Ⓑ  E1

⊘ **G9055** Oncology; primary focus of visit; other, unspecified service not otherwise listed (for use in a Medicare-approved demonstration project) Ⓑ  E1

⊘ **G9056** Oncology; practice guidelines; management adheres to guidelines (for use in a Medicare-approved demonstration project) Ⓑ  E1

⊘ **G9057** Oncology; practice guidelines; management differs from guidelines as a result of patient enrollment in an institutional review board approved clinical trial (for use in a Medicare-approved demonstration project) Ⓑ  E1

⊘ **G9058** Oncology; practice guidelines; management differs from guidelines because the treating physician disagrees with guideline recommendations (for use in a Medicare-approved demonstration project) Ⓑ  E1

⊘ **G9059** Oncology; practice guidelines; management differs from guidelines because the patient, after being offered treatment consistent with guidelines, has opted for alternative treatment or management, including no treatment (for use in a Medicare-approved demonstration project) Ⓑ  E1

⊘ **G9060** Oncology; practice guidelines; management differs from guidelines for reason(s) associated with patient comorbid illness or performance status not factored into guidelines (for use in a Medicare-approved demonstration project) Ⓑ  E1

⊘ **G9061** Oncology; practice guidelines; patient's condition not addressed by available guidelines (for use in a Medicare-approved demonstration project) Ⓑ  E1

⊘ **G9062** Oncology; practice guidelines; management differs from guidelines for other reason(s) not listed (for use in a Medicare-approved demonstration project) Ⓑ  E1

✱ **G9063** Oncology; disease status; limited to non-small cell lung cancer; extent of disease initially established as stage I (prior to neo-adjuvant therapy, if any) with no evidence of disease progression, recurrence, or metastases (for use in a Medicare-approved demonstration project) Ⓑ  M

---

🐾 MIPS  ⬢ Quantity Physician  ⬢ Quantity Hospital  ♀ Female only

♂ Male only  Ⓐ Age  ♿ DMEPOS  A2-Z3 ASC Payment Indicator  A-Y ASC Status Indicator  Coding Clinic

* **G9064** Oncology; disease status; limited to non-small cell lung cancer; extent of disease initially established as stage II (prior to neo-adjuvant therapy, if any) with no evidence of disease progression, recurrence, or metastases (for use in a Medicare-approved demonstration project) Ⓑ    M

* **G9065** Oncology; disease status; limited to non-small cell lung cancer; extent of disease initially established as stage IIIA (prior to neo-adjuvant therapy, if any) with no evidence of disease progression, recurrence, or metastases (for use in a Medicare-approved demonstration project) Ⓑ    M

* **G9066** Oncology; disease status; limited to non-small cell lung cancer; stage IIIB-IV at diagnosis, metastatic, locally recurrent, or progressive (for use in a Medicare-approved demonstration project) Ⓑ    M

* **G9067** Oncology; disease status; limited to non-small cell lung cancer; extent of disease unknown, staging in progress, or not listed (for use in a Medicare-approved demonstration project) Ⓑ    M

* **G9068** Oncology; disease status; limited to small cell and combined small cell/non-small cell; extent of disease initially established as limited with no evidence of disease progression, recurrence, or metastases (for use in a Medicare-approved demonstration project) Ⓑ    M

* **G9069** Oncology; disease status; small cell lung cancer, limited to small cell and combined small cell/non-small cell; extensive stage at diagnosis, metastatic, locally recurrent, or progressive (for use in a Medicare-approved demonstration project) Ⓑ    M

* **G9070** Oncology; disease status; small cell lung cancer, limited to small cell and combined small cell/non-small cell; extent of disease unknown, staging in progress, or not listed (for use in a Medicare-approved demonstration project) Ⓑ    M

* **G9071** Oncology; disease status; invasive female breast cancer (does not include ductal carcinoma in situ); adenocarcinoma as predominant cell type; stage I or stage IIA-IIB; or T3, N1, M0; and ER and/or PR positive; with no evidence of disease progression, recurrence, or metastases (for use in a Medicare-approved demonstration project) Ⓑ ♀    M

* **G9072** Oncology; disease status; invasive female breast cancer (does not include ductal carcinoma in situ); adenocarcinoma as predominant cell type; stage I, or stage IIA-IIB; or T3, N1, M0; and ER and PR negative; with no evidence of disease progression, recurrence, or metastases (for use in a Medicare-approved demonstration project) Ⓑ ♀    M

* **G9073** Oncology; disease status; invasive female breast cancer (does not include ductal carcinoma in situ); adenocarcinoma as predominant cell type; stage IIIA-IIIB; and not T3, N1, M0; and ER and/or PR positive; with no evidence of disease progression, recurrence, or metastases (for use in a Medicare-approved demonstration project) Ⓑ ♀    M

* **G9074** Oncology; disease status; invasive female breast cancer (does not include ductal carcinoma in situ); adenocarcinoma as predominant cell type; stage IIIA-IIIB; and not T3, N1, M0; and ER and PR negative; with no evidence of disease progression, recurrence, or metastases (for use in a Medicare-approved demonstration project) Ⓑ ♀    M

* **G9075** Oncology; disease status; invasive female breast cancer (does not include ductal carcinoma in situ); adenocarcinoma as predominant cell type; M1 at diagnosis, metastatic, locally recurrent, or progressive (for use in a Medicare-approved demonstration project) Ⓑ ♀    M

* **G9077** Oncology; disease status; prostate cancer, limited to adenocarcinoma as predominant cell type; T1-T2c and Gleason 2-7 and PSA < or equal to 20 at diagnosis with no evidence of disease progression, recurrence, or metastases (for use in a Medicare-approved demonstration project) Ⓑ ♂    M

* **G9078** Oncology; disease status; prostate cancer, limited to adenocarcinoma as predominant cell type; T2 or T3a Gleason 8-10 or PSA >20 at diagnosis with no evidence of disease progression, recurrence, or metastases (for use in a Medicare-approved demonstration project) Ⓑ ♂    M

▶ New    ↻ Revised    ✔ Reinstated    ~~deleted~~ Deleted    ⊘ Not covered or valid by Medicare

⊙ Special coverage instructions    * Carrier discretion    Ⓑ Bill Part B MAC    Ⓑ Bill DME MAC

✻ **G9079**  Oncology; disease status; prostate cancer, limited to adenocarcinoma as predominant cell type; T3b-T4, any N; any T, N1 at diagnosis with no evidence of disease progression, recurrence, or metastases (for use in a Medicare-approved demonstration project) ⑧ ♂M

✻ **G9080**  Oncology; disease status; prostate cancer, limited to adenocarcinoma; after initial treatment with rising PSA or failure of PSA decline (for use in a Medicare-approved demonstration project) ⑧ ♂        M

✻ **G9083**  Oncology; disease status; prostate cancer, limited to adenocarcinoma; extent of disease unknown, staging in progress, or not listed (for use in a Medicare-approved demonstration project) ⑧ ♂        M

✻ **G9084**  Oncology; disease status; colon cancer, limited to invasive cancer, adenocarcinoma as predominant cell type; extent of disease initially established as T1-3, N0, M0 with no evidence of disease progression, recurrence, or metastases (for use in a Medicare-approved demonstration project) ⑧        M

✻ **G9085**  Oncology; disease status; colon cancer, limited to invasive cancer, adenocarcinoma as predominant cell type; extent of disease initially established as T4, N0, M0 with no evidence of disease progression, recurrence, or metastases (for use in a Medicare-approved demonstration project) ⑧        M

✻ **G9086**  Oncology; disease status; colon cancer, limited to invasive cancer, adenocarcinoma as predominant cell type; extent of disease initially established as T1-4, N1-2, M0 with no evidence of disease progression, recurrence, or metastases (for use in a Medicare-approved demonstration project) ⑧        M

✻ **G9087**  Oncology; disease status; colon cancer, limited to invasive cancer, adenocarcinoma as predominant cell type; M1 at diagnosis, metastatic, locally recurrent, or progressive with current clinical, radiologic, or biochemical evidence of disease (for use in a Medicare-approved demonstration project) ⑧        M

✻ **G9088**  Oncology; disease status; colon cancer, limited to invasive cancer, adenocarcinoma as predominant cell type; M1 at diagnosis, metastatic, locally recurrent, or progressive without current clinical, radiologic, or biochemical evidence of disease (for use in a Medicare-approved demonstration project) ⑧        M

✻ **G9089**  Oncology; disease status; colon cancer, limited to invasive cancer, adenocarcinoma as predominant cell type; extent of disease unknown, staging in progress, or not listed (for use in a Medicare-approved demonstration project) ⑧        M

✻ **G9090**  Oncology; disease status; rectal cancer, limited to invasive cancer, adenocarcinoma as predominant cell type; extent of disease initially established as T1-2, N0, M0 (prior to neo-adjuvant therapy, if any) with no evidence of disease progression, recurrence, or metastases (for use in a Medicare-approved demonstration project) ⑧        M

✻ **G9091**  Oncology; disease status; rectal cancer, limited to invasive cancer, adenocarcinoma as predominant cell type; extent of disease initially established as T3, N0, M0 (prior to neo-adjuvant therapy, if any) with no evidence of disease progression, recurrence, or metastases (for use in a Medicare-approved demonstration project) ⑧        M

✻ **G9092**  Oncology; disease status; rectal cancer, limited to invasive cancer, adenocarcinoma as predominant cell type; extent of disease initially established as T1-3, N1-2, M0 (prior to neo-adjuvant therapy, if any) with no evidence of disease progression, recurrence or metastases (for use in a Medicare-approved demonstration project) ⑧        M

✻ **G9093**  Oncology; disease status; rectal cancer, limited to invasive cancer, adenocarcinoma as predominant cell type; extent of disease initially established as T4, any N, M0 (prior to neo-adjuvant therapy, if any) with no evidence of disease progression, recurrence, or metastases (for use in a Medicare-approved demonstration project) ⑧        M

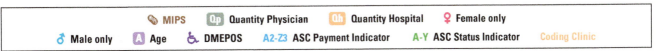

* **G9094** Oncology; disease status; rectal cancer, limited to invasive cancer, adenocarcinoma as predominant cell type; M1 at diagnosis, metastatic, locally recurrent, or progressive (for use in a Medicare-approved demonstration project) Ⓑ  M

* **G9095** Oncology; disease status; rectal cancer, limited to invasive cancer, adenocarcinoma as predominant cell type; extent of disease unknown, staging in progress, or not listed (for use in a Medicare-approved demonstration project) Ⓑ  M

* **G9096** Oncology; disease status; esophageal cancer, limited to adenocarcinoma or squamous cell carcinoma as predominant cell type; extent of disease initially established as T1-T3, N0-N1 or NX (prior to neo-adjuvant therapy, if any) with no evidence of disease progression, recurrence, or metastases (for use in a Medicare-approved demonstration project) Ⓑ  M

* **G9097** Oncology; disease status; esophageal cancer, limited to adenocarcinoma or squamous cell carcinoma as predominant cell type; extent of disease initially established as T4, any N, M0 (prior to neo-adjuvant therapy, if any) with no evidence of disease progression, recurrence, or metastases (for use in a Medicare-approved demonstration project) Ⓑ  M

* **G9098** Oncology; disease status; esophageal cancer, limited to adenocarcinoma or squamous cell carcinoma as predominant cell type; M1 at diagnosis, meta-static, locally recurrent, or progressive (for use in a Medicare-approved demonstration project) Ⓑ  M

* **G9099** Oncology; disease status; esophageal cancer, limited to adenocarcinoma or squamous cell carcinoma as predominant cell type; extent of disease unknown, staging in progress, or not listed (for use in a Medicare-approved demonstration project) Ⓑ  M

* **G9100** Oncology; disease status; gastric cancer, limited to adenocarcinoma as predominant cell type; post R0 resection (with or without neoadjuvant therapy) with no evidence of disease recurrence, progression, or metastases (for use in a Medicare-approved demonstration project) Ⓑ  M

* **G9101** Oncology; disease status; gastric cancer, limited to adenocarcinoma as predominant cell type; post R1 or R2 resection (with or without neoadjuvant therapy) with no evidence of disease progression, or metastases (for use in a Medicare-approved demonstration project) Ⓑ  M

* **G9102** Oncology; disease status; gastric cancer, limited to adenocarcinoma as predominant cell type; clinical or pathologic M0, unresectable with no evidence of disease progression, or metastases (for use in a Medicare-approved demonstration project Ⓑ  M

* **G9103** Oncology; disease status; gastric cancer, limited to adenocarcinoma as predominant cell type; clinical or pathologic M1 at diagnosis, metastatic, locally recurrent, or progressive (for use in a Medicare-approved demonstration project) Ⓑ  M

* **G9104** Oncology; disease status; gastric cancer, limited to adenocarcinoma as predominant cell type; extent of disease unknown, staging in progress, or not listed (for use in a Medicare-approved demonstration project Ⓑ  M

* **G9105** Oncology; disease status; pancreatic cancer, limited to adenocarcinoma as predominant cell type; post R0 resection without evidence of disease progression, recurrence, or metastases (for use in a Medicare-approved demonstration project) Ⓑ  M

* **G9106** Oncology; disease status; pancreatic cancer, limited to adenocarcinoma; post R1 or R2 resection with no evidence of disease progression or metastases (for use in a Medicare-approved demonstration project) Ⓑ  M

* **G9107** Oncology; disease status; pancreatic cancer, limited to adenocarcinoma; unresectable at diagnosis, M1 at diagnosis, metastatic, locally recurrent, or progressive (for use in a Medicare-approved demonstration project) Ⓑ  M

* **G9108** Oncology; disease status; pancreatic cancer, limited to adenocarcinoma; extent of disease unknown, staging in progress, or not listed (for use in a Medicare-approved demonstration project) Ⓑ  M

---

▶ New    ↻ Revised    ✔ Reinstated    ~~deleted~~ Deleted    ⊘ Not covered or valid by Medicare

⊛ Special coverage instructions    ✳ Carrier discretion    Ⓑ Bill Part B MAC    Ⓓ Bill DME MAC

✳ **G9109** Oncology; disease status; head and neck cancer, limited to cancers of oral cavity, pharynx and larynx with squamous cell as predominant cell type; extent of disease initially established as T1-T2 and N0, M0 (prior to neo-adjuvant therapy, if any) with no evidence of disease progression, recurrence, or metastases (for use in a Medicare-approved demonstration project) Ⓑ **M**

✳ **G9110** Oncology; disease status; head and neck cancer, limited to cancers of oral cavity, pharynx, and larynx with squamous cell as predominant cell type; extent of disease initially established as T3-4 and/ or N1-3, M0 (prior to neo-adjuvant therapy, if any) with no evidence of disease progression, recurrence, or metastases (for use in a Medicare-approved demonstration project) Ⓑ **M**

✳ **G9111** Oncology; disease status; head and neck cancer, limited to cancers of oral cavity, pharynx and larynx with squamous cell as predominant cell type; M1 at diagnosis, metastatic, locally recurrent, or progressive (for use in a Medicare-approved demonstration project) Ⓑ **M**

✳ **G9112** Oncology; disease status; head and neck cancer, limited to cancers of oral cavity, pharynx and larynx with squamous cell as predominant cell type; extent of disease unknown, staging in progress, or not listed (for use in a Medicare-approved demonstration project) Ⓑ **M**

✳ **G9113** Oncology; disease status; ovarian cancer, limited to epithelial cancer; pathologic stage IA-B (grade 1) without evidence of disease progression, recurrence, or metastases (for use in a Medicare-approved demonstration project) Ⓑ ♀ **M**

✳ **G9114** Oncology; disease status; ovarian cancer, limited to epithelial cancer; pathologic stage IA-B (grade 2-3); or stage IC (all grades); or stage II; without evidence of disease progression, recurrence, or metastases (for use in a Medicare-approved demonstration project) Ⓑ ♀ **M**

✳ **G9115** Oncology; disease status; ovarian cancer, limited to epithelial cancer; pathologic stage III-IV; without evidence of progression, recurrence, or metastases (for use in a Medicare-approved demonstration project) Ⓑ ♀ **M**

✳ **G9116** Oncology; disease status; ovarian cancer, limited to epithelial cancer; evidence of disease progression, or recurrence and/or platinum resistance (for use in a Medicare-approved demonstration project) Ⓑ ♀ **M**

✳ **G9117** Oncology; disease status; ovarian cancer, limited to epithelial cancer; extent of disease unknown, staging in progress, or not listed (for use in a Medicare-approved demonstration project) Ⓑ ♀ **M**

✳ **G9123** Oncology; disease status; chronic myelogenous leukemia, limited to Philadelphia chromosome positive and/ or BCR-ABL positive; chronic phase not in hematologic, cytogenetic, or molecular remission (for use in a Medicare-approved demonstration project) Ⓑ **M**

✳ **G9124** Oncology; disease status; chronic myelogenous leukemia, limited to Philadelphia chromosome positive and/ or BCR-ABL positive; accelerated phase not in hematologic cytogenetic, or molecular remission (for use in a Medicare-approved demonstration project) Ⓑ **M**

✳ **G9125** Oncology; disease status; chronic myelogenous leukemia, limited to Philadelphia chromosome positive and/ or BCR-ABL positive; blast phase not in hematologic, cytogenetic, or molecular remission (for use in a Medicare-approved demonstration project) Ⓑ **M**

✳ **G9126** Oncology; disease status; chronic myelogenous leukemia, limited to Philadelphia chromosome positive and/ or BCR-ABL positive; in hematologic, cytogenetic, or molecular remission (for use in a Medicare-approved demonstration project) Ⓑ **M**

✳ **G9128** Oncology: disease status; limited to multiple myeloma, systemic disease; smouldering, stage I (for use in a Medicare-approved demonstration project) Ⓑ **M**

✳ **G9129** Oncology; disease status; limited to multiple myeloma, systemic disease; stage II or higher (for use in a Medicare-approved demonstration project) Ⓑ **M**

✳ **G9130** Oncology; disease status; limited to multiple myeloma, systemic disease; extent of disease unknown, staging in progress, or not listed (for use in a Medicare-approved demonstration project) Ⓑ **M**

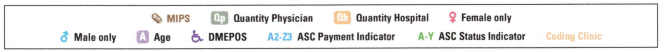

| 🝆 MIPS | Ⓠp Quantity Physician | Ⓠh Quantity Hospital | ♀ Female only |
|---|---|---|---|
| ♂ Male only | Ⓐ Age | ♿ DMEPOS | A2-Z3 ASC Payment Indicator | A-Y ASC Status Indicator | Coding Clinic |

\* **G9131**   Oncology; disease status; invasive female breast cancer (does not include ductal carcinoma in situ); adenocarcinoma as predominant cell type; extent of disease unknown, staging in progress, or not listed (for use in a Medicare-approved demonstration project) Ⓑ ♀      **M**

\* **G9132**   Oncology; disease status; prostate cancer, limited to adenocarcinoma; hormone-refractory/androgen-independent (e.g., rising PSA on anti-androgen therapy or post-orchiectomy); clinical metastases (for use in a Medicare-approved demonstration project) Ⓑ ♂      **M**

\* **G9133**   Oncology; disease status; prostate cancer, limited to adenocarcinoma; hormone-responsive; clinical metastases or M1 at diagnosis (for use in a Medicare-approved demonstration project) Ⓑ ♂      **M**

\* **G9134**   Oncology; disease status; non-Hodgkin's lymphoma, any cellular classification; stage I, II at diagnosis, not relapsed, not refractory (for use in a Medicare-approved demonstration project) Ⓑ      **M**

\* **G9135**   Oncology; disease status; non-Hodgkin's lymphoma, any cellular classification; stage III, IV, not relapsed, not refractory (for use in a Medicare-approved demonstration project) Ⓑ      **M**

\* **G9136**   Oncology; disease status; non-Hodgkin's lymphoma, transformed from original cellular diagnosis to a second cellular classification (for use in a Medicare-approved demonstration project) Ⓑ      **M**

\* **G9137**   Oncology; disease status; non-Hodgkin's lymphoma, any cellular classification; relapsed/refractory (for use in a Medicare-approved demonstration project) Ⓑ      **M**

\* **G9138**   Oncology; disease status; non-Hodgkin's lymphoma, any cellular classification; diagnostic evaluation, stage not determined, evaluation of possible relapse or non-response to therapy, or not listed (for use in a Medicare-approved demonstration project) Ⓑ      **M**

\* **G9139**   Oncology; disease status; chronic myelogenous leukemia, limited to Philadelphia chromosome positive and/or BCR-ABL positive; extent of disease unknown, staging in progress, not listed (for use in a Medicare-approved demonstration project) Ⓑ      **M**

\* **G9140**   Frontier extended stay clinic demonstration; for a patient stay in a clinic approved for the CMS demonstration project; the following measures should be present: the stay must be equal to or greater than 4 hours; weather or other conditions must prevent transfer or the case falls into a category of monitoring and observation cases that are permitted by the rules of the demonstration; there is a maximum frontier extended stay clinic (FESC) visit of 48 hours, except in the case when weather or other conditions prevent transfer; payment is made on each period up to 4 hours, after the first 4 hours Ⓑ      **A**

## Warfarin Responsiveness Testing

\* **G9143**   Warfarin responsiveness testing by genetic technique using any method, any number of specimen(s) Ⓑ ⓆⓅ ⓆⒽ      **N**

This would be a once-in-a-lifetime test unless there is a reason to believe that the patient's personal genetic characteristics would change over time. (https://www.cms.gov/ContractorLearningResources/downloads/JA6715.pdf)

*Laboratory Certification: General immunology, Hematology*

**Coding Clinic: 2010, Q2, P10**

## Outpatient IV Insulin Treatment

⊘ **G9147**   Outpatient intravenous insulin treatment (OIVIT) either pulsatile or continuous, by any means, guided by the results of measurements for: respiratory quotient; and/or, urine urea nitrogen (UUN); and/or, arterial, venous or capillary glucose; and/or potassium concentration Ⓑ      **E1**

On December 23, 2009, CMS issued a national non-coverage decision on the use of OIVIT. CR 6775.

Not covered on Physician Fee Schedule

**Coding Clinic: 2010, Q2, P10**

## Quality Assurance

\* **G9148**   National committee for quality assurance - level 1 medical home Ⓑ      **M**

---

▶ New      ⮂ Revised      ✔ Reinstated      ~~deleted~~ Deleted      ⊘ Not covered or valid by Medicare
⊙ Special coverage instructions      \* Carrier discretion      Ⓑ Bill Part B MAC      Ⓑ Bill DME MAC

\* **G9149** National committee for quality assurance - level 2 medical home ⓑ M

\* **G9150** National committee for quality assurance - level 3 medical home ⓑ M

\* **G9151** MAPCP demonstration - state provided services ⓑ M

\* **G9152** MAPCP demonstration - community health teams ⓑ M

\* **G9153** MAPCP demonstration - physician incentive pool ⓑ M

## Wheelchair Evaluation

\* **G9156** Evaluation for wheelchair requiring face to face visit with physician ⓑ Qp Qh M

## Cardiac Monitoring

\* **G9157** Transesophageal doppler measurement of cardiac output (including probe placement, image acquisition, and interpretation per course of treatment) for monitoring purposes ⓑ Qp Qh B

## ~~Functional Limitation~~

~~G9158~~ ~~Motor speech functional limitation, discharge status, at discharge from therapy or to end reporting~~ ✖

~~G9159~~ ~~Spoken language comprehension functional limitation, current status at therapy episode outset and at reporting intervals~~ ✖

~~G9160~~ ~~Spoken language comprehension functional limitation, projected goal status at therapy episode outset, at reporting intervals, and at discharge or to end reporting~~ ✖

~~G9161~~ ~~Spoken language comprehension functional limitation, discharge status at discharge from therapy or to end reporting~~ ✖

~~G9162~~ ~~Spoken language expression functional limitation, current status at therapy episode outset and at reporting intervals~~ ✖

~~G9163~~ ~~Spoken language expression functional limitation, projected goal status at therapy episode outset, at reporting intervals, and at discharge or to end reporting~~ ✖

~~G9164~~ ~~Spoken language expression functional limitation, discharge status at discharge from therapy or to end reporting~~ ✖

~~G9165~~ ~~Attention functional limitation, current status at therapy episode outset and at reporting intervals~~ ✖

~~G9166~~ ~~Attention functional limitation, projected goal status at therapy episode outset, at reporting intervals, and at discharge or to end reporting~~ ✖

~~G9167~~ ~~Attention functional limitation, discharge status at discharge from therapy or to end reporting~~ ✖

~~G9168~~ ~~Memory functional limitation, current status at therapy episode outset and at reporting intervals~~ ✖

~~G9169~~ ~~Memory functional limitation, projected goal status at therapy episode outset, at reporting intervals, and at discharge or to end reporting~~ ✖

~~G9170~~ ~~Memory functional limitation, discharge status at discharge from therapy or to end reporting~~ ✖

~~G9171~~ ~~Voice functional limitation, current status at therapy episode outset and at reporting intervals~~ ✖

~~G9172~~ ~~Voice functional limitation, projected goal status at therapy episode outset, at reporting intervals, and at discharge or to end reporting~~ ✖

~~G9173~~ ~~Voice functional limitation, discharge status at discharge from therapy or to end reporting~~ ✖

~~G9174~~ ~~Other speech language pathology functional limitation, current status at therapy episode outset and at reporting intervals~~ ✖

~~G9175~~ ~~Other speech language pathology functional limitation, projected goal status at therapy episode outset, at reporting intervals, and at discharge or to end reporting~~ ✖

~~G9176~~ ~~Other speech language pathology functional limitation, discharge status at discharge from therapy or to end reporting~~ ✖

~~G9186~~ ~~Motor speech functional limitation, projected goal status at therapy episode outset, at reporting intervals, and at discharge or to end reporting~~ ✖

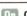 **MIPS**  **Quantity Physician**  **Quantity Hospital** ♀ **Female only**

♂ **Male only**  **Age**  **DMEPOS** **A2-Z3** **ASC Payment Indicator** **A-Y** **ASC Status Indicator** **Coding Clinic**

## Bundled Payment Care Improvement

\* **G9187** Bundled payments for care improvement initiative home visit for patient assessment performed by a qualified health care professional for individuals not considered homebound including, but not limited to, assessment of safety, falls, clinical status, fluid status, medication reconciliation/management, patient compliance with orders/plan of care, performance of activities of daily living, appropriateness of care setting; (for use only in the Medicare-approved bundled payments for care improvement initiative); may not be billed for a 30-day period covered by a transitional care management code Ⓑ 🅠ᵖ 🅠ʰ    E1

## Quality Measures: Miscellaneous

\* **G9188** Beta-blocker therapy not prescribed, reason not given Ⓑ    M

\* **G9189** Beta-blocker therapy prescribed or currently being taken Ⓑ    M

\* **G9190** Documentation of medical reason(s) for not prescribing beta-blocker therapy (e.g., allergy, intolerance, other medical reasons) Ⓑ    M

\* **G9191** Documentation of patient reason(s) for not prescribing beta-blocker therapy (e.g., patient declined, other patient reasons) Ⓑ    M

\* **G9192** Documentation of system reason(s) for not prescribing beta-blocker therapy (e.g., other reasons attributable to the health care system) Ⓑ    M

\* **G9196** Documentation of medical reason(s) for not ordering a first or second generation cephalosporin for antimicrobial prophylaxis (e.g., patients enrolled in clinical trials, patients with documented infection prior to surgical procedure of interest, patients who were receiving antibiotics more than 24 hours prior to surgery [except colon surgery patients taking oral prophylactic antibiotics], patients who were receiving antibiotics within 24 hours prior to arrival [except colon surgery patients taking oral prophylactic antibiotics], other medical reason(s)) Ⓑ    M

\* **G9197** Documentation of order for first or second generation cephalosporin for antimicrobial prophylaxis Ⓑ    M

\* **G9198** Order for first or second generation cephalosporin for antimicrobial prophylaxis was not documented, reason not given Ⓑ    M

\* **G9212** DSM-IVTM criteria for major depressive disorder documented at the initial evaluation Ⓑ    M

\* **G9213** DSM-IV-TR criteria for major depressive disorder not documented at the initial evaluation, reason not otherwise specified Ⓑ    M

\* **G9223** Pneumocystis jiroveci pneumonia prophylaxis prescribed within 3 months of low CD4+ cell count below 500 cells/mm3 or a CD4 percentage below 15% Ⓑ    M

\* **G9225** Foot exam was not performed, reason not given Ⓑ    M

\* **G9226** Foot examination performed (includes examination through visual inspection, sensory exam with 10-g monofilament plus testing any one of the following: vibration using 128-hz tuning fork, pinprick sensation, ankle reflexes, or vibration perception threshold, and pulse exam; report when all of the 3 components are completed) Ⓑ    M

\* **G9227** Functional outcome assessment documented, care plan not documented, documentation the patient is not eligible for a care plan at the time of the encounter Ⓑ    M

\* **G9228** Chlamydia, gonorrhea and syphilis screening results documented (report when results are present for all of the 3 screenings) Ⓑ    M

\* **G9229** Chlamydia, gonorrhea, and syphilis screening results not documented (patient refusal is the only allowed exception) Ⓑ    M

\* **G9230** Chlamydia, gonorrhea, and syphilis not screened, reason not given Ⓑ    M

\* **G9231** Documentation of end stage renal disease (ESRD), dialysis, renal transplant before or during the measurement period or pregnancy during the measurement period Ⓑ    M

---

▶ New    ↻ Revised    ✔ Reinstated    ~~deleted~~ Deleted    ⊘ Not covered or valid by Medicare
✸ Special coverage instructions    \* Carrier discretion    Ⓑ Bill Part B MAC    Ⓓ Bill DME MAC

* **G9232** Clinician treating major depressive disorder did not communicate to clinician treating comorbid condition for specified patient reason (e.g., patient is unable to communicate the diagnosis of a comorbid condition; the patient is unwilling to communicate the diagnosis of a comorbid condition; or the patient is unaware of the comorbid condition, or any other specified patient reason) Ⓑ    M

↺ * **G9239** Documentation of reasons for patient initiating maintenance hemodialysis with a catheter as the mode of vascular access (e.g., patient has a maturing arteriovenous fistula (AVF)/arteriovenous graft (AVG), time-limited trial of hemodialysis, other medical reasons, patient declined AVF/AVG, other patient reasons, patient followed by reporting nephrologist for fewer than 90 days, other system reasons) Ⓑ    M

* **G9240** Patient whose mode of vascular access is a catheter at the time maintenance hemodialysis is initiated Ⓑ    M

* **G9241** Patient whose mode of vascular access is not a catheter at the time maintenance hemodialysis is initiated Ⓑ    M

* **G9242** Documentation of viral load equal to or greater than 200 copies/ml or viral load not performed Ⓑ    M

* **G9243** Documentation of viral load less than 200 copies/ml Ⓑ    M

* **G9246** Patient did not have at least one medical visit in each 6 month period of the 24 month measurement period, with a minimum of 60 days between medical visits Ⓑ    M

* **G9247** Patient had at least one medical visit in each 6 month period of the 24 month measurement period, with a minimum of 60 days between medical visits Ⓑ    M

* **G9250** Documentation of patient pain brought to a comfortable level within 48 hours from initial assessment Ⓑ    M

* **G9251** Documentation of patient with pain not brought to a comfortable level within 48 hours from initial assessment Ⓑ    M

* **G9254** Documentation of patient discharged to home later than post-operative day 2 following CAS Ⓑ    M

* **G9255** Documentation of patient discharged to home no later than post operative day 2 following CAS Ⓑ    M

* **G9256** Documentation of patient death following CAS Ⓑ    M

* **G9257** Documentation of patient stroke following CAS Ⓑ    M

* **G9258** Documentation of patient stroke following CEA Ⓑ    M

* **G9259** Documentation of patient survival and absence of stroke following CAS Ⓑ    M

* **G9260** Documentation of patient death following CEA Ⓑ    M

* **G9261** Documentation of patient survival and absence of stroke following CEA Ⓑ    M

* **G9262** Documentation of patient death in the hospital following endovascular AAA repair Ⓑ    M

* **G9263** Documentation of patient discharged alive following endovascular AAA repair Ⓑ    M

↺ * **G9264** Documentation of patient receiving maintenance hemodialysis for greater than or equal to 90 days with a catheter for documented reasons (e.g., other medical reasons, patient declined arteriovenous fistula (AVF)/arteriovenous graft (AVG), other patient reasons) Ⓑ    M

* **G9265** Patient receiving maintenance hemodialysis for greater than or equal to 90 days with a catheter as the mode of vascular access Ⓑ    M

* **G9266** Patient receiving maintenance hemodialysis for greater than or equal to 90 days without a catheter as the mode of vascular access Ⓑ    M

* **G9267** Documentation of patient with one or more complications or mortality within 30 days Ⓑ    M

* **G9268** Documentation of patient with one or more complications within 90 days Ⓑ M

* **G9269** Documentation of patient without one or more complications and without mortality within 30 days Ⓑ    M

* **G9270** Documentation of patient without one or more complications within 90 days Ⓑ    M

* **G9273** Blood pressure has a systolic value of <140 and a diastolic value of <90 Ⓑ    M

* **G9274** Blood pressure has a systolic value of = 140 and a diastolic value of = 90 or systolic value <140 and diastolic value = 90 or systolic value = 140 and diastolic value <90 Ⓑ    M

* **G9275** Documentation that patient is a current non-tobacco user Ⓑ    M

* **G9276** Documentation that patient is a current tobacco user Ⓑ    M

---

🐾 MIPS   🅞🅟 Quantity Physician   🅞🅗 Quantity Hospital   ♀ Female only
♂ Male only   🅐 Age   ♿ DMEPOS   A2-Z3 ASC Payment Indicator   A-Y ASC Status Indicator   Coding Clinic

\* **G9277** Documentation that the patient is on daily aspirin or anti-platelet or has documentation of a valid contraindication or exception to aspirin/anti-platelet; contraindications/exceptions include anti-coagulant use, allergy to aspirin or anti-platelets, history of gastrointestinal bleed and bleeding disorder; additionally, the following exceptions documented by the physician as a reason for not taking daily aspirin or anti-platelet are acceptable (use of non-steroidal anti-inflammatory agents, documented risk for drug interaction, uncontrolled hypertension defined as >180 systolic or >110 diastolic or gastroesophageal reflux) Ⓑ   M

\* **G9278** Documentation that the patient is not on daily aspirin or anti-platelet regimen Ⓑ   M

\* **G9279** Pneumococcal screening performed and documentation of vaccination received prior to discharge Ⓑ   M

\* **G9280** Pneumococcal vaccination not administered prior to discharge, reason not specified Ⓑ   M

\* **G9281** Screening performed and documentation that vaccination not indicated/patient refusal Ⓑ   M

\* **G9282** Documentation of medical reason(s) for not reporting the histological type or NSCLC-NOS classification with an explanation (e.g., biopsy taken for other purposes in a patient with a history of non-small cell lung cancer or other documented medical reasons) Ⓑ   M

\* **G9283** Non small cell lung cancer biopsy and cytology specimen report documents classification into specific histologic type or classified as NSCLC-NOS with an explanation Ⓑ   M

\* **G9284** Non small cell lung cancer biopsy and cytology specimen report does not document classification into specific histologic type or classified as NSCLC-NOS with an explanation Ⓑ   M

\* **G9285** Specimen site other than anatomic location of lung or is not classified as non small cell lung cancer Ⓑ   M

Ⓜ \* **G9286** Antibiotic regimen prescribed within 10 days after onset of symptoms Ⓑ   M

Ⓜ \* **G9287** Antibiotic regimen not prescribed within 10 days after onset of symptoms Ⓑ   M

\* **G9288** Documentation of medical reason(s) for not reporting the histological type or NSCLC-NOS classification with an explanation (e.g., a solitary fibrous tumor in a person with a history of non-small cell carcinoma or other documented medical reasons ) Ⓑ   M

\* **G9289** Non-small cell lung cancer biopsy and cytology specimen report documents classification into specific histologic type or classified as NSCLC-NOS with an explanation Ⓑ

\* **G9290** Non-small cell lung cancer biopsy and cytology specimen report does not document classification into specific histologic type or classified as NSCLC-NOS with an explanation Ⓑ   M

\* **G9291** Specimen site other than anatomic location of lung, is not classified as non small cell lung cancer or classified as NSCLC-NOS Ⓑ   M

\* **G9292** Documentation of medical reason(s) for not reporting PT category and a statement on thickness and ulceration and for PT1, mitotic rate (e.g., negative skin biopsies in a patient with a history of melanoma or other documented medical reasons) Ⓑ   M

\* **G9293** Pathology report does not include the PT category and a statement on thickness and ulceration and for PT1, mitotic rate Ⓑ   M

\* **G9294** Pathology report includes the PT category and a statement on thickness and ulceration and for PT1, mitotic rate Ⓑ   M

\* **G9295** Specimen site other than anatomic cutaneous location Ⓑ   M

Ⓜ \* **G9296** Patients with documented shared decision-making including discussion of conservative (non-surgical) therapy (e.g., NSAIDs, analgesics, weight loss, exercise, injections) prior to the procedure   M

Ⓜ \* **G9297** Shared decision-making including discussion of conservative (non-surgical) therapy (e.g., NSAIDs, analgesics, weight loss, exercise, injections) prior to the procedure not documented, reason not given Ⓑ   M

Ⓜ \* **G9298** Patients who are evaluated for venous thromboembolic and cardiovascular risk factors within 30 days prior to the procedure (e.g., history of DVT, PE, MI, arrhythmia and stroke) Ⓑ   M

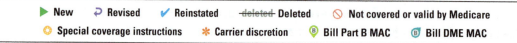
▶ New    ↻ Revised    ✔ Reinstated    ‑deleted‑ Deleted    ⊘ Not covered or valid by Medicare
✪ Special coverage instructions    \* Carrier discretion    Ⓑ Bill Part B MAC    Ⓓ Bill DME MAC

* **G9299** Patients who are not evaluated for venous thromboembolic and cardiovascular risk factors within 30 days prior to the procedure (e.g., history of DVT, PE, MI, arrhythmia and stroke, reason not given) Ⓑ **M**

* **G9300** Documentation of medical reason(s) for not completely infusing the prophylactic antibiotic prior to the inflation of the proximal tourniquet (e.g., a tourniquet was not used) Ⓑ **M**

* **G9301** Patients who had the prophylactic antibiotic completely infused prior to the inflation of the proximal tourniquet Ⓑ **M**

* **G9302** Prophylactic antibiotic not completely infused prior to the inflation of the proximal tourniquet, reason not given Ⓑ **M**

* **G9303** Operative report does not identify the prosthetic implant specifications including the prosthetic implant manufacturer, the brand name of the prosthetic implant and the size of each prosthetic implant, reason not given Ⓑ **M**

* **G9304** Operative report identifies the prosthetic implant specifications including the prosthetic implant manufacturer, the brand name of the prosthetic implant and the size of each prosthetic implant Ⓑ **M**

* **G9305** Intervention for presence of leak of endoluminal contents through an anastomosis not required Ⓑ **M**

* **G9306** Intervention for presence of leak of endoluminal contents through an anastomosis required Ⓑ **M**

* **G9307** No return to the operating room for a surgical procedure, for complications of the principal operative procedure, within 30 days of the principal operative procedure Ⓟ **M**

* **G9308** Unplanned return to the operating room for a surgical procedure, for complications of the principal operative procedure, within 30 days of the principal operative procedure Ⓟ **M**

* **G9309** No unplanned hospital readmission within 30 days of principal procedure Ⓑ **M**

* **G9310** Unplanned hospital readmission within 30 days of principal procedure Ⓑ **M**

* **G9311** No surgical site infection Ⓑ **M**

* **G9312** Surgical site infection Ⓑ **M**

* **G9313** Amoxicillin, with or without clavulanate, not prescribed as first line antibiotic at the time of diagnosis for documented reason Ⓑ **M**

* **G9314** Amoxicillin, with or without clavulanate, not prescribed as first line antibiotic at the time of diagnosis, reason not given Ⓑ **M**

* **G9315** Documentation amoxicillin, with or without clavulanate, prescribed as a first line antibiotic at the time of diagnosis Ⓑ **M**

* **G9316** Documentation of patient-specific risk assessment with a risk calculator based on multi-institutional clinical data, the specific risk calculator used, and communication of risk assessment from risk calculator with the patient or family Ⓑ **M**

* **G9317** Documentation of patient-specific risk assessment with a risk calculator based on multi-institutional clinical data, the specific risk calculator used, and communication of risk assessment from risk calculator with the patient or family not completed Ⓑ **M**

* **G9318** Imaging study named according to standardized nomenclature Ⓑ **M**

* **G9319** Imaging study not named according to standardized nomenclature, reason not given Ⓑ **M**

* **G9321** Count of previous CT (any type of CT) and cardiac nuclear medicine (myocardial perfusion) studies documented in the 12-month period prior to the current study Ⓟ **M**

* **G9322** Count of previous CT and cardiac nuclear medicine (myocardial perfusion) studies not documented in the 12-month period prior to the current study, reason not given Ⓟ **M**

* **G9326** CT studies performed not reported to a radiation dose index registry that is capable of collecting at a minimum all necessary data elements, reason not given Ⓑ **M**

* **G9327** CT studies performed reported to a radiation dose index registry that is capable of collecting at a minimum all necessary data elements Ⓟ **M**

* **G9329** DICOM format image data available to non-affiliated external healthcare facilities or entities on a secure, media free, reciprocally searchable basis with patient authorization for at least a 12-month period after the study not documented in final report, reason not given Ⓑ **M**

---

\* **G9340** Final report documented that DICOM format image data available to non-affiliated external healthcare facilities or entities on a secure, media free, reciprocally searchable basis with patient authorization for at least a 12-month period after the study Ⓑ M

\* **G9341** Search conducted for prior patient CT studies completed at non-affiliated external healthcare facilities or entities within the past 12-months and are available through a secure, authorized, media-free, shared archive prior to an imaging study being performed Ⓑ M

\* **G9342** Search not conducted prior to an imaging study being performed for prior patient CT studies completed at non-affiliated external healthcare facilities or entities within the past 12-months and are available through a secure, authorized, media-free, shared archive, reason not given Ⓑ M

\* **G9344** Due to system reasons search not conducted for DICOM format images for prior patient CT imaging studies completed at non-affiliated external healthcare facilities or entities within the past 12 months that are available through a secure, authorized, media-free, shared archive (e.g., non-affiliated external healthcare facilities or entities does not have archival abilities through a shared archival system) Ⓑ M

\* **G9345** Follow-up recommendations documented according to recommended guidelines for incidentally detected pulmonary nodules (e.g., follow-up CT imaging studies needed or that no follow-up is needed) based at a minimum on nodule size and patient risk factors Ⓑ M

\* **G9347** Follow-up recommendations not documented according to recommended guidelines for incidentally detected pulmonary nodules, reason not given Ⓑ M

\* **G9348** CT scan of the paranasal sinuses ordered at the time of diagnosis for documented reasons Ⓑ M

↻ \* **G9349** CT scan of the paranasal sinuses ordered at the time of diagnosis or received within 28 days after date of diagnosis Ⓑ M

\* **G9350** CT scan of the paranasal sinuses not ordered at the time of diagnosis or received within 28 days after date of diagnosis Ⓑ M

\* **G9351** More than one CT scan of the paranasal sinuses ordered or received within 90 days after diagnosis Ⓑ M

\* **G9352** More than one CT scan of the paranasal sinuses ordered or received within 90 days after the date of diagnosis, reason not given Ⓑ M

\* **G9353** More than one CT scan of the paranasal sinuses ordered or received within 90 days after the date of diagnosis for documented reasons (e.g., patients with complications, second CT obtained prior to surgery, other medical reasons) Ⓑ M

\* **G9354** One CT scan or no CT scan of the paranasal sinuses ordered within 90 days after the date of diagnosis Ⓑ M

↻ \* **G9355** Early elective delivery or early induction not performed (less than 39 weeks gestation) Ⓑ M

↻ \* **G9356** Early elective delivery or early induction performed (less than 39 weeks gestation) Ⓑ M

\* **G9357** Post-partum screenings, evaluations and education performed Ⓑ M

\* **G9358** Post-partum screenings, evaluations and education not performed Ⓑ M

↻ \* **G9359** Documentation of negative or managed positive TB screen with further evidence that TB is not active prior to the treatment with a biologic immune response modifier Ⓑ M

\* **G9360** No documentation of negative or managed positive TB screen Ⓑ M

\* **G9361** Medical indication for induction [documentation of reason(s) for elective delivery (c-section) or early induction (e.g., hemorrhage and placental complications, hypertension, preeclampsia and eclampsia, rupture of membranes-premature or prolonged, maternal conditions complicating pregnancy/delivery, fetal conditions complicating pregnancy/delivery, late pregnancy, prior uterine surgery, or participation in clinical trial)] Ⓑ M

\* **G9364** Sinusitis caused by, or presumed to be caused by, bacterial infection Ⓑ M

\* **G9365** One high-risk medication ordered Ⓑ M

\* **G9366** One high-risk medication not ordered Ⓑ M

\* **G9367** At least two different high-risk medications ordered Ⓑ M

\* **G9368** At least two different high-risk medications not ordered Ⓑ M

---

▶ New ↻ Revised ✔ Reinstated ~~deleted~~ Deleted ⊘ Not covered or valid by Medicare
Ⓢ Special coverage instructions \* Carrier discretion Ⓑ Bill Part B MAC Ⓓ Bill DME MAC

* **G9380** Patient offered assistance with end of life issues during the measurement period ⓑ  M

* **G9382** Patient not offered assistance with end of life issues during the measurement period ⓑ  M

* **G9383** Patient received screening for HCV infection within the 12 month reporting period ⓑ  M

* **G9384** Documentation of medical reason(s) for not receiving annual screening for HCV infection (e.g., decompensated cirrhosis indicating advanced disease [i.e., ascites, esophageal variceal bleeding, hepatic encephalopathy], hepatocellular carcinoma, waitlist for organ transplant, limited life expectancy, other medical reasons) ⓑ  M

* **G9385** Documentation of patient reason(s) for not receiving annual screening for HCV infection (e.g., patient declined, other patient reasons) ⓑ  M

* **G9386** Screening for HCV infection not received within the 12 month reporting period, reason not given ⓑ  M

* **G9389** Unplanned rupture of the posterior capsule requiring vitrectomy during cataract surgery ⓑ  M

* **G9390** No unplanned rupture of the posterior capsule requiring vitrectomy during cataract surgery ⓑ  M

* **G9393** Patient with an initial PHQ-9 score greater than nine who achieves remission at 12 months as demonstrated by a 12 month (+/- 30 days) PHQ-9 score of less than five ⓑ  M

* **G9394** Patient who had a diagnosis of bipolar disorder or personality disorder, death, permanent nursing home resident or receiving hospice or palliative care any time during the measurement or assessment period ⓑ  M

* **G9395** Patient with an initial PHQ-9 score greater than nine who did not achieve remission at 12 months as demonstrated by a 12 month (+/- 30 days) PHQ-9 score greater than or equal to five ⓑ  M

* **G9396** Patient with an initial PHQ-9 score greater than nine who was not assessed for remission at 12 months (+/- 30 days) ⓑ  M

* **G9399** Documentation in the patient record of a discussion between the physician/clinician and the patient that includes all of the following: treatment choices appropriate to genotype, risks and benefits, evidence of effectiveness, and patient preferences toward the outcome of the treatment ⓑ  M

* **G9400** Documentation of medical or patient reason(s) for not discussing treatment options; medical reasons: patient is not a candidate for treatment due to advanced physical or mental health comorbidity (including active substance use); currently receiving antiviral treatment; successful antiviral treatment (with sustained virologic response) prior to reporting period; other documented medical reasons; patient reasons: patient unable or unwilling to participate in the discussion or other patient reasons ⓑ M

* **G9401** No documentation of a discussion in the patient record of a discussion between the physician or other qualified health care professional and the patient that includes all of the following: treatment choices appropriate to genotype, risks and benefits, evidence of effectiveness, and patient preferences toward treatment ⓑ  M

* **G9402** Patient received follow-up on the date of discharge or within 30 days after discharge ⓑ  M

* **G9403** Clinician documented reason patient was not able to complete 30 day follow-up from acute inpatient setting discharge (e.g., patient death prior to follow-up visit, patient non-compliant for visit follow-up) ⓑ  M

* **G9404** Patient did not receive follow-up on the date of discharge or within 30 days after discharge ⓑ  M

↩ * **G9405** Patient received follow-up within 7 days after discharge ⓑ  M

* **G9406** Clinician documented reason patient was not able to complete 7 day follow-up from acute inpatient setting discharge (i.e patient death prior to follow-up visit, patient non-compliance for visit follow-up) ⓑ  M

* **G9407** Patient did not receive follow-up on or within 7 days after discharge ⓑ  M

* **G9408** Patients with cardiac tamponade and/or pericardiocentesis occurring within 30 days ⓑ  M

* **G9409** Patients without cardiac tamponade and/or pericardiocentesis occurring within 30 days ⓑ M

* **G9410** Patient admitted within 180 days, status post CIED implantation, replacement, or revision with an infection requiring device removal or surgical revision ⓑ M

* **G9411** Patient not admitted within 180 days, status post CIED implantation, replacement, or revision with an infection requiring device removal or surgical revision ⓑ M

* **G9412** Patient admitted within 180 days, status post CIED implantation, replacement, or revision with an infection requiring device removal or surgical revision ⓑ M

* **G9413** Patient not admitted within 180 days, status post CIED implantation, replacement, or revision with an infection requiring device removal or surgical revision ⓑ M

↻ * **G9414** Patient had one dose of meningococcal vaccine (serogroups a, c, w, y) on or between the patient's 11th and 13th birthdays ⓑ M

* **G9415** Patient did not have one dose of meningococcal vaccine on or between the patient's 11th and 13th birthdays ⓑ M

* **G9416** Patient had one tetanus, diphtheria toxoids and acellular pertussis vaccine (Tdap) or one tetanus, diphtheria toxoids vaccine (Td) on or between the patient's 10th and 13th birthdays ⓑ M

* **G9417** Patient did not have one tetanus, diphtheria toxoids and acellular pertussis vaccine (Tdap) on or between the patient's 10th and 13th birthdays ⓑ M

* **G9418** Primary non-small cell lung cancer biopsy and cytology specimen report documents classification into specific histologic type or classified as NSCLC-NOS with an explanation ⓑ M

* **G9419** Documentation of medical reason(s) for not including the histological type or NSCLC-NOS classification with an explanation (e.g., biopsy taken for other purposes in a patient with a history of primary non-small cell lung cancer or other documented medical reasons) ⓑ M

* **G9420** Specimen site other than anatomic location of lung or is not classified as primary non-small cell lung cancer ⓑ M

* **G9421** Primary non-small cell lung cancer biopsy and cytology specimen report does not document classification into specific histologic type or classified as NSCLC-NOS with an explanation ⓑ M

* **G9422** Primary lung carcinoma resection report documents pT category, pN category and for non-small cell lung cancer, histologic type (squamous cell carcinoma, adenocarcinoma and not nsclc-nos) ⓑ M

* **G9423** Documentation of medical reason for not including pT category, pN category and histologic type [for patient with appropriate exclusion criteria (e.g., metastatic disease, benign tumors, malignant tumors other than carcinomas, inadequate surgical specimens)] ⓑ M

* **G9424** Specimen site other than anatomic location of lung, or classified as NSCLC-NOS ⓑ M

* **G9425** Primary lung carcinoma resection report does not document pT category, pN category and for non-small cell lung cancer, histologic type (squamous cell carcinoma,adenocarcinoma) ⓑ M

* **G9426** Improvement in median time from ED arrival to initial ED oral or parenteral pain medication administration performed for ED admitted patients ⓑ M

* **G9427** Improvement in median time from ED arrival to initial ED oral or parenteral pain medication administration not performed for ED admitted patients ⓑ M

* **G9428** Pathology report includes the pT category and a statement on thickness, ulceration and mitotic rate ⓑ M

* **G9429** Documentation of medical reason(s) for not including pT category and a statement on thickness, ulceration and mitotic rate (e.g., negative skin biopsies in a patient with a history of melanoma or other documented medical reasons) ⓑ M

* **G9430** Specimen site other than anatomic cutaneous location ⓑ M

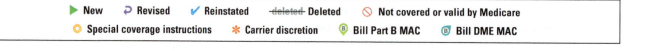

▶ New   ↻ Revised   ✔ Reinstated   ̶d̶e̶l̶e̶t̶e̶d̶ Deleted   ⊘ Not covered or valid by Medicare
⊙ Special coverage instructions   * Carrier discretion   ⓑ Bill Part B MAC   ⓑ Bill DME MAC

* **G9431** Pathology report does not include the pT category and a statement on thickness, ulceration and mitotic rate Ⓑ M

* **G9432** Asthma well-controlled based on the ACT, C-ACT, ACQ, or ATAQ score and results documented Ⓑ M

* **G9434** Asthma not well-controlled based on the ACT, C-ACT, ACQ, or ATAQ score, or specified asthma control tool not used, reason not given Ⓑ M

* **G9448** Patients who were born in the years 1945-1965 Ⓑ M

* **G9449** History of receiving blood transfusions prior to 1992 Ⓑ M

* **G9450** History of injection drug use Ⓑ M

* **G9451** Patient received one-time screening for HCV infection Ⓑ M

* **G9452** Documentation of medical reason(s) for not receiving one-time screening for HCV infection (e.g., decompensated cirrhosis indicating advanced disease [i.e., ascites, esophageal variceal bleeding, hepatic encephalopathy], hepatocellular carcinoma, waitlist for organ transplant, limited life expectancy, other medical reasons) Ⓑ M

* **G9453** Documentation of patient reason(s) for not receiving one-time screening for HCV infection (e.g., patient declined, other patient reasons) Ⓑ M

* **G9454** One-time screening for HCV infection not received within 12 month reporting period and no documentation of prior screening for HCV infection, reason not given Ⓑ M

* **G9455** Patient underwent abdominal imaging with ultrasound, contrast enhanced CT or contrast MRI for HCC Ⓑ M

* **G9456** Documentation of medical or patient reason(s) for not ordering or performing screening for HCC. medical reason: comorbid medical conditions with expected survival <5 years, hepatic decompensation and not a candidate for liver transplantation, or other medical reasons; patient reasons: patient declined or other patient reasons (e.g., cost of tests, time related to accessing testing equipment) Ⓑ M

* **G9457** Patient did not undergo abdominal imaging and did not have a documented reason for not undergoing abdominal imaging in the submission period Ⓑ M

* **G9458** Patient documented as tobacco user and received tobacco cessation intervention (must include at least one of the following: advice given to quit smoking or tobacco use, counseling on the benefits of quitting smoking or tobacco use, assistance with or referral to external smoking or tobacco cessation support programs, or current enrollment in smoking or tobacco use cessation program) if identified as a tobacco user Ⓑ M

* **G9459** Currently a tobacco non-user Ⓑ M

* **G9460** Tobacco assessment or tobacco cessation intervention not performed, reason not given Ⓑ M

* **G9468** Patient not receiving corticosteroids greater than or equal to 10 mg/day of prednisone equivalents for 60 or greater consecutive days or a single prescription equating to 600 mg prednisone or greater for all fills Ⓑ M

↻ * **G9469** Patients who have received or are receiving corticosteroids greater than or equal to 10 mg/day of prednisone equivalents for 90 or greater consecutive days or a single prescription equating to 900 mg prednisone or greater for all fills Ⓑ M

* **G9470** Patients not receiving corticosteroids greater than or equal to 10 mg/day of prednisone equivalents for 60 or greater consecutive days or a single prescription equating to 600 mg prednisone or greater for all fills Ⓑ M

* **G9471** Within the past 2 years, central dual-energy x-ray absorptiometry (DXA) not ordered or documented Ⓑ M

~~G9472~~ ~~Within the past 2 years, central dual-energy x-ray absorptiometry (DXA) not ordered and documented, no review of systems and no medication history or pharmacologic therapy (other than minerals/vitamins) for osteoporosis prescribed~~ ✖

* **G9473** Services performed by chaplain in the hospice setting, each 15 minutes Ⓑ B

* **G9474** Services performed by dietary counselor in the hospice setting, each 15 minutes Ⓑ B

* **G9475** Services performed by other counselor in the hospice setting, each 15 minutes Ⓑ B

* **G9476** Services performed by volunteer in the hospice setting, each 15 minutes Ⓑ B

| 🐾 MIPS | 🅞🅟 Quantity Physician | 🅞🅗 Quantity Hospital | ♀ Female only |
| ♂ Male only | 🅐 Age | ♿ DMEPOS | A2-Z3 ASC Payment Indicator | A-Y ASC Status Indicator | Coding Clinic |

TEMPORARY PROCEDURES/PROFESSIONAL SERVICES    G9431 — G9476

271

\* **G9477** Services performed by care coordinator in the hospice setting, each 15 minutes Ⓑ      **B**

\* **G9478** Services performed by other qualified therapist in the hospice setting, each 15 minutes Ⓑ      **B**

\* **G9479** Services performed by qualified pharmacist in the hospice setting, each 15 minutes Ⓑ      **B**

\* **G9480** Admission to Medicare Care Choice Model program (MCCM) Ⓑ **Qp** **Qh**      **B**

\* **G9481** Remote in-home visit for the evaluation and management of a new patient for use only in the Medicare-approved comprehensive care for joint replacement model, which requires these 3 key components: a problem focused history; a problem focused examination; and straightforward medical decision making, furnished in real time using interactive audio and video technology. Counseling and coordination of care with other physicians, other qualified health care professionals or agencies are provided consistent with the nature of the problem(s) and the needs of the patient or the family or both. Usually, the presenting problem(s) are self limited or minor. Typically, 10 minutes are spent with the patient or family or both via real time, audio and video intercommunications technology Ⓑ      **B**

\* **G9482** Remote in-home visit for the evaluation and management of a new patient for use only in the Medicare-approved comprehensive care for joint replacement model, which requires these 3 key components: an expanded problem focused history; an expanded problem focused examination; straightforward medical decision making, furnished in real time using interactive audio and video technology. Counseling and coordination of care with other physicians, other qualified health care professionals or agencies are provided consistent with the nature of the problem(s) and the needs of the patient or the family or both. Usually, the presenting problem(s) are of low to moderate severity. Typically, 20 minutes are spent with the patient or family or both via real time, audio and video intercommunications technology Ⓑ      **B**

\* **G9483** Remote in-home visit for the evaluation and management of a new patient for use only in the Medicare-approved comprehensive care for joint replacement model, which requires these 3 key components: a detailed history; a detailed examination; medical decision making of low complexity, furnished in real time using interactive audio and video technology. Counseling and coordination of care with other physicians, other qualified health care professionals or agencies are provided consistent with the nature of the problem(s) and the needs of the patient or the family or both. Usually, the presenting problem(s) are of moderate severity. Typically, 30 minutes are spent with the patient or family or both via real time, audio and video intercommunications technology Ⓑ      **B**

\* **G9484** Remote in-home visit for the evaluation and management of a new patient for use only in the Medicare-approved comprehensive care for joint replacement model, which requires these 3 key components: a comprehensive history; a comprehensive examination; medical decision making of moderate complexity, furnished in real time using interactive audio and video technology. Counseling and coordination of care with other physicians, other qualified health care professionals or agencies are provided consistent with the nature of the problem(s) and the needs of the patient or the family or both. Usually, the presenting problem(s) are of moderate to high severity. Typically, 45 minutes are spent with the patient or family or both via real time, audio and video intercommunications technology Ⓑ      **B**

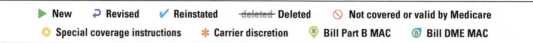

▶ New    ↻ Revised    ✔ Reinstated    ~~deleted~~ Deleted    ⊘ Not covered or valid by Medicare
⊕ Special coverage instructions    \* Carrier discretion    Ⓑ Bill Part B MAC    Ⓓ Bill DME MAC

✳ **G9485** Remote in-home visit for the evaluation and management of a new patient for use only in the Medicare-approved comprehensive care for joint replacement model, which requires these 3 key components: a comprehensive history; a comprehensive examination; medical decision making of high complexity, furnished in real time using interactive audio and video technology. Counseling and coordination of care with other physicians, other qualified health care professionals or agencies are provided consistent with the nature of the problem(s) and the needs of the patient or the family or both. Usually, the presenting problem(s) are of moderate to high severity. Typically, 60 minutes are spent with the patient or family or both via real time, audio and video intercommunications technology ⓑ **B**

✳ **G9486** Remote in-home visit for the evaluation and management of an established patient for use only in the Medicare-approved comprehensive care for joint replacement model, which requires at least 2 of the following 3 key components: a problem focused history; a problem focused examination; straightforward medical decision making, furnished in real time using interactive audio and video technology. Counseling and coordination of care with other physicians, other qualified health care professionals or agencies are provided consistent with the nature of the problem(s) and the needs of the patient or the family or both. Usually, the presenting problem(s) are self limited or minor. Typically, 10 minutes are spent with the patient or family or both via real time, audio and video intercommunications technology ⓑ **B**

✳ **G9487** Remote in-home visit for the evaluation and management of an established patient for use only in the Medicare-approved comprehensive care for joint replacement model, which requires at least 2 of the following 3 key components: an expanded problem focused history; an expanded problem focused examination; medical decision making of low complexity, furnished in real time using interactive audio and video technology. Counseling and coordination of care with other physicians, other qualified health care professionals or agencies are provided consistent with the nature of the problem(s) and the needs of the patient or the family or both. Usually, the presenting problem(s) are of low to moderate severity. Typically, 15 minutes are spent with the patient or family or both via real time, audio and video intercommunications technology ⓑ **B**

✳ **G9488** Remote in-home visit for the evaluation and management of an established patient for use only in the Medicare-approved comprehensive care for joint replacement model, which requires at least 2 of the following 3 key components: a detailed history; a detailed examination; medical decision making of moderate complexity, furnished in real time using interactive audio and video technology. Counseling and coordination of care with other physicians, other qualified health care professionals or agencies are provided consistent with the nature of the problem(s) and the needs of the patient or the family or both. Usually, the presenting problem(s) are of moderate to high severity. Typically, 25 minutes are spent with the patient or family or both via real time, audio and video intercommunications technology ⓑ **B**

| 🦊 MIPS | ⓠ Quantity Physician | ⓠ Quantity Hospital | ♀ Female only |
| ♂ Male only | Ⓐ Age | ♿ DMEPOS | A2-Z3 ASC Payment Indicator | A-Y ASC Status Indicator | Coding Clinic |

* **G9489** Remote in-home visit for the evaluation and management of an established patient for use only in the Medicare-approved comprehensive care for joint replacement model, which requires at least 2 of the following 3 key components: a comprehensive history; a comprehensive examination; medical decision making of high complexity, furnished in real time using interactive audio and video technology. Counseling and coordination of care with other physicians, other qualified health care professionals or agencies are provided consistent with the nature of the problem(s) and the needs of the patient or the family or both. Usually, the presenting problem(s) are of moderate to high severity. Typically, 40 minutes are spent with the patient or family or both via real time, audio and video intercommunications technology ⓑ **B**

* **G9490** Comprehensive care for joint replacement model, home visit for patient assessment performed by clinical staff for an individual not considered homebound, including, but not necessarily limited to patient assessment of clinical status, safety/fall prevention, functional status/ambulation, medication reconciliation/management, compliance with orders/plan of care, performance of activities of daily living, and ensuring beneficiary connections to community and other services. (for use only in the Medicare-approved CJR model); may not be billed for a 30 day period covered by a transitional care management code ⓑ **B**

* **G9497** Received instruction from the anesthesiologist or proxy prior to the day of surgery to abstain from smoking on the day of surgery ⓑ **M**

* **G9498** Antibiotic regimen prescribed ⓑ **M**

* **G9500** Radiation exposure indices, or exposure time and number of fluorographic images in final report for procedures using fluoroscopy, documented ⓑ **M**

* **G9501** Radiation exposure indices, or exposure time and number of fluorographic images not documented in final report for procedure using fluoroscopy, reason not given ⓑ **M**

* **G9502** Documentation of medical reason for not performing foot exam (i.e., patients who have had either a bilateral amputation above or below the knee, or both a left and right amputation above or below the knee before or during the measurement period) ⓑ **M**

* **G9503** Patient taking tamsulosin hydrochloride ⓑ **M**

* **G9504** Documented reason for not assessing Hepatitis B virus (HBV) status (e.g. patient not initiating anti-TNF therapy, patient declined) prior to initiating anti-TNF therapy ⓑ **M**

* **G9505** Antibiotic regimen prescribed within 10 days after onset of symptoms for documented medical reason ⓑ **M**

* **G9506** Biologic immune response modifier prescribed ⓑ **M**

* **G9507** Documentation that the patient is on a statin medication or has documentation of a valid contraindication or exception to statin medications; contraindications/exceptions that can be defined by diagnosis codes include pregnancy during the measurement period, active liver disease, rhabdomyolysis, end stage renal disease on dialysis and heart failure; provider documented contraindications/exceptions include breastfeeding during the measurement period, woman of child-bearing age not actively taking birth control, allergy to statin, drug interaction (HIV protease inhibitors, nefazodone, cyclosporine, gemfibrozil, and danazol) and intolerance (with supporting documentation of trying a statin at least once within the last 5 years or diagnosis codes for myostitis or toxic myopathy related to drugs) ⓑ**M**

* **G9508** Documentation that the patient is not on a statin medication ⓑ **M**

* **G9509** Adult patients 18 years of age or older with major depression or dysthymia who reached remission at 12 months as demonstrated by a 12 month (+/-60 days) PHQ-9 or PHQ-9m score of less than 5 ⓑ **M**

↻ * **G9510** Adult patients 18 years of age or older with major depression or dysthymia who did not reach remission at twelve months as demonstrated by a twelve month (+/-60 days) PHQ-9 or PHQ-9m score of less than 5. Either PHQ-9 or PHQ-9m score was not assessed or is greater than or equal to 5 ⓑ **M**

▶ New    ↻ Revised    ✔ Reinstated    ~~deleted~~ Deleted    ⊘ Not covered or valid by Medicare
✪ Special coverage instructions    * Carrier discretion    ⓑ Bill Part B MAC    ⓑ Bill DME MAC

* **G9511** Index event date PHQ-9 score greater than 9 documented during the 12 month denominator identification period Ⓑ M

* **G9512** Individual had a PDC of 0.8 or greater Ⓑ M

* **G9513** Individual did not have a PDC of 0.8 or greater Ⓑ M

* **G9514** Patient required a return to the operating room within 90 days of surgery Ⓑ M

* **G9515** Patient did not require a return to the operating room within 90 days of surgery Ⓑ M

* **G9516** Patient achieved an improvement in visual acuity, from their preoperative level, within 90 days of surgery Ⓑ M

* **G9517** Patient did not achieve an improvement in visual acuity, from their preoperative level, within 90 days of surgery, reason not given Ⓑ M

* **G9518** Documentation of active injection drug use Ⓑ M

↻ * **G9519** Patient achieves final refraction (spherical equivalent) +/-1.0 diopters of their planned refraction within 90 days of surgery Ⓑ M

↻ * **G9520** Patient does not achieve final refraction (spherical equivalent) +/-1.0 diopters of their planned refraction within 90 days of surgery Ⓑ M

* **G9521** Total number of emergency department visits and inpatient hospitalizations less than two in the past 12 months Ⓑ M

* **G9522** Total number of emergency department visits and inpatient hospitalizations equal to or greater than two in the past 12 months or patient not screened, reason not given Ⓑ M

* **G9523** Patient discontinued from hemodialysis or peritoneal dialysis Ⓑ M

* **G9524** Patient was referred to hospice care Ⓑ M

* **G9525** Documentation of patient reason(s) for not referring to hospice care (e.g., patient declined, other patient reasons) Ⓑ M

* **G9526** Patient was not referred to hospice care, reason not given Ⓑ M

* **G9529** Patient with minor blunt head trauma had an appropriate indication(s) for a head CT Ⓑ M

* **G9530** Patient presented within a minor blunt head trauma and had a head CT ordered for trauma by an emergency care provider Ⓑ M

↻ * **G9531** Patient has documentation of ventricular shunt, brain tumor, multisystem trauma, or is currently taking an antiplatelet medication including: abciximab, anagrelide, cangrelor, cilostazol, clopidogrel, dipyridamole, eptifibatide, prasugrel, ticlopidine, ticagrelor, tirofiban, or vorapaxar Ⓑ M

* **G9532** Patient had a head CT for trauma ordered by someone other than an emergency care provider, or was ordered for a reason other than trauma Ⓑ M

* **G9533** Patient with minor blunt head trauma did not have an appropriate indication(s) for a head CT Ⓑ M

* **G9537** Documentation of system reason(s) for obtaining imaging of the head (CT or MRI) (i.e., needed as part of a clinical trial; other clinician ordered the study) Ⓑ M

* **G9539** Intent for potential removal at time of placement Ⓑ M

* **G9540** Patient alive 3 months post procedure Ⓑ M

* **G9541** Filter removed within 3 months of placement Ⓑ M

* **G9542** Documented re-assessment for the appropriateness of filter removal within 3 months of placement Ⓑ M

* **G9543** Documentation of at least two attempts to reach the patient to arrange a clinical re-assessment for the appropriateness of filter removal within 3 months of placement Ⓑ M

* **G9544** Patients that do not have the filter removed, documented re-assessment for the appropriateness of filter removal, or documentation of at least two attempts to reach the patient to arrange a clinical re-assessment for the appropriateness of filter removal within 3 months of placement Ⓑ M

↻ * **G9547** Cystic renal lesion that is simple appearing (Bosniak I or II), or adrenal lesion less than or equal to 1.0 cm or adrenal lesion greater than 1.0 cm but less than or equal to 4.0 cm classified as likely benign by unenhanced CT or washout protocol CT, or MRI with in- and opposed-phase sequences or other equivalent institutional imaging protocols Ⓑ M

↻ * **G9548** Final reports for imaging studies stating no follow-up imaging is recommended Ⓑ M

---

| 🐾 MIPS | Qp Quantity Physician | Qh Quantity Hospital | ♀ Female only |
|---|---|---|---|
| ♂ Male only | Ⓐ Age | ♿ DMEPOS | A2-Z3 ASC Payment Indicator | A-Y ASC Status Indicator | Coding Clinic |

**G9549** Documentation of medical reason(s) that follow-up imaging is indicated (e.g., patient has lymphadenopathy, signs of metastasis or an active diagnosis or history of cancer, and other medical reason(s)) Ⓑ M

**G9550** Final reports for imaging studies with follow-up imaging recommended Ⓑ M

**G9551** Final reports for imaging studies without an incidentally found lesion noted Ⓑ M

**G9552** Incidental thyroid nodule <1.0 cm noted in report Ⓑ M

**G9553** Prior thyroid disease diagnosis Ⓑ M

**G9554** Final reports for CT, CTA, MRI or MRA of the chest or neck or ultrasound of the neck with follow-up imaging recommended Ⓑ M

**G9555** Documentation of medical reason(s) for recommending follow up imaging (e.g., patient has multiple endocrine neoplasia, patient has cervical lymphadenopathy, other medical reason(s)) Ⓑ M

**G9556** Final reports for CT, CTA, MRI or MRA of the chest or neck or ultrasound of the neck with follow-up imaging not recommended Ⓑ M

**G9557** Final reports for CT, CTA, MRI or MRA studies of the chest or neck or ultrasound of the neck without an incidentally found thyroid nodule <1.0 cm noted or no nodule found Ⓑ M

**G9558** Patient treated with a beta-lactam antibiotic as definitive therapy Ⓑ M

**G9559** Documentation of medical reason(s) for not prescribing a beta-lactam antibiotic (e.g., allergy, intolerance to beta-lactam antibiotics) Ⓑ M

**G9560** Patient not treated with a beta-lactam antibiotic as definitive therapy, reason not given Ⓑ M

**G9561** Patients prescribed opiates for longer than six weeks Ⓑ M

**G9562** Patients who had a follow-up evaluation conducted at least every three months during opioid therapy Ⓑ M

**G9563** Patients who did not have a follow-up evaluation conducted at least every three months during opioid therapy Ⓑ M

**G9573** Adult patients 18 years of age or older with major depression or dysthymia who did not reach remission at six months as demonstrated by a six month (+/-60 days) PHQ-9 or PHQ-9m score of less than five Ⓑ M

**G9574** Adult patients 18 years of age or older with major depression or dysthymia who did not reach remission at six months as demonstrated by a six month (+/-60 days) PHQ-9 or PHQ-9m score of less than five; either PHQ-9 or PHQ-9m score was not assessed or is greater than or equal to five Ⓑ M

**G9577** Patients prescribed opiates for longer than six weeks Ⓑ M

**G9578** Documentation of signed opioid treatment agreement at least once during opioid therapy Ⓑ M

**G9579** No documentation of signed an opioid treatment agreement at least once during opioid therapy Ⓑ M

**G9580** Door to puncture time of less than 2 hours Ⓑ M

**G9582** Door to puncture time of greater than 2 hours, no reason given Ⓑ M

**G9583** Patients prescribed opiates for longer than 6 weeks Ⓑ M

**G9584** Patient evaluated for risk of misuse of opiates by using a brief validated instrument (e.g., opioid risk tool, SOAPP-R) or patient interviewed at least once during opioid therapy Ⓑ M

**G9585** Patient not evaluated for risk of misuse of opiates by using a brief validated instrument (e.g., opioid risk tool, SOAPP-R) or patient not interviewed at least once during opioid therapy Ⓑ M

**G9593** Pediatric patient with minor blunt head trauma classified as low risk according to the pecarn Prediction Rules Ⓑ Ⓐ M

**G9594** Patient presented with a minor blunt head trauma and had a head CT ordered for trauma by an emergency care provider Ⓑ M

**G9595** Patient has documentation of ventricular shunt, brain tumor, or coagulopathy Ⓑ M

**G9596** Pediatric patient had a head CT for trauma ordered by someone other than an emergency care provider, or was ordered for a reason other than trauma Ⓑ Ⓐ M

▶ New  ↵ Revised  ✔ Reinstated  ~~deleted~~ Deleted  ⊘ Not covered or valid by Medicare
Ⓞ Special coverage instructions  ✳ Carrier discretion  Ⓑ Bill Part B MAC  Ⓑ Bill DME MAC

✻ **G9597** Pediatric patient with minor blunt head trauma not classified as low risk according to the pecarn Prediction Rules ⑧ Ⓐ M

✻ **G9598** Aortic aneurysm 5.5-5.9 cm maximum diameter on centerline formatted CT or minor diameter on axial formatted CT ⑧ M

✻ **G9599** Aortic aneurysm 6.0 cm or greater maximum diameter on centerline formatted CT or minor diameter on axial formatted CT ⑧ M

✻ **G9600** Symptomatic AAAS that required urgent/emergent (non-elective) repair ⑧ M

✻ **G9601** Patient discharge to home no later than post-operative day #7 ⑧ M

✻ **G9602** Patient not discharged to home by post-operative day #7 ⑧ M

✻ **G9603** Patient survey score improved from baseline following treatment ⑧ M

✻ **G9604** Patient survey results not available ⑧ M

✻ **G9605** Patient survey score did not improve from baseline following treatment ⑧ M

✻ **G9606** Intraoperative cystoscopy performed to evaluate for lower tract injury ⑧ M

✻ **G9607** Documented medical reasons for not performing intraoperative cystoscopy (e.g., urethral pathology precluding cystoscopy, any patient who has a congenital or acquired absence of the urethra) or in the case of patient death ⑧ M

✻ **G9608** Intraoperative cystoscopy not performed to evaluate for lower tract injury ⑧ M

✻ **G9609** Documentation of an order for anti-platelet agents ⑧ M

✻ **G9610** Documentation of medical reason(s) in the patient's record for not ordering anti-platelet agents ⑧ M

✻ **G9611** Order for anti-platelet agents was not documented in the patient's record, reason not given ⑧ M

✻ **G9612** Photodocumentation of two or more cecal landmarks to establish a complete examination ⑧ M

✻ **G9613** Documentation of post-surgical anatomy (e.g., right hemicolectomy, ileocecal resection, etc.) ⑧ M

✻ **G9614** Photodocumentation of less than two cecal landmarks (i.e., no cecal landmarks or only one cecal landmark) to establish a complete examination ⑧ M

✻ **G9615** Preoperative assessment documented ⑧ M

✻ **G9616** Documentation of reason(s) for not documenting a preoperative assessment (e.g., patient with a gynecologic or other pelvic malignancy noted at the time of surgery) ⑧ M

✻ **G9617** Preoperative assessment not documented, reason not given ⑧ M

✻ **G9618** Documentation of screening for uterine malignancy or those that had an ultrasound and/or endometrial sampling of any kind ⑧ M

✻ **G9620** Patient not screened for uterine malignancy, or those that have not had an ultrasound and/or endometrial sampling of any kind, reason not given ⑧ M

✻ **G9621** Patient identified as an unhealthy alcohol user when screened for unhealthy alcohol use using a systematic screening method and received brief counseling ⑧ M

✻ **G9622** Patient not identified as an unhealthy alcohol user when screened for unhealthy alcohol use using a systematic screening method ⑧ M

✻ **G9623** Documentation of medical reason(s) for not screening for unhealthy alcohol use (e.g., limited life expectancy, other medical reasons) ⑧ M

✻ **G9624** Patient not screened for unhealthy alcohol use using a systematic screening method or patient did not receive brief counseling if identified as an unhealthy alcohol user, reason not given ⑧ M

✻ **G9625** Patient sustained bladder injury at the time of surgery or discovered subsequently up to 30 days post-surgery ⑧ M

✻ **G9626** Documented medical reason for reporting bladder injury (e.g., gynecologic or other pelvic malignancy documented, concurrent surgery involving bladder pathology, injury that occurs during urinary incontinence procedure, patient death from non-medical causes not related to surgery, patient died during procedure without evidence of bladder injury) ⑧ M

🐾 MIPS  Ⓠp Quantity Physician  Ⓠh Quantity Hospital  ♀ Female only
♂ Male only  Ⓐ Age  DMEPOS  A2-Z3 ASC Payment Indicator  A-Y ASC Status Indicator  Coding Clinic

* **G9627** Patient did not sustain bladder injury at the time of surgery nor discovered subsequently up to 30 days post-surgery ⑧ M

* **G9628** Patient sustained bowel injury at the time of surgery or discovered subsequently up to 30 days post-surgery ⑧ M

* **G9629** Documented medical reasons for not reporting bowel injury (e.g., gynecologic or other pelvic malignancy documented, planned (e.g., not due to an unexpected bowel injury) resection and/or re-anastomosis of bowel, or patient death from non-medical causes not related to surgery, patient died during procedure without evidence of bowel injury) ⑧ M

* **G9630** Patient did not sustain a bowel injury at the time of surgery nor discovered subsequently up to 30 days post-surgery ⑧ M

* **G9631** Patient sustained ureter injury at the time of surgery or discovered subsequently up to 30 days post-surgery ⑧ M

* **G9632** Documented medical reasons for not reporting ureter injury (e.g., gynecologic or other pelvic malignancy documented, concurrent surgery involving bladder pathology, injury that occurs during a urinary incontinence procedure, patient death from non-medical causes not related to surgery, patient died during procedure without evidence of ureter injury) ⑧ M

* **G9633** Patient did not sustain ureter injury at the time of surgery nor discovered subsequently up to 30 days post-surgery ⑧ M

* **G9634** Health-related quality of life assessed with tool during at least two visits and quality of life score remained the same or improved ⑧ M

* **G9635** Health-related quality of life not assessed with tool for documented reason(s) (e.g., patient has a cognitive or neuropsychiatric impairment that impairs his/her ability to complete the HRQOL survey, patient has the inability to read and/or write in order to complete the HRQOL questionnaire) ⑧ M

* **G9636** Health-related quality of life not assessed with tool during at least two visits or quality of life score declined ⑧ M

* **G9637** At least two orders for the same high-risk medications ⑧ M

* **G9638** At least two orders for the same high-risk medications not ordered ⑧ M

* **G9639** Major amputation or open surgical bypass not required within 48 hours of the index endovascular lower extremity revascularization procedure ⑧ M

* **G9640** Documentation of planned hybrid or staged procedure ⑧ M

* **G9641** Major amputation or open surgical bypass required within 48 hours of the index endovascular lower extremity revascularization procedure ⑧ M

* **G9642** Current smokers (e.g., cigarette, cigar, pipe, e-cigarette or marijuana) ⑧ M

* **G9643** Elective surgery ⑧ M

* **G9644** Patients who abstained from smoking prior to anesthesia on the day of surgery or procedure ⑧ M

* **G9645** Patients who did not abstain from smoking prior to anesthesia on the day of surgery or procedure ⑧ M

* **G9646** Patients with 90 day MRS score of 0 to 2 ⑧ M

* **G9647** Patients in whom MRS score could not be obtained at 90 day follow-up ⑧ M

* **G9648** Patients with 90 day MRS score greater than 2 ⑧ M

* **G9649** Psoriasis assessment tool documented meeting any one of the specified benchmarks (e.g., PGA; 5-point or 6-point scale), body surface area (BSA), psoriasis area and severity index (PASI) and/or dermatology life quality index) (DLQI)) ⑧ M

* **G9651** Psoriasis assessment tool documented not meeting any one of the specified benchmarks (e.g., (pga; 5-point or 6-point scale), body surface area (bsa), psoriasis area and severity index (pasi) and/or dermatology life quality index) (dlqi)) or psoriasis assessment tool not documented ⑧ M

* **G9654** Monitored anesthesia care (mac) ⑧ M

* **G9655** A transfer of care protocol or handoff tool/checklist that includes the required key handoff elements is used ⑧ M

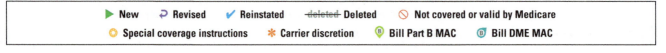

▶ New   ↩ Revised   ✔ Reinstated   ~~deleted~~ Deleted   ⃠ Not covered or valid by Medicare

⊙ Special coverage instructions   ✳ Carrier discretion   Ⓑ Bill Part B MAC   Ⓑ Bill DME MAC

✱ **G9656** Patient transferred directly from anesthetizing location to PACU or other non-ICU location ⓑ     M

✱ **G9658** A transfer of care protocol or handoff tool/checklist that includes the required key handoff elements is not used ⓑ   M

✱ **G9659** Patients greater than 85 years of age who did not have a history of colorectal cancer or valid medical reason for the colonoscopy, including: iron deficiency anemia, lower gastrointestinal bleeding, Crohn's Disease (i.e., regional enteritis), familial adenomatous polyposis, lynch syndrome (i.e., hereditary non-polyposis colorectal cancer), inflammatory bowel disease, ulcerative colitis, abnormal finding of gastrointestinal tract, or changes in bowel habits ⓑ   M

✱ **G9660** Documentation of medical reason(s) for a colonoscopy performed on a patient greater than 85 years of age (e.g., last colonoscopy incomplete, last colonoscopy had inadequate prep, iron deficiency anemia, lower gastrointestinal bleeding, Crohn's Disease (i.e., regional enteritis), familial history of adenomatous polyposis, lynch syndrome (i.e., hereditary non-polyposis colorectal cancer), inflammatory bowel disease, ulcerative colitis, abnormal finding of gastrointestinal tract, or changes in bowel habits) ⓑ   M

✱ **G9661** Patients greater than 85 years of age who received a routine colonoscopy for a reason other than the following: an assessment of signs/symptoms of GI tract illness, and/or the patient is considered high risk, and/or to follow-up on previously diagnosed advance lesions ⓑ   M

✱ **G9662** Previously diagnosed or have an active diagnosis of clinical ascvd ⓟ   M

↻ ✱ **G9663** Any fasting or direct ldl-c laboratory test result <=190 mg/dL ⓑ   M

✱ **G9664** Patients who are currently statin therapy users or received an order (prescription) for statin therapy ⓑ   M

✱ **G9665** Patients who are not currently statin therapy users or did not receive an order (prescription) for statin therapy ⓟ   M

✱ **G9666** The highest fasting or direct ldl-c laboratory test result of 70-189 mg/dL in the measurement period or two years prior to the beginning of the measurement period ⓟ   M

✱ **G9674** Patients with clinical ascvd diagnosis ⓟ   M

✱ **G9675** Patients who have ever had a fasting or direct laboratory result of ldl-c = 190 mg/dl ⓑ   M

✱ **G9676** Patients aged 40 to 75 years at the beginning of the measurement period with type 1 or type 2 diabetes and with an ldl-c result of 70-189 mg/dl recorded as the highest fasting or direct laboratory test result in the measurement year or during the two years prior to the beginning of the measurement period ⓑ   M

✱ **G9678** Oncology care model (OCM) monthly enhanced oncology services (MEOS) payment for OCM enhanced services. G9678 payments may only be made to OCM practitioners for ocm beneficiaries for the furnishment of enhanced services as defined in the OCM participation agreement ⓑ Qp Qh   B

✱ **G9679** This code is for onsite acute care treatment of a nursing facility resident with pneumonia; may only be billed once per day per beneficiary ⓟ   B

✱ **G9680** This code is for onsite acute care treatment of a nursing facility resident with CHF; may only be billed once per day per beneficiary ⓑ   B

✱ **G9681** This code is for onsite acute care treatment of a resident with COPD or asthma; may only be billed once per day per beneficiary ⓟ   B

✱ **G9682** This code is for the onsite acute care treatment a nursing facility resident with a skin infection; may only be billed once per day per beneficiary ⓟ   B

✱ **G9683** Facility service(s) for the onsite acute care treatment of a nursing facility resident with fluid or electrolyte disorder. (May only be billed once per day per beneficiary). This service is for a demonstration project. ⓑ   B

✱ **G9684** This code is for the onsite acute care treatment of a nursing facility resident for a UTI; may only be billed once per day per beneficiary ⓟ   B

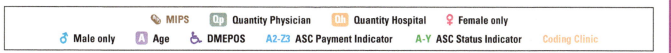

🐾 MIPS    Qp Quantity Physician    Qh Quantity Hospital    ♀ Female only

♂ Male only    Ⓐ Age    ♿ DMEPOS    A2-Z3 ASC Payment Indicator    A-Y ASC Status Indicator    Coding Clinic

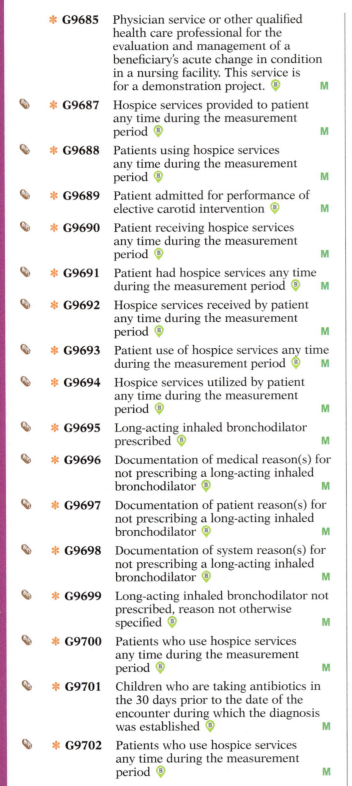

* **G9685** Physician service or other qualified health care professional for the evaluation and management of a beneficiary's acute change in condition in a nursing facility. This service is for a demonstration project. Ⓑ M

* **G9687** Hospice services provided to patient any time during the measurement period Ⓑ M

* **G9688** Patients using hospice services any time during the measurement period Ⓑ M

* **G9689** Patient admitted for performance of elective carotid intervention Ⓑ M

* **G9690** Patient receiving hospice services any time during the measurement period Ⓑ M

* **G9691** Patient had hospice services any time during the measurement period Ⓑ M

* **G9692** Hospice services received by patient any time during the measurement period Ⓑ M

* **G9693** Patient use of hospice services any time during the measurement period Ⓑ M

* **G9694** Hospice services utilized by patient any time during the measurement period Ⓑ M

* **G9695** Long-acting inhaled bronchodilator prescribed Ⓑ M

* **G9696** Documentation of medical reason(s) for not prescribing a long-acting inhaled bronchodilator Ⓑ M

* **G9697** Documentation of patient reason(s) for not prescribing a long-acting inhaled bronchodilator Ⓑ M

* **G9698** Documentation of system reason(s) for not prescribing a long-acting inhaled bronchodilator Ⓑ M

* **G9699** Long-acting inhaled bronchodilator not prescribed, reason not otherwise specified Ⓑ M

* **G9700** Patients who use hospice services any time during the measurement period Ⓑ M

* **G9701** Children who are taking antibiotics in the 30 days prior to the date of the encounter during which the diagnosis was established Ⓑ M

* **G9702** Patients who use hospice services any time during the measurement period Ⓑ M

* **G9703** Children who are taking antibiotics in the 30 days prior to the diagnosis of pharyngitis Ⓑ M

* **G9704** AJCC breast cancer stage I: T1 mic or T1a documented Ⓑ M

* **G9705** AJCC breast cancer stage I: T1b (tumor >0.5 cm but <=1 cm in greatest dimension) documented Ⓑ M

* **G9706** Low (or very low) risk of recurrence, prostate cancer Ⓑ M

* **G9707** Patient received hospice services any time during the measurement period Ⓑ M

* **G9708** Women who had a bilateral mastectomy or who have a history of a bilateral mastectomy or for whom there is evidence of a right and a left unilateral mastectomy Ⓑ M

* **G9709** Hospice services used by patient any time during the measurement period Ⓑ M

* **G9710** Patient was provided hospice services any time during the measurement period Ⓑ M

* **G9711** Patients with a diagnosis or past history of total colectomy or colorectal cancer Ⓑ M

* **G9712** Documentation of medical reason(s) for prescribing or dispensing antibiotic (e.g., intestinal infection, pertussis, bacterial infection, Lyme disease, otitis media, acute sinusitis, acute pharyngitis, acute tonsillitis, chronic sinusitis, infection of the pharynx/larynx/tonsils/adenoids, prostatitis, cellulitis/ mastoiditis/bone infections, acute lymphadenitis, impetigo, skin staph infections, pneumonia, gonococcal infections/venereal disease/ syphilis, chlamydia, inflammatory diseases, female reproductive organs), infections of the kidney, cystitis/UTI, acne, HIV disease/asymptomatic HIV, cystic fibrosis, disorders of the immune system, malignancy neoplasms, chronic bronchitis, emphysema, bronchiectasis, extrinsic allergic alveolitis, chronic airway obstruction, chronic obstructive asthma, pneumoconiosis and other lung disease due to external agents, other diseases of the respiratory system, and tuberculosis Ⓑ M

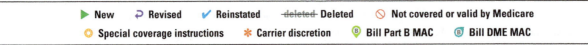

▶ New    ↻ Revised    ✓ Reinstated    ~~deleted~~ Deleted    ⊘ Not covered or valid by Medicare

⬡ Special coverage instructions    * Carrier discretion    Ⓑ Bill Part B MAC    Ⓑ Bill DME MAC

**G9713** Patients who use hospice services any time during the measurement period ⓑ M

**G9714** Patient is using hospice services any time during the measurement period ⓑ M

**G9715** Patients who use hospice services any time during the measurement period ⓑ M

**G9716** BMI is documented as being outside of normal limits, follow-up plan is not completed for documented reason ⓑ M

**G9717** Documentation stating the patient has an active diagnosis of depression or has a diagnosed bipolar disorder, therefore screening or follow-up not required ⓑ M

**G9718** Hospice services for patient provided any time during the measurement period ⓑ M

**G9719** Patient is not ambulatory, bed ridden, immobile, confined to chair, wheelchair bound, dependent on helper pushing wheelchair, independent in wheelchair or minimal help in wheelchair ⓑ M

**G9720** Hospice services for patient occurred any time during the measurement period ⓑ M

**G9721** Patient not ambulatory, bed ridden, immobile, confined to chair, wheelchair bound, dependent on helper pushing wheelchair, independent in wheelchair or minimal help in wheelchair ⓑ M

**G9722** Documented history of renal failure or baseline serum creatinine = 4.0 mg/dl; renal transplant recipients are not considered to have preoperative renal failure, unless, since transplantation the CR has been or is 4.0 or higher ⓑ M

**G9723** Hospice services for patient received any time during the measurement period ⓑ M

**G9724** Patients who had documentation of use of anticoagulant medications overlapping the measurement year ⓑ M

**G9725** Patients who use hospice services any time during the measurement period ⓑ M

**G9726** Patient refused to participate ⓑ M

**G9727** Patient unable to complete the knee FS prom at initial evaluation and/or discharge due to blindness, illiteracy, severe mental incapacity or language incompatibility and an adequate proxy is not available ⓑ M

**G9728** Patient refused to participate ⓑ M

**G9729** Patient unable to complete the hip FS prom at initial evaluation and/or discharge due to blindness, illiteracy, severe mental incapacity or language incompatibility and an adequate proxy is not available ⓑ M

**G9730** Patient refused to participate ⓑ M

**G9731** Patient unable to complete the foot/ankle FS prom at initial evaluation and/or discharge due to blindness, illiteracy, severe mental incapacity or language incompatibility and an adequate proxy is not available ⓑ M

**G9732** Patient refused to participate ⓑ M

**G9733** Patient unable to complete the low back FS prom at initial evaluation and/or discharge due to blindness, illiteracy, severe mental incapacity or language incompatibility and an adequate proxy is not available ⓑ M

**G9734** Patient refused to participate ⓑ M

**G9735** Patient unable to complete the shoulder FS prom at initial evaluation and/or discharge due to blindness, illiteracy, severe mental incapacity or language incompatibility and an adequate proxy is not available ⓑ M

**G9736** Patient refused to participate ⓑ M

**G9737** Patient unable to complete the elbow/wrist/hand FS prom at initial evaluation and/or discharge due to blindness, illiteracy, severe mental incapacity or language incompatibility and an adequate proxy is not available ⓑ M

**G9738** Patient refused to participate ⓑ M

**G9739** Patient unable to complete the general orthopedic FS prom at initial evaluation and/or discharge due to blindness, illiteracy, severe mental incapacity or language incompatibility and an adequate proxy is not available ⓑ M

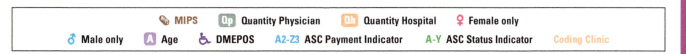

🐾 MIPS  Qp Quantity Physician  Qh Quantity Hospital  ♀ Female only  ♂ Male only  A Age  ♿ DMEPOS  A2-Z3 ASC Payment Indicator  A-Y ASC Status Indicator  Coding Clinic

* G9740 Hospice services given to patient any time during the measurement period Ⓑ M

* G9741 Patients who use hospice services any time during the measurement period Ⓑ M

~~G9742 Psychiatric symptoms assessed~~ ✖

~~G9743 Psychiatric symptoms not assessed, reason not otherwise specified~~ ✖

* G9744 Patient not eligible due to active diagnosis of hypertension Ⓑ M

* G9745 Documented reason for not screening or recommending a follow-up for high blood pressure Ⓑ M

* G9746 Patient has mitral stenosis or prosthetic heart valves or patient has transient or reversible cause of AF (e.g., pneumonia, hyperthyroidism, pregnancy, cardiac surgery) Ⓑ M

* G9747 Patient is undergoing palliative dialysis with a catheter Ⓑ M

* G9748 Patient approved by a qualified transplant program and scheduled to receive a living donor kidney transplant Ⓑ M

* G9749 Patient is undergoing palliative dialysis with a catheter Ⓑ M

* G9750 Patient approved by a qualified transplant program and scheduled to receive a living donor kidney transplant Ⓑ M

* G9751 Patient died at any time during the 24-month measurement period Ⓑ M

* G9752 Emergency surgery Ⓑ M

* G9753 Documentation of medical reason for not conducting a search for DICOM format images for prior patient CT imaging studies completed at non-affiliated external healthcare facilities or entities within the past 12 months that are available through a secure, authorized, media-free, shared archive (e.g., trauma, acute myocardial infarction, stroke, aortic aneurysm where time is of the essence) Ⓑ M

* G9754 A finding of an incidental pulmonary nodule Ⓑ M

* G9755 Documentation of medical reason(s) for not including a recommended interval and modality for follow-up or for no follow-up, and source of recommendations (e.g., patients with unexplained fever, immunocompromised patients who are at risk for infection) Ⓑ M

* G9756 Surgical procedures that included the use of silicone oil Ⓑ M

* G9757 Surgical procedures that included the use of silicone oil Ⓑ M

* G9758 Patient in hospice at any time during the measurement period Ⓑ M

* G9759 History of preoperative posterior capsule rupture Ⓑ M

* G9760 Patients who use hospice services any time during the measurement period Ⓑ M

* G9761 Patients who use hospice services any time during the measurement period Ⓑ M

* G9762 Patient had at least two HPV vaccines (with at least 146 days between the two) or three HPV vaccines on or between the patient's 9th and 13th birthdays Ⓑ M

* G9763 Patient did not have at least two HPV vaccines (with at least 146 days between the two) or three HPV vaccines on or between the patient's 9th and 13th birthdays Ⓑ M

* G9764 Patient has been treated with systemic medication for psoriasis vulgaris Ⓑ M

* G9765 Documentation that the patient declined change in medication or alternative therapies were unavailable, has documented contraindications, or has not been treated with systemic for at least six consecutive months (e.g., experienced adverse effects or lack of efficacy with all other therapy options) in order to achieve better disease control as measured by PGA, BSA, PASI, or DLQI Ⓑ M

* G9766 Patients who are transferred from one institution to another with a known diagnosis of CVA for endovascular stroke treatment Ⓑ M

* G9767 Hospitalized patients with newly diagnosed CVA considered for endovascular stroke treatment Ⓑ M

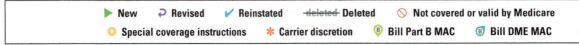

▶ New   ↻ Revised   ✔ Reinstated   ~~deleted~~ Deleted   ⊘ Not covered or valid by Medicare
✪ Special coverage instructions   * Carrier discretion   Ⓑ Bill Part B MAC   Ⓓ Bill DME MAC

* **G9768** Patients who utilize hospice services any time during the measurement period Ⓑ M

* **G9769** Patient had a bone mineral density test in the past two years or received osteoporosis medication or therapy in the past 12 months Ⓑ M

* **G9770** Peripheral nerve block (PNB) Ⓑ M

* **G9771** At least 1 body temperature measurement equal to or greater than 35.5 degrees Celsius (or 95.9 degrees Fahrenheit) achieved within the 30 minutes immediately before or the 15 minutes immediately after anesthesia end time Ⓑ M

↻ * **G9772** Documentation of medical reason(s) for not achieving at least 1 body temperature measurement equal to or greater than 35.5 degrees Celsius (or 95.9 degrees Fahrenheit) within the 30 minutes immediately before or the 15 minutes immediately after anesthesia end time (e.g., emergency cases, intentional hypothermia, etc.) Ⓑ M

* **G9773** At least 1 body temperature measurement equal to or greater than 35.5 degrees Celsius (or 95.9 degrees Fahrenheit) not achieved within the 30 minutes immediately before or the 15 minutes immediately after anesthesia end time, reason not given Ⓑ M

* **G9774** Patients who have had a hysterectomy Ⓑ M

* **G9775** Patient received at least 2 prophylactic pharmacologic anti-emetic agents of different classes preoperatively and/or intraoperatively Ⓑ M

* **G9776** Documentation of medical reason for not receiving at least 2 prophylactic pharmacologic anti-emetic agents of different classes preoperatively and/or intraoperatively (e.g., intolerance or other medical reason) Ⓑ M

* **G9777** Patient did not receive at least 2 prophylactic pharmacologic anti-emetic agents of different classes preoperatively and/or intraoperatively Ⓑ M

* **G9778** Patients who have a diagnosis of pregnancy Ⓑ M

* **G9779** Patients who are breastfeeding Ⓑ M

* **G9780** Patients who have a diagnosis of rhabdomyolysis Ⓑ M

↻ * **G9781** Documentation of medical reason(s) for not currently being a statin therapy user or receive an order (prescription) for statin therapy (e.g., patient with adverse effect, allergy or intolerance to statin medication therapy, patients who are receiving palliative care or hospice care, patients with active liver disease or hepatic disease or insufficiency, and patients with end stage renal disease [ESRD]) Ⓑ M

* **G9782** History of or active diagnosis of familial or pure hypercholesterolemia Ⓑ M

* **G9783** Documentation of patients with diabetes who have a most recent fasting or direct LDL-C laboratory test result <70 mg/dl and are not taking statin therapy Ⓑ M

* **G9784** Pathologists/dermatopathologists providing a second opinion on a biopsy Ⓑ M

↻ * **G9785** Pathology report diagnosing cutaneous basal cell carcinoma, squamous cell carcinoma, or melanoma (to include in situ disease) sent from the pathologist/dermatopathologist to the biopsying clinician for review within 7 days from the time when the tissue specimen was received by the pathologist Ⓑ M

↻ * **G9786** Pathology report diagnosing cutaneous basal cell carcinoma, squamous cell carcinoma, or melanoma (to include in situ disease) was not sent from the pathologist/dermatopathologist to the biopsying clinician for review within 7 days from the time when the tissue specimen was received by the pathologist Ⓑ M

* **G9787** Patient alive as of the last day of the measurement year Ⓑ M

* **G9788** Most recent bp is less than or equal to 140/90 mm hg Ⓑ M

* **G9789** Blood pressure recorded during inpatient stays, emergency room visits, urgent care visits, and patient self-reported BP's (home and health fair BP results) Ⓑ M

* **G9790** Most recent BP is greater than 140/90 mm hg, or blood pressure not documented Ⓑ M

* **G9791** Most recent tobacco status is tobacco free Ⓑ M

🏷 MIPS    Ⓞᵖ Quantity Physician    Ⓞₕ Quantity Hospital    ♀ Female only
♂ Male only    Ⓐ Age    ♿ DMEPOS    A2-Z3 ASC Payment Indicator    A-Y ASC Status Indicator    Coding Clinic

* **G9792** Most recent tobacco status is not tobacco free ⓑ M

* **G9793** Patient is currently on a daily aspirin or other antiplatelet ⓑ M

* **G9794** Documentation of medical reason(s) for not on a daily aspirin or other antiplatelet (e.g., history of gastrointestinal bleed, intra-cranial bleed, idiopathic thrombocytopenic purpura (ITP), gastric bypass or documentation of active anticoagulant use during the measurement period) ⓑ M

* **G9795** Patient is not currently on a daily aspirin or other antiplatelet ⓑ M

* **G9796** Patient is currently on a statin therapy ⓑ M

* **G9797** Patient is not on a statin therapy ⓑ M

↻ * **G9798** Discharge(s) for AMI between July 1 of the year prior measurement period year to June 30 of the measurement period ⓑ M

* **G9799** Patients with a medication dispensing event indicator of a history of asthma any time during the patient's history through the end of the measure period ⓑ M

* **G9800** Patients who are identified as having an intolerance or allergy to beta-blocker therapy ⓑ M

* **G9801** Hospitalizations in which the patient was transferred directly to a non-acute care facility for any diagnosis ⓑ M

* **G9802** Patients who use hospice services any time during the measurement period ⓑ M

* **G9803** Patient prescribed at least a 135 day treatment within the 180-day course of treatment with beta-blockers post discharge for AMI ⓑ M

* **G9804** Patient was not prescribed at least a 135 day treatment within the 180-day course of treatment with beta-blockers post discharge for AMI ⓑ M

* **G9805** Patients who use hospice services any time during the measurement period ⓑ M

* **G9806** Patients who received cervical cytology or an HPV test ⓑ M

* **G9807** Patients who did not receive cervical cytology or an HPV test ⓑ M

* **G9808** Any patients who had no asthma controller medications dispensed during the measurement year ⓑ M

* **G9809** Patients who use hospice services any time during the measurement period ⓑ M

* **G9810** Patient achieved a pDC of at least 75% for their asthma controller medication ⓑ M

* **G9811** Patient did not achieve a pDC of at least 75% for their asthma controller medication ⓑ M

* **G9812** Patient died including all deaths occurring during the hospitalization in which the operation was performed, even if after 30 days, and those deaths occurring after discharge from the hospital, but within 30 days of the procedure ⓟ M

* **G9813** Patient did not die within 30 days of the procedure or during the index hospitalization ⓑ M

* **G9814** Death occurring during the index acute care hospitalization ⓑ M

* **G9815** Death did not occur during the index acute care hospitalization ⓑ M

* **G9816** Death occurring after discharge from the hospital but within 30 days post procedure ⓑ M

* **G9817** Death did not occur after discharge from the hospital within 30 days post procedure ⓟ M

* **G9818** Documentation of sexual activity ⓑ M

* **G9819** Patients who use hospice services any time during the measurement period ⓑ M

* **G9820** Documentation of a chlamydia screening test with proper follow-up ⓑ M

* **G9821** No documentation of a chlamydia screening test with proper follow-up ⓑ M

* **G9822** Women who had an endometrial ablation procedure during the year prior to the index date (exclusive of the index date) ⓟ M

* **G9823** Endometrial sampling or hysteroscopy with biopsy and results documented ⓟ M

* **G9824** Endometrial sampling or hysteroscopy with biopsy and results not documented ⓑ M

---

| ▶ New | ↻ Revised | ✔ Reinstated | deleted Deleted | ⊘ Not covered or valid by Medicare |
| Special coverage instructions | * Carrier discretion | ⓟ Bill Part B MAC | ⓑ Bill DME MAC |

* **G9825** HER-2/neu negative or undocumented/unknown Ⓑ M

* **G9826** Patient transferred to practice after initiation of chemotherapy Ⓑ M

* **G9827** HER2-targeted therapies not administered during the initial course of treatment Ⓑ M

* **G9828** HER2-targeted therapies administered during the initial course of treatment Ⓑ M

* **G9829** Breast adjuvant chemotherapy administered Ⓑ M

* **G9830** HER-2/neu positive Ⓑ M

* **G9831** AJCC stage at breast cancer diagnosis = II or III Ⓑ M

* **G9832** AJCC stage at breast cancer diagnosis = I (Ia or Ib) and T-stage at breast cancer diagnosis does not equal = T1, T1a, T1b Ⓑ M

* **G9833** Patient transfer to practice after initiation of chemotherapy Ⓑ M

* **G9834** Patient has metastatic disease at diagnosis Ⓑ M

* **G9835** Trastuzumab administered within 12 months of diagnosis Ⓑ M

* **G9836** Reason for not administering trastuzumab documented (e.g., patient declined, patient died, patient transferred, contraindication or other clinical exclusion, neoadjuvant chemotherapy or radiation not complete) Ⓑ M

* **G9837** Trastuzumab not administered within 12 months of diagnosis Ⓑ M

* **G9838** Patient has metastatic disease at diagnosis Ⓑ M

* **G9839** Anti-EGFR monoclonal antibody therapy Ⓑ M

* **G9840** Ras (KRas and NRas) gene mutation testing performed before initiation of anti-EGFR MoAb Ⓑ M

* **G9841** Ras (KRas and NRas) gene mutation testing not performed before initiation of anti-EGFR MoAb Ⓑ M

* **G9842** Patient has metastatic disease at diagnosis Ⓑ M

* **G9843** Ras (KRas and NRas) gene mutation Ⓑ M

* **G9844** Patient did not receive anti-EGFR monoclonal antibody therapy Ⓑ M

* **G9845** Patient received anti-EGFR monoclonal antibody therapy Ⓑ M

* **G9846** Patients who died from cancer Ⓑ M

* **G9847** Patient received chemotherapy in the last 14 days of life Ⓑ M

* **G9848** Patient did not receive chemotherapy in the last 14 days of life Ⓑ M

* **G9849** Patients who died from cancer Ⓑ M

* **G9850** Patient had more than one emergency department visit in the last 30 days of life Ⓑ M

* **G9851** Patient had one or less emergency department visits in the last 30 days of life Ⓑ M

* **G9852** Patients who died from cancer Ⓑ M

* **G9853** Patient admitted to the ICU in the last 30 days of life Ⓑ M

* **G9854** Patient was not admitted to the ICU in the last 30 days of life Ⓑ M

* **G9855** Patients who died from cancer Ⓑ M

* **G9856** Patient was not admitted to hospice Ⓑ M

* **G9857** Patient admitted to hospice Ⓑ M

* **G9858** Patient enrolled in hospice Ⓑ M

* **G9859** Patients who died from cancer Ⓑ M

* **G9860** Patient spent less than three days in hospice care Ⓑ M

* **G9861** Patient spent greater than or equal to three days in hospice care Ⓑ M

* **G9862** Documentation of medical reason(s) for not recommending at least a 10 year follow-up interval (e.g., inadequate prep, familial or personal history of colonic polyps, patient had no adenoma and age is = 66 years old, or life expectancy <10 years old, other medical reasons) Ⓑ M

* **G9873** First Medicare diabetes prevention program (MDPP) core session was attended by an MDPP beneficiary under the MDPP expanded model (EM). A core session is an MDPP service that: (1) is furnished by an MDPP supplier during months 1 through 6 of the MDPP services period; (2) is approximately 1 hour in length; and (3) adheres to a CDC-approved DPP curriculum for core sessions. M

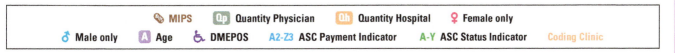

🅜 MIPS   🆀🅿 Quantity Physician   🆀🅷 Quantity Hospital   ♀ Female only
♂ Male only   🅐 Age   ♿ DMEPOS   A2-Z3 ASC Payment Indicator   A-Y ASC Status Indicator   Coding Clinic

* **G9874** Four total Medicare diabetes prevention program (MDPP) core sessions were attended by an MDPP beneficiary under the mdpp expanded model (EM). A core session is an MDPP service that: (1) is furnished by an MDPP supplier during months 1 through 6 of the MDPP services period; (2) is approximately 1 hour in length; and (3) adheres to a CDC-approved DPP curriculum for core sessions. **M**

* **G9875** Nine total Medicare diabetes prevention program (MDPP) core sessions were attended by an MDPP beneficiary under the MDPP expanded model (EM). A core session is an MDPP service that: (1) is furnished by an MDPP supplier during months 1 through 6 of the MDPP services period; (2) is approximately 1 hour in length; and (3) adheres to a CDC-approved DPP curriculum for core sessions. **M**

* **G9876** Two Medicare diabetes prevention program (MDPP) core maintenance sessions (MS) were attended by an MDPP beneficiary in months (mo) 7-9 under the mdpp expanded model (EM). A core maintenance session is an MDPP service that: (1) is furnished by an MDPP supplier during months 7 through 12 of the MDPP services period; (2) is approximately 1 hour in length; and (3) adheres to a CDC-approved DPP curriculum for maintenance sessions. The beneficiary did not achieve at least 5% weight loss (WL) from his/her baseline weight, as measured by at least one in-person weight measurement at a core maintenance session in months 7-9. **M**

* **G9877** Two Medicare diabetes prevention program (MDPP) core maintenance sessions (MS) were attended by an MDPP beneficiary in months (mo) 10-12 under the MDPP expanded model (EM). A core maintenance session is an MDPP service that: (1) is furnished by an MDPP supplier during months 7 through 12 of the MDPP services period; (2) is approximately 1 hour in length; and (3) adheres to a CDC-approved DPP curriculum for maintenance sessions. The beneficiary did not achieve at least 5% weight loss (WL) from his/her baseline weight, as measured by at least one in-person weight measurement at a core maintenance session in months 10-12. **M**

* **G9878** Two Medicare diabetes prevention program (MDPP) core maintenance sessions (MS) were attended by an MDPP beneficiary in months (mo) 7-9 under the MDPP expanded model (EM). A core maintenance session is an MDPP service that: (1) is furnished by an MDPP supplier during months 7 through 12 of the MDPP services period; (2) is approximately 1 hour in length; and (3) adheres to a CDC-approved DPP curriculum for maintenance sessions. The beneficiary achieved at least 5% weight loss (WL) from his/her baseline weight, as measured by at least one in-person weight measurement at a core maintenance session in months 7-9. **M**

* **G9879** Two Medicare diabetes prevention program (MDPP) core maintenance sessions (MS) were attended by an MDPP beneficiary in months (mo) 10-12 under the MDPP expanded model (EM). A core maintenance session is an MDPP service that: (1) is furnished by an MDPP supplier during months 7 through 12 of the MDPP services period; (2) is approximately 1 hour in length; and (3) adheres to a CDC-approved DPP curriculum for maintenance sessions. The beneficiary achieved at least 5% weight loss (WL) from his/her baseline weight, as measured by at least one in-person weight measurement at a core maintenance session in months 10-12. **M**

* **G9880** The MDPP beneficiary achieved at least 5% weight loss (WL) from his/her baseline weight in months 1-12 of the MDPP services period under the MDPP expanded model (EM). This is a one-time payment available when a beneficiary first achieves at least 5% weight loss from baseline as measured by an in-person weight measurement at a core session or core maintenance session. **M**

* **G9881** The MDPP beneficiary achieved at least 9% weight loss (WL) from his/her baseline weight in months 1-24 under the MDPP expanded model (EM). This is a one-time payment available when a beneficiary first achieves at least 9% weight loss from baseline as measured by an in-person weight measurement at a core session, core maintenance session, or ongoing maintenance session. **M**

---

▶ New    ↻ Revised    ✔ Reinstated    ~~deleted~~ Deleted    ⊘ Not covered or valid by Medicare

⊛ Special coverage instructions    ✳ Carrier discretion    Ⓑ Bill Part B MAC    Ⓑ Bill DME MAC

✱ **G9882** Two Medicare diabetes prevention program (MDPP) ongoing maintenance sessions (MS) were attended by an MDPP beneficiary in months (mo) 13-15 under the MDPP expanded model (EM). An ongoing maintenance session is an MDPP service that: (1) is furnished by an MDPP supplier during months 13 through 24 of the MDPP services period; (2) is approximately 1 hour in length; and (3) adheres to a CDC-approved DPP curriculum for maintenance sessions. The beneficiary maintained at least 5% weight loss (WL) from his/her baseline weight, as measured by at least one in-person weight measurement at an ongoing maintenance session in months 13-15. **M**

✱ **G9883** Two Medicare diabetes prevention program (MDPP) ongoing maintenance sessions (MS) were attended by an MDPP beneficiary in months (mo) 16-18 under the MDPP expanded model (EM). An ongoing maintenance session is an MDPP service that: (1) is furnished by an MDPP supplier during months 13 through 24 of the MDPP services period; (2) is approximately 1 hour in length; and (3) adheres to a CDC-approved DPP curriculum for maintenance sessions. The beneficiary maintained at least 5% weight loss (WL) from his/her baseline weight, as measured by at least one in-person weight measurement at an ongoing maintenance session in months 16-18. **M**

✱ **G9884** Two Medicare diabetes prevention program (MDPP) ongoing maintenance sessions (MS) were attended by an MDPP beneficiary in months (mo) 19-21 under the MDPP expanded model (EM). An ongoing maintenance session is an MDPP service that: (1) is furnished by an MDPP supplier during months 13 through 24 of the MDPP services period; (2) is approximately 1 hour in length; and (3) adheres to a CDC-approved DPP curriculum for maintenance sessions. The beneficiary maintained at least 5% weight loss (WL) from his/her baseline weight, as measured by at least one in-person weight measurement at an ongoing maintenance session in months 19-21. **M**

✱ **G9885** Two Medicare diabetes prevention program (MDPP) ongoing maintenance sessions (MS) were attended by an MDPP beneficiary in months (mo) 22-24 under the MDPP expanded model (EM). An ongoing maintenance session is an MDPP service that: (1) is furnished by an MDPP supplier during months 13 through 24 of the MDPP services period; (2) is approximately 1 hour in length; and (3) adheres to a CDC-approved DPP curriculum for maintenance sessions. The beneficiary maintained at least 5% weight loss (WL) from his/her baseline weight, as measured by at least one in-person weight measurement at an ongoing maintenance session in months 22-24. **M**

**NOTE:** The following codes do not imply that codes in other sections are necessarily covered.

## Quality Measures: Miscellaneous

✱ **G9890** Bridge payment: a one-time payment for the first Medicare diabetes prevention program (MDPP) core session, core maintenance session, or ongoing maintenance session furnished by an MDPP supplier to an MDPP beneficiary during months 1-24 of the MDPP expanded model (EM) who has previously received MDPP services from a different MDPP supplier under the MDPP expanded model. A supplier may only receive one bridge payment per MDPP beneficiary. **M**

✱ **G9891** MDPP session reported as a line-item on a claim for a payable MDPP expanded model (EM) HCPCS code for a session furnished by the billing supplier under the MDPP expanded model and counting toward achievement of the attendance performance goal for the payable MDPP expanded model HCPCS code (this code is for reporting purposes only) **M**

✱ **G9890** Dilated macular exam performed, including documentation of the presence or absence of macular thickening or geographic atrophy or hemorrhage and the level of macular degeneration severity Ⓑ **M**

🏵 MIPS   🆀🅿 Quantity Physician   🅀🅷 Quantity Hospital   ♀ Female only
♂ Male only   🅰 Age   ♿ DMEPOS   A2-Z3 ASC Payment Indicator   A-Y ASC Status Indicator   Coding Clinic

* **G9891** Documentation of medical reason(s) for not performing a dilated macular examination Ⓑ M

* **G9892** Documentation of patient reason(s) for not performing a dilated macular examination Ⓑ M

* **G9893** Dilated macular exam was not performed, reason not otherwise specified Ⓑ M

* **G9894** Androgen deprivation therapy prescribed/administered in combination with external beam radiotherapy to the prostate Ⓑ M

* **G9895** Documentation of medical reason(s) for not prescribing/administering androgen deprivation therapy in combination with external beam radiotherapy to the prostate (e.g., salvage therapy) Ⓑ M

* **G9896** Documentation of patient reason(s) for not prescribing/administering androgen deprivation therapy in combination with external beam radiotherapy to the prostate Ⓑ M

* **G9897** Patients who were not prescribed/administered androgen deprivation therapy in combination with external beam radiotherapy to the prostate, reason not given Ⓑ M

↩ * **G9898** Patient age 65 or older in institutional special needs plans (SNP) or residing in long-term care with POS code 32, 33, 34, 54, or 56 for more than 90 days during the measurement period Ⓑ M

* **G9899** Screening, diagnostic, film, digital or digital breast tomosynthesis (3D) mammography results documented and reviewed Ⓑ M

* **G9900** Screening, diagnostic, film, digital or digital breast tomosynthesis (3D) mammography results were not documented and reviewed, reason not otherwise specified Ⓑ M

↩ * **G9901** Patient age 65 or older in institutional special needs plans (SNP) or residing in long-term care with pos code 32, 33, 34, 54, or 56 for more than 90 days during the measurement period Ⓑ M

* **G9902** Patient screened for tobacco use and identified as a tobacco user Ⓑ M

* **G9903** Patient screened for tobacco use and identified as a tobacco non-user Ⓑ M

* **G9904** Documentation of medical reason(s) for not screening for tobacco use (e.g., limited life expectancy, other medical reason) Ⓑ M

* **G9905** Patient not screened for tobacco use, reason not given Ⓑ M

* **G9906** Patient identified as a tobacco user received tobacco cessation intervention (counseling and/or pharmacotherapy) Ⓑ M

* **G9907** Documentation of medical reason(s) for not providing tobacco cessation intervention (e.g., limited life expectancy, other medical reason) Ⓑ M

* **G9908** Patient identified as tobacco user did not receive tobacco cessation intervention (counseling and/or pharmacotherapy), reason not given Ⓑ M

* **G9909** Documentation of medical reason(s) for not providing tobacco cessation intervention if identified as a tobacco user (e.g., limited life expectancy, other medical reason) Ⓑ M

↩ * **G9910** Patients age 65 or older in institutional special needs plans (SNP) or residing in long-term care with pos code 32, 33, 34, 54, or 56 for more than 90 days during the measurement period Ⓑ M

* **G9911** Clinically node negative (t1n0m0 or t2n0m0) invasive breast cancer before or after neoadjuvant systemic therapy Ⓑ M

* **G9912** Hepatitis B virus (HBV) status assessed and results interpreted prior to initiating anti-TNF (tumor necrosis factor) therapy Ⓑ M

* **G9913** Hepatitis B virus (HBV) status not assessed and results interpreted prior to initiating anti-TNF (tumor necrosis factor) therapy, reason not given Ⓑ M

* **G9914** Patient receiving an anti-TNF agent Ⓑ M

* **G9915** No record of HBV results documented Ⓑ M

* **G9916** Functional status performed once in the last 12 months Ⓑ M

↩ * **G9917** Documentation of advanced stage dementia and caregiver knowledge is limited Ⓑ M

* **G9918** Functional status not performed, reason not otherwise specified Ⓑ M

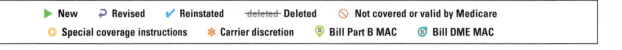
▶ New   ↩ Revised   ✔ Reinstated   ~~deleted~~ Deleted   ⊘ Not covered or valid by Medicare   ⊙ Special coverage instructions   * Carrier discretion   Ⓑ Bill Part B MAC   Ⓑ Bill DME MAC

\* **G9919** Screening performed and positive and provision of recommendations Ⓑ M

\* **G9920** Screening performed and negative Ⓑ M

\* **G9921** No screening performed, partial screening performed or positive screen without recommendations and reason is not given or otherwise specified Ⓑ M

\* **G9922** Safety concerns screen provided and if positive then documented mitigation recommendations Ⓑ M

\* **G9923** Safety concerns screen provided and negative Ⓑ M

\* **G9924** Documentation of medical reason(s) for not providing safety concerns screen or for not providing recommendations, orders or referrals for positive screen (e.g., patient in palliative care, other medical reason) Ⓑ M

\* **G9925** Safety concerns screening not provided, reason not otherwise specified Ⓑ M

\* **G9926** Safety concerns screening positive screen is without provision of mitigation recommendations, including but not limited to referral to other resources Ⓑ M

\* **G9927** Documentation of system reason(s) for not prescribing warfarin or another FDA-approved anticoagulation due to patient being currently enrolled in a clinical trial related to af/atrial flutter treatment Ⓑ M

\* **G9928** Warfarin or another FDA-approved anticoagulant not prescribed, reason not given Ⓑ M

\* **G9929** Patient with transient or reversible cause of AF (e.g., pneumonia, hyperthyroidism, pregnancy, cardiac surgery) Ⓑ M

\* **G9930** Patients who are receiving comfort care only Ⓑ M

\* **G9931** Documentation of CHA2DS2-VASc risk score of 0 or 1 Ⓑ M

\* **G9932** Documentation of patient reason(s) for not having records of negative or managed positive TB screen (e.g., patient does not return for mantoux (ppd) skin test evaluation) Ⓑ M

\* **G9933** Adenoma(s) or colorectal cancer detected during screening colonoscopy Ⓑ M

\* **G9934** Documentation that neoplasm detected is only diagnosed as traditional serrated adenoma, sessile serrated polyp, or sessile serrated adenoma Ⓑ M

\* **G9935** Adenoma(s) or colorectal cancer not detected during screening colonoscopy Ⓑ M

\* **G9936** Surveillance colonoscopy - personal history of colonic polyps, colon cancer, or other malignant neoplasm of rectum, rectosigmoid junction, and anus Ⓑ M

\* **G9937** Diagnostic colonoscopy Ⓑ M

↻ \* **G9938** Patients age 65 or older in institutional special needs plans (SNP) or residing in long-term care with POS code 32, 33, 34, 54, or 56 for more than 90 days during the measurement period Ⓑ M

\* **G9939** Pathologists/dermatopathologists is the same clinician who performed the biopsy Ⓑ M

\* **G9940** Documentation of medical reason(s) for not on a statin (e.g., pregnancy, in vitro fertilization, clomiphene rx, esrd, cirrhosis, muscular pain and disease during the measurement period or prior year) M

~~G9941 Back pain was measured by the visual analog scale (VAS) within 3 months preoperatively and at 3 months (6-20 weeks) postoperatively~~ ✖

↻ \* **G9942** Patient had any additional spine procedures performed on the same date as the lumbar discectomy/laminectomy Ⓑ M

\* **G9943** Back pain was not measured by the visual analog scale (VAS) within three months preoperatively and at three months (6-20 weeks) postoperatively Ⓑ M

~~G9944 Back pain was measured by the visual analog scale (VAS) within three months preoperatively and at one year (9 to 15 months) postoperatively~~ ✖

\* **G9945** Patient had cancer, fracture or infection related to the lumbar spine or patient had idiopathic or congenital scoliosis Ⓑ M

\* **G9946** Back pain was not measured by the visual analog scale (VAS) within three months preoperatively and at one year (9 to 15 months) postoperatively Ⓑ M

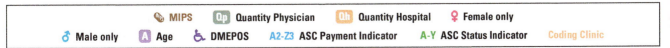

🐾 MIPS    Ⓠⓟ Quantity Physician    Ⓠⓗ Quantity Hospital    ♀ Female only    ♂ Male only    Ⓐ Age    ♿ DMEPOS    A2-Z3 ASC Payment Indicator    A-Y ASC Status Indicator    Coding Clinic

~~G9947~~ ~~Leg pain was measured by the visual~~ ✖
~~analog scale (VAS) within three months~~
~~preoperatively and at three months~~
~~(6 to 20 weeks) postoperatively~~

↻ ✳ **G9948** Patient had any additional spine
procedures performed on the same
date as the lumbar discectomy/
laminectomy Ⓑ M

↻ ✳ **G9949** Leg pain was not measured by
the visual analog scale (VAS) at
three months (6 to 20 weeks)
postoperatively Ⓑ M

✳ **G9954** Patient exhibits 2 or more risk factors
for post-operative vomiting Ⓑ M

✳ **G9955** Cases in which an inhalational
anesthetic is used only for
induction Ⓑ M

✳ **G9956** Patient received combination therapy
consisting of at least two prophylactic
pharmacologic anti-emetic agents of
different classes preoperatively and/or
intraoperatively Ⓑ M

✳ **G9957** Documentation of medical reason for
not receiving combination therapy
consisting of at least two prophylactic
pharmacologic anti-emetic agents of
different classes preoperatively and/
or intraoperatively (e.g., intolerance or
other medical reason) Ⓑ M

✳ **G9958** Patient did not receive combination
therapy consisting of at least two
prophylactic pharmacologic anti-emetic
agents of different classes preoperatively
and/or intraoperatively Ⓑ M

✳ **G9959** Systemic antimicrobials not
prescribed Ⓑ M

✳ **G9960** Documentation of medical
reason(s) for prescribing systemic
antimicrobials Ⓑ M

✳ **G9961** Systemic antimicrobials
prescribed Ⓑ M

✳ **G9962** Embolization endpoints are
documented separately for each
embolized vessel and ovarian artery
angiography or embolization
performed in the presence of
variant uterine artery anatomy Ⓑ M

✳ **G9963** Embolization endpoints are not
documented separately for each
embolized vessel or ovarian artery
angiography or embolization not
performed in the presence of variant
uterine artery anatomy Ⓑ M

✳ **G9964** Patient received at least one
well-child visit with a PCP during
the performance period Ⓑ M

✳ **G9965** Patient did not receive at least one
well-child visit with a PCP during the
performance period Ⓑ M

✳ **G9966** Children who were screened for risk of
developmental, behavioral and social
delays using a standardized tool with
interpretation and report Ⓑ M

✳ **G9967** Children who were not screened for
risk of developmental, behavioral and
social delays using a standardized tool
with interpretation and report Ⓑ M

✳ **G9968** Patient was referred to another
provider or specialist during the
performance period Ⓑ M

✳ **G9969** Provider who referred the patient to
another provider received a report from
the provider to whom the patient was
referred Ⓑ M

✳ **G9970** Provider who referred the patient to
another provider did not receive a
report from the provider to whom the
patient was referred Ⓑ M

✳ **G9974** Dilated macular exam performed,
including documentation of the
presence or absence of macular
thickening or geographic atrophy or
hemorrhage and the level of macular
degeneration severity Ⓑ M

✳ **G9975** Documentation of medical reason(s)
for not performing a dilated macular
examination Ⓑ M

✳ **G9976** Documentation of patient reason(s)
for not performing a dilated macular
examination Ⓑ M

✳ **G9977** Dilated macular exam was not
performed, reason not otherwise
specified Ⓑ M

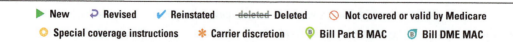

▶ New    ↻ Revised    ✔ Reinstated    ~~deleted~~ Deleted    ⊘ Not covered or valid by Medicare
⊙ Special coverage instructions    ✳ Carrier discretion    Ⓑ Bill Part B MAC    Ⓑ Bill DME MAC

\* **G9978** Remote in-home visit for the evaluation and management of a new patient for use only in a Medicare-approved bundled payments for care improvement advanced (BCPI advanced) model episode of care, which requires these 3 key components: a problem focused history; a problem focused examination; and straightforward medical decision making, furnished in real time using interactive audio and video technology. Counseling and coordination of care with other physicians, other qualified health care professionals or agencies are provided consistent with the nature of the problem(s) and the needs of the patient or the family or both. Usually, the presenting problem(s) are self limited or minor. Typically, 10 minutes are spent with the patient or family or both via real time, audio and video intercommunications technology. Ⓑ B

\* **G9979** Remote in-home visit for the evaluation and management of a new patient for use only in a Medicare-approved bundled payments for care improvement advanced (BCPI advanced) model episode of care, which requires these 3 key components: an expanded problem focused history; an expanded problem focused examination; straightforward medical decision making, furnished in real time using interactive audio and video technology. Counseling and coordination of care with other physicians, other qualified health care professionals or agencies are provided consistent with the nature of the problem(s) and the needs of the patient or the family or both. Usually, the presenting problem(s) are of low to moderate severity. Typically, 20 minutes are spent with the patient or family or both via real time, audio and video intercommunications technology. Ⓑ B

\* **G9980** Remote in-home visit for the evaluation and management of a new patient for use only in a Medicare-approved bundled payments for care improvement advanced (BCPI advanced) model episode of care, which requires these 3 key components: a detailed history; a detailed examination; medical decision making of low complexity, furnished in real time using interactive audio and video technology. Counseling and coordination of care with other physicians, other qualified health care professionals or agencies are provided consistent with the nature of the problem(s) and the needs of the patient or the family or both. Usually, the presenting problem(s) are of moderate severity. Typically, 30 minutes are spent with the patient or family or both via real time, audio and video intercommunications technology. Ⓑ B

\* **G9981** Remote in-home visit for the evaluation and management of a new patient for use only in a Medicare-approved bundled payments for care improvement advanced (BCPI advanced) model episode of care, which requires these 3 key components: a comprehensive history; a comprehensive examination; medical decision making of moderate complexity, furnished in real time using interactive audio and video technology. Counseling and coordination of care with other physicians, other qualified health care professionals or agencies are provided consistent with the nature of the problem(s) and the needs of the patient or the family or both. Usually, the presenting problem(s) are of moderate to high severity. Typically, 45 minutes are spent with the patient or family or both via real time, audio and video intercommunications technology. Ⓑ B

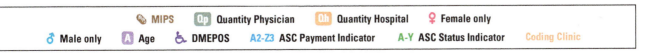

🔖 MIPS    Ⓠp Quantity Physician    Ⓠh Quantity Hospital    ♀ Female only

♂ Male only    Ⓐ Age    ♿ DMEPOS    A2-Z3 ASC Payment Indicator    A-Y ASC Status Indicator    Coding Clinic

* **G9982** Remote in-home visit for the evaluation and management of a new patient for use only in a Medicare-approved bundled payments for care improvement advanced (BCPI advanced) model episode of care, which requires these 3 key components: a comprehensive history; a comprehensive examination; medical decision making of high complexity, furnished in real time using interactive audio and video technology. Counseling and coordination of care with other physicians, other qualified health care professionals or agencies are provided consistent with the nature of the problem(s) and the needs of the patient or the family or both. Usually, the presenting problem(s) are of moderate to high severity. Typically, 60 minutes are spent with the patient or family or both via real time, audio and video intercommunications technology. Ⓑ **B**

* **G9983** Remote in-home visit for the evaluation and management of an established patient for use only in a Medicare-approved bundled payments for care improvement advanced (BCPI advanced) model episode of care, which requires at least 2 of the following 3 key components: a problem focused history; a problem focused examination; straightforward medical decision making, furnished in real time using interactive audio and video technology. Counseling and coordination of care with other physicians, other qualified health care professionals or agencies are provided consistent with the nature of the problem(s) and the needs of the patient or the family or both. Usually, the presenting problem(s) are self limited or minor. Typically, 10 minutes are spent with the patient or family or both via real time, audio and video intercommunications technology. Ⓑ **B**

* **G9984** Remote in-home visit for the evaluation and management of an established patient for use only in a Medicare-approved bundled payments for care improvement advanced (BCPI advanced) model episode of care, which requires at least 2 of the following 3 key components: an expanded problem focused history; an expanded problem focused examination; medical decision making of low complexity, furnished in real time using interactive audio and video technology. Counseling and coordination of care with other physicians, other qualified health care professionals or agencies are provided consistent with the nature of the problem(s) and the needs of the patient or the family or both. Usually, the presenting problem(s) are of low to moderate severity. Typically, 15 minutes are spent with the patient or family or both via real time, audio and video intercommunications technology. Ⓑ **B**

* **G9985** Remote in-home visit for the evaluation and management of an established patient for use only in a Medicare-approved bundled payments for care improvement advanced (BCPI advanced) model episode of care, which requires at least 2 of the following 3 key components: a detailed history; a detailed examination; medical decision making of moderate complexity, furnished in real time using interactive audio and video technology. Counseling and coordination of care with other physicians, other qualified health care professionals or agencies are provided consistent with the nature of the problem(s) and the needs of the patient or the family or both. Usually, the presenting problem(s) are of moderate to high severity. Typically, 25 minutes are spent with the patient or family or both via real time, audio and video intercommunications technology. Ⓑ **B**

▶ New   ↻ Revised   ✔ Reinstated   ~~deleted~~ Deleted   ⊘ Not covered or valid by Medicare
⊙ Special coverage instructions   * Carrier discretion   Ⓑ Bill Part B MAC   Ⓓ Bill DME MAC

\* **G9986** Remote in-home visit for the evaluation and management of an established patient for use only in a Medicare-approved bundled payments for care improvement advanced (BCPI advanced) model episode of care, which requires at least 2 of the following 3 key components: a comprehensive history; a comprehensive examination; medical decision making of high complexity, furnished in real time using interactive audio and video technology. Counseling and coordination of care with other physicians, other qualified health care professionals or agencies are provided consistent with the nature of the problem(s) and the needs of the patient or the family or both. Usually, the presenting problem(s) are of moderate to high severity. Typically, 40 minutes are spent with the patient or family or both via real time, audio and video intercommunications technology. Ⓑ B

\* **G9987** Bundled payments for care improvement advanced (BCPI advanced) model home visit for patient assessment performed by clinical staff for an individual not considered homebound, including, but not necessarily limited to patient assessment of clinical status, safety/fall prevention, functional status/ambulation, medication reconciliation/management, compliance with orders/plan of care, performance of activities of daily living, and ensuring beneficiary connections to community and other services; for use only for a BCPI advanced model episode of care; may not be billed for a 30-day period covered by a transitional care management code. Ⓑ B

| 👜 MIPS | Ⓠ𝐩 Quantity Physician | Ⓠ𝐡 Quantity Hospital | ♀ Female only |
|---|---|---|---|
| ♂ Male only | Ⓐ Age | ♿ DMEPOS | A2-Z3 ASC Payment Indicator | A-Y ASC Status Indicator | Coding Clinic |

TEMPORARY PROCEDURES/PROFESSIONAL SERVICES  G9986 — G9987

293

## BEHAVIORAL HEALTH AND/OR SUBSTANCE ABUSE TREATMENT SERVICES (H0001-H9999)

**Note:** Used by Medicaid state agencies because no national code exists to meet the reporting needs of these agencies.

⃠ **H0001** Alcohol and/or drug assessment

⃠ **H0002** Behavioral health screening to determine eligibility for admission to treatment program

⃠ **H0003** Alcohol and/or drug screening; laboratory analysis of specimens for presence of alcohol and/or drugs

⃠ **H0004** Behavioral health counseling and therapy, per 15 minutes

⃠ **H0005** Alcohol and/or drug services; group counseling by a clinician

⃠ **H0006** Alcohol and/or drug services; case management

⃠ **H0007** Alcohol and/or drug services; crisis intervention (outpatient)

⃠ **H0008** Alcohol and/or drug services; sub-acute detoxification (hospital inpatient)

⃠ **H0009** Alcohol and/or drug services; acute detoxification (hospital inpatient)

⃠ **H0010** Alcohol and/or drug services; sub-acute detoxification (residential addiction program inpatient)

⃠ **H0011** Alcohol and/or drug services; acute detoxification (residential addiction program inpatient)

⃠ **H0012** Alcohol and/or drug services; sub-acute detoxification (residential addiction program outpatient)

⃠ **H0013** Alcohol and/or drug services; acute detoxification (residential addiction program outpatient)

⃠ **H0014** Alcohol and/or drug services; ambulatory detoxification

⃠ **H0015** Alcohol and/or drug services; intensive outpatient (treatment program that operates at least 3 hours/day and at least 3 days/week and is based on an individualized treatment plan), including assessment, counseling; crisis intervention, and activity therapies or education

⃠ **H0016** Alcohol and/or drug services; medical/somatic (medical intervention in ambulatory setting)

⃠ **H0017** Behavioral health; residential (hospital residential treatment program), without room and board, per diem

⃠ **H0018** Behavioral health; short-term residential (non-hospital residential treatment program), without room and board, per diem

⃠ **H0019** Behavioral health; long-term residential (non-medical, non-acute care in a residential treatment program where stay is typically longer than 30 days), without room and board, per diem

⃠ **H0020** Alcohol and/or drug services; methadone administration and/or service (provision of the drug by a licensed program)

⃠ **H0021** Alcohol and/or drug training service (for staff and personnel not employed by providers)

⃠ **H0022** Alcohol and/or drug intervention service (planned facilitation)

⃠ **H0023** Behavioral health outreach service (planned approach to reach a targeted population)

⃠ **H0024** Behavioral health prevention information dissemination service (one-way direct or non-direct contact with service audiences to affect knowledge and attitude)

⃠ **H0025** Behavioral health prevention education service (delivery of services with target population to affect knowledge, attitude and/or behavior)

⃠ **H0026** Alcohol and/or drug prevention process service, community-based (delivery of services to develop skills of impactors)

⃠ **H0027** Alcohol and/or drug prevention environmental service (broad range of external activities geared toward modifying systems in order to mainstream prevention through policy and law)

⃠ **H0028** Alcohol and/or drug prevention problem identification and referral service (e.g., student assistance and employee assistance programs), does not include assessment

⃠ **H0029** Alcohol and/or drug prevention alternatives service (services for populations that exclude alcohol and other drug use, e.g., alcohol-free social events)

⃠ **H0030** Behavioral health hotline service

⃠ **H0031** Mental health assessment, by non-physician

⃠ **H0032** Mental health service plan development by non-physician

⃠ **H0033** Oral medication administration, direct observation

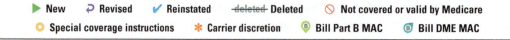

▶ New    ↻ Revised    ✔ Reinstated    ~~deleted~~ Deleted    ⃠ Not covered or valid by Medicare
   ⊙ Special coverage instructions    ✳ Carrier discretion    Ⓑ Bill Part B MAC    Ⓑ Bill DME MAC

**H0034** Medication training and support, per 15 minutes

**H0035** Mental health partial hospitalization, treatment, less than 24 hours

**H0036** Community psychiatric supportive treatment, face-to-face, per 15 minutes

**H0037** Community psychiatric supportive treatment program, per diem

**H0038** Self-help/peer services, per 15 minutes

**H0039** Assertive community treatment, face-to-face, per 15 minutes

**H0040** Assertive community treatment program, per diem

**H0041** Foster care, child, non-therapeutic, per diem Ⓐ

**H0042** Foster care, child, non-therapeutic, per month Ⓐ

**H0043** Supported housing, per diem

**H0044** Supported housing, per month

**H0045** Respite care services, not in the home, per diem

**H0046** Mental health services, not otherwise specified

**H0047** Alcohol and/or other drug abuse services, not otherwise specified

**H0048** Alcohol and/or other drug testing: collection and handling only, specimens other than blood

**H0049** Alcohol and/or drug screening

**H0050** Alcohol and/or drug services, brief intervention, per 15 minutes

**H1000** Prenatal care, at-risk assessment ♀

**H1001** Prenatal care, at-risk enhanced service; antepartum management ♀

**H1002** Prenatal care, at-risk enhanced service; care coordination ♀

**H1003** Prenatal care, at-risk enhanced service; education ♀

**H1004** Prenatal care, at-risk enhanced service; follow-up home visit ♀

**H1005** Prenatal care, at-risk enhanced service package (includes H1001-H1004) ♀

**H1010** Non-medical family planning education, per session

**H1011** Family assessment by licensed behavioral health professional for state defined purposes

**H2000** Comprehensive multidisciplinary evaluation

**H2001** Rehabilitation program, per 1/2 day

**H2010** Comprehensive medication services, per 15 minutes

**H2011** Crisis intervention service, per 15 minutes

**H2012** Behavioral health day treatment, per hour

**H2013** Psychiatric health facility service, per diem

**H2014** Skills training and development, per 15 minutes

**H2015** Comprehensive community support services, per 15 minutes

**H2016** Comprehensive community support services, per diem

**H2017** Psychosocial rehabilitation services, per 15 minutes

**H2018** Psychosocial rehabilitation services, per diem

**H2019** Therapeutic behavioral services, per 15 minutes

**H2020** Therapeutic behavioral services, per diem

**H2021** Community-based wrap-around services, per 15 minutes

**H2022** Community-based wrap-around services, per diem

**H2023** Supported employment, per 15 minutes

**H2024** Supported employment, per diem

**H2025** Ongoing support to maintain employment, per 15 minutes

**H2026** Ongoing support to maintain employment, per diem

**H2027** Psychoeducational service, per 15 minutes

**H2028** Sexual offender treatment service, per 15 minutes

**H2029** Sexual offender treatment service, per diem

**H2030** Mental health clubhouse services, per 15 minutes

**H2031** Mental health clubhouse services, per diem

**H2032** Activity therapy, per 15 minutes

**H2033** Multisystemic therapy for juveniles, per 15 minutes Ⓐ

**H2034** Alcohol and/or drug abuse halfway house services, per diem

**H2035** Alcohol and/or other drug treatment program, per hour

**H2036** Alcohol and/or other drug treatment program, per diem

**H2037** Developmental delay prevention activities, dependent child of client, per 15 minutes Ⓐ

---

🐚 MIPS   Ⓠp Quantity Physician   Ⓠh Quantity Hospital   ♀ Female only

♂ Male only   Ⓐ Age   ♿ DMEPOS   A2-Z3 ASC Payment Indicator   A-Y ASC Status Indicator   Coding Clinic

## DRUGS OTHER THAN CHEMOTHERAPY DRUGS (J0100-J8999)

### Injection

⊛ **J0120** Injection, tetracycline, up to 250 mg Ⓑ Ⓓ Qp Qh  N1 N

*Other: Achromycin*

*IOM: 100-02, 15, 50*

▶ ✳ **J0121** Injection, omadacycline, 1 mg  K2 G

▶ ✳ **J0122** Injection, eravacycline, 1 mg  K2 K

✳ **J0129** Injection, abatacept, 10 mg (Code may be used for medicare when drug administered under the direct supervision of a physician, not for use when drug is self-administered) Ⓑ Ⓓ Qp Qh  K2 K

*Other: Orencia*

⊛ **J0130** Injection, abciximab, 10 mg Ⓑ Ⓓ Qp Qh  N1 N

*Other: ReoPro*

*IOM: 100-02, 15, 50*

✳ **J0131** Injection, acetaminophen, 10 mg Ⓑ Ⓓ Qp Qh  N1 N

*Other: Ofirmev*

**Coding Clinic: 2012, Q1, P9**

✳ **J0132** Injection, acetylcysteine, 100 mg Ⓑ Ⓓ Qp Qh  N1 N

*Other: Acetadote*

✳ **J0133** Injection, acyclovir, 5 mg Ⓓ Ⓑ Qp Qh  N1 N

✳ **J0135** Injection, adalimumab, 20 mg Ⓑ Ⓓ Qp Qh  K2 K

*Other: Humira*

*IOM: 100-02, 15, 50*

⊛ **J0153** Injection, adenosine, 1 mg (not to be used to report any adenosine phosphate compounds) Ⓑ Ⓓ Qp Qh  N1 N

*Other: Adenocard, Adenoscan*

⊛ **J0171** Injection, adrenalin, epinephrine, 0.1 mg Ⓓ Ⓑ Qp Qh  N1 N

*Other: AUVI-Q, Sus-Phrine*

*IOM: 100-02, 15, 50*

**Coding Clinic: 2011, Q1, P8**

✳ **J0178** Injection, aflibercept, 1 mg Ⓓ Ⓑ Qp Qh  K2 K

*Other: Eylea*

▶ ✳ **J0179** Injection, brolucizumab-dbll, 1 mg  K2 K

✳ **J0180** Injection, agalsidase beta, 1 mg Ⓑ Ⓓ Qp Qh  K2 K

*Other: Fabrazyme*

*IOM: 100-02, 15, 50*

✳ **J0185** Injection, aprepitant, 1 mg  G

*Other: Emend*

⊛ **J0190** Injection, biperiden lactate, per 5 mg Ⓑ Ⓓ Qp Qh  E2

*Other: Akineton*

*IOM: 100-02, 15, 50*

⊛ **J0200** Injection, alatrofloxacin mesylate, 100 mg Ⓑ Ⓓ Qp Qh  E2

*Other: Trovan*

*IOM: 100-02, 15, 50*

✳ **J0202** Injection, alemtuzumab, 1 mg Ⓑ Ⓓ Qp Qh  K2 K

*Other: Lemtrada*

⊛ **J0205** Injection, alglucerase, per 10 units Ⓓ Ⓑ Qp Qh  E2

*Other: Ceredase*

*IOM: 100-02, 15, 50*

⊛ **J0207** Injection, amifostine, 500 mg Ⓓ Ⓑ Qp Qh  K2 K

*Other: Ethyol*

*IOM: 100-02, 15, 50*

⊛ **J0210** Injection, methyldopate HCL, up to 250 mg Ⓓ Ⓑ Qp Qh  N1 N

*Other: Aldomet*

*IOM: 100-02, 15, 50*

✳ **J0215** Injection, alefacept, 0.5 mg Ⓓ Ⓑ Qp Qh  E2

✳ **J0220** Injection, alglucosidase alfa, not otherwise specified, 10 mg Ⓓ Ⓑ Qp Qh  K2 K

**Coding Clinic: 2013, Q2, P5; 2012, Q1, P9**

✳ **J0221** Injection, alglucosidase alfa, (lumizyme), 10 mg Ⓓ Ⓑ Qp Qh  K2 K

**Coding Clinic: 2013, Q2, P5**

▶ ✳ **J0222** Injection, patisiran, 0.1 mg  K2 G

⊛ **J0256** Injection, alpha 1-proteinase inhibitor (human), not otherwise specified, 10 mg Ⓓ Ⓑ Qp Qh  K2 K

*Other: Prolastin, Zemaira*

*IOM: 100-02, 15, 50*

**Coding Clinic: 2012, Q1, P9**

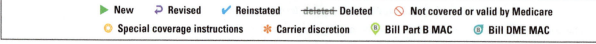

▶ New   ↻ Revised   ✔ Reinstated   ~~deleted~~ Deleted   ⊘ Not covered or valid by Medicare
⊛ Special coverage instructions   ✳ Carrier discretion   Ⓑ Bill Part B MAC   Ⓓ Bill DME MAC

⚙ **J0257** Injection, alpha 1 proteinase inhibitor (human), (glassia), 10 mg Ⓑ Ⓑ Qp Qh    K2 K

*IOM: 100-02, 15, 50*

**Coding Clinic: 2012, Q1, P8**

⚙ **J0270** Injection, alprostadil, per 1.25 mcg (Code may be used for Medicare when drug administered under the direct supervision of a physician, not for use when drug is self-administered) Ⓑ Ⓑ Qp Qh    B

*Other: Caverject, Prostaglandin E1, Prostin VR Pediatric*

*IOM: 100-02, 15, 50*

⚙ **J0275** Alprostadil urethral suppository (Code may be used for Medicare when drug administered under the direct supervision of a physician, not for use when drug is self-administered) Ⓑ Ⓑ Qp Qh    B

*Other: Muse*

*IOM: 100-02, 15, 50*

＊ **J0278** Injection, amikacin sulfate, 100 mg Ⓑ Ⓑ Qp Qh    N1 N

⚙ **J0280** Injection, aminophylline, up to 250 mg Ⓑ Ⓑ Qp Qh    N1 N

*IOM: 100-02, 15, 50*

⚙ **J0282** Injection, amiodarone hydrochloride, 30 mg Ⓑ Ⓑ Qp Qh    N1 N

*Other: Cordarone*

*IOM: 100-02, 15, 50*

⚙ **J0285** Injection, amphotericin B, 50 mg Ⓑ Ⓑ Qp Qh    N1 N

*Other: ABLC, Amphocin, Fungizone*

*IOM: 100-02, 15, 50*

⚙ **J0287** Injection, amphotericin B lipid complex, 10 mg Ⓑ Ⓑ Qp Qh    K2 K

*Other: Abelcet*

*IOM: 100-02, 15, 50*

⚙ **J0288** Injection, amphotericin B cholesteryl sulfate complex, 10 mg Ⓑ Ⓑ Qp Qh    E2

*IOM: 100-02, 15, 50*

⚙ **J0289** Injection, amphotericin B liposome, 10 mg Ⓑ Ⓑ Qp Qh    K2 K

*Other: AmBisome*

*IOM: 100-02, 15, 50*

⚙ **J0290** Injection, ampicillin sodium, 500 mg Ⓑ Ⓑ Qp Qh    N1 N

*Other: Omnipen-N, Polycillin-N, Totacillin-N*

*IOM: 100-02, 15, 50*

▶ ＊ **J0291** Injection, plazomicin, 5 mg    K2 G

⚙ **J0295** Injection, ampicillin sodium/sulbactam sodium, per 1.5 gm Ⓑ Ⓑ Qp Qh    N1 N

*Other: Omnipen-N, Polycillin-N, Totacillin-N, Unasyn*

*IOM: 100-02, 15, 50*

⚙ **J0300** Injection, amobarbital, up to 125 mg Ⓑ Ⓑ Qp Qh    K2 K

*Other: Amytal*

*IOM: 100-02, 15, 50*

⚙ **J0330** Injection, succinylcholine chloride, up to 20 mg Ⓑ Ⓑ Qp Qh    N1 N

*Other: Anectine, Quelicin, Surostrin*

*IOM: 100-02, 15, 50*

＊ **J0348** Injection, anidulafungin, 1 mg Ⓑ Ⓑ Qp Qh    N1 N

*Other: Eraxis*

⚙ **J0350** Injection, anistreplase, per 30 units Ⓑ Ⓑ Qp Qh    E2

*Other: Eminase*

*IOM: 100-02, 15, 50*

⚙ **J0360** Injection, hydralazine hydrochloride, up to 20 mg Ⓑ Ⓑ Qp Qh    N1 N

*Other: Apresoline*

*IOM: 100-02, 15, 50*

＊ **J0364** Injection, apomorphine hydrochloride, 1 mg Ⓑ Ⓑ Qp Qh    E2

⚙ **J0365** Injection, aprotinin, 10,000 KIU Ⓑ Ⓑ Qp Qh    E2

*IOM: 100-02, 15, 50*

⚙ **J0380** Injection, metaraminol bitartrate, per 10 mg Ⓑ Ⓑ Qp Qh    N1 N

*Other: Aramine*

*IOM: 100-02, 15, 50*

⚙ **J0390** Injection, chloroquine hydrochloride, up to 250 mg Ⓑ Ⓑ Qp Qh    N1 N

Benefit only for diagnosed malaria or amebiasis

*Other: Aralen*

*IOM: 100-02, 15, 50*

⚙ **J0395** Injection, arbutamine HCL, 1 mg Ⓑ Ⓑ Qp Qh    E2

*IOM: 100-02, 15, 50*

---

🅜 MIPS    Qp Quantity Physician    Qh Quantity Hospital    ♀ Female only

♂ Male only    🅐 Age    ♿ DMEPOS    A2-Z3 ASC Payment Indicator    A-Y ASC Status Indicator    Coding Clinic

* **J0400** Injection, aripiprazole, intramuscular, 0.25 mg ⑧ ⑧ **Qp** **Qh**    K2 K

* **J0401** Injection, aripiprazole, extended release, 1 mg ⑧ ⑧ **Qp** **Qh**    K2 K

    *Other: Abilify Maintena*

⚙ **J0456** Injection, azithromycin, 500 mg ⑧ ⑧ **Qp** **Qh**    N1 N

    *Other: Zithromax*

    *IOM: 100-02, 15, 50*

⚙ **J0461** Injection, atropine sulfate, 0.01 mg ⑧ ⑧ **Qp** **Qh**    N1 N

    *IOM: 100-02, 15, 50*

⚙ **J0470** Injection, dimercaprol, per 100 mg ⑧ ⑧ **Qp** **Qh**    K2 K

    *Other: BAL In Oil*

    *IOM: 100-02, 15, 50*

⚙ **J0475** Injection, baclofen, 10 mg ⑧ ⑧ **Qp** **Qh**    K2 K

    *Other: Gablofen, Lioresal*

    *IOM: 100-02, 15, 50*

⚙ **J0476** Injection, baclofen 50 mcg for intrathecal trial ⑧ ⑧ **Qp** **Qh**    K2 K

    *Other: Gablofen, Lioresal*

    *IOM: 100-02, 15, 50*

⚙ **J0480** Injection, basiliximab, 20 mg ⑧ ⑧ **Qp** **Qh**    K2 K

    *Other: Simulect*

    *IOM: 100-02, 15, 50*

* **J0485** Injection, belatacept, 1 mg ⑧ ⑧ **Qp** **Qh**    K2 K

    *Other: Nulojix*

* **J0490** Injection, belimumab, 10 mg ⑧ ⑧ **Qp** **Qh**    K2 K

    *Other: Benlysta*

    **Coding Clinic: 2012, Q1, P9**

⚙ **J0500** Injection, dicyclomine HCL, up to 20 mg ⑧ ⑧ **Qp** **Qh**    N1 N

    *Other: Antispas, Bentyl, Dibent, Dilomine, Di-Spaz, Neoquess, Or-Tyl, Spasmoject*

    *IOM: 100-02, 15, 50*

⚙ **J0515** Injection, benztropine mesylate, per 1 mg ⑧ ⑧ **Qp** **Qh**    N1 N

    *Other: Cogentin*

    *IOM: 100-02, 15, 50*

* **J0517** Injection, benralizumab, 1 mg    G

    *Other: Fasenra*

⚙ **J0520** Injection, bethanechol chloride, myotonachol or urecholine, up to 5 mg ⑧ ⑧ **Qp** **Qh**    E2

    *IOM: 100-02, 15, 50*

* **J0558** Injection, penicillin G benzathine and penicillin G procaine,100,000 units ⑧ ⑧ **Qp** **Qh**    N1 N

    *Other: Bicillin C-R*

    **Coding Clinic: 2011, Q1, P8**

⚙ **J0561** Injection, penicillin G benzathine, 100,000 units ⑧ ⑧ **Qp** **Qh**    K2 K

    *Other: Bicillin L-A, Permapen*

    *IOM: 100-02, 15, 50*

    **Coding Clinic: 2013, Q2, P3; 2011, Q1, P8**

* **J0565** Injection, bezlotoxumab, 10 mg    K2 G

* **J0567** Injection, cerliponase alfa, 1 mg    G

    *Other: Brineura*

* **J0570** Buprenorphine implant, 74.2 mg **Qp** **Qh**    K2 G

    *Other: Probuphine System Kit*

    **Coding Clinic: 2017, Q1, P9**

⚙ **J0571** Buprenorphine, oral, 1 mg ⑧ ⑧ **Qp** **Qh**    E1

⚙ **J0572** Buprenorphine/naloxone, oral, less than or equal to 3 mg buprenorphine ⑧ ⑧ **Qp** **Qh**    E1

⚙ **J0573** Buprenorphine/naloxone, oral, greater than 3 mg, but less than or equal to 6 mg buprenorphine ⑧ ⑧ **Qp** **Qh**    E1

⚙ **J0574** Buprenorphine/naloxone, oral, greater than 6 mg, but less than or equal to 10 mg buprenorphine ⑧ ⑧ **Qp** **Qh**    E1

⚙ **J0575** Buprenorphine/naloxone, oral, greater than 10 mg buprenorphine ⑧ ⑧ **Qp** **Qh**    E1

* **J0583** Injection, bivalirudin, 1 mg ⑧ ⑧ **Qp** **Qh**    N1 N

    *Other: Angiomax*

* **J0584** Injection, burosumab-twza 1 mg    K

    *Other: Crysvita*

⚙ **J0585** Injection, onabotulinumtoxinA, 1 unit ⑧ ⑧ **Qp** **Qh**    K2 K

    *Other: Botox, Botox Cosmetic, Oculinum*

    *IOM: 100-02, 15, 50*

* **J0586** Injection, abobotulinumtoxinA, 5 units ⑧ ⑧ **Qp** **Qh**    K2 K

⚙ **J0587** Injection, rimabotulinumtoxinB, 100 units ⑧ ⑧ **Qp** **Qh**    K2 K

    *Other: Myobloc, Nplate*

    *IOM: 100-02, 15, 50*

---

▶ New    ↩ Revised    ✔ Reinstated    ~~deleted~~ Deleted    ⊘ Not covered or valid by Medicare
⚙ Special coverage instructions    * Carrier discretion    ⑧ Bill Part B MAC    ⑧ Bill DME MAC

* **J0588** Injection, incobotulinumtoxin A, 1 unit ⓥ ⓑ Qp Qh — K2 K

*Other: Xeomin*

Coding Clinic: 2012, Q1, P9

☼ **J0592** Injection, buprenorphine hydrochloride, 0.1 mg ⓥ ⓑ Qp Qh — N1 N

*Other: Buprenex*

*IOM: 100-02, 15, 50*

▶ * **J0593** Injection, lanadelumab-flyo, 1 mg (Code may be used for Medicare when drug administered under direct supervision of a physician, not for use when drug is self-administered) — K2 K

* **J0594** Injection, busulfan, 1 mg ⓑ ⓑ Qp Qh — K2 K

*Other: Myleran*

* **J0595** Injection, butorphanol tartrate, 1 mg ⓑ ⓑ Qp Qh — N1 N

* **J0596** Injection, C1 esterase inhibitor (recombinant), ruconest, 10 units ⓑ ⓑ Qp Qh — K2 K

* **J0597** Injection, C-1 esterase inhibitor (human), Berinert, 10 units ⓑ ⓑ Qp Qh — K2 K

Coding Clinic: 2011, Q1, P7

* **J0598** Injection, C1 esterase inhibitor (human), cinryze, 10 units ⓑ ⓑ Qp Qh — K2 K

* **J0599** Injection, c-1 esterase inhibitor (human), (haegarda), 10 units — G

*Other: Berinert*

☼ **J0600** Injection, edetate calcium disodium, up to 1000 mg ⓑ ⓑ Qp Qh — K2 K

*Other: Calcium Disodium Versenate*

*IOM: 100-02, 15, 50*

☼ **J0604** Cinacalcet, oral, 1 mg, (for ESRD on dialysis) — B

☼ **J0606** Injection, etelcalcetide, 0.1 mg — K2 K

☼ **J0610** Injection, calcium gluconate, per 10 ml ⓑ ⓑ Qp Qh — N1 N

*Other: Kaleinate*

*IOM: 100-02, 15, 50*

☼ **J0620** Injection, calcium glycerophosphate and calcium lactate, per 10 ml ⓑ ⓑ Qp Qh — N1 N

*Other: Calphosan*

*MCM: 2049*

*IOM: 100-02, 15, 50*

☼ **J0630** Injection, calcitonin (salmon), up to 400 units ⓑ ⓑ Qp Qh — K2 K

*Other: Calcimar, Calcitonin-salmon, Miacalcin*

*IOM: 100-02, 15, 50*

☼ **J0636** Injection, calcitriol, 0.1 mcg ⓥ ⓑ Qp Qh — N1 N

Non-dialysis use

*Other: Calcijex*

*IOM: 100-02, 15, 50*

* **J0637** Injection, caspofungin acetate, 5 mg ⓑ ⓑ Qp Qh — K2 K

*Other: Cancidas, Caspofungin*

* **J0638** Injection, canakinumab, 1 mg ⓥ Qp Qh — K2 K

*Other: Ilaris*

☼ **J0640** Injection, leucovorin calcium, per 50 mg ⓥ ⓑ Qp Qh — N1 N

*Other: Wellcovorin*

*IOM: 100-02, 15, 50*

Coding Clinic: 2009, Q1, P10

↩☼ **J0641** Injection, levoleucovorin not otherwise specified, 0.5 mg ⓑ ⓑ Qp Qh — K2 K

Part of treatment regimen for osteosarcoma

▶ * **J0642** Injection, levoleucovorin (khapzory), 0.5 mg — K2 G

☼ **J0670** Injection, mepivacaine HCL, per 10 ml ⓥ ⓑ Qp Qh — N1 N

*Other: Carbocaine, Isocaine HCl, Polocaine*

*IOM: 100-02, 15, 50*

☼ **J0690** Injection, cefezolin sodium, 500 mg ⓥ ⓑ Qp Qh — N1 N

*Other: Ancef, Kefzol, Zolicef*

*IOM: 100-02, 15, 50*

* **J0692** Injection, cefepime HCL, 500 mg ⓥ ⓑ Qp Qh — N1 N

*Other: Maxipime*

☼ **J0694** Injection, cefoxitin sodium, 1 gm ⓥ ⓑ Qp Qh — N1 N

*Other: Mefoxin*

*IOM: 100-02, 15, 50,*

Cross Reference Q0090

* **J0695** Injection, ceftolozane 50 mg and tazobactam 25 mg ⓥ ⓑ Qp Qh — K2 K

*Other: Zerbaxa*

☼ **J0696** Injection, ceftriaxone sodium, per 250 mg ⓥ ⓑ Qp Qh — N1 N

*Other: Rocephin*

*IOM: 100-02, 15, 50*

☼ **J0697** Injection, sterile cefuroxime sodium, per 750 mg ⓥ ⓑ Qp Qh — N1 N

*Other: Kefurox, Zinacef*

*IOM: 100-02, 15, 50*

🏷 MIPS    Qp Quantity Physician    Qh Quantity Hospital    ♀ Female only
♂ Male only    Ⓐ Age    ♿ DMEPOS    A2-Z3 ASC Payment Indicator    A-Y ASC Status Indicator    Coding Clinic

**⚙ J0698** Injection, cefotaxime sodium, per gm ⓑ ⓑ Qp Qh    N1 N

*Other: Claforan*

*IOM: 100-02, 15, 50*

**⚙ J0702** Injection, betamethasone acetate 3 mg and betamethasone sodium phosphate 3 mg ⓑ ⓑ Qp Qh   N1 N

*Other: Betameth, Celestone Soluspan, Selestoject*

*IOM: 100-02, 15, 50*

Coding Clinic: 2018, Q4, P6

**✳ J0706** Injection, caffeine citrate, 5 mg ⓑ ⓑ Qp Qh    N1 N

*Other: Cafcit, Cipro IV, Ciprofloxacin*

**⚙ J0710** Injection, cephapirin sodium, up to 1 gm ⓑ ⓑ Qp Qh    E2

*Other: Cefadyl*

*IOM: 100-02, 15, 50*

**✳ J0712** Injection, ceftaroline fosamil, 10 mg ⓑ ⓑ Qp Qh    K2 K

*Other: Teflaro*

Coding Clinic: 2012, Q1, P9

**⚙ J0713** Injection, ceftazidime, per 500 mg ⓑ ⓑ Qp Qh    N1 N

*Other: Fortaz, Tazicef*

*IOM: 100-02, 15, 50*

**✳ J0714** Injection, ceftazidime and avibactam, 0.5 g/0.125 g ⓑ ⓑ Qp Qh   K2 K

**⚙ J0715** Injection, ceftizoxime sodium, per 500 mg ⓑ ⓑ Qp Qh    N1 N

*IOM: 100-02, 15, 50*

**✳ J0716** Injection, centruroides immune F(ab)2, up to 120 milligrams ⓑ ⓑ Qp Qh K2 K

*Other: Anascorp*

**✳ J0717** Injection, certolizumab pegol, 1 mg (Code may be used for Medicare when drug administered under the direct supervision of a physician, not for use when drug is self-administered) ⓑ ⓑ Qp Qh   K2 K

*Other: Cimzia*

**⚙ J0720** Injection, chloramphenicol sodium succinate, up to 1 gm ⓑ ⓑ Qp Qh    N1 N

*Other: Chloromycetin Sodium Succinate*

*IOM: 100-02, 15, 50*

**⚙ J0725** Injection, chorionic gonadotropin, per 1,000 USP units ⓑ ⓑ Qp Qh   N1 N

*Other: A.P.L., Chorex-5, Chorex-10, Chorignon, Choron-10, Chorionic Gonadotropin, Choron 10, Corgonject-5, Follutein, Glukor, Gonic, Novarel, Pregnyl, Profasi HP*

*IOM: 100-02, 15, 50*

**⚙ J0735** Injection, clonidine hydrochloride (HCL), 1 mg ⓑ ⓑ Qp Qh   N1 N

*Other: Duraclon*

*IOM: 100-02, 15, 50*

**⚙ J0740** Injection, cidofovir, 375 mg ⓑ ⓑ Qp Qh    K2 K

*Other: Vistide*

*IOM: 100-02, 15, 50*

**⚙ J0743** Injection, cilastatin sodium; imipenem, per 250 mg ⓑ ⓑ Qp Qh   N1 N

*Other: Primaxin*

*IOM: 100-02, 15, 50*

**✳ J0744** Injection, ciprofloxacin for intravenous infusion, 200 mg ⓑ ⓑ Qp Qh   N1 N

**⚙ J0745** Injection, codeine phosphate, per 30 mg ⓑ ⓑ Qp Qh    N1 N

*IOM: 100-02, 15, 50*

**⚙ J0770** Injection, colistimethate sodium, up to 150 mg ⓑ ⓑ Qp Qh   N1 N

*Other: Coly-Mycin M*

*IOM: 100-02, 15, 50*

**✳ J0775** Injection, collagenase, clostridium histolyticum, 0.01 mg ⓑ ⓑ Qp Qh   K2 K

*Other: Xiaflex*

Coding Clinic: 2011, Q1, P7

**⚙ J0780** Injection, prochlorperazine, up to 10 mg ⓑ ⓑ Qp Qh   N1 N

*Other: Compa-Z, Compazine, Cotranzine, Ultrazine-10*

*IOM: 100-02, 15, 50*

**⚙ J0795** Injection, corticorelin ovine triflutate, 1 mcg ⓑ ⓑ Qp Qh   K2 K

*Other: Acthrel*

*IOM: 100-02, 15, 50*

**⚙ J0800** Injection, corticotropin, up to 40 units ⓑ ⓑ Qp Qh   K2 K

*Other: ACTH, Acthar*

*IOM: 100-02, 15, 50*

**✳ J0834** Injection, cosyntropin, 0.25 mg ⓑ ⓑ Qp Qh   N1 N

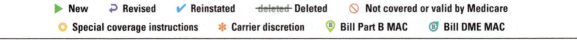

▶ New    ↩ Revised    ✔ Reinstated    ~~deleted~~ Deleted    ⊘ Not covered or valid by Medicare
⚙ Special coverage instructions    ✳ Carrier discretion    ⓑ Bill Part B MAC    ⓑ Bill DME MAC

* **J0840** Injection, crotalidae polyvalent immune fab (ovine), up to 1 gram ⑱ ⑱ Qp Qh   K2 K

*Other: Crofab*

Coding Clinic: 2012, Q1, P9

* **J0841** Injection, crotalidae immune f(ab')2 (equine), 120 mg   K

*Other: Anavip*

⚙ **J0850** Injection, cytomegalovirus immune globulin intravenous (human), per vial ⑱ ⑱ Qp Qh   K2 K

Prophylaxis to prevent cytomegalovirus disease associated with transplantation of kidney, lung, liver, pancreas, and heart.

*Other: Cytogam*

*IOM: 100-02, 15, 50*

* **J0875** Injection, dalbavancin, 5 mg ⑱ ⑱ Qp Qh   K2 K

*Other: Dalvance*

* **J0878** Injection, daptomycin, 1 mg ⑱ ⑱ Qp Qh   K2 K

*Other: Cubicin*

⚙ **J0881** Injection, darbepoetin alfa, 1 mcg (non-ESRD use) ⑱ ⑱ Qp Qh   K2 K

*Other: Aranesp*

⚙ **J0882** Injection, darbepoetin alfa, 1 mcg (for ESRD on dialysis) ⑱ ⑱ Qp Qh   K2 K

*Other: Aranesp*

*IOM: 100-02, 6, 10; 100-04, 4, 240*

⚙ **J0883** Injection, argatroban, 1 mg (for non-ESRD use) Qp Qh   K2 K

*IOM: 100-02, 15, 50*

⚙ **J0884** Injection, argatroban, 1 mg (for ESRD on dialysis) Qp Qh   K2 K

*IOM: 100-02, 15, 50*

⚙ **J0885** Injection, epoetin alfa, (for non-ESRD use), 1000 units ⑱ ⑱ Qp Qh   K2 K

*Other: Epogen, Procrit*

*IOM: 100-02, 15, 50*

Coding Clinic: 2006, Q2, P5

⚙ **J0887** Injection, epoetin beta, 1 mcg, (for ESRD on dialysis) ⑱ ⑱ Qp Qh   N1 N

*Other: Mircera*

⚙ **J0888** Injection, epoetin beta, 1 mcg, (for non ESRD use) ⑱ ⑱ Qp Qh   K2 K

*Other: Mircera*

* **J0890** Injection, peginesatide, 0.1 mg (for ESRD on dialysis) ⑱ ⑱ Qp Qh   E1

*Other: Omontys*

* **J0894** Injection, decitabine, 1 mg ⑱ ⑱ Qp Qh   K2 K

Indicated for treatment of myelodysplastic syndromes (MDS)

*Other: Dacogen*

⚙ **J0895** Injection, deferoxamine mesylate, 500 mg ⑱ ⑱ Qp Qh   N1 N

*Other: Desferal, Desferal mesylate*

*IOM: 100-02, 15, 50,*

*Cross Reference Q0087*

* **J0897** Injection, denosumab, 1 mg ⑱ ⑱ Qp Qh   K2 K

*Other: Prolia, Xgeva*

Coding Clinic: 2016, Q1, P5; 2012, Q1, P9

⚙ **J0945** Injection, brompheniramine maleate, per 10 mg ⑱ ⑱ Qp Qh   N1 N

*Other: Codimal-A, Cophene-B, Dehist, Histaject, Nasahist B, ND Stat, Oraminic II, Sinusol-B*

*IOM: 100-02, 15, 50*

⚙ **J1000** Injection, depo-estradiol cypionate, up to 5 mg ⑱ ⑱ Qp Qh   N1 N

*Other: DepGynogen, Depogen, Dura-Estrin, Estra-D, Estro-Cyp, Estroject LA, Estronol-LA*

*IOM: 100-02, 15, 50*

⚙ **J1020** Injection, methylprednisolone acetate, 20 mg ⑱ ⑱ Qp Qh   N1 N

*Other: DepMedalone, Depoject, Depo-Medrol, Depopred, D-Med 80, Duralone, Medralone, M-Prednisol, Rep-Pred*

*IOM: 100-02, 15, 50*

Coding Clinic: 2019, Q3, P14; 2018, Q4, P5-6; 2005, Q3, P10

⚙ **J1030** Injection, methylprednisolone acetate, 40 mg ⑱ ⑱ Qp Qh   N1 N

*Other: DepMedalone, Depoject, Depo-Medrol, Depropred, D-Med 80, Duralone, Medralone, M-Prednisol, Rep-Pred*

*IOM: 100-02, 15, 50*

Coding Clinic: 2019, Q3, P14; 2018, Q4, P6; 2005, Q3, P10

⚙ **J1040** Injection, methylprednisolone acetate, 80 mg ⑱ ⑱ Qp Qh   N1 N

*Other: DepMedalone, Depoject, Depo-Medrol, Depropred, D-Med 80, Duralone, Medralone, M-Prednisol, Rep-Pred*

*IOM: 100-02, 15, 50*

Coding Clinic: 2018, Q4, P6

| ✎ MIPS | Qp Quantity Physician | Qh Quantity Hospital | ♀ Female only |
|---|---|---|---|
| ♂ Male only | Ⓐ Age | ♿ DMEPOS | A2-Z3 ASC Payment Indicator | A-Y ASC Status Indicator | Coding Clinic |

✳ **J1050** Injection, medroxyprogesterone acetate, 1 mg Ⓑ Ⓑ Qp Qh    N1 N

*Other: Depo-Provera Contraceptive*

✿ **J1071** Injection, testosterone cypionate, 1 mg Qp Qh    N1 N

*Other: Andro-Cyp, Andro/Fem, Andronaq-LA, Andronate, De-Comberol, DepAndro, DepAndrogyn, Depotest, Depo-Testadiol, Depo-Testosterone, Depotestrogen, Duratest, Duratestrin, Menoject LA, Testa-C, Testadiate-Depo, Testaject-LA, Test-Estro Cypionates, Testoject-LA,*

Coding Clinic: 2015, Q2, P7

✿ **J1094** Injection, dexamethasone acetate, 1 mg Ⓑ Ⓑ Qp Qh    N1 N

*Other: Dalalone LA, Decadron LA, Decaject LA, Dexacen-LA-8, Dexasone L.A., Dexone-LA, Solurex LA*

*IOM: 100-02, 15, 50*

✿ **J1095** Injection, dexamethasone 9% Ⓑ

▶ ✳ **J1096** Dexamethasone, lacrimal ophthalmic insert, 0.1 mg    K2 G

▶ ✳ **J1097** Phenylephrine 10.16 mg/ml and ketorolac 2.88 mg/ml ophthalmic irrigation solution, 1 ml    K2 G

✿ **J1100** Injection, dexamethasone sodium phosphate, 1 mg Ⓑ Ⓑ Qp Qh    N1 N

*Other: Dalalone, Decadron Phosphate, Decaject, Dexacen-4, Dexone, Hexadrol Phosphate, Solurex*

*IOM: 100-02, 15, 50*

✿ **J1110** Injection, dihydroergotamine mesylate, per 1 mg Ⓑ Ⓑ Qp Qh    K2 K

*Other: D.H.E. 45*

*IOM: 100-02, 15, 50*

✿ **J1120** Injection, acetazolamide sodium, up to 500 mg Ⓑ Ⓑ Qp Qh    N1 N

*Other: Diamox*

*IOM: 100-02, 15, 50*

✳ **J1130** Injection, diclofenac sodium, 0.5 mg Qp Qh    K2 K

Coding Clinic: 2017, Q1, P9

✿ **J1160** Injection, digoxin, up to 0.5 mg Ⓑ Ⓑ Qp Qh    N1 N

*Other: Lanoxin*

*IOM: 100-02, 15, 50*

✿ **J1162** Injection, digoxin immune Fab (ovine), per vial Ⓑ Ⓑ Qp Qh    K2 K

*Other: DigiFab*

*IOM: 100-02, 15, 50*

✿ **J1165** Injection, phenytoin sodium, per 50 mg Ⓑ Ⓑ Qp Qh    N1 N

*Other: Dilantin*

*IOM: 100-02, 15, 50*

✿ **J1170** Injection, hydromorphone, up to 4 mg Ⓑ Ⓑ Qp Qh    N1 N

*Other: Dilaudid*

*IOM: 100-02, 15, 50*

✿ **J1180** Injection, dyphylline, up to 500 mg Ⓑ Ⓑ Qp Qh    E2

*Other: Dilor, Lufyllin*

*IOM: 100-02, 15, 50*

✿ **J1190** Injection, dexrazoxane hydrochloride, per 250 mg Ⓑ Ⓑ Qp Qh    K2 K

*Other: Totect, Zinecard*

*IOM: 100-02, 15, 50*

✿ **J1200** Injection, diphenhydramine HCL, up to 50 mg Ⓑ Ⓑ Qp Qh    N1 N

*Other: Bena-D, Benadryl, Benahist, Ben-Allergin, Benoject, Chlorothiazide sodium, Dihydrex, Diphenacen-50, Hyrexin-50, Nordryl, Wehdryl*

*IOM: 100-02, 15, 50*

✿ **J1205** Injection, chlorothiazide sodium, per 500 mg Ⓑ Ⓑ Qp Qh    N1 N

*Other: Diuril*

*IOM: 100-02, 15, 50*

✿ **J1212** Injection, DMSO, dimethyl sulfoxide, 50%, 50 ml Ⓑ Ⓑ Qp Qh    K2 K

*Other: Rimso-50*

*IOM: 100-02, 15, 50; 100-03, 4, 230.12*

✿ **J1230** Injection, methadone HCL, up to 10 mg Ⓑ Ⓑ Qp Qh    N1 N

*Other: Dolophine HCl*

*MCM: 2049*

*IOM: 100-02, 15, 50*

✿ **J1240** Injection, dimenhydrinate, up to 50 mg Ⓑ Ⓑ Qp Qh    N1 N

*Other: Dinate, Dommanate, Dramamine, Dramanate, Dramilin, Dramocen, Dramoject, Dymenate, Hydrate, Marmine, Wehamine*

*IOM: 100-02, 15, 50*

✿ **J1245** Injection, dipyridamole, per 10 mg Ⓑ Ⓑ Qp Qh    N1 N

*Other: Persantine*

*IOM: 100-04, 15, 50; 100-04, 12, 30.6*

---

▶ New   ↻ Revised   ✔ Reinstated   ~~deleted~~ Deleted   ⊘ Not covered or valid by Medicare
✿ Special coverage instructions   ✳ Carrier discretion   Ⓑ Bill Part B MAC   Ⓑ Bill DME MAC

✿ **J1250** Injection, dobutamine HCL, per 250 mg ⦿ Ⓑ Qp Qh    N1 N

*Other: Dobutrex*

*IOM: 100-02, 15, 50*

✿ **J1260** Injection, dolasetron mesylate, 10 mg ⦿ Ⓑ Qp Qh    N1 N

*Other: Anzemet*

*IOM: 100-02, 15, 50*

＊ **J1265** Injection, dopamine HCL, 40 mg ⦿ Ⓑ Qp Qh    N1 N

＊ **J1267** Injection, doripenem, 10 mg ⦿ Ⓑ Qp Qh    N1 N

*Other: Donbax, Doribax*

＊ **J1270** Injection, doxercalciferol, 1 mcg ⦿ Ⓑ Qp Qh    N1 N

*Other: Hectorol*

＊ **J1290** Injection, ecallantide, 1 mg Ⓑ Ⓑ Qp Qh    K2 K

*Other: Kalbitor*

**Coding Clinic: 2011, Q1, P7**

＊ **J1300** Injection, eculizumab, 10 mg ⦿ Ⓑ Qp Qh    K2 K

*Other: Soliris*

＊ **J1301** Injection, edaravone, 1 mg ⦿    G

*Other: Radicava*

▶ ＊ **J1303** Injection, ravulizumab-cwvz, 10 mg    K2 G

✿ **J1320** Injection, amitriptyline HCL, up to 20 mg ⦿ Ⓑ Qp Qh    N1 N

*Other: Elavil, Enovil*

*IOM: 100-02, 15, 50*

＊ **J1322** Injection, elosulfase alfa, 1 mg Ⓑ Ⓑ Qp Qh    K2 K

＊ **J1324** Injection, enfuvirtide, 1 mg ⦿ Ⓑ Qp Qh    E2

✿ **J1325** Injection, epoprostenol, 0.5 mg ⦿ Qp Qh    N1 N

*Other: Flolan, Veletri*

*IOM: 100-02, 15, 50*

✿ **J1327** Injection, eptifibatide, 5 mg ⦿ Ⓑ Qp Qh    K2 K

*Other: Integrilin*

*IOM: 100-02, 15, 50*

✿ **J1330** Injection, ergonovine maleate, up to 0.2 mg ⦿ Ⓑ Qp Qh    N1 N

Benefit limited to obstetrical diagnosis

*IOM: 100-02, 15, 50*

＊ **J1335** Injection, ertapenem sodium, 500 mg Ⓑ Ⓑ Qp Qh    N1 N

*Other: Invanz*

✿ **J1364** Injection, erythromycin lactobionate, per 500 mg ⦿ Ⓑ Qp Qh    K2 K

*IOM: 100-02, 15, 50*

✿ **J1380** Injection, estradiol valerate, up to 10 mg ⦿ Ⓑ Qp Qh    N1 N

*Other: Delestrogen, Dioval, Duragen, Estra-L, Gynogen L.A., L.A.E. 20, Valergen*

*IOM: 100-02, 15, 50*

**Coding Clinic: 2011, Q1, P8**

✿ **J1410** Injection, estrogen conjugated, per 25 mg ⦿ Ⓑ Qp Qh    K2 K

*Other: Premarin*

*IOM: 100-02, 15, 50*

＊ **J1428** Injection, eteplirsen, 10 mg    K2 G

✿ **J1430** Injection, ethanolamine oleate, 100 mg ⦿ Ⓑ Qp Qh    K2 K

*Other: Ethamolin*

*IOM: 100-02, 15, 50*

✿ **J1435** Injection, estrone, per 1 mg ⦿ Ⓑ Qp Qh    E2

*Other: Estronol, Kestrone 5, Theelin Aqueous*

*IOM: 100-02, 15, 50*

✿ **J1436** Injection, etidronate disodium, per 300 mg ⦿ Ⓑ Qp Qh    E1

*Other: Didronel*

*IOM: 100-02, 15, 50*

✿ **J1438** Injection, etanercept, 25 mg (Code may be used for Medicare when drug administered under the direct supervision of a physician, not for use when drug is self-administered) ⦿ Ⓑ Qp Qh    K2 K

*Other: Enbrel*

*IOM: 100-02, 15, 50*

＊ **J1439** Injection, ferric carboxymaltose, 1 mg ⦿ Ⓑ Qp Qh    K2 K

*Other: Injectafer*

✿ **J1442** Injection, filgrastim (G-CSF), excludes biosimilars, 1 mcg ⦿ Ⓑ Qp Qh    K2 K

*Other: Neupogen*

＊ **J1443** Injection, ferric pyrophosphate citrate solution, 0.1 mg of iron Ⓑ Ⓑ Qp Qh    N1 N

▶ ✿ **J1444** Injection, ferric pyrophosphate citrate powder, 0.1 mg of iron    N

✿ **J1447** Injection, TBO-filgrastim, 1 mcg ⦿ Ⓑ Qp Qh    K2 K

*Other: GRANIX*

*IOM: 100-02, 15, 50*

| 🖐 MIPS | Qp Quantity Physician | Qh Quantity Hospital | ♀ Female only |
| --- | --- | --- | --- |
| ♂ Male only | Ⓐ Age | ♿ DMEPOS | A2-Z3 ASC Payment Indicator    A-Y ASC Status Indicator    Coding Clinic |

⚙ **J1450** Injection, fluconazole, 200 mg Ⓑ Ⓑ Qp Qh  N1 N

*Other: Diflucan*

*IOM: 100-02, 15, 50*

⚙ **J1451** Injection, fomepizole, 15 mg Ⓑ Ⓑ Qp Qh  K2 K

*IOM: 100-02, 15, 50*

⚙ **J1452** Injection, fomivirsen sodium, intraocular, 1.65 mg Ⓑ Ⓑ Qp Qh  E2

*IOM: 100-02, 15, 50*

✳ **J1453** Injection, fosaprepitant, 1 mg Ⓑ Ⓑ Qp Qh  K2 K

Prevents chemotherapy-induced nausea and vomiting

*Other: Emend*

✳ **J1454** Injection, fosnetupitant 235 mg and palonosetron 0.25 mg Ⓑ Ⓑ  G

*Other: Akynzeo and Aloxi*

⚙ **J1455** Injection, foscarnet sodium, per 1000 mg Ⓑ Ⓑ Qp Qh  K2 K

*Other: Foscavir*

*IOM: 100-02, 15, 50*

✳ **J1457** Injection, gallium nitrate, 1 mg Ⓑ Ⓑ Qp Qh  E2

✳ **J1458** Injection, galsulfase, 1 mg Ⓑ Ⓑ Qp Qh  K2 K

*Other: Naglazyme*

✳ **J1459** Injection, immune globulin (Privigen), intravenous, non-lyophilized (e.g., liquid), 500 mg Ⓑ Ⓑ Qp Qh  K2 K

⚙ **J1460** Injection, gamma globulin, intramuscular, 1 cc Ⓑ Ⓑ Qp Qh  K2 K

*Other: Gammar, GamaSTAN*

*IOM: 100-02, 15, 50*

Coding Clinic: 2011, Q1, P8

✳ **J1555** Injection, immune globulin (cuvitru), 100 mg  K2 K

✳ **J1556** Injection, immune globulin (Bivigam), 500 mg Ⓑ Ⓑ Qp Qh  K2 K

✳ **J1557** Injection, immune globulin, (gammaplex), intravenous, non-lyophilized (e.g., liquid), 500 mg Ⓑ Ⓑ Qp Qh  K2 K

Coding Clinic: 2012, Q1, P9

✳ **J1559** Injection, immune globulin (hizentra), 100 mg Ⓑ Ⓑ Qp Qh  K2 K

Coding Clinic: 2011, Q1, P6

⚙ **J1560** Injection, gamma globulin, intramuscular, over 10 cc Ⓑ Ⓑ Qp Qh  K2 K

*Other: Gammar, GamaSTAN*

*IOM: 100-02, 15, 50*

⚙ **J1561** Injection, immune globulin, (Gamunex-C/Gammaked), non-lyophilized (e.g., liquid), 500 mg Ⓑ Ⓑ Qp Qh  K2 K

*IOM: 100-02, 15, 50*

Coding Clinic: 2012, Q1, P9

✳ **J1562** Injection, immune globulin (Vivaglobin), 100 mg Ⓑ Ⓑ Qp Qh  E2

⚙ **J1566** Injection, immune globulin, intravenous, lyophilized (e.g., powder), not otherwise specified, 500 mg Ⓑ Ⓑ Qp Qh  K2 K

*Other: Carimune, Gammagard S/D, Polygam*

*IOM: 100-02, 15, 50*

✳ **J1568** Injection, immune globulin, (Octagam), intravenous, non-lyophilized (e.g., liquid), 500 mg Ⓑ Ⓑ Qp Qh  K2 K

⚙ **J1569** Injection, immune globulin, (Gammagard Liquid), non-lyophilized (e.g., liquid), 500 mg Ⓑ Ⓑ Qp Qh  K2 K

*IOM: 100-02, 15, 50*

⚙ **J1570** Injection, ganciclovir sodium, 500 mg Ⓑ Ⓑ Qp Qh  N1 N

*Other: Cytovene*

*IOM: 100-02, 15, 50*

⚙ **J1571** Injection, hepatitis B immune globulin (HepaGam B), intramuscular, 0.5 ml Ⓑ Ⓑ Qp Qh  K2 K

*IOM: 100-02, 15, 50*

Coding Clinic: 2008, Q3, P7-8

⚙ **J1572** Injection, immune globulin, (flebogamma/flebogamma DIF) intravenous, non-lyophilized (e.g., liquid), 500 mg Ⓑ Ⓑ Qp Qh  K2 K

*IOM: 100-02, 15, 50*

✳ **J1573** Injection, hepatitis B immune globulin (HepaGam B), intravenous, 0.5 ml Ⓑ Ⓑ Qp Qh  K2 K

Coding Clinic: 2008, Q3, P8

✳ **J1575** Injection, immune globulin/ hyaluronidase (HYQVIA), 100 mg immunoglobulin Ⓑ Ⓑ Qp Qh  K2 K

⚙ **J1580** Injection, Garamycin, gentamicin, up to 80 mg Ⓑ Ⓑ Qp Qh  N1 N

*Other: Gentamicin Sulfate, Jenamicin*

*IOM: 100-02, 15, 50*

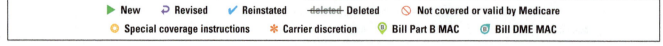

▶ New ↻ Revised ✔ Reinstated ~~deleted~~ Deleted ⊘ Not covered or valid by Medicare
⚙ Special coverage instructions ✳ Carrier discretion Ⓑ Bill Part B MAC Ⓑ Bill DME MAC

**J1595** Injection, glatiramer acetate, 20 mg ⊙ Ⓑ Qp Qh  K2 K

*Other: Copaxone*

*IOM: 100-02, 15, 50*

**✱ J1599** Injection, immune globulin, intravenous, non-lyophilized (e.g., liquid), not otherwise specified, 500 mg ⊙ Ⓑ Qp Qh  N1 N

Coding Clinic: 2011, P1, Q6

**J1600** Injection, gold sodium thiomalate, up to 50 mg Ⓑ Ⓑ Qp Qh  E2

*Other: Myochrysine*

*IOM: 100-02, 15, 50*

**✱ J1602** Injection, golimumab, 1 mg, for intravenous use Ⓑ Ⓑ Qp Qh  K2 K

*Other: Simponi Aria*

**J1610** Injection, glucagon hydrochloride, per 1 mg ⊙ Ⓑ Qp Qh  K2 K

*Other: GlucaGen, Glucagon Emergency*

*IOM: 100-02, 15, 50*

**J1620** Injection, gonadorelin hydrochloride, per 100 mcg Ⓑ Ⓑ Qp Qh  E2

*Other: Factrel*

*IOM: 100-02, 15, 50*

**J1626** Injection, granisetron hydrochloride, 100 mcg Ⓑ Ⓑ Qp Qh  N1 N

*Other: Kytril*

*IOM: 100-02, 15, 50*

**✱ J1627** Injection, granisetron, extended-release, 0.1 mg  K2 G

**✱ J1628** Injection, guselkumab, 1 mg Ⓑ Ⓑ  G

*Other: Tremfya*

**J1630** Injection, haloperidol, up to 5 mg Ⓑ Ⓑ Qp Qh  N1 N

*Other: Haldol, Haloperidol Lactate*

*IOM: 100-02, 15, 50*

**J1631** Injection, haloperidol decanoate, per 50 mg ⊙ Ⓑ Qp Qh  N1 N

*IOM: 100-02, 15, 50*

**J1640** Injection, hemin, 1 mg Ⓑ Ⓑ Qp Qh  K2 K

*Other: Panhematin*

*IOM: 100-02, 15, 50*

**J1642** Injection, heparin sodium, (heparin lock flush), per 10 units Ⓑ Ⓑ Qp Qh  N1 N

*Other: Hep-Lock U/P, Vasceze*

*IOM: 100-02, 15, 50*

**J1644** Injection, heparin sodium, per 1000 units Ⓑ Ⓑ Qp Qh  N1 N

*Other: Heparin Sodium (Porcine), Liquaemin Sodium*

*IOM: 100-02, 15, 50*

**J1645** Injection, dalteparin sodium, per 2500 IU Ⓑ Ⓑ Qp Qh  N1 N

*Other: Fragmin*

*IOM: 100-02, 15, 50*

**✱ J1650** Injection, enoxaparin sodium, 10 mg Ⓑ Ⓑ Qp Qh  N1 N

*Other: Lovenox*

**J1652** Injection, fondaparinux sodium, 0.5 mg ⊙ Ⓑ Qp Qh  N1 N

*Other: Arixtra*

*IOM: 100-02, 15, 50*

**✱ J1655** Injection, tinzaparin sodium, 1000 IU Ⓑ Ⓑ Qp Qh  N1 N

*Other: Innohep*

**J1670** Injection, tetanus immune globulin, human, up to 250 units Ⓑ Ⓑ Qp Qh  K2 K

Indicated for transient protection against tetanus post-exposure to tetanus (Z23).

*Other: Hyper-Tet*

*IOM: 100-02, 15, 50*

**J1675** Injection, histrelin acetate, 10 mcg Ⓑ Ⓑ Qp Qh  B

*IOM: 100-02, 15, 50*

**J1700** Injection, hydrocortisone acetate, up to 25 mg ⊙ Ⓑ Qp Qh  N1 N

*Other: Hydrocortone Acetate*

*IOM: 100-02, 15, 50*

**J1710** Injection, hydrocortisone sodium phosphate, up to 50 mg Ⓑ Ⓑ Qp Qh  N1 N

*Other: A-hydroCort, Hydrocortone phosphate, Solu-Cortef*

*IOM: 100-02, 15, 50*

**J1720** Injection, hydrocortisone sodium succinate, up to 100 mg Ⓑ Ⓑ Qp Qh  N1 N

*Other: A-HydroCort, Solu-Cortef*

*IOM: 100-02, 15, 50*

**✱ J1726** Injection, hydroxyprogesterone caproate (makena), 10 mg  K2 K

**✱ J1729** Injection, hydroxyprogesterone caproate, not otherwise specified, 10 mg  N1 N

---

🖐 MIPS   Qp Quantity Physician   Qh Quantity Hospital   ♀ Female only

♂ Male only   Ⓐ Age   ♿ DMEPOS   A2-Z3 ASC Payment Indicator   A-Y ASC Status Indicator   Coding Clinic

⊛ **J1730** Injection, diazoxide, up to
300 mg Ⓑ Ⓑ Qp Qh  E2

*Other:* Hyperstat

*IOM: 100-02, 15, 50*

✳ **J1740** Injection, ibandronate sodium,
1 mg Ⓑ Ⓑ Qp Qh  K2 K

*Other:* Boniva

✳ **J1741** Injection, ibuprofen,
100 mg Ⓑ Ⓑ Qp Qh  N1 N

*Other:* Caldolor

⊛ **J1742** Injection, ibutilide fumarate,
1 mg Ⓑ Ⓑ Qp Qh  K2 K

*Other:* Corvert

*IOM: 100-02, 15, 50*

✳ **J1743** Injection, idursulfase,
1 mg Ⓑ Ⓑ Qp Qh  K2 K

*Other:* Elaprase

✳ **J1744** Injection, icatibant,
1 mg Ⓑ Ⓑ Qp Qh  K2 K

*Other:* Firazyr

⊛ **J1745** Injection, infliximab, excludes
biosimilar, 10 mg Ⓑ Ⓑ Qp Qh  K2 K

Report total number of 10 mg
increments administered

For biosimilar, Inflectra, report Q5102

*Other:* Remicade

*IOM: 100-02, 15, 50*

✳ **J1746** Injection, ibalizumab-uiyk,
10 mg Ⓑ Ⓑ  K

*Other:* Trogarzo

⊛ **J1750** Injection, iron dextran,
50 mg Ⓑ Ⓑ Qp Qh  K2 K

*Other:* Dexferrum, Imferon, Infed

*IOM: 100-02, 15, 50*

✳ **J1756** Injection, iron sucrose,
1 mg Ⓑ Ⓑ Qp Qh  N1 N

*Other:* Venofer

⊛ **J1786** Injection, imiglucerase,
10 units Ⓑ Ⓑ Qp Qh  K2 K

*Other:* Cerezyme

*IOM: 100-02, 15, 50*

**Coding Clinic: 2011, Q1, P8**

⊛ **J1790** Injection, droperidol, up to
5 mg Ⓑ Ⓑ Qp Qh  N1 N

*Other:* Inapsine

*IOM: 100-02, 15, 50*

⊛ **J1800** Injection, propranolol HCL,
up to 1 mg Ⓑ Ⓑ Qp Qh  N1 N

*Other:* Inderal

*IOM: 100-02, 15, 50*

⊛ **J1810** Injection, droperidol and
fentanyl citrate, up to 2 ml
ampule Ⓑ Ⓑ Qp Qh  E1

*Other:* Innovar

*IOM: 100-02, 15, 50*

⊛ **J1815** Injection, insulin, per
5 units Ⓑ Ⓑ Qp Qh  N1 N

*Other:* Humalog, Humulin, Lantus,
Novolin, Novolog

*IOM: 100-02, 15, 50; 100-03, 4, 280.14*

✳ **J1817** Insulin for administration through
DME (i.e., insulin pump) per
50 units Ⓑ Ⓑ Qp Qh  N1 N

*Other:* Apidra Solostar, Insulin Lispro,
Humalog, Humulin, Novolin, Novolog

✳ **J1826** Injection, interferon beta-1a,
30 mcg Ⓑ Ⓑ  K2 K

*Other:* Avonex

**Coding Clinic: 2011, Q2, P9; Q1, P8**

⊛ **J1830** Injection, interferon beta-1b, 0.25 mg
(Code may be used for Medicare
when drug administered under the
direct supervision of a physician,
not for use when drug is
self-administered) Ⓑ Ⓑ Qp Qh  K2 K

*Other:* Betaseron

*IOM: 100-02, 15, 50*

✳ **J1833** Injection, isavuconazonium,
1 mg Ⓑ Ⓑ Qp Qh  K2 K

✳ **J1835** Injection, itraconazole,
50 mg Ⓑ Ⓑ Qp Qh  E2

*Other:* Sporanox

⊛ **J1840** Injection, kanamycin sulfate,
up to 500 mg Ⓑ Ⓑ Qp Qh  N1 N

*Other:* Kantrex, Klebcil

*IOM: 100-02, 15, 50*

⊛ **J1850** Injection, kanamycin sulfate,
up to 75 mg Ⓑ Ⓑ Qp Qh  N1 N

*Other:* Kantrex, Klebcil

*IOM: 100-02, 15, 50*

**Coding Clinic: 2013: Q2, P3**

⊛ **J1885** Injection, ketorolac tromethamine,
per 15 mg Ⓑ Ⓑ Qp Qh  N1 N

*Other:* Toradol

*IOM: 100-02, 15, 50*

---

▶ New  ↻ Revised  ✔ Reinstated  ~~deleted~~ Deleted  ⊘ Not covered or valid by Medicare
⊛ Special coverage instructions  ✳ Carrier discretion  Ⓑ Bill Part B MAC  Ⓑ Bill DME MAC

**J1890** Injection, cephalothin sodium, up to 1 gram ⓥ ⑧ Qp Qh   N1 N

*Other: Keflin*

*IOM: 100-02, 15, 50*

**J1930** Injection, lanreotide, 1 mg ⓥ ⑧ Qp Qh   K2 K

Treats acromegaly and symptoms caused by neuroendocrine tumors

*Other: Somatuline Depot*

**J1931** Injection, laronidase, 0.1 mg ⑧ ⓖ Qp Qh   K2 K

*Other: Aldurazyme*

**J1940** Injection, furosemide, up to 20 mg ⑧ ⓖ Qp Qh   N1 N

*Other: Furomide M.D., Lasix*

*MCM: 2049*

*IOM: 100-02, 15, 50*

~~J1942   Injection, aripiprazole lauroxil, 1 mg~~ ✖

▶ **J1943** Injection, aripiprazole lauroxil, (aristada initio), 1 mg   K2 G

▶ **J1944** Injection, aripiprazole lauroxil, (aristada), 1 mg   K2 K

**J1945** Injection, lepirudin, 50 mg ⑧ ⑧ Qp Qh   E2

*IOM: 100-02, 15, 50*

**J1950** Injection, leuprolide acetate (for depot suspension), per 3.75 mg ⓥ ⑧ Qp Qh   K2 K

*Other: Lupron, Lupron Depot, Lupron Depot-Ped*

*IOM: 100-02, 15, 50*

**Coding Clinic: 2019, Q2, P11-12**

**J1953** Injection, levetiracetam, 10 mg ⑧ ⓖ Qp Qh   N1 N

*Other: Keppra*

**J1955** Injection, levocarnitine, per 1 gm ⓥ ⑧ Qp Qh   B

*Other: Carnitor*

*IOM: 100-02, 15, 50*

**J1956** Injection, levofloxacin, 250 mg ⓥ ⑧ Qp Qh   N1 N

*Other: Levaquin*

*IOM: 100-02, 15, 50*

**J1960** Injection, levorphanol tartrate, up to 2 mg ⓥ ⑧ Qp Qh   N1 N

*Other: Levo-Dromoran*

*MCM: 2049*

*IOM: 100-02, 15, 50*

**J1980** Injection, hyoscyamine sulfate, up to 0.25 mg ⓥ ⑧ Qp Qh   N1 N

*Other: Levsin*

*IOM: 100-02, 15, 50*

**J1990** Injection, chlordiazepoxide HCL, up to 100 mg ⓥ ⑧ Qp Qh   N1 N

*Other: Librium*

*IOM: 100-02, 15, 50*

**J2001** Injection, lidocaine HCL for intravenous infusion, 10 mg ⓥ ⑧ Qp Qh   N1 N

*Other: Caine-1, Caine-2, Dilocaine, L-Caine, Lidocaine in D5W, Lidoject, Nervocaine, Nulicaine, Xylocaine*

*IOM: 100-02, 15, 50*

**J2010** Injection, lincomycin HCL, up to 300 mg ⑧ Qp Qh   N1 N

*Other: Lincocin*

*IOM: 100-02, 15, 50*

**J2020** Injection, linezolid, 200 mg ⓥ ⑧ Qp Qh   N1 N

*Other: Zyvox*

**J2060** Injection, lorazepam, 2 mg ⓥ ⑧ Qp Qh   N1 N

*Other: Ativan*

*IOM: 100-02, 15, 50*

**J2062** Loxapine for inhalation, 1 mg ⓥ ⑧   K

*Other: Adasuve*

**J2150** Injection, mannitol, 25% in 50 ml ⓥ ⑧ Qp Qh   N1 N

*Other: Aridol*

*MCM: 2049*

*IOM: 100-02, 15, 50*

**J2170** Injection, mecasermin, 1 mg ⓥ ⑧ Qp Qh   N1 N

*Other: Increlex*

**J2175** Injection, meperidine hydrochloride, per 100 mg ⓥ ⑧ Qp Qh   N1 N

*Other: Demerol*

*IOM: 100-02, 15, 50*

**J2180** Injection, meperidine and promethazine HCL, up to 50 mg ⓥ ⑧ Qp Qh   N1 N

*Other: Mepergan*

*IOM: 100-02, 15, 50*

**J2182** Injection, mepolizumab, 1 mg Qp Qh   K2 G

---

| 🐾 MIPS | Qp Quantity Physician | Qh Quantity Hospital | ♀ Female only |
|---|---|---|---|
| ♂ Male only | Ⓐ Age | ⚕ DMEPOS | A2-Z3 ASC Payment Indicator | A-Y ASC Status Indicator | Coding Clinic |

* **J2185** Injection, meropenem, 100 mg Ⓑ Ⓑ Qp Qh    N1 N

*Other: Merrem*

* **J2186** Inj., meropenem, vaborbactam Ⓑ Ⓑ    G

*Other: Vabomere*

*Medicare Statute 1833(t)*

⊛ **J2210** Injection, methylergonovine maleate, up to 0.2 mg Ⓑ Ⓑ Qp Qh    N1 N

Benefit limited to obstetrical diagnoses for prevention and control of post-partum hemorrhage

*Other: Methergine*

*IOM: 100-02, 15, 50*

* **J2212** Injection, methylnaltrexone, 0.1 mg Ⓑ Ⓑ Qp Qh    N1 N

*Other: Relistor*

* **J2248** Injection, micafungin sodium, 1 mg Ⓑ Ⓑ Qp Qh    N1 N

*Other: Mycamine*

⊛ **J2250** Injection, midazolam hydrochloride, per 1 mg Ⓑ Ⓑ Qp Qh    N1 N

*Other: Versed*

*IOM: 100-02, 15, 50*

⊛ **J2260** Injection, milrinone lactate, 5 mg Ⓑ Ⓑ Qp Qh    N1 N

*Other: Primacor*

*IOM: 100-02, 15, 50*

* **J2265** Injection, minocycline hydrochloride, 1 mg Ⓑ Ⓑ Qp Qh    K2 K

*Other: Minocine*

⊛ **J2270** Injection, morphine sulfate, up to 10 mg Ⓑ Ⓑ Qp Qh    N1 N

*Other: Astramorph PF, Duramorph*

*IOM: 100-02, 15, 50*

*Coding Clinic: 2013, Q2, P4*

⊛ **J2274** Injection, morphine sulfate, preservative-free for epidural or intrathecal use, 10 mg Ⓑ Ⓑ Qp Qh    N1 N

*Other: Duramorph, Infumorph*

*IOM: 100-03, 4, 280.1; 100-02, 15, 50*

⊛ **J2278** Injection, ziconotide, 1 mcg Ⓑ Ⓑ Qp Qh    K2 K

*Other: Prialt*

* **J2280** Injection, moxifloxacin, 100 mg Ⓑ Ⓑ Qp Qh    N1 N

*Other: Avelox*

⊛ **J2300** Injection, nalbuphine hydrochloride, per 10 mg Ⓑ Ⓑ Qp Qh    N1 N

*Other: Nubain*

*IOM: 100-02, 15, 50*

⊛ **J2310** Injection, naloxone hydrochloride, per 1 mg Ⓑ Ⓑ Qp Qh    N1 N

*Other: Narcan*

*IOM: 100-02, 15, 50*

* **J2315** Injection, naltrexone, depot form, 1 mg Ⓑ Ⓑ Qp Qh    K2 K

*Other: Vivitrol*

⊛ **J2320** Injection, nandrolone decanoate, up to 50 mg Ⓑ Ⓑ Qp Qh    K2 K

*Other: Anabolin LA 100, Androlone, Deca-Durabolin, Decolone, Hybolin Decanoate, Nandrobolic LA, Neo-Durabolic*

*IOM: 100-02, 15, 50*

*Coding Clinic: 2011, Q1, P8*

* **J2323** Injection, natalizumab, 1 mg Ⓑ Ⓑ Qp Qh    K2 K

*Other: Tysabri*

⊛ **J2325** Injection, nesiritide, 0.1 mg Ⓑ Ⓑ Qp Qh    K2 K

*Other: Natrecor*

*IOM: 100-02, 15, 50*

* **J2326** Injection, nusinersen, 0.1 mg    K2 G

* **J2350** Injection, ocrelizumab, 1 mg    K2 G

* **J2353** Injection, octreotide, depot form for intramuscular injection, 1 mg Ⓑ Ⓑ Qp Qh    K2 K

*Other: Sandostatin LAR Depot*

* **J2354** Injection, octreotide, non-depot form for subcutaneous or intravenous injection, 25 mcg Ⓑ Ⓑ Qp Qh    N1 N

*Other: Sandostatin LAR Depot*

⊛ **J2355** Injection, oprelvekin, 5 mg Ⓑ Ⓑ Qp Qh    K2 K

*Other: Neumega*

*IOM: 100-02, 15, 50*

* **J2357** Injection, omalizumab, 5 mg Ⓑ Ⓑ Qp Qh    K2 K

*Other: Xolair*

* **J2358** Injection, olanzapine, long-acting, 1 mg Ⓑ Ⓑ Qp Qh    N1 N

*Other: Zyprexa Relprevv*

*Coding Clinic: 2011, Q1, P6*

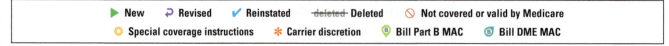

▶ New    ↻ Revised    ✔ Reinstated    ~~deleted~~ Deleted    ⊘ Not covered or valid by Medicare
⊛ Special coverage instructions    * Carrier discretion    Ⓑ Bill Part B MAC    Ⓑ Bill DME MAC

⚙ **J2360** Injection, orphenadrine citrate, up to 60 mg 📍 Ⓑ Qp Qh N1 N

*Other: Antiflex, Banflex, Flexoject, Flexon, K-Flex, Myolin, Neocyten, Norflex, O-Flex, Orphenate*

*IOM: 100-02, 15, 50*

⚙ **J2370** Injection, phenylephrine HCL, up to 1 ml 📍 Ⓑ Qp Qh N1 N

*Other: Neo-Synephrine*

*IOM: 100-02, 15, 50*

⚙ **J2400** Injection, chloroprocaine hydrochloride, per 30 ml Ⓑ Ⓑ Qp Qh N1 N

*Other: Nesacaine, Nesacaine-MPF*

*IOM: 100-02, 15, 50*

⚙ **J2405** Injection, ondansetron hydrochloride, per 1 mg Ⓑ Ⓑ Qp Qh N1 N

*Other: Zofran*

*IOM: 100-02, 15, 50*

⚙ **J2407** Injection, oritavancin, 10 mg Ⓑ Ⓑ Qp Qh K2 K

*Other: Orbactiv*

*IOM: 100-02, 15, 50*

⚙ **J2410** Injection, oxymorphone HCL, up to 1 mg Ⓑ Ⓑ Qp Qh N1 N

*Other: Numorphan, Opana*

*IOM: 100-02, 15, 50*

✳ **J2425** Injection, palifermin, 50 mcg Ⓑ Ⓑ Qp Qh K2 K

*Other: Kepivance*

✳ **J2426** Injection, paliperidone palmitate extended release, 1 mg Ⓑ Ⓑ Qp Qh K2 K

*Other: Invega Sustenna*

**Coding Clinic: 2011, Q1, P7**

⚙ **J2430** Injection, pamidronate disodium, per 30 mg 📍 Ⓑ Qp Qh N1 N

*Other: Aredia*

*IOM: 100-02, 15, 50*

⚙ **J2440** Injection, papaverine HCL, up to 60 mg 📍 Ⓑ Qp Qh N1 N

*IOM: 100-02, 15, 50*

⚙ **J2460** Injection, oxytetracycline HCL, up to 50 mg Ⓑ Ⓑ Qp Qh E2

*Other: Terramycin IM*

*IOM: 100-02, 15, 50*

✳ **J2469** Injection, palonosetron HCL, 25 mcg 📍 Ⓑ Qp Qh K2 K

Example: 0.25 mgm dose = 10 units Example of use is acute, delayed, nausea and vomiting due to chemotherapy

*Other: Aloxi*

⚙ **J2501** Injection, paricalcitol, 1 mcg Ⓑ Ⓑ Qp Qh N1 N

*Other: Zemplar*

*IOM: 100-02, 15, 50*

✳ **J2502** Injection, pasireotide long acting, 1 mg Ⓑ Ⓑ Qp Qh K2 K

*Other: Signifor LAR*

✳ **J2503** Injection, pegaptanib sodium, 0.3 mg Ⓑ Ⓑ Qp Qh K2 K

*Other: Macugen*

⚙ **J2504** Injection, pegademase bovine, 25 IU Ⓑ Ⓑ Qp Qh K2 K

*Other: Adagen*

*IOM: 100-02, 15, 50*

✳ **J2505** Injection, pegfilgrastim, 6 mg 📍 Ⓑ Qp Qh K2 K

Report 1 unit per 6 mg.

*Other: Neulasta*

✳ **J2507** Injection, pegloticase, 1 mg 📍 Ⓑ Qp Qh K2 K

*Other: Krystexxa*

**Coding Clinic: 2012, Q1, P9**

⚙ **J2510** Injection, penicillin G procaine, aqueous, up to 600,000 units Ⓑ Ⓑ Qp Qh N1 N

*Other: Crysticillin, Duracillin AS, Pfizerpen AS, Wycillin*

*IOM: 100-02, 15, 50*

⚙ **J2513** Injection, pentastarch, 10% solution, 100 ml Ⓑ Ⓑ Qp Qh E2

*IOM: 100-02, 15, 50*

⚙ **J2515** Injection, pentobarbital sodium, per 50 mg Ⓑ Ⓑ Qp Qh K2 K

*Other: Nembutal sodium solution*

*IOM: 100-02, 15, 50*

⚙ **J2540** Injection, penicillin G potassium, up to 600,000 units Ⓑ Ⓑ Qp Qh N1 N

*Other: Pfizerpen-G*

*IOM: 100-02, 15, 50*

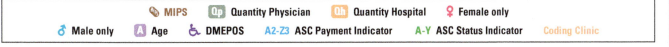

🖐 MIPS   Qp Quantity Physician   Qh Quantity Hospital   ♀ Female only
♂ Male only   Ⓐ Age   ♿ DMEPOS   A2-Z3 ASC Payment Indicator   A-Y ASC Status Indicator   Coding Clinic

✿ **J2543** Injection, piperacillin sodium/ tazobactam sodium, 1 gram/0.125 grams (1.125 grams) Ⓑ Ⓓ Qp Qh    N1 N

*Other: Zosyn*

*IOM: 100-02, 15, 50*

✿ **J2545** Pentamidine isethionate, inhalation solution, FDA-approved final product, non-compounded, administered through DME, unit dose form, per 300 mg Ⓑ Ⓓ Qp Qh    B

*Other: Nebupent*

✳ **J2547** Injection, peramivir, 1 mg Ⓑ Ⓓ Qp Qh    K2 K

✿ **J2550** Injection, promethazine HCL, up to 50 mg Ⓑ Ⓓ Qp Qh    N1 N

Administration of phenergan suppository considered part of E/M encounter

*Other: Anergan, Phenazine, Phenergan, Prorex, Prothazine, V-Gan*

*IOM: 100-02, 15, 50*

✿ **J2560** Injection, phenobarbital sodium, up to 120 mg Ⓑ Ⓓ Qp Qh    N1 N

*Other: Luminal Sodium*

*IOM: 100-02, 15, 50*

✳ **J2562** Injection, plerixafor, 1 mg Ⓑ Ⓓ Qp Qh    K2 K

FDA approved for non-Hodgkin lymphoma and multiple myeloma in 2008.

*Other: Mozobil*

✿ **J2590** Injection, oxytocin, up to 10 units Ⓑ Ⓓ Qp Qh    N1 N

*Other: Pitocin, Syntocinon*

*IOM: 100-02, 15, 50*

✿ **J2597** Injection, desmopressin acetate, per 1 mcg Ⓑ Ⓓ Qp Qh    K2 K

*Other: DDAVP*

*IOM: 100-02, 15, 50*

✿ **J2650** Injection, prednisolone acetate, up to 1 ml Ⓑ Ⓓ Qp Qh    N1 N

*Other: Key-Pred, Predalone, Predcor, Predicort, Predoject*

*IOM: 100-02, 15, 50*

✿ **J2670** Injection, tolazoline HCL, up to 25 mg Ⓑ Ⓓ Qp Qh    N1 N

*Other: Priscoline HCl*

*IOM: 100-02, 15, 50*

✿ **J2675** Injection, progesterone, per 50 mg Ⓥ Ⓑ Qp Qh    N1 N

*Other: Gesterol 50, Progestaject*

*IOM: 100-02, 15, 50*

✿ **J2680** Injection, fluphenazine decanoate, up to 25 mg Ⓥ Ⓑ Qp Qh    N1 N

*Other: Prolixin Decanoate*

*MCM: 2049*

*IOM: 100-02, 15, 50*

✿ **J2690** Injection, procainamide HCL, up to 1 gm Ⓥ Ⓑ Qp Qh ♀    N1 N

Benefit limited to obstetrical diagnoses

*Other: Pronestyl, Prostaphlin*

*IOM: 100-02, 15, 50*

✿ **J2700** Injection, oxacillin sodium, up to 250 mg Ⓥ Ⓑ Qp Qh    N1 N

*Other: Bactocill*

*IOM: 100-02, 15, 50*

✳ **J2704** Injection, propofol, 10 mg Ⓥ Ⓑ Qp Qh    N1 N

*Other: Diprivan*

✿ **J2710** Injection, neostigmine methylsulfate, up to 0.5 mg Ⓥ Ⓑ Qp Qh    N1 N

*Other: Prostigmin*

*IOM: 100-02, 15, 50*

✿ **J2720** Injection, protamine sulfate, per 10 mg Ⓥ Ⓑ Qp Qh    N1 N

*IOM: 100-02, 15, 50*

✳ **J2724** Injection, protein C concentrate, intravenous, human, 10 IU Ⓥ Ⓑ Qp Qh    K2 K

*Other: Ceprotin*

✿ **J2725** Injection, protirelin, per 250 mcg Ⓥ Ⓑ Qp Qh    E2

*Other: Relefact TRH, Thypinone*

*IOM: 100-02, 15, 50*

✿ **J2730** Injection, pralidoxime chloride, up to 1 gm Ⓥ Ⓑ Qp Qh    N1 N

*Other: Protopam Chloride*

*IOM: 100-02, 15, 50*

✿ **J2760** Injection, phentolamine mesylate, up to 5 mg Ⓥ Ⓑ Qp Qh    K2 K

*Other: Regitine*

*IOM: 100-02, 15, 50*

✿ **J2765** Injection, metoclopramide HCL, up to 10 mg Ⓥ Ⓑ Qp Qh    N1 N

*Other: Reglan*

*IOM: 100-02, 15, 50*

---

▶ New    ↩ Revised    ✔ Reinstated    ~~deleted~~ Deleted    ⃠ Not covered or valid by Medicare
✿ Special coverage instructions    ✳ Carrier discretion    Ⓑ Bill Part B MAC    Ⓓ Bill DME MAC

⚙ **J2770** Injection, quinupristin/dalfopristin, 500 mg (150/350) Ⓑ Ⓑ Qp Qh    K2 K

*Other: Synercid*

*IOM: 100-02, 15, 50*

✳ **J2778** Injection, ranibizumab, 0.1 mg Ⓥ Ⓑ Qp Qh    K2 K

May be reported for exudative senile macular degeneration (wet AMD) with 67028 (RT or LT)

*Other: Lucentis*

⚙ **J2780** Injection, ranitidine hydrochloride, 25 mg Ⓑ Ⓑ Qp Qh    N1 N

*Other: Zantac*

*IOM: 100-02, 15, 50*

✳ **J2783** Injection, rasburicase, 0.5 mg Ⓥ Ⓑ Qp Qh    K2 K

*Other: Elitek*

✳ **J2785** Injection, regadenoson, 0.1 mg Ⓑ Ⓑ Qp Qh    N1 N

One billing unit equal to 0.1 mg of regadenoson

*Other: Lexiscan*

✳ **J2786** Injection, reslizumab, 1 mg Qp Qh    K2 G

**Coding Clinic: 2016, Q4, P9**

✳ **J2787** Riboflavin 5'-phosphate, ophthalmic solution, up to 3 mL Ⓑ

*Other: Photrexa Viscous*

⚙ **J2788** Injection, Rho D immune globulin, human, minidose, 50 mcg (250 IU) Ⓥ Ⓑ Qp Qh    N1 N

*Other: HypRho-D, MicRhoGAM, Rhesonativ, RhoGam*

*IOM: 100-02, 15, 50*

⚙ **J2790** Injection, Rho D immune globulin, human, full dose, 300 mcg (1500 IU) Ⓑ Ⓑ Qp Qh    N1 N

Administered to pregnant female to prevent hemolistic disease of newborn. Report 90384 to private payer

*Other: Gamulin Rh, Hyperrho S/D, HypRho-D, Rhesonativ, RhoGAM*

*IOM: 100-02, 15, 50*

⚙ **J2791** Injection, Rho(D) immune globulin (human), (Rhophylac), intramuscular or intravenous, 100 IU Ⓑ Ⓑ Qp Qh    N1 N

Agent must be billed per 100 IU in both physician office and hospital outpatient settings

*Other: HypRho-D*

*IOM: 100-02, 15, 50*

⚙ **J2792** Injection, Rho D immune globulin intravenous, human, solvent detergent, 100 IU Ⓥ Ⓑ Qp Qh    K2 K

*Other: Gamulin Rh, Hyperrho S/D, WinRHo-SDF*

*IOM: 100-02, 15, 50*

⚙ **J2793** Injection, rilonacept, 1 mg Ⓑ Ⓑ Qp Qh    K2 K

*Other: Arcalyst*

*IOM: 100-02, 15, 50*

↻ ✳ **J2794** Injection, risperidone (risperdal consta), 0.5 mg Ⓥ Ⓑ Qp Qh    K2 K

*Other: Risperdal Costa*

✳ **J2795** Injection, ropivacaine hydrochloride, 1 mg Ⓑ Ⓑ Qp Qh    N1 N

*Other: Naropin*

✳ **J2796** Injection, romiplostim, 10 mcg Ⓑ Ⓑ Qp Qh    K2 K

Stimulates bone marrow megakarocytes to produce platelets (i.e., ITP)

*Other: Nplate*

⚙ **J2797** Injection, rolapitant, 0.5 mg    G

*Other: Varubi*

▶ ✳ **J2798** Injection, risperidone, (perseris), 0.5 mg    K2 G

⚙ **J2800** Injection, methocarbamol, up to 10 ml Ⓑ Ⓑ Qp Qh    N1 N

*Other: Robaxin*

*IOM: 100-02, 15, 50*

✳ **J2805** Injection, sincalide, 5 mcg Ⓑ Ⓑ Qp Qh    N1 N

*Other: Kinevac*

⚙ **J2810** Injection, theophylline, per 40 mg Ⓑ Ⓑ Qp Qh    N1 N

*IOM: 100-02, 15, 50*

⚙ **J2820** Injection, sargramostim (GM-CSF), 50 mcg Ⓑ Ⓑ Qp Qh    K2 K

*Other: Leukine, Prokine*

*IOM: 100-02, 15, 50*

✳ **J2840** Injection, sebelipase alfa, 1 mg Qp Qh    K2 G

⚙ **J2850** Injection, secretin, synthetic, human, 1 mcg Ⓑ Ⓑ Qp Qh    K2 K

*Other: Chirhostim*

*IOM: 100-02, 15, 50*

✳ **J2860** Injection, siltuximab, 10 mg Ⓑ Ⓑ Qp Qh    K2 K

---

🐾 MIPS    Qp **Quantity Physician**    Qh **Quantity Hospital**    ♀ **Female only**

♂ **Male only**    Ⓐ **Age**    ♿ **DMEPOS**    A2-Z3 **ASC Payment Indicator**    A-Y **ASC Status Indicator**    **Coding Clinic**

○ **J2910**   Injection, aurothioglucose, up to 50 mg ⊕ ⓑ Qp Qh                E2

*Other: Solganal*

*IOM: 100-02, 15, 50*

○ **J2916**   Injection, sodium ferric gluconate complex in sucrose injection, 12.5 mg ⊕ ⓑ Qp Qh          N1 N

*Other: Ferrlecit, Nulecit*

*IOM: 100-02, 15, 50*

○ **J2920**   Injection, methylprednisolone sodium succinate, up to 40 mg ⓑ ⓑ Qp Qh          N1 N

*Other: A-MethaPred, Solu-Medrol*

*IOM: 100-02, 15, 50*

○ **J2930**   Injection, methylprednisolone sodium succinate, up to 125 mg ⓑ ⓑ Qp Qh          N1 N

*Other: A-MethaPred, Solu-Medrol*

*IOM: 100-02, 15, 50*

○ **J2940**   Injection, somatrem, 1 mg ⓑ ⓑ Qp Qh                E2

*IOM: 100-02, 15, 50,*

*Medicare Statute 1861s2b*

○ **J2941**   Injection, somatropin, 1 mg ⓑ ⓑ Qp Qh          K2 K

*Other: Genotropin, Humatrope, Nutropin, Omnitrope, Saizen, Serostim, Zorbtive*

*IOM: 100-02, 15, 50,*

*Medicare Statute 1861s2b*

○ **J2950**   Injection, promazine HCL, up to 25 mg ⊕ ⓑ Qp Qh          N1 N

*Other: Prozine-50, Sparine*

*IOM: 100-02, 15, 50*

○ **J2993**   Injection, reteplase, 18.1 mg ⊕ ⓑ Qp Qh          K2 K

*Other: Retavase*

*IOM: 100-02, 15, 50*

○ **J2995**   Injection, streptokinase, per 250,000 IU ⊕ ⓑ Qp Qh          N1 N

Bill 1 unit for each 250,000 IU

*Other: Kabikinase, Streptase*

*IOM: 100-02, 15, 50*

○ **J2997**   Injection, alteplase recombinant, 1 mg ⊕ ⓑ Qp Qh          K2 K

Thrombolytic agent, treatment of occluded catheters. Bill units of 1 mg administered.

*Other: Activase, Cathflo Activase*

*IOM: 100-02, 15, 50*

**Coding Clinic: 2014, Q1, P4**

○ **J3000**   Injection, streptomycin, up to 1 gm ⓑ ⓑ Qp Qh          N1 N

*IOM: 100-02, 15, 50*

○ **J3010**   Injection, fentanyl citrate, 0.1 mg ⊕ ⓑ Qp Qh          N1 N

*Other: Sublimaze*

*IOM: 100-02, 15, 50*

○ **J3030**   Injection, sumatriptan succinate, 6 mg (Code may be used for Medicare when drug administered under the direct supervision of a physician, not for use when drug is self-administered) ⊕ ⓑ Qp Qh          N1 N

*Other: Imitrex, Sumarel Dosepro*

*IOM: 100-02, 15, 150*

▶ ✳ **J3031**   Injection, fremanezumab-vfrm, 1 mg (Code may be used for Medicare when drug administered under the direct supervision of a physician, not for use when drug is self-administered)          K2 G

✳ **J3060**   Injection, taliglucerase alfa, 10 units ⊕ ⓑ Qp Qh          K2 K

*Other: Elelyso*

○ **J3070**   Injection, pentazocine, 30 mg ⊕ ⓑ Qp Qh          K2 K

*Other: Talwin*

*IOM: 100-02, 15, 50*

✳ **J3090**   Injection, tedizolid phosphate, 1 mg ⓑ ⓑ Qp Qh          K2 K

*Other: Sivextro*

✳ **J3095**   Injection, televancin, 10 mg ⊕ ⓑ Qp Qh          K2 K

Prescribed for the treatment of adults with complicated skin and skin structure infections (cSSSI) of the following Gram-positive microorganisms: Staphylococcus aureus; Streptococcus pyogenes, Streptococcus agalactiae, Streptococcus anginosusgroup. Separately payable under the ASC payment system.

*Other: Vibativ*

**Coding Clinic: 2011, Q1, P7**

---

▶ New    ↻ Revised    ✔ Reinstated    deleted Deleted    ⊘ Not covered or valid by Medicare
○ Special coverage instructions    ✳ Carrier discretion    ⓑ Bill Part B MAC    ⓑ Bill DME MAC

**312**

* **J3101** Injection, tenecteplase, 1 mg ⓥ Ⓑ Qp Qh    K2 K

    *Other: TNKase*

✿ **J3105** Injection, terbutaline sulfate, up to 1 mg ⓥ Ⓑ Qp Qh    N1 N

    *Other: Brethine*

    *IOM: 100-02, 15, 50*

✿ **J3110** Injection, teriparatide, 10 mcg ⓥ Ⓑ Qp Qh    B

▶ * **J3111** Injection, romosozumab-aqqg, 1 mg    K2 G

✿ **J3121** Injection, testosterone enanthate, 1 mg ⓥ Ⓑ Qp Qh    N1 N

    *Other: Andrest 90-4, Andro L.A. 200, Andro-Estro 90-4, Androgyn L.A, Andropository 100, Andryl 200, Deladumone, Deladumone OB, Delatest, Delatestadiol, Delatestryl, Ditate-DS, Dua-Gen L.A., Duoval P.A., Durathate-200, Estra-Testrin, Everone, TEEV, Testadiate, Testone LA, Testradiol 90/4, Testrin PA, Valertest*

✿ **J3145** Injection, testosterone undecanoate, 1 mg ⓥ Ⓑ Qp Qh    K2 K

✿ **J3230** Injection, chlorpromazine HCL, up to 50 mg ⓥ Ⓑ Qp Qh    N1 N

    *Other: Ornazine, Thorazine*

    *IOM: 100-02, 15, 50*

✿ **J3240** Injection, thyrotropin alfa, 0.9 mg provided in 1.1 mg vial ⓥ Ⓑ Qp Qh    K2 K

    *Other: Thyrogen*

    *IOM: 100-02, 15, 50*

* **J3243** Injection, tigecycline, 1 mg ⓥ Ⓑ Qp Qh    K2 K

* **J3245** Injection, tildrakizumab, 1 mg ⓥ Ⓑ    E2

    *Other: Ilumya*

* **J3246** Injection, tirofiban HCL, 0.25 mg ⓥ Ⓑ Qp Qh    K2 K

    *Other: Aggrastat*

✿ **J3250** Injection, trimethobenzamide HCL, up to 200 mg ⓥ Ⓑ Qp Qh    N1 N

    *Other: Arrestin, Ticon, Tigan, Tiject 20*

    *IOM: 100-02, 15, 50*

✿ **J3260** Injection, tobramycin sulfate, up to 80 mg ⓥ Ⓑ Qp Qh    N1 N

    *Other: Nebcin*

    *IOM: 100-02, 15, 50*

* **J3262** Injection, tocilizumab, 1 mg ⓥ Ⓑ Qp Qh    K2 K

    Indicated for the treatment of adult patients with moderately to severely active rheumatoid arthritis (RA) who have had an inadequate response to one or more tumor necrosis factor (TNF) antagonist therapies.

    *Other: Actemra*

    **Coding Clinic: 2011, Q1, P7**

✿ **J3265** Injection, torsemide, 10 mg/ml ⓥ Ⓑ Qp Qh    N1 N

    *Other: Demadex*

    *IOM: 100-02, 15, 50*

✿ **J3280** Injection, thiethylperazine maleate, up to 10 mg ⓥ Ⓑ Qp Qh    E2

    *Other: Norzine, Torecan*

    *IOM: 100-02, 15, 50*

* **J3285** Injection, treprostinil, 1 mg ⓥ Ⓑ Qp Qh    K2 K

    *Other: Remodulin*

✿ **J3300** Injection, triamcinolone acetonide, preservative free, 1 mg ⓥ Ⓑ Qp Qh    K2 K

    *Other: Cenacort A-40, Kenaject-40, Kenalog, Triam-A, Triesence, Tri-Kort, Trilog*

✿ **J3301** Injection, triamcinolone acetonide, not otherwise specified, 10 mg ⓥ Ⓑ Qp Qh    N1 N

    *Other: Cenacort A-40, Kenaject-40, Kenalog, Triam A, Triesence, Tri-Kort, Trilog*

    *IOM: 100-02, 15, 50*

    **Coding Clinic: 2018, Q4, P7; 2013, Q2, P4**

✿ **J3302** Injection, triamcinolone diacetate, per 5 mg ⓥ Ⓑ Qp Qh    N1 N

    *Other: Amcort, Aristocort , Cenacort Forte, Trilone*

    *IOM: 100-02, 15, 50*

✿ **J3303** Injection, triamcinolone hexacetonide, per 5 mg ⓥ Ⓑ Qp Qh    N1 N

    *Other: Aristospan*

    *IOM: 100-02, 15, 50*

✿ **J3304** Injection, triamcinolone acetonide, preservative-free, extended-release, microsphere formulation, 1 mg ⓥ Ⓑ    G

    *Other: Zilretta*

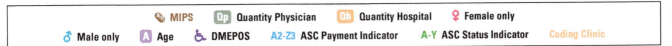

   🖘 MIPS    Qp Quantity Physician    Qh Quantity Hospital    ♀ Female only

   ♂ Male only    Ⓐ Age    ♿ DMEPOS    A2-Z3 ASC Payment Indicator    A-Y ASC Status Indicator    Coding Clinic

○ **J3305** Injection, trimetrexate glucuronate, per 25 mg Ⓑ Ⓑ Ⓠp Ⓠh      E2

*Other: NeuTrexin*

*IOM: 100-02, 15, 50*

○ **J3310** Injection, perphenazine, up to 5 mg Ⓑ Ⓑ Ⓠp Ⓠh      N1 N

*Other: Trilafon*

*IOM: 100-02, 15, 50*

○ **J3315** Injection, triptorelin pamoate, 3.75 mg Ⓑ Ⓑ Ⓠp Ⓠh      K2 K

*Other: Trelstar*

*IOM: 100-02, 15, 50*

○ **J3316** Injection, triptorelin, extended-release, 3.75 mg Ⓑ Ⓑ      G

*Other: Trelstar, Trelstar Depot, Trelstar LA*

○ **J3320** Injection, spectinomycin dihydrochloride, up to 2 gm Ⓟ Ⓑ Ⓠp Ⓠh      E2

*Other: Trobicin*

*IOM: 100-02, 15, 50*

○ **J3350** Injection, urea, up to 40 gm Ⓟ Ⓑ Ⓠp Ⓠh      N1 N

*Other: Ureaphil*

*IOM: 100-02, 15, 50*

○ **J3355** Injection, urofollitropin, 75 IU Ⓟ Ⓑ Ⓠp Ⓠh      E2

*Other: Bravelle, Metrodin*

*IOM: 100-02, 15, 50*

＊ **J3357** Ustekinumab, for subcutaneous injection, 1 mg Ⓟ Ⓑ Ⓠp Ⓠh      K2 K

*Other: Stelara*

Coding Clinic: 2017, Q1, P3; 2016, Q4, P10; 2011, Q1, P7

＊ **J3358** Ustekinumab, for intravenous injection, 1 mg      K2 G

*Cross Reference Q9989*

○ **J3360** Injection, diazepam, up to 5 mg Ⓑ Ⓑ Ⓠp Ⓠh      N1 N

*Other: Valium, Zetran*

*IOM: 100-02, 15, 50*

Coding Clinic: 2007, Q2, P6-7

○ **J3364** Injection, urokinase, 5000 IU vial Ⓑ Ⓑ Ⓠp Ⓠh      N1 N

*Other: Abbokinase*

*IOM: 100-02, 15, 50*

○ **J3365** Injection, IV, urokinase, 250,000 IU vial Ⓑ Ⓑ Ⓠp Ⓠh      E2

*Other: Abbokinase*

*IOM: 100-02, 15, 50,*

*Cross Reference Q0089*

○ **J3370** Injection, vancomycin HCL, 500 mg Ⓟ Ⓑ Ⓠp Ⓠh      N1 N

*Other: Vancocin, Vancoled*

*IOM: 100-02, 15, 50; 100-03, 4, 280.14*

○ **J3380** Injection, vedolizumab, 1 mg Ⓟ Ⓑ Ⓠp Ⓠh      K2 K

*Other: Entyvio*

＊ **J3385** Injection, velaglucerase alfa, 100 units Ⓑ Ⓑ Ⓠp Ⓠh      K2 K

Enzyme replacement therapy in Gaucher Disease that results from a specific enzyme deficiency in the body, caused by a genetic mutation received from both parents. Type 1 is the most prevalent Ashkenazi Jewish genetic disease, occurring in one in every 1,000.

*Other: VPRIV*

Coding Clinic: 2011, Q1, P7

○ **J3396** Injection, verteporfin, 0.1 mg Ⓑ Ⓑ Ⓠp Ⓠh      K2 K

*Other: Visudyne*

*IOM: 100-03, 1, 80.2; 100-03, 1, 80.3*

＊ **J3397** Injection, vestronidase alfa-vjbk, 1 mg Ⓟ Ⓑ      K

*Other: Mepsevii*

＊ **J3398** Injection, voretigene neparvovec-rzyl, 1 billion vector genomes Ⓟ Ⓑ      G

*Other: Luxturna*

○ **J3400** Injection, triflupromazine HCL, up to 20 mg Ⓑ Ⓑ Ⓠp Ⓠh      E2

*Other: Vesprin*

*IOM: 100-02, 15, 50*

○ **J3410** Injection, hydroxyzine HCL, up to 25 mg Ⓟ Ⓑ Ⓠp Ⓠh      N1 N

*Other: Hyzine-50, Vistaject 25, Vistaril*

*IOM: 100-02, 15, 50*

＊ **J3411** Injection, thiamine HCL, 100 mg Ⓟ Ⓑ Ⓠp Ⓠh      N1 N

＊ **J3415** Injection, pyridoxine HCL, 100 mg Ⓟ Ⓑ Ⓠp Ⓠh      N1 N

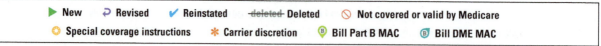

▶ New    ↻ Revised    ✔ Reinstated    ~~deleted~~ Deleted    ⊘ Not covered or valid by Medicare
○ Special coverage instructions    ＊ Carrier discretion    Ⓑ Bill Part B MAC    Ⓑ Bill DME MAC

**J3420** Injection, vitamin B-12 cyanocobalamin, up to 1000 mcg Ⓑ Ⓑ Ⓠp Ⓠh    N1 N

Medicare carriers may have local coverage decisions regarding vitamin B12 injections that provide reimbursement only for patients with certain types of anemia and other conditions.

*Other: Berubigen, Betalin 12, Cobex, Redisol, Rubramin PC, Sytobex*

*IOM: 100-02, 15, 50; 100-03, 2, 150.6*

**J3430** Injection, phytonadione (vitamin K), per 1 mg Ⓑ Ⓑ Ⓠp Ⓠh    N1 N

*Other: AquaMephyton, Konakion, Menadione, Synkavite, Vitamin K1*

*IOM: 100-02, 15, 50*

**J3465** Injection, voriconazole, 10 mg Ⓑ Ⓑ Ⓠp Ⓠh    K2 K

*Other: VFEND*

*IOM: 100-02, 15, 50*

**J3470** Injection, hyaluronidase, up to 150 units Ⓑ Ⓑ Ⓠp Ⓠh    N1 N

*Other: Amphadase, Wydase*

*IOM: 100-02, 15, 50*

**J3471** Injection, hyaluronidase, ovine, preservative free, per 1 USP unit (up to 999 USP units) Ⓑ Ⓑ Ⓠp Ⓠh    N1 N

*Other: Vitrase*

**J3472** Injection, hyaluronidase, ovine, preservative free, per 1000 USP units Ⓑ Ⓑ Ⓠp Ⓠh    N1 N

**J3473** Injection, hyaluronidase, recombinant, 1 USP unit Ⓑ Ⓑ Ⓠp Ⓠh    N1 N

*Other: Hylenex*

*IOM: 100-02, 15, 50*

**J3475** Injection, magnesium sulfate, per 500 mg Ⓑ Ⓑ Ⓠp Ⓠh    N1 N

*IOM: 100-02, 15, 50*

**J3480** Injection, potassium chloride, per 2 meq Ⓑ Ⓑ Ⓠp Ⓠh    N1 N

*IOM: 100-02, 15, 50*

**J3485** Injection, zidovudine, 10 mg Ⓑ Ⓑ Ⓠp Ⓠh    N1 N

*Other: Retrovir*

*IOM: 100-02, 15, 50*

**\* J3486** Injection, ziprasidone mesylate, 10 mg Ⓑ Ⓑ Ⓠp Ⓠh    N1 N

*Other: Geodon*

**\* J3489** Injection, zoledronic acid, 1 mg Ⓑ Ⓑ Ⓠp Ⓠh    N1 N

*Other: Reclast, Zometra*

**J3490** Unclassified drugs Ⓑ Ⓑ    N1 N

Bill on paper. Bill one unit. Identify drug and total dosage in "Remarks" field.

*Other: Acthib, Aminocaproic Acid, Baciim, Bacitracin, Benzocaine, Bumetanide, Bupivacaine, Cefotetan, Ciprofloxacin, Cleocin Phosphate, Clindamycin, Cortisone Acetate Micronized, Definity, Diprivan, Doxy, Engerix-B, Ethanolamine, Famotidine, Ganirelix, Gonal-F, Hyaluronic Acid, Marcaine, Metronidazole, Nafcillin, Naltrexone, Ovidrel, Pegasys, Peg-Intron, Penicillin G Sodium, Propofol, Protonix, Recombivax, Rifadin, Rifampin, Sensorcaine-MPF, Smz-TMP, Sufentanil Citrate, Testopel Pellets, Testosterone, Treanda, Valcyte, Veritas Collagen Matrix*

*IOM: 100-02, 15, 50*

Coding Clinic: 2017, Q1, P1-3, P8; 2014, Q2, P6; 2013, Q2, P3-4

**⊘ J3520** Edetate disodium, per 150 mg Ⓑ Ⓑ Ⓠp Ⓠh    E1

*Other: Chealamide, Disotate, Endrate ethylenediamine-tetra-acetic*

*IOM: 100-03, 1, 20.21; 100-03, 1, 20.22*

**J3530** Nasal vaccine inhalation Ⓑ Ⓑ Ⓠp Ⓠh    N1 N

*IOM: 100-02, 15, 50*

**⊘ J3535** Drug administered through a metered dose inhaler Ⓑ Ⓑ    E1

*Other: Ipratropium bromide*

*IOM: 100-02, 15, 50*

**⊘ J3570** Laetrile, amygdalin, vitamin B-17 Ⓑ Ⓑ    E1

*IOM: 100-03, 1, 30.7*

**\* J3590** Unclassified biologics Ⓑ    N1 N

Bill on paper. Bill one unit. Identify drug and total dosage in "Remarks" field.

Coding Clinic: 2017, Q1, P1-3; 2016, Q4, P10

**\* J3591** Unclassified drug or biological used for ESRD on dialysis Ⓑ    B

**J7030** Infusion, normal saline solution, 1000 cc Ⓑ Ⓑ Ⓠp Ⓠh    N1 N

*Other: Sodium Chloride*

*IOM: 100-02, 15, 50*

**J7040** Infusion, normal saline solution, sterile (500 ml = 1 unit) Ⓑ Ⓑ Ⓠp Ⓠh    N1 N

*Other: Sodium Chloride*

*IOM: 100-02, 15, 50*

---

| 🏷 MIPS | Ⓠp Quantity Physician | Ⓠh Quantity Hospital | ♀ Female only |
|---|---|---|---|
| ♂ Male only | Ⓐ Age | ♿ DMEPOS | A2-Z3 ASC Payment Indicator    A-Y ASC Status Indicator    Coding Clinic |

⊗ **J7042** 5% dextrose/normal saline
(500 ml = 1 unit) Ⓑ Ⓓ Qp Qh    N1 N

*Other: Dextrose-Nacl*

*IOM: 100-02, 15, 50*

⊗ **J7050** Infusion, normal saline solution,
250 cc Ⓑ Ⓓ Qp Qh    N1 N

*Other: Sodium Chloride*

*IOM: 100-02, 15, 50*

⊗ **J7060** 5% dextrose/water
(500 ml = 1 unit) Ⓑ Ⓓ Qp Qh    N1 N

*IOM: 100-02, 15, 50*

⊗ **J7070** Infusion, D 5 W,
1000 cc Ⓑ Ⓓ Qp Qh    N1 N

*Other: Dextrose*

*IOM: 100-02, 15, 50*

⊗ **J7100** Infusion, dextran 40,
500 ml Ⓥ Ⓑ Qp Qh    N1 N

*Other: Gentran, LMD, Rheomacrodex*

*IOM: 100-02, 15, 50*

⊗ **J7110** Infusion, dextran 75,
500 ml Ⓥ Ⓑ Qp Qh    N1 N

*Other: Gentran 75*

*IOM: 100-02, 15, 50*

⊗ **J7120** Ringer's lactate infusion, up to
1000 cc Ⓥ Ⓑ Qp Qh    N1 N

Replacement fluid or electrolytes.

*Other: Potassium Chloride*

*IOM: 100-02, 15, 50*

⊗ **J7121** 5% dextrose in lactated
ringers infusion, up to
1000 cc Ⓥ Ⓑ Qp Qh    N1 N

*IOM: 100-02, 15, 50*

⊗ **J7131** Hypertonic saline solution,
1 ml Ⓥ Ⓑ Qp Qh    N1 N

*IOM: 100-02, 15, 50*

**Coding Clinic: 2012, Q1, P9**

## Clotting Factors

✳ **J7170** Injection, emicizumab-kxwh,
0.5 mg Ⓑ    G

*Other: Hemlibra*

✳ **J7175** Injection, Factor X, (human),
1 IU Ⓥ Qp Qh    K2 K

**Coding Clinic: 2017, Q1, P9**

✳ **J7177** Injection, human fibrinogen
concentrate (fibryga), 1 mg Ⓑ    K

✳ **J7178** Injection, human fibrinogen
concentrate, not otherwise
specified, 1 mg Ⓥ Qp Qh    K2 K

*Other: Riastap*

⊗ **J7179** Injection, von Willebrand factor
(recombinant), (vonvendi),
1 IU VWF:RCo Ⓥ Qp Qh    K2 G

**Coding Clinic: 2017, Q1, P9**

✳ **J7180** Injection, factor XIII (antihemophilic
factor, human), 1 IU Ⓑ Qp Qh    K2 K

*Other: Corifact*

**Coding Clinic: 2012, Q1, P8**

✳ **J7181** Injection, factor XIII a-subunit,
(recombinant), per IU Ⓥ Qp Qh    K2 K

✳ **J7182** Injection, factor VIII, (antihemophilic
factor, recombinant), (novoeight),
per IU Ⓑ Qp Qh    K2 K

⊗ **J7183** Injection, von Willebrand factor
complex (human), wilate,
1 IU VWF:RCo Ⓥ Qp Qh    K2 K

*IOM: 100-02, 15, 50*

**Coding Clinic: 2012, Q1, P9**

✳ **J7185** Injection, Factor VIII (antihemophilic
factor, recombinant) (Xyntha),
per IU Ⓑ Qp Qh    K2 K

⊗ **J7186** Injection, anti-hemophilic
factor VIII/von Willebrand
factor complex (human),
per factor VIII IU Ⓥ Qp Qh    K2 K

*Other: Alphanate*

*IOM: 100-02, 15, 50*

⊗ **J7187** Injection, von Willebrand factor
complex (HUMATE-P), per IU
VWF:RCo Ⓥ Qp Qh    K2 K

*Other: Humate-P Low Dilutent*

*IOM: 100-02, 15, 50*

⊗ **J7188** Injection, factor VIII (antihemophilic
factor, recombinant), (obizur), per
IU Ⓥ Qp Qh    K2 K

*IOM: 100-02, 15, 50*

⊗ **J7189** Factor VIIa (anti-hemophilic
factor, recombinant), per
1 mcg Ⓑ Qp Qh    K2 K

*Other: NovoSeven*

*IOM: 100-02, 15, 50*

⊗ **J7190** Factor VIII anti-hemophilic factor,
human, per IU Ⓥ Qp Qh    K2 K

*Other: Alphanate/von Willebrand factor
complex, Hemofil M, Koate DVI,
Koate-HP, Kogenate, Monoclate-P,
Recombinate*

*IOM: 100-02, 15, 50*

---

▶ New    ↩ Revised    ✔ Reinstated    ~~deleted~~ Deleted    ⊘ Not covered or valid by Medicare
⊗ Special coverage instructions    ✳ Carrier discretion    Ⓑ Bill Part B MAC    Ⓓ Bill DME MAC

**J7191** Factor VIII, anti-hemophilic factor (porcine), per IU ⑧ Qp Qh  E2

*Other: Hyate:C, Koate-HP, Kogenate, Monoclate-P, Recombinate*

*IOM: 100-02, 15, 50*

**J7192** Factor VIII (anti-hemophilic factor, recombinant) per IU, not otherwise specified ⑧ Qp Qh  K2 K

*Other: Advate, Helixate FS, Kogenate FS, Koate-HP, Recombinate, Xyntha*

*IOM: 100-02, 15, 50*

**J7193** Factor IX (anti-hemophilic factor, purified, non-recombinant) per IU ⑧ Qp Qh  K2 K

*Other: AlphaNine SD, Mononine, Proplex*

*IOM: 100-02, 15, 50*

**J7194** Factor IX, complex, per IU ⑧ Qp Qh  K2 K

*Other: Bebulin, Konyne-80, Profilnine Heat-treated, Profilnine SD, Proplex SX-T, Proplex T*

*IOM: 100-02, 15, 50*

**J7195** Injection, Factor IX (anti-hemophilic factor, recombinant) per IU, not otherwise specified ⑧ Qp Qh  K2 K

*Other: Benefix, Profiline, Proplex T*

*IOM: 100-02, 15, 50*

**J7196** Injection, antithrombin recombinant, 50 IU ⑧ Qp Qh  E2

*Other: ATryn,  Feiba VH Immuno*

**Coding Clinic: 2011, Q1, P6**

**J7197** Anti-thrombin III (human), per IU ⑧ Qp Qh  K2 K

*Other: Thrombate III*

*IOM: 100-02, 15, 50*

**J7198** Anti-inhibitor, per IU ⑧ Qp Qh  K2 K

Diagnosis examples: D66 Congenital Factor VIII disorder; D67 Congenital Factor IX disorder; D68.0 VonWillebrand's disease

*Other: Autoplex T, Feiba NF, Hemophilia clotting factors*

*IOM: 100-02, 15, 50; 100-03, 2, 110.3*

**J7199** Hemophilia clotting factor, not otherwise classified ⑧  B

*Other: Autoplex T*

*IOM: 100-02, 15, 50; 100-03, 2, 110.3*

**J7200** Injection, factor IX, (antihemophilic factor, recombinant), rixubis, per IU ⑧ Qp Qh  K2 K

*IOM: 100-02, 15, 50*

**J7201** Injection, factor IX, fc fusion protein (recombinant), alprolix, 1 IU ⑧ Qp Qh  K2 K

*IOM: 100-02, 15, 50*

**J7202** Injection, Factor IX, albumin fusion protein, (recombinant), idelvion, 1 IU Qp Qh  K2 G

**Coding Clinic: 2016, Q4, P9**

**J7203** Injection factor ix, (antihemophilic factor, recombinant), glycopegylated, (rebinyn), 1 iu  G

*Other: Profilnine SD, Bebulin VH, Bebulin, Proplex T*

**J7205** Injection, factor VIII Fc fusion protein (recombinant), per IU ⑧ Qp Qh  K2 K

*Other: Eloctate*

**J7207** Injection, Factor VIII, (antihemophilic factor, recombinant), PEGylated, 1 IU Qp Qh  K2 G

*Other: Adynovate*

▶ **J7208** Injection, Factor VIII, (antihemophilic factor, recombinant), pegylated-aucl, (jivi), 1 i.u.  K2 G

✱ **J7209** Injection, Factor VIII, (antihemophilic factor, recombinant), (Nuwiq), 1 IU Qp Qh  K2 G

✱ **J7210** Injection, Factor VIII, (antihemophilic factor, recombinant), (afstyla), 1 i.u. ⑧  K2 G

✱ **J7211** Injection, Factor VIII, (antihemophilic factor, recombinant), (kovaltry), 1 i.u. ⑧  K2 K

## Contraceptives

**J7296** Levonorgestrel-releasing intrauterine contraceptive system (Kyleena), 19.5 mg ⑧ ♀  E1

*Medicare Statute 1862(a)(1)*

*Cross Reference Q9984*

**J7297** Levonorgestrel-releasing intrauterine contraceptive system (Liletta), 52 mg ⑧ Qp Qh ♀  E1

*Medicare Statute 1862(a)(1)*

○ **J7298** Levonorgestrel-releasing intrauterine contraceptive system (Mirena), 52 mg ⦿ Qp Qh ♀ **E1**

*Medicare Statute 1862(a)(1)*

○ **J7300** Intrauterine copper contraceptive Ⓑ ♀ **E1**

Report IUD insertion with 58300. Bill usual and customary charge.

*Other: Paragard T 380 A*

*Medicare Statute 1862a1*

○ **J7301** Levonorgestrel-releasing intrauterine contraceptive system (Skyla), 13.5 mg ⦿ Qp Qh ♀ **E1**

*Medicare Statute 1862(a)(1)*

○ **J7303** Contraceptive supply, hormone containing vaginal ring, each Ⓑ ♀ **E1**

*Medicare Statute 1862.1*

○ **J7304** Contraceptive supply, hormone containing patch, each Ⓑ ♀ **E1**

Only billed by Family Planning Clinics

*Medicare Statute 1862.1*

○ **J7306** Levonorgestrel (contraceptive) implant system, including implants and supplies Ⓑ ♀ **E1**

○ **J7307** Etonogestrel (contraceptive) implant system, including implant and supplies Ⓑ ♀ **E1**

## Aminolevulinic Acid HCL

✱ **J7308** Aminolevulinic acid HCL for topical administration, 20%, single unit dosage form (354 mg) Ⓑ Qp Qh **K2 K**

*Other: Levulan Kerastick*

✿ **J7309** Methyl aminolevulinate (MAL) for topical administration, 16.8%, 1 gram Ⓑ Qp Qh **N1 N**

*Other: Metvixia*

*Coding Clinic: 2011, Q1, P6*

## Ganciclovir

✿ **J7310** Ganciclovir, 4.5 mg, long-acting implant Ⓑ Qp Qh **E2**

*IOM: 100-02, 15, 50*

## Ophthalmic Drugs

⤴ ✱ **J7311** Injection, fluocinolone acetonide, intravitreal implant (retisert), 0.01 mg ⦿ Qp Qh **K2 K**

Treatment of chronic noninfectious posterior segment uveitis

*Other: Retisert*

✱ **J7312** Injection, dexamethasone, intravitreal implant, 0.1 mg ⦿ Qp Qh **K2 K**

To bill for Ozurdex services submit the following codes: J7312 and 67028 with the modifier -22 (for the increased work difficulty and increased risk). Indicated for the treatment of macular edema occurring after branch retinal vein occlusion (BRVO) or central retinal vein occlusion (CRVO) and non-infectious uveitis affecting the posterior segment of the eye.

*Other: Ozurdex*

*Coding Clinic: 2011, Q1, P7*

⤴ ✱ **J7313** Injection, fluocinolone acetonide, intravitreal implant (iluvien), 0.01 mg Ⓑ Qp Qh **K2 K**

*Other: Iluvien*

▶ ✱ **J7314** Injection, fluocinolone acetonide, intravitreal implant (yutiq), 0.01 mg **K2 G**

✱ **J7315** Mitomycin, ophthalmic, 0.2 mg ⦿ Qp Qh **N1 N**

*Other: Mitosol, Mutamycin*

*Coding Clinic: 2016, Q4, P8; 2014, Q2, P6*

✱ **J7316** Injection, ocriplasmin, 0.125 mg Ⓑ Qp Qh **K2 K**

*Other: Jetrea*

## Hyaluronan

✱ **J7318** Hyaluronan or derivative, durolane, for intra-articular injection, 1 mg Ⓑ **G**

*Other: Morisu*

✱ **J7320** Hyaluronan or derivitive, genvisc 850, for intra-articular injection, 1 mg Ⓑ Qp Qh **K2 K**

✱ **J7321** Hyaluronan or derivative, Hyalgan, Supartz or Visco-3, for intra-articular injection, per dose ⦿ Qp Qh **K2 K**

Therapeutic goal is to restore visco-elasticity of synovial hyaluronan, thereby decreasing pain, improving mobility and restoring natural protective functions of hyaluronan in joint

---

▶ New    ⤴ Revised    ✔ Reinstated    ~~deleted~~ Deleted    ○ Not covered or valid by Medicare

✿ Special coverage instructions    ✱ Carrier discretion    Ⓑ Bill Part B MAC    Ⓓ Bill DME MAC

* **J7322** Hyaluronan or derivative, hymovis, for intra-articular injection, 1 mg Qp Qh K2 G

* **J7323** Hyaluronan or derivative, Euflexxa, for intra-articular injection, per dose B Qp Qh K2 K

* **J7324** Hyaluronan or derivative, Orthovisc, for intra-articular injection, per dose B Qp Qh K2 K

* **J7325** Hyaluronan or derivative, Synvisc or Synvisc-One, for intra-articular injection, 1 mg B Qp Qh K2 K

* **J7326** Hyaluronan or derivative, Gel-One, for intra-articular injection, per dose B Qp Qh K2 K

    Coding Clinic: 2012, Q1, P8

* **J7327** Hyaluronan or derivative, monovisc, for intra-articular injection, per dose B Qp Qh K2 K

* **J7328** Hyaluronan or derivative, gelsyn-3, for intra-articular injection, 0.1 mg B Qp Qh K2 G

* **J7329** Hyaluronan or derivative, trivisc, for intra-articular injection, 1 mg B E2

## Miscellaneous Drugs

* **J7330** Autologous cultured chondrocytes, implant B Qp Qh B

    *Other: Carticel*

    Coding Clinic: 2010, Q4, P3

▶ * **J7331** Hyaluronan or derivative, synojoynt, for intra-articular injection, 1 mg K

▶ * **J7332** Hyaluronan or derivative, triluron, for intra-articular injection, 1 mg K

* **J7336** Capsaicin 8% patch, per square centimeter Qp Qh K2 K

    *Other: Qutenza*

* **J7340** Carbidopa 5 mg/levodopa 20 mg enteral suspension, 100 ml B Qp Qh K2 K

    *Other: Duopa*

* **J7342** Instillation, ciprofloxacin otic suspension, 6 mg B Qp Qh K2 G

* **J7345** Aminolevulinic acid HCL for topical administration, 10% gel, 10 mg B K2 G

▶ * **J7401** Mometasone furoate sinus implant, 10 micrograms N

## Immunosuppressive Drugs (Includes Non-injectibles)

* **J7500** Azathioprine, oral, 50 mg B Qp Qh N1 N

    *Other: Azasan, Imuran*

    IOM: 100-02, 15, 50

* **J7501** Azathioprine, parenteral, 100 mg B B Qp Qh K2 K

    *Other: Imuran*

    IOM: 100-02, 15, 50

* **J7502** Cyclosporine, oral, 100 mg B B Qp Qh N1 N

    *Other: Gengraf, Neoral, Sandimmune*

    IOM: 100-02, 15, 50

* **J7503** Tacrolimus, extended release, (Envarsus XR), oral, 0.25 mg B B Qp Qh K2 G

    IOM: 100-02, 15, 50

* **J7504** Lymphocyte immune globulin, antithymocyte globulin, equine, parenteral, 250 mg B B Qp Qh K2 K

    *Other: Atgam*

    IOM: 100-02, 15, 50; 100-03, 2, 110.3

* **J7505** Muromonab-CD3, parenteral, 5 mg B B Qp Qh K2 K

    *Other: Monoclonal antibodies (parenteral)*

    IOM: 100-02, 15, 50

* **J7507** Tacrolimus, immediate release, oral, 1 mg B B Qp Qh N1 N

    *Other: Prograf*

    IOM: 100-02, 15, 50

* **J7508** Tacrolimus, extended release, (Astagraf XL), oral, 0.1 mg B B Qp Qh N1 N

    IOM: 100-02, 15, 50

* **J7509** Methylprednisolone oral, per 4 mg B B Qp Qh N1 N

    *Other: Medrol*

    IOM: 100-02, 15, 50

* **J7510** Prednisolone oral, per 5 mg B B Qp Qh N1 N

    *Other: Delta-Cortef, Flo-Pred, Orapred*

    IOM: 100-02, 15, 50

* **J7511** Lymphocyte immune globulin, antithymocyte globulin, rabbit, parenteral, 25 mg B B Qp Qh K2 K

    *Other: Thymoglobulin*

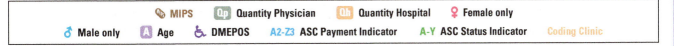
MIPS    Qp Quantity Physician    Qh Quantity Hospital    ♀ Female only
♂ Male only    A Age    DMEPOS    A2-Z3 ASC Payment Indicator    A-Y ASC Status Indicator    Coding Clinic

○ **J7512** Prednisone, immediate release or delayed release, oral, 1 mg ⑧ ⑧ **Qp** **Qh**     N1 N

*Other: Cyclosporine*

*IOM: 100-02, 15, 50*

○ **J7513** Daclizumab, parenteral, 25 mg ⑧ ⑧ **Qp** **Qh**     E2

*Other: Zenapax*

*IOM: 100-02, 15, 50*

\* **J7515** Cyclosporine, oral, 25 mg ⑧ ⑧ **Qp** **Qh**     N1 N

*Other: Gengraf, Neoral, Sandimmune*

\* **J7516** Cyclosporin, parenteral, 250 mg ⑧ ⑧ **Qp** **Qh**     N1 N

*Other: Sandimmune*

\* **J7517** Mycophenolate mofetil, oral, 250 mg ⑧ ⑧ **Qp** **Qh**     N1 N

*Other: CellCept*

○ **J7518** Mycophenolic acid, oral, 180 mg ⑧ ⑧ **Qp** **Qh**     N1 N

*Other: Myfortic*

*IOM: 100-04, 4, 240; 100-4, 17, 80.3.1*

○ **J7520** Sirolimus, oral, 1 mg ⑧ ⑧ **Qp** **Qh**     N1 N

*Other: Rapamune*

*IOM: 100-02, 15, 50*

○ **J7525** Tacrolimus, parenteral, 5 mg ⑧ ⑧ **Qp** **Qh**     K2 K

*Other: Prograf*

*IOM: 100-02, 15, 50*

○ **J7527** Everolimus, oral, 0.25 mg ⑧ ⑧ **Qp** **Qh**     N1 N

*Other: Zortress*

*IOM: 100-02, 15, 50*

○ **J7599** Immunosuppressive drug, not otherwise classified ⑧ ⑧     N1 N

Bill on paper. Bill one unit. Identify drug and total dosage in "Remarks" field.

*IOM: 100-02, 15, 50*

## Inhalation Solutions

\* **J7604** Acetylcysteine, inhalation solution, compounded product, administered through DME, unit dose form, per gram ⑧ ⑧ **Qp** **Qh**     M

*Other: Mucomyst (unit dose form), Mucosol*

\* **J7605** Arformoterol, inhalation solution, FDA approved final product, non-compounded, administered through DME, unit dose form, 15 mcg ⑧ ⑧ **Qp** **Qh**     M

Maintenance treatment of bronchoconstriction in patients with chronic obstructive pulmonary disease (COPD).

*Other: Brovana*

\* **J7606** Formoterol fumarate, inhalation solution, FDA approved final product, non-compounded, administered through DME, unit dose form, 20 mcg ⑧ ⑧ **Qp** **Qh**     M

*Other: Perforomist*

\* **J7607** Levalbuterol, inhalation solution, compounded product, administered through DME, concentrated form, 0.5 mg ⑧ ⑧ **Qp** **Qh**     M

○ **J7608** Acetylcysteine, inhalation solution, FDA-approved final product, non-compounded, administered through DME, unit dose form, per gram ⑧ ⑧ **Qp** **Qh**     M

*Other: Mucomyst, Mucosol*

\* **J7609** Albuterol, inhalation solution, compounded product, administered through DME, unit dose, 1 mg ⑧ ⑧ **Qp** **Qh**     M

Patient's home, medications—such as a albuterol when administered through a nebulizer—are considered DME and are payable under Part B.

*Other: Proventil, Ventolin, Xopenex*

\* **J7610** Albuterol, inhalation solution, compounded product, administered through DME, concentrated form, 1 mg ⑧ ⑧ **Qp** **Qh**     M

*Other: Proventil, Ventolin, Xopenex*

○ **J7611** Albuterol, inhalation solution, FDA-approved final product, non-compounded, administered through DME, concentrated form, 1 mg ⑧ ⑧ **Qp** **Qh**     M

Report once for each milligram administered. For example, 2 mg of concentrated albuterol (usually diluted with saline), reported with J7611×2.

*Other: Proventil, Ventolin, Xopenex*

○ **J7612** Levalbuterol, inhalation solution, FDA-approved final product, non-compounded, administered through DME, concentrated form, 0.5 mg ⑧ ⑧ **Qp** **Qh**     M

*Other: Xopenex*

| ▶ New | ↩ Revised | ✔ Reinstated | ~~deleted~~ Deleted | ⊘ Not covered or valid by Medicare |
|---|---|---|---|---|
| ○ Special coverage instructions | | \* Carrier discretion | ⑧ Bill Part B MAC | ⑧ Bill DME MAC |

○ **J7613** Albuterol, inhalation solution, FDA-approved final product, non-compounded, administered through DME, unit dose, 1 mg ⓥ ⓑ Qp Qh    M

*Other: Accuneb, Proventil, Ventolin, Xopenex*

○ **J7614** Levalbuterol, inhalation solution, FDA-approved final product, non-compounded, administered through DME, unit dose, 0.5 mg ⓑ ⓑ Qp Qh    M

*Other: Xopenex*

✳ **J7615** Levalbuterol, inhalation solution, compounded product, administered through DME, unit dose, 0.5 mg ⓑ ⓑ Qp Qh    M

○ **J7620** Albuterol, up to 2.5 mg and ipratropium bromide, up to 0.5 mg,FDA-approved final product, non-compounded, administered through DME ⓥ ⓑ Qp Qh    M

*Other: DuoNeb*

✳ **J7622** Beclomethasone, inhalation solution, compounded product, administered through DME, unit dose form, per mg ⓥ ⓑ Qp Qh    M

✳ **J7624** Betamethasone, inhalation solution, compounded product, administered through DME, unit dose form, per mg ⓥ ⓑ Qp Qh    M

✳ **J7626** Budesonide inhalation solution, FDA-approved final product, non-compounded, administered through DME, unit dose form, up to 0.5 mg ⓥ ⓑ Qp Qh    M

*Other: Pulmicort*

✳ **J7627** Budesonide, inhalation solution, compounded product, administered through DME, unit dose form, up to 0.5 mg ⓑ ⓑ Qp Qh    M

*Other: Pulmicort Respules*

○ **J7628** Bitolterol mesylate, inhalation solution, compounded product, administered through DME, concentrated form, per milligram ⓥ ⓑ Qp Qh    M

*Other: Tornalate*

○ **J7629** Bitolterol mesylate, inhalation solution, compounded product, administered through DME, unit dose form, per milligram ⓑ ⓑ Qp Qh    M

*Other: Tornalate*

○ **J7631** Cromolyn sodium, inhalation solution, FDA-approved final product, non-compounded, administered through DME, unit dose form, per 10 mg ⓥ ⓑ Qp Qh    M

*Other: Intal*

✳ **J7632** Cromolyn sodium, inhalation solution, compounded product, administered through DME, unit dose form, per 10 mg ⓑ ⓑ Qp Qh    M

*Other: Intal*

✳ **J7633** Budesonide, inhalation solution, FDA-approved final product, non-compounded, administered through DME, concentrated form, per 0.25 mg ⓥ ⓑ Qp Qh    M

*Other: Pulmicort Respules*

✳ **J7634** Budesonide, inhalation solution, compounded product, administered through DME, concentrated form, per 0.25 mg ⓥ ⓑ Qp Qh    M

*Other: Pulmicort Respules*

○ **J7635** Atropine, inhalation solution, compounded product, administered through DME, concentrated form, per milligram ⓥ ⓑ Qp Qh    M

○ **J7636** Atropine, inhalation solution, compounded product, administered through DME, unit dose form, per milligram ⓥ ⓑ Qp Qh    M

○ **J7637** Dexamethasone, inhalation solution, compounded product, administered through DME, concentrated form, per milligram ⓥ ⓑ Qp Qh    M

○ **J7638** Dexamethasone, inhalation solution, compounded product, administered through DME, unit dose form, per milligram ⓥ ⓑ Qp Qh    M

○ **J7639** Dornase alfa, inhalation solution, FDA-approved final product, non-compounded, administered through DME, unit dose form, per milligram ⓥ ⓑ Qp Qh    M

*Other: Pulmozyme*

✳ **J7640** Formoterol, inhalation solution, compounded product, administered through DME, unit dose form, 12 mcg ⓥ ⓑ Qp Qh    E1

✳ **J7641** Flunisolide, inhalation solution, compounded product, administered through DME, unit dose, per milligram ⓥ ⓑ Qp Qh    M

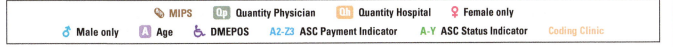

🖐 **MIPS**    Qp **Quantity Physician**    Qh **Quantity Hospital**    ♀ **Female only**

♂ **Male only**    A **Age**    ♿ **DMEPOS**    A2-Z3 **ASC Payment Indicator**    A-Y **ASC Status Indicator**    *Coding Clinic*

⚙ **J7642** Glycopyrrolate, inhalation solution, compounded product, administered through DME, concentrated form, per milligram Ⓑ Ⓑ Qp Qh    M

⚙ **J7643** Glycopyrrolate, inhalation solution, compounded product, administered through DME, unit dose form, per milligram Ⓑ Ⓑ Qp Qh    M

⚙ **J7644** Ipratropium bromide, inhalation solution, FDA-approved final product, non-compounded, administered through DME, unit dose form, per milligram Ⓑ Ⓑ Qp Qh    M

*Other: Atrovent*

✱ **J7645** Ipratropium bromide, inhalation solution, compounded product, administered through DME, unit dose form, per milligram Ⓥ Ⓑ Qp Qh    M

*Other: Atrovent*

✱ **J7647** Isoetharine HCL, inhalation solution, compounded product, administered through DME, concentrated form, per milligram Ⓑ Ⓑ Qp Qh    M

*Other: Bronkosol*

⚙ **J7648** Isoetharine HCL, inhalation solution, FDA-approved final product, non-compounded, administered through DME, concentrated form, per milligram Ⓑ Ⓑ Qp Qh    M

*Other: Bronkosol*

⚙ **J7649** Isoetharine HCL, inhalation solution, FDA-approved final product, non-compounded, administered through DME, unit dose form, per milligram Ⓑ Ⓑ Qp Qh    M

*Other: Bronkosol*

✱ **J7650** Isoetharine HCL, inhalation solution, compounded product, administered through DME, unit dose form, per milligram Ⓑ Ⓑ Qp Qh    M

*Other: Bronkosol*

✱ **J7657** Isoproterenol HCL, inhalation solution, compounded product, administered through DME, concentrated form, per milligram Ⓑ Ⓑ Qp Qh    M

*Other: Isuprel*

⚙ **J7658** Isoproterenol HCL inhalation solution, FDA-approved final product, non-compounded, administered through DME, concentrated form, per milligram Ⓑ Ⓑ Qp Qh    M

*Other: Isuprel*

⚙ **J7659** Isoproterenol HCL, inhalation solution, FDA-approved final product, non-compounded, administered through DME, unit dose form, per milligram Ⓑ Ⓑ Qp Qh    M

*Other: Isuprel*

✱ **J7660** Isoproterenol HCL, inhalation solution, compounded product, administered through DME, unit dose form, per milligram Ⓑ Ⓑ Qp Qh    M

*Other: Isuprel*

✱ **J7665** Mannitol, administered through an inhaler, 5 mg Ⓥ Ⓑ Qp Qh    N1 N

*Other: Aridol*

✱ **J7667** Metaproterenol sulfate, inhalation solution, compounded product, concentrated form, per 10 mg Ⓑ Ⓑ Qp Qh    M

*Other: Alupent, Metaprel*

⚙ **J7668** Metaproterenol sulfate, inhalation solution, FDA-approved final product, non-compounded, administered through DME, concentrated form, per 10 mg Ⓥ Ⓑ Qp Qh    M

*Other: Alupent, Metaprel*

⚙ **J7669** Metaproterenol sulfate, inhalation solution, FDA-approved final product, non-compounded, administered through DME, unit dose form, per 10 mg Ⓥ Ⓑ Qp Qh    M

*Other: Alupent, Metaprel*

✱ **J7670** Metaproterenol sulfate, inhalation solution, compounded product, administered through DME, unit dose form, per 10 mg Ⓥ Ⓑ Qp Qh    M

*Other: Alupent, Metaprel*

✱ **J7674** Methacholine chloride administered as inhalation solution through a nebulizer, per 1 mg Ⓥ Ⓑ Qp Qh    N1 N

*Other: Provocholine*

✱ **J7676** Pentamidine isethionate, inhalation solution, compounded product, administered through DME, unit dose form, per 300 mg Ⓥ Ⓑ Qp Qh    M

*Other: NebuPent, Pentam*

▶ ✱ **J7677** Revefenacin inhalation solution, FDA-approved final product, non-compounded, administered through DME, 1 microgram    M

⚙ **J7680** Terbutaline sulfate, inhalation solution, compounded product, administered through DME, concentrated form, per milligram Ⓑ Ⓑ Qp Qh    M

*Other: Brethine*

▶ New  ↻ Revised  ✔ Reinstated  ~~deleted~~ Deleted  ⊘ Not covered or valid by Medicare
⚙ Special coverage instructions  ✱ Carrier discretion  Ⓑ Bill Part B MAC  Ⓑ Bill DME MAC

✿ **J7681** Terbutaline sulfate, inhalation solution, compounded product, administered through DME, unit dose form, per milligram 📍 Ⓑ **Qp** **Qh** **M**

*Other: Brethine*

✿ **J7682** Tobramycin, inhalation solution, FDA-approved final product, non-compounded unit dose form, administered through DME, per 300 mg Ⓑ Ⓔ **Qp** **Qh** **M**

*Other: Bethkis, Kitabis PAK, Tobi*

✿ **J7683** Triamcinolone, inhalation solution, compounded product, administered through DME, concentrated form, per milligram 📍 Ⓑ **Qp** **Qh** **M**

✿ **J7684** Triamcinolone, inhalation solution, compounded product, administered through DME, unit dose form, per milligram Ⓑ Ⓑ **Qp** **Qh** **M**

*Other: Triamcinolone acetonide*

✱ **J7685** Tobramycin, inhalation solution, compounded product, administered through DME, unit dose form, per 300 mg 📍 Ⓑ **Qp** **Qh** **M**

*Other: Tobi*

✱ **J7686** Treprostinil, inhalation solution, FDA-approved final product, non-compounded, administered through DME, unit dose form, 1.74 mg 📍 Ⓑ **Qp** **Qh** **M**

*Other: Tyvaso*

## Not Otherwise Classified/Specified

✿ **J7699** NOC drugs, inhalation solution administered through DME Ⓑ Ⓔ **M**

*Other: Gentamicin Sulfate*

✿ **J7799** NOC drugs, other than inhalation drugs, administered through DME Ⓑ Ⓔ **N1 N**

Bill on paper. Bill one unit and identify drug and total dosage in the "Remark" field.

*Other: Cuvitru, Epinephrine, Mannitol, Osmitrol, Phenylephrine, Resectisol, Sodium chloride*

*IOM: 100-02, 15, 110.3*

✿ **J7999** Compounded drug, not otherwise classified Ⓑ Ⓔ **N1 N**

**Coding Clinic: 2017, Q1, P1-2; 2016, Q4, P8**

✿ **J8498** Antiemetic drug, rectal/suppository, not otherwise specified Ⓑ **B**

*Other: Compazine, Compro, Phenadoz, Phenergan, Prochlorperazine, Promethazine, Promethegan*

*Medicare Statute 1861(s)2t*

🚫 **J8499** Prescription drug, oral, non chemotherapeutic, NOS Ⓔ Ⓑ **E1**

*Other: Acyclovir, Calcitrol, Cromolyn Sodium, OFEV, Valganciclovir HCL, Zovirax*

*IOM: 100-02, 15, 50*

**Coding Clinic: 2013, Q2, P4**

## Oral Anti-Cancer Drugs

✿ **J8501** Aprepitant, oral, 5 mg Ⓑ **Qp** **Qh** **K2 K**

*Other: Emend*

✿ **J8510** Busulfan; oral, 2 mg Ⓑ **Qp** **Qh** **N1 N**

*Other: Myleran*

*IOM: 100-02, 15, 50; 100-04, 4, 240; 100-04, 17, 80.1.1*

🚫 **J8515** Cabergoline, oral, 0.25 mg Ⓑ **E1**

*IOM: 100-02, 15, 50; 100-04, 4, 240*

✿ **J8520** Capecitabine, oral, 150 mg Ⓑ **Qp** **Qh** **N1 N**

*Other: Xeloda*

*IOM: 100-02, 15, 50; 100-04, 4, 240; 100-04, 17, 80.1.1*

✿ **J8521** Capecitabine, oral, 500 mg Ⓑ **Qp** **Qh** **N1 N**

*Other: Xeloda*

*IOM: 100-02, 15, 50; 100-04, 4, 240; 100-04, 17, 80.1.1*

✿ **J8530** Cyclophosphamide; oral, 25 mg Ⓑ **Qp** **Qh** **N1 N**

*Other: Cytoxan*

*IOM: 100-02, 15, 50; 100-04, 4, 240; 100-04, 17, 80.1.1*

✿ **J8540** Dexamethasone, oral, 0.25 mg Ⓑ **Qp** **Qh** **N1 N**

*Other: Decadron, Dexone, Dexpak, Locort*

*Medicare Statute 1861(s)2t*

✿ **J8560** Etoposide; oral, 50 mg Ⓑ **Qp** **Qh** **K2 K**

*Other: VePesid*

*IOM: 100-02, 15, 50; 100-04, 4, 230.1; 100-04, 4, 240; 100-04, 17, 80.1.1*

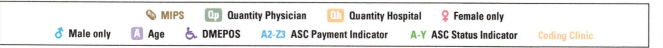

🏷 **MIPS**   **Qp** Quantity Physician   **Qh** Quantity Hospital   ♀ Female only   ♂ Male only   Ⓐ Age   ♿ DMEPOS   **A2-Z3** ASC Payment Indicator   **A-Y** ASC Status Indicator   Coding Clinic

✳ **J8562** Fludarabine phosphate, oral, 10 mg Ⓠ Ⓠp Ⓠh  E2

*Other: Fludara, Oforta*

Coding Clinic: 2011, Q1, P9

✷ **J8565** Gefitinib, oral, 250 mg Ⓠ  E2

*Other: Iressa*

✷ **J8597** Antiemetic drug, oral, not otherwise specified Ⓑ  N1 N

*Medicare Statute 1861(s)2t*

✷ **J8600** Melphalan; oral, 2 mg Ⓑ Ⓠp Ⓠh  N1 N

*Other: Alkeran*

*IOM: 100-02, 15, 50; 100-04, 4, 240; 100-04, 17, 80.1.1*

✷ **J8610** Methotrexate; oral, 2.5 mg Ⓑ Ⓠp Ⓠh  N1 N

*Other: Rheumatrex, Trexall*

*IOM: 100-02, 15, 50; 100-04, 4, 240; 100-04, 17, 80.1.1*

✳ **J8650** Nabilone, oral, 1 mg Ⓑ Ⓠp Ⓠh  E2

✷ **J8655** Netupitant 300 mg and palonosetron 0.5 mg, oral Ⓠ Ⓠp Ⓠh  K2 K

*Other: Akynzeo*

Coding Clinic: 2015, Q4, P4

✷ **J8670** Rolapitant, oral, 1 mg Ⓠp Ⓠh  K2 K

*Other: Varubi*

✷ **J8700** Temozolomide, oral, 5 mg Ⓑ Ⓠp Ⓠh  N1 N

*Other: Temodar*

*IOM: 100-02, 15, 50; 100-04, 4, 240*

✳ **J8705** Topotecan, oral, 0.25 mg Ⓑ Ⓠp Ⓠh  K2 K

Treatment for ovarian and lung cancers, etc. Report J9350 (Topotecan, 4 mg) for intravenous version

*Other: Hycamtin*

✷ **J8999** Prescription drug, oral, chemotherapeutic, NOS Ⓑ  B

*Other: Anastrozole, Arinidex, Aromasin, Droxia, Erivedge, Flutamide, Gleevec, Hydrea, Hydroxyurea, Leukeran, Matulane, Megestrol Acetate, Mercaptopurine, Nolvadex, Tamoxifen Citrate*

*IOM: 100-02, 15, 50; 100-04, 4, 250; 100-04, 17, 80.1.1; 100-04, 17, 80.1.2*

## CHEMOTHERAPY DRUGS (J9000-J9999)

**NOTE:** These codes cover the cost of the chemotherapy drug only, not to include the administration

✷ **J9000** Injection, doxorubicin hydrochloride, 10 mg Ⓑ Ⓑ Ⓠp Ⓠh  N1 N

*Other: Adriamycin, Rubex*

*IOM: 100-02, 15, 50*

Coding Clinic: 2007, Q4, P5

✷ **J9015** Injection, aldesleukin, per single use vial Ⓑ Ⓑ Ⓠp Ⓠh  K2 K

*Other: Proleukin*

*IOM: 100-02, 15, 50*

✳ **J9017** Injection, arsenic trioxide, 1 mg Ⓑ Ⓑ Ⓠp Ⓠh  K2 K

*Other: Trisenox*

✷ **J9019** Injection, asparaginase (Erwinaze), 1,000 IU Ⓑ Ⓑ Ⓠp Ⓠh  K2 K

*IOM: 100-02, 15, 50*

✷ **J9020** Injection, asparaginase, not otherwise specified 10,000 units Ⓑ Ⓑ Ⓠp Ⓠh  N1 N

*IOM: 100-02, 15, 50*

✳ **J9022** Injection, atezolizumab, 10 mg  K2 G

✳ **J9023** Injection, avelumab, 10 mg  K2 G

✳ **J9025** Injection, azacitidine, 1 mg Ⓑ Ⓑ Ⓠp Ⓠh  K2 K

✳ **J9027** Injection, clofarabine, 1 mg Ⓑ Ⓑ Ⓠp Ⓠh  K2 K

*Other: Clolar*

▶ ✷ **J9030** BCG live intravesical instillation, 1 mg  K2 K

~~J9031 BCG (intravesical), per instillation~~  ✖

✳ **J9032** Injection, belinostat, 10 mg Ⓑ Ⓑ Ⓠp Ⓠh  K2 K

*Other: Beleodaq*

✳ **J9033** Injection, bendamustine HCL (treanda), 1 mg Ⓑ Ⓑ Ⓠp Ⓠh  K2 K

Treatment for form of non-Hodgkin's lymphoma; standard administration time is as an intravenous infusion over 30 minutes

*Other: Treanda*

✳ **J9034** Injection, bendamustine HCL (bendeka), 1 mg Ⓠp Ⓠh  K2 G

Coding Clinic: 2017, Q1, P10

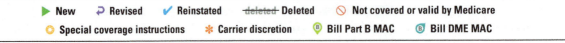

▶ **New**    ↩ **Revised**    ✔ **Reinstated**    ~~deleted~~ **Deleted**    ⊘ **Not covered or valid by Medicare**
✷ **Special coverage instructions**    ✳ **Carrier discretion**    Ⓑ **Bill Part B MAC**    Ⓑ **Bill DME MAC**

* **J9035** Injection, bevacizumab, 10 mg Ⓑ Ⓑ ⓆⓅ Ⓠⓗ **K2 K**

For malignant neoplasm of breast, considered J9207.

*Other: Avastin*

Coding Clinic: 2013, Q3, P9, Q2, P8

▶ * **J9036** Injection, bendamustine hydrochloride, (belrapzo/bendamustine), 1 mg **K2 G**

* **J9039** Injection, blinatumomab, 1 mcg Ⓑ Ⓑ ⓆⓅ Ⓠⓗ **K2 K**

*Other: Blincyto*

✿ **J9040** Injection, bleomycin sulfate, 15 units Ⓑ Ⓑ ⓆⓅ Ⓠⓗ **N1 N**

*Other: Blenoxane*

IOM: 100-02, 15, 50

* **J9041** Injection, bortezomib (velcade), 0.1 mg Ⓑ Ⓑ ⓆⓅ Ⓠⓗ **K2 K**

*Other: Velcade*

* **J9042** Injection, brentuximab vedotin, 1 mg Ⓑ Ⓑ ⓆⓅ Ⓠⓗ **K2 K**

*Other: Adcetris*

* **J9043** Injection, cabazitaxel, 1 mg Ⓑ Ⓑ ⓆⓅ Ⓠⓗ **K2 K**

*Other: Jevtana*

Coding Clinic: 2012, Q1, P9

* **J9044** Injection, bortezomib, not otherwise specified, 0.1 mg **K**

*Other: Velcade*

✿ **J9045** Injection, carboplatin, 50 mg Ⓑ Ⓑ ⓆⓅ Ⓠⓗ **N1 N**

*Other: Paraplatin*

IOM: 100-02, 15, 50

* **J9047** Injection, carfilzomib, 1 mg Ⓑ Ⓑ ⓆⓅ Ⓠⓗ **K2 K**

*Other: Kyprolis*

✿ **J9050** Injection, carmustine, 100 mg Ⓑ Ⓑ ⓆⓅ Ⓠⓗ **K2 K**

*Other: BiCNU*

IOM: 100-02, 15, 50

* **J9055** Injection, cetuximab, 10 mg Ⓑ Ⓑ ⓆⓅ Ⓠⓗ **K2 K**

*Other: Erbitux*

* **J9057** Injection, copanlisib, 1 mg **G**

*Other: Aliqopa*

✿ **J9060** Injection, cisplatin, powder or solution, 10 mg Ⓑ Ⓑ ⓆⓅ Ⓠⓗ **N1 N**

*Other: Plantinol AQ*

IOM: 100-02, 15, 50

Coding Clinic: 2013, Q2, P6; 2011, Q1, P8

✿ **J9065** Injection, cladribine, per 1 mg Ⓑ Ⓑ ⓆⓅ Ⓠⓗ **K2 K**

*Other: Leustatin*

IOM: 100-02, 15, 50

✿ **J9070** Cyclophosphamide, 100 mg Ⓑ Ⓑ ⓆⓅ Ⓠⓗ **K2 K**

*Other: Cytoxan, Neosar*

IOM: 100-02, 15, 50

Coding Clinic: 2011, Q1, P8-9

* **J9098** Injection, cytarabine liposome, 10 mg Ⓑ Ⓑ ⓆⓅ Ⓠⓗ **K2 K**

*Other: DepoCyt*

✿ **J9100** Injection, cytarabine, 100 mg Ⓑ Ⓑ ⓆⓅ Ⓠⓗ **N1 N**

*Other: Cytosar-U*

IOM: 100-02, 15, 50

Coding Clinic: 2011, Q1, P9

▶ * **J9118** Injection, calaspargase pegol-mknl, 10 units **E2**

▶ * **J9119** Injection, cemiplimab-rwlc, 1 mg **K2 G**

✿ **J9120** Injection, dactinomycin, 0.5 mg Ⓑ Ⓑ ⓆⓅ Ⓠⓗ **K2 K**

*Other: Cosmegen*

IOM: 100-02, 15, 50

✿ **J9130** Dacarbazine, 100 mg Ⓑ Ⓑ ⓆⓅ Ⓠⓗ **N1 N**

*Other: DTIC-Dome*

IOM: 100-02, 15, 50

Coding Clinic: 2011, Q1, P9

✿ **J9145** Injection, daratumumab, 10 mg ⓆⓅ Ⓠⓗ **K2 G**

*Other: Darzalex*

IOM: 100-02, 15, 50

✿ **J9150** Injection, daunorubicin, 10 mg Ⓑ Ⓑ ⓆⓅ Ⓠⓗ **K2 K**

*Other: Cerubidine*

IOM: 100-02, 15, 50

✿ **J9151** Injection, daunorubicin citrate, liposomal formulation, 10 mg Ⓑ Ⓑ ⓆⓅ Ⓠⓗ **E2**

*Other: Daunoxome*

IOM: 100-02, 15, 50

---

🐾 MIPS    ⓆⓅ Quantity Physician    Ⓠⓗ Quantity Hospital    ♀ Female only

♂ Male only    Ⓐ Age    ♿ DMEPOS    A2-Z3 ASC Payment Indicator    A-Y ASC Status Indicator    Coding Clinic

✳ **J9153**   njection, liposomal, 1 mg daunorubicin
and 2.27 mg cytarabine   G
*Other: Vyxeos*

✳ **J9155**   Injection, degarelix,
1 mg Ⓑ Ⓓ Qp Qh   K2 K
Report 1 unit for every 1 mg.
*Other: Firmagon*

✳ **J9160**   Injection, denileukin diftitox,
300 mcg Ⓑ Ⓓ Qp Qh   E2

✿ **J9165**   Injection, diethylstilbestrol
diphosphate, 250 mg Ⓑ Ⓓ Qp Qh   E2
*Other: Stilphostrol*
*IOM: 100-02, 15, 50*

✿ **J9171**   Injection, docetaxel,
1 mg Ⓑ Ⓓ Qp Qh   K2 K
Report 1 unit for every 1 mg.
*Other: Docefrez, Taxotere*
*IOM: 100-02, 15, 50*
**Coding Clinic: 2012, Q1, P9**

✳ **J9173**   Injection, durvalumab, 10 mg   G
*Other: Imfinzi*

✿ **J9175**   Injection, Elliott's B solution,
1 ml Ⓑ Ⓓ Qp Qh   N1 N
*IOM: 100-02, 15, 50*

✳ **J9176**   Injection, elotuzumab,
1 mg Qp Qh   K2 G
*Other: Empliciti*

✳ **J9178**   Injection, epirubicin HCL,
2 mg Ⓑ Ⓓ Qp Qh   N1 N
*Other: Ellence*

✳ **J9179**   Injection, eribulin mesylate,
0.1 mg Ⓑ Ⓓ Qp Qh   K2 K
*Other: Halaven*

✿ **J9181**   Injection, etoposide,
10 mg Ⓑ Ⓓ Qp Qh   N1 N
*Other: Etopophos, Toposar*

✿ **J9185**   Injection, fludarabine phosphate,
50 mg Ⓑ Ⓓ Qp Qh   K2 K
*Other: Fludara*
*IOM: 100-02, 15, 50*

✿ **J9190**   Injection, fluorouracil,
500 mg Ⓑ Ⓓ Qp Qh   N1 N
*Other: Adrucil*
*IOM: 100-02, 15, 50*

▶ ✳ **J9199**   Injection, gemcitabine hydrochloride
(infugem), 200 mg   N

✿ **J9200**   Injection, floxuridine,
500 mg Ⓑ Ⓓ Qp Qh   N1 N
*Other: FUDR*
*IOM: 100-02, 15, 50*

↻ ✿ **J9201**   Injection, gemcitabine
hydrochloride, not otherwise
specified, 200 mg Ⓑ Ⓓ Qp Qh   N1 N
*Other: Gemzar*
*IOM: 100-02, 15, 50*

✿ **J9202**   Goserelin acetate implant, per
3.6 mg Ⓑ Ⓓ Qp Qh   K2 K
*Other: Zoladex*
*IOM: 100-02, 15, 50*

✳ **J9203**   Injection, gemtuzumab ozogamicin,
0.1 mg   K2 G

▶ ✳ **J9204**   Injection, mogamulizumab-kpkc,
1 mg   K2 G

✿ **J9205**   Injection, irinotecan liposome,
1 mg Qp Qh   K2 G
*Other: ONIVYDE*
*IOM: 100-02, 15, 50*

✿ **J9206**   Injection, irinotecan,
20 mg Ⓑ Ⓓ Qp Qh   N1 N
*Other: Camptosar*
*IOM: 100-02, 15, 50*

✳ **J9207**   Injection, ixabepilone,
1 mg Ⓑ Ⓓ Qp Qh   K2 K
*Other: Ixempra Kit*

✿ **J9208**   Injection, ifosfamide,
1 gm Ⓑ Ⓓ Qp Qh   N1 N
*Other: Ifex*
*IOM: 100-02, 15, 50*

✿ **J9209**   Injection, mesna,
200 mg Ⓑ Ⓓ Qp Qh   N1 N
*Other: Mesnex*
*IOM: 100-02, 15, 50*

▶ ✳ **J9210**   Injection, emapalumab-lzsg, 1 mg   K2 G

✿ **J9211**   Injection, idarubicin hydrochloride,
5 mg Ⓑ Ⓓ Qp Qh   K2 K
*Other: Idamycin PFS*
*IOM: 100-02, 15, 50*

✿ **J9212**   Injection, interferon alfacon-1,
recombinant, 1 mcg Ⓑ Ⓓ Qp Qh   N1 N
*Other: Amgen, Infergen*
*IOM: 100-02, 15, 50*

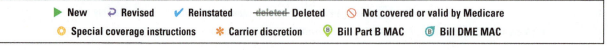

▶ New   ↻ Revised   ✔ Reinstated   ~~deleted~~ Deleted   ⊘ Not covered or valid by Medicare
✿ Special coverage instructions   ✳ Carrier discretion   Ⓑ Bill Part B MAC   Ⓓ Bill DME MAC

⚙ **J9213** Injection, interferon, alfa-2a, recombinant, 3 million units Ⓑ Ⓑ Qp Qh **N1 N**

*Other: Roferon-A*

*IOM: 100-02, 15, 50*

⚙ **J9214** Injection, interferon, alfa-2b, recombinant, 1 million units Ⓑ Ⓑ Qp Qh **K2 K**

*Other: Intron-A*

*IOM: 100-02, 15, 50*

⚙ **J9215** Injection, interferon, alfa-n3 (human leukocyte derived), 250,000 IU Ⓑ Ⓑ Qp Qh **E2**

*Other: Alferon N*

*IOM: 100-02, 15, 50*

⚙ **J9216** Injection, interferon, gamma-1B, 3 million units Ⓑ Ⓑ Qp Qh **K2 K**

*Other: Actimmune*

*IOM: 100-02, 15, 50*

⚙ **J9217** Leuprolide acetate (for depot suspension), 7.5 mg Ⓑ Ⓑ Qp Qh **K2 K**

*Other: Eligard, Lupron Depot*

*IOM: 100-02, 15, 50*

**Coding Clinic: 2019, Q2, P11; 2015, Q3, P3**

⚙ **J9218** Leuprolide acetate, per 1 mg Ⓑ Ⓑ Qp Qh **K2 K**

*Other: Lupron*

*IOM: 100-02, 15, 50*

**Coding Clinic: 2019, Q2, P11; 2015, Q3, P3**

⚙ **J9219** Leuprolide acetate implant, 65 mg Ⓑ Ⓑ Qp Qh **E2**

*Other: Viadur*

*IOM: 100-02, 15, 50*

⚙ **J9225** Histrelin implant (Vantas), 50 mg Ⓑ Ⓑ Qp Qh **K2 K**

*IOM: 100-02, 15, 50*

⚙ **J9226** Histrelin implant (Supprelin LA), 50 mg Ⓑ Ⓑ Qp Qh **K2 K**

*Other: Vantas*

*IOM: 100-02, 15, 50*

✳ **J9228** Injection, ipilimumab, 1 mg Ⓑ Ⓑ Qp Qh **K2 K**

*Other: Yervoy*

**Coding Clinic: 2012, Q1, P9**

✳ **J9229** Injection, inotuzumab ozogamicin, 0.1 mg **G**

*Other: Besponsa*

⚙ **J9230** Injection, mechlorethamine hydrochloride, (nitrogen mustard), 10 mg Ⓑ Ⓑ Qp Qh **K2 K**

*Other: Mustargen*

*IOM: 100-02, 15, 50*

⚙ **J9245** Injection, melphalan hydrochloride, 50 mg Ⓑ Ⓑ Qp Qh **K2 K**

*Other: Alkeran, Evomela*

*IOM: 100-02, 15, 50*

⚙ **J9250** Methotrexate sodium, 5 mg Ⓑ Ⓑ Qp Qh **N1 N**

*Other: Folex*

*IOM: 100-02, 15, 50*

⚙ **J9260** Methotrexate sodium, 50 mg Ⓑ Ⓑ Qp Qh **N1 N**

*Other: Folex*

*IOM: 100-02, 15, 50*

✳ **J9261** Injection, nelarabine, 50 mg Ⓑ Ⓑ Qp Qh **K2 K**

*Other: Arranon*

✳ **J9262** Injection, omacetaxine mepesuccinate, 0.01 mg Ⓑ Qp Qh **K2 K**

*Other: Synribo*

✳ **J9263** Injection, oxaliplatin, 0.5 mg Ⓑ Ⓑ Qp Qh **N1 N**

Eloxatin, platinum-based anticancer drug that destroys cancer cells

*Other: Eloxatin*

**Coding Clinic: 2009, Q1, P10**

✳ **J9264** Injection, paclitaxel protein-bound particles, 1 mg Ⓑ Ⓑ **K2 K**

*Other: Abraxane*

⚙ **J9266** Injection, pegaspargase, per single dose vial Ⓑ Ⓑ Qp Qh **K2 K**

*Other: Oncaspar*

*IOM: 100-02, 15, 50*

⚙ **J9267** Injection, paclitaxel, 1 mg Ⓑ Ⓑ Qp Qh **N1 N**

*Other: Taxol*

⚙ **J9268** Injection, pentostatin, 10 mg Ⓑ Ⓑ Qp Qh **K2 K**

*Other: Nipent*

*IOM: 100-02, 15, 50*

▶ ✳ **J9269** Injection, tagraxofusp-erzs, 10 micrograms **K2 G**

⚙ **J9270** Injection, plicamycin, 2.5 mg Ⓑ Ⓑ Qp Qh **N1 N**

*Other: Mithracin*

*IOM: 100-02, 15, 50*

🐾 MIPS     Qp Quantity Physician     Qh Quantity Hospital     ♀ Female only
♂ Male only     Ⓐ Age     ♿ DMEPOS     A2-Z3 ASC Payment Indicator     A-Y ASC Status Indicator     Coding Clinic

* **J9271** Injection, pembrolizumab, 1 mg Ⓑ Ⓑ Qp Qh    K2 K

  *Other: Keytruda*

☼ **J9280** Injection, mitomycin, 5 mg Ⓑ Ⓑ Qp Qh    K2 K

  *Other: Mitosol, Mutamycin*

  *IOM: 100-02, 15, 50*

  Coding Clinic: 2016, Q4, P8; 2014, Q2, P6; 2011, Q1, P9

* **J9285** Injection, olaratumab, 10 mg    K2 G

☼ **J9293** Injection, mitoxantrone hydrochloride, per 5 mg Ⓑ Ⓑ Qp Qh    K2 K

  *Other: Novantrone*

  *IOM: 100-02, 15, 50*

* **J9295** Injection, necitumumab, 1 mg Qp Qh    K2 G

  *Other: Portrazza*

☼ **J9299** Injection, nivolumab, 1 mg Ⓑ Ⓑ Qp Qh    K2 K

  *Other: Opdivo*

* **J9301** Injection, obinutuzumab, 10 mg Ⓑ Ⓑ Qp Qh    K2 K

  *Other: Gazyva*

* **J9302** Injection, ofatumumab, 10 mg Ⓑ Ⓑ Qp Qh    K2 K

  *Other: Arzerra*

  Coding Clinic: 2011, Q1, P7

* **J9303** Injection, panitumumab, 10 mg Ⓑ Ⓑ Qp Qh    K2 K

  *Other: Vectibix*

* **J9305** Injection, pemetrexed, 10 mg Ⓑ Ⓑ Qp Qh    K2 K

  *Other: Alimta*

* **J9306** Injection, pertuzumab, 1 mg Ⓑ Ⓑ Qp Qh    K2 K

  *Other: Perjeta*

* **J9307** Injection, pralatrexate, 1 mg Ⓑ Ⓑ Qp Qh    K2 K

  *Other: Folotyn*

  Coding Clinic: 2011, Q1, P7

* **J9308** Injection, ramucirumab, 5 mg Ⓑ Ⓑ Qp Qh    K2 K

  *Other: Cyramza*

▶ * **J9309** Injection, polatuzumab vedotin-piiq, 1 mg    K2 G

☼ **J9311** Injection, rituximab 10 mg and hyaluronidase    G

  *Other: Rituxan*

☼ **J9312** Injection, rituximab, 10 mg    K

  *Other: Rituxan*

▶ * **J9313** Injection, moxetumomab pasudotox-tdfk, 0.01 mg    K2 G

* **J9315** Injection, romidepsin, 1 mg Ⓑ Ⓑ Qp Qh    K2 K

  *Other: Istodax*

  Coding Clinic: 2011, Q1, P7

☼ **J9320** Injection, streptozocin, 1 gram Ⓑ Ⓑ Qp Qh    K2 K

  *Other: Zanosar*

  *IOM: 100-02, 15, 50*

* **J9325** Injection, talimogene laherparepvec, per 1 million plaque forming units Qp Qh    K2 G

  *Other: Imlygic*

  Coding Clinic: 2019, Q2, P12

* **J9328** Injection, temozolomide, 1 mg Ⓑ Ⓑ Qp Qh    K2 K

  Intravenous formulation, not for oral administration

  *Other: Temodar*

* **J9330** Injection, temsirolimus, 1 mg Ⓑ Ⓑ Qp Qh    K2 K

  Treatment for advanced renal cell carcinoma; standard administration is intravenous infusion greater than 30-60 minutes

  *Other: Torisel*

☼ **J9340** Injection, thiotepa, 15 mg Ⓑ Ⓑ Qp Qh    K2 K

  *Other: Tepadina, Triethylene thio Phosphoramide/T*

  *IOM: 100-02, 15, 50*

* **J9351** Injection, topotecan, 0.1 mg Ⓑ Ⓑ Qp Qh    N1 N

  *Other: Hycamtin*

  Coding Clinic: 2011, Q1, P9

* **J9352** Injection, trabectedin, 0.1 mg Qp Qh    K2 G

  *Other: Yondelis*

* **J9354** Injection, ado-trastuzumab emtansine, 1 mg Ⓑ Ⓑ Qp Qh    K2 K

  *Other: Kadcyla*

↻ * **J9355** Injection, trastuzumab, excludes biosimilar, 10 mg Ⓑ Ⓑ Qp Qh    K2 K

  *Other: Herceptin*

▶ * **J9356** Injection, trastuzumab, 10 mg and hyaluronidase-oysk    K2 G

---

| ▶ New | ↻ Revised | ✔ Reinstated | ~~deleted~~ Deleted | ⊘ Not covered or valid by Medicare |
|---|---|---|---|---|
| ☼ Special coverage instructions | | * Carrier discretion | Ⓑ Bill Part B MAC | Ⓑ Bill DME MAC |

**J9357**   Injection, valrubicin, intravesical, 200 mg ⑨ ⑧ **Qp** **Qh**            K2  K

*Other: Valstar*

*IOM: 100-02, 15, 50*

**J9360**   Injection, vinblastine sulfate, 1 mg ⑨ ⑧ **Qp** **Qh**            N1  N

*Other: Alkaban-AQ, Velban, Velsar*

*IOM: 100-02, 15, 50*

**J9370**   Vincristine sulfate, 1 mg ⑨ ⑧ **Qp** **Qh**            N1  N

*Other: Oncovin, Vincasar PFS*

*IOM: 100-02, 15, 50*

Coding Clinic: 2011, Q1, P9

**✳ J9371**   Injection, vincristine sulfate liposome, 1 mg ⑨ ⑧ **Qp** **Qh**            K2  K

**J9390**   Injection, vinorelbine tartrate, 10 mg ⑨ ⑧ **Qp** **Qh**            N1  N

*Other: Navelbine*

*IOM: 100-02, 15, 50*

**✳ J9395**   Injection, fulvestrant, 25 mg ⑨ ⑧ **Qp** **Qh**            K2  K

*Other: Faslodex*

**✳ J9400**   Injection, ziv-aflibercept, 1 mg ⑨ ⑧ **Qp** **Qh**            K2  K

*Other: Zaltrap*

**J9600**   Injection, porfimer sodium, 75 mg ⑨ ⑧ **Qp** **Qh**            K2  K

*Other: Photofrin*

*IOM: 100-02, 15, 50*

**J9999**   Not otherwise classified, antineoplastic drugs ⑨ ⑧            N1  N

Bill on paper, bill one unit, and identify drug and total dosage in "Remarks" field. Include invoice of cost or NDC number in "Remarks" field.

*Other: Imlygic, Yondelis*

*IOM: 100-02, 15, 50; 100-03, 2, 110.2*

Coding Clinic: 2017, Q1, P3; 2013, Q2, P3

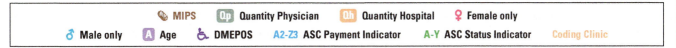

🖐 **MIPS**   **Qp** Quantity Physician   **Qh** Quantity Hospital   ♀ Female only
♂ **Male only**   Ⓐ **Age**   ♿ **DMEPOS**   A2-Z3 **ASC Payment Indicator**   A-Y **ASC Status Indicator**   Coding Clinic

## TEMPORARY CODES ASSIGNED TO DME REGIONAL CARRIERS (K0000-K9999)

**NOTE:** This section contains national codes assigned by CMS on a temporary basis and for the exclusive use of the durable medical equipment regional carriers (DMERC).

### Wheelchairs and Accessories

✳ **K0001** Standard wheelchair Ⓑ Qp Qh ♿ Y
Capped rental

✳ **K0002** Standard hemi (low seat) wheelchair Ⓑ Qp Qh ♿ Y
Capped rental

✳ **K0003** Lightweight wheelchair Ⓑ Qp Qh ♿ Y
Capped rental

✳ **K0004** High strength, lightweight wheelchair Ⓑ Qp Qh ♿ Y
Capped rental

✳ **K0005** Ultralightweight wheelchair Ⓑ Qp Qh ♿ Y
Capped rental. Inexpensive and routinely purchased DME

✳ **K0006** Heavy duty wheelchair Ⓑ Qp Qh ♿ Y
Capped rental

✳ **K0007** Extra heavy duty wheelchair Ⓑ Qp Qh ♿ Y
Capped rental

✪ **K0008** Custom manual wheelchair/base Ⓑ Qh Y

✳ **K0009** Other manual wheelchair/base Ⓑ Qp Qh ♿ Y
Not otherwise classified

✳ **K0010** Standard - weight frame motorized/power wheelchair Ⓑ ♿ Y
Capped rental. Codes K0010-K0014 are not for manual wheelchairs with add-on power packs. Use the appropriate code for the manual wheelchair base provided (K0001-K0009) and code K0460.

✳ **K0011** Standard - weight frame motorized/power wheelchair with programmable control parameters for speed adjustment, tremor dampening, acceleration control and braking Ⓑ ♿ Y
Capped rental. A patient who requires a power wheelchair usually is totally nonambulatory and has severe weakness of the upper extremities due to a neurologic or muscular disease/condition.

✳ **K0012** Lightweight portable motorized/power wheelchair Ⓑ ♿ Y
Capped rental

✪ **K0013** Custom motorized/power wheelchair base Ⓑ Qh Y

✳ **K0014** Other motorized/power wheelchair base Ⓑ Y
Capped rental

✳ **K0015** Detachable, non-adjustable height armrest, replacement only, each Ⓑ Qp Qh ♿ Y
Inexpensive and routinely purchased DME

✳ **K0017** Detachable, adjustable height armrest, base, replacement only, each Ⓑ Qp Qh ♿ Y
Inexpensive and routinely purchased DME

✳ **K0018** Detachable, adjustable height armrest, upper portion, replacement only, each Ⓑ Qp Qh ♿ Y
Inexpensive and routinely purchased DME

✳ **K0019** Arm pad, replacement only, each Ⓑ Qp Qh ♿ Y
Inexpensive and routinely purchased DME

✳ **K0020** Fixed, adjustable height armrest, pair Ⓑ Qp Qh ♿ Y
Inexpensive and routinely purchased DME

✳ **K0037** High mount flip-up footrest, each Ⓑ Qp Qh ♿ Y
Inexpensive and routinely purchased DME

✳ **K0038** Leg strap, each Ⓑ Qp Qh ♿ Y
Inexpensive and routinely purchased DME

✳ **K0039** Leg strap, H style, each Ⓑ Qp Qh ♿ Y
Inexpensive and routinely purchased DME

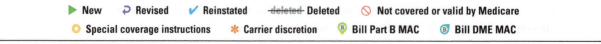

▶ New   ↻ Revised   ✔ Reinstated   ~~deleted~~ Deleted   ⊘ Not covered or valid by Medicare   ✪ Special coverage instructions   ✳ Carrier discretion   Ⓑ Bill Part B MAC   Ⓓ Bill DME MAC

✳ **K0040** Adjustable angle footplate,
each ⑥ Qp Qh ♿     Y

*Inexpensive and routinely purchased DME*

✳ **K0041** Large size footplate,
each ⑥ Qp Qh ♿     Y

*Inexpensive and routinely purchased DME*

✳ **K0042** Standard size footplate, replacement
only, each ⑥ Qp Qh ♿     Y

*Inexpensive and routinely purchased DME*

✳ **K0043** Footrest, lower extension tube,
replacement only, each ⑥ Qp Qh ♿ Y

*Inexpensive and routinely purchased DME*

✳ **K0044** Footrest, upper hanger bracket,
replacement only, each ⑥ Qp Qh ♿ Y

*Inexpensive and routinely purchased DME*

✳ **K0045** Footrest, complete assembly,
replacement only, each ⑥ Qp Qh ♿ Y

*Inexpensive and routinely purchased DME*

✳ **K0046** Elevating legrest, lower extension tube,
replacement only, each ⑥ Qp Qh ♿ Y

*Inexpensive and routinely purchased DME*

✳ **K0047** Elevating legrest, upper hanger bracket,
replacement only, each ⑥ Qp Qh ♿ Y

*Inexpensive and routinely purchased DME*

✳ **K0050** Ratchet assembly, replacement
only ⑥ Qp Qh ♿     Y

*Inexpensive and routinely purchased DME*

✳ **K0051** Cam release assembly, footrest or
legrests, replacement only,
each ⑥ Qp Qh ♿     Y

*Inexpensive and routinely purchased DME*

✳ **K0052** Swing-away, detachable footrests,
replacement only, each ⑥ Qp Qh ♿ Y

*Inexpensive and routinely purchased DME*

✳ **K0053** Elevating footrests, articulating
(telescoping), each ⑥ Qp Qh ♿     Y

*Inexpensive and routinely purchased DME*

✳ **K0056** Seat height less than 17" or equal to or
greater than 21" for a high strength,
lightweight, or ultralightweight
wheelchair ⑥ Qp Qh ♿     Y

*Inexpensive and routinely purchased DME*

✳ **K0065** Spoke protectors, each ⑥ Qp Qh ♿ Y

*Inexpensive and routinely purchased DME*

✳ **K0069** Rear wheel assembly, complete, with
solid tire, spokes or molded,
replacement only, each Qp Qh ♿ Y

*Inexpensive and routinely purchased DME*

✳ **K0070** Rear wheel assembly, complete, with
pneumatic tire, spokes or molded,
replacement only, each ⑥ Qp Qh ♿ Y

*Inexpensive and routinely purchased DME*

✳ **K0071** Front caster assembly, complete, with
pneumatic tire, replacement only,
each ⑥ Qp Qh ♿     Y

*Caster assembly includes a caster fork
(E2396), wheel rim, and tire.
Inexpensive and routinely purchased DME*

✳ **K0072** Front caster assembly, complete, with
semi-pneumatic tire, replacement only,
each ⑥ Qp Qh ♿     Y

*Inexpensive and routinely purchased DME*

✳ **K0073** Caster pin lock, each ⑥ Qp Qh ♿ Y

*Inexpensive and routinely purchased DME*

✳ **K0077** Front caster assembly, complete, with
solid tire, replacement only,
each ⑥ Qp Qh ♿     Y

✳ **K0098** Drive belt for power wheelchair,
replacement only ⑥ ♿     Y

*Inexpensive and routinely purchased DME*

✳ **K0105** IV hanger, each ⑥ Qp Qh ♿     Y

*Inexpensive and routinely purchased DME*

✳ **K0108** Wheelchair component or accessory,
not otherwise specified ⑥     Y

✿ **K0195** Elevating leg rests, pair (for use with
capped rental wheelchair
base) ⑥ Qp Qh ♿     Y

*Medically necessary replacement items
are covered if rollabout chair or
transport chair covered*

*IOM: 100-03, 4, 280.1*

| 🐭 MIPS | Qp Quantity Physician | Qh Quantity Hospital | ♀ Female only |
| ♂ Male only | A Age | & DMEPOS | A2-Z3 ASC Payment Indicator | A-Y ASC Status Indicator | Coding Clinic |

## Infusion Pump, Supplies, and Batteries

⚙ **K0455** Infusion pump used for uninterrupted parenteral administration of medication (e.g., epoprostenol or treprostinol) ⑧ **Qp** **Qh** 👤    Y

An EIP may also be referred to as an external insulin pump, ambulatory pump, or mini-infuser. CMN/DIF required. Frequent and substantial service DME.

*IOM: 100-03, 1, 50.3*

⚙ **K0462** Temporary replacement for patient owned equipment being repaired, any type ⑧ **Qp** **Qh**    Y

Only report for maintenance and service for an item for which initial claim was paid. The term power mobility device (PMD) includes power operated vehicles (POVs) and power wheelchairs (PWCs). Not Otherwise Classified.

*IOM: 100-04, 20, 40.1*

⚙ **K0552** Supplies for external non-insulin drug infusion pump, syringe type cartridge, sterile, each ⑧ **Qh** 👤    Y

Supplies

*IOM: 100-03, 1, 50.3*

⚙ **K0553** Supply allowance for therapeutic continuous glucose monitor (CGM), includes all supplies and accessories, 1 month supply = 1 unit of service ⑧ 👤    Y

⚙ **K0554** Receiver (monitor), dedicated, for use with therapeutic glucose continuous monitor system ⑧ 👤    Y

✳ **K0601** Replacement battery for external infusion pump owned by patient, silver oxide, 1.5 volt, each ⑧ **Qh** 👤    Y

Inexpensive and routinely purchased DME

✳ **K0602** Replacement battery for external infusion pump owned by patient, silver oxide, 3 volt, each ⑧ **Qp** **Qh** 👤    Y

Inexpensive and routinely purchased DME

✳ **K0603** Replacement battery for external infusion pump owned by patient, alkaline, 1.5 volt, each ⑧ **Qh** 👤    Y

Inexpensive and routinely purchased DME

✳ **K0604** Replacement battery for external infusion pump owned by patient, lithium, 3.6 volt, each ⑧ **Qh** 👤    Y

Inexpensive and routinely purchased DME

✳ **K0605** Replacement battery for external infusion pump owned by patient, lithium, 4.5 volt, each ⑧ **Qp** **Qh** 👤    Y

Inexpensive and routinely purchased DME

## Defibrillator and Accessories

✳ **K0606** Automatic external defibrillator, with integrated electrocardiogram analysis, garment type ⑧ **Qp** **Qh** 👤    Y

Capped rental

✳ **K0607** Replacement battery for automated external defibrillator, garment type only, each ⑧ **Qp** **Qh** 👤    Y

Inexpensive and routinely purchased DME

✳ **K0608** Replacement garment for use with automated external defibrillator, each ⑧ **Qp** **Qh** 👤    Y

Inexpensive and routinely purchased DME

✳ **K0609** Replacement electrodes for use with automated external defibrillator, garment type only, each ⑧ **Qp** **Qh** 👤 Y

Supplies

## Miscellaneous

✳ **K0669** Wheelchair accessory, wheelchair seat or back cushion, does not meet specific code criteria or no written coding verification from DME PDAC ⑧    Y

Inexpensive and routinely purchased DME

✳ **K0672** Addition to lower extremity orthosis, removable soft interface, all components, replacement only, each ⑧ **Qp** 👤    A

Prosthetics/Orthotics

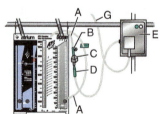

**Figure 18** Infusion pump.

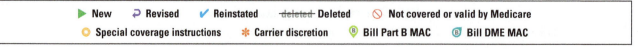

✳ **K0730** Controlled dose inhalation drug delivery system Ⓑ Qp Qh 🦽   Y

*Inexpensive and routinely purchased DME*

✳ **K0733** Power wheelchair accessory, 12 to 24 amp hour sealed lead acid battery, each (e.g., gel cell, absorbed glassmat) Ⓑ Qp Qh 🦽   Y

*Inexpensive and routinely purchased DME*

✳ **K0738** Portable gaseous oxygen system, rental; home compressor used to fill portable oxygen cylinders; includes portable containers, regulator, flowmeter, humidifier, cannula or mask, and tubing Ⓑ Qp Qh 🦽   Y

*Oxygen and oxygen equipment*

✳ **K0739** Repair or nonroutine service for durable medical equipment other than oxygen equipment requiring the skill of a technician, labor component, per 15 minutes Ⓑ Ⓑ   Y

🚫 **K0740** Repair or nonroutine service for oxygen equipment requiring the skill of a technician, labor component, per 15 minutes Ⓑ Qp Qh   E1

✳ **K0743** Suction pump, home model, portable, for use on wounds Ⓑ Qp Qh   Y

✳ **K0744** Absorptive wound dressing for use with suction pump, home model, portable, pad size 16 square inches or less Qp   A

✳ **K0745** Absorptive wound dressing for use with suction pump, home model, portable, pad size more than 16 square inches but less than or equal to 48 square inches Ⓑ Qp   A

✳ **K0746** Absorptive wound dressing for use with suction pump, home model, portable, pad size greater than 48 square inches Ⓑ Qp   A

## Power Mobility Devices

✳ **K0800** Power operated vehicle, group 1 standard, patient weight capacity up to and including 300 pounds Ⓑ Qp Qh 🦽   Y

*Power mobility device (PMD) includes power operated vehicles (POVs) and power wheelchairs (PWCs). Inexpensive and routinely purchased DME*

✳ **K0801** Power operated vehicle, group 1 heavy duty, patient weight capacity 301 to 450 pounds Ⓑ Qp Qh 🦽   Y

*Inexpensive and routinely purchased DME*

✳ **K0802** Power operated vehicle, group 1 very heavy duty, patient weight capacity 451 to 600 pounds Ⓑ Qp Qh 🦽   Y

*Inexpensive and routinely purchased DME*

✳ **K0806** Power operated vehicle, group 2 standard, patient weight capacity up to and including 300 pounds Ⓑ Qp Qh 🦽   Y

*Inexpensive and routinely purchased DME*

✳ **K0807** Power operated vehicle, group 2 heavy duty, patient weight capacity 301 to 450 pounds Ⓑ Qp Qh 🦽   Y

*Inexpensive and routinely purchased DME*

✳ **K0808** Power operated vehicle, group 2 very heavy duty, patient weight capacity 451 to 600 pounds Ⓑ Qp Qh 🦽   Y

*Inexpensive and routinely purchased DME*

✳ **K0812** Power operated vehicle, not otherwise classified Ⓑ Qp Qh   Y

*Not Otherwise Classified.*

✳ **K0813** Power wheelchair, group 1 standard, portable, sling/solid seat and back, patient weight capacity up to and including 300 pounds Ⓑ Qp Qh 🦽   Y

*Capped rental*

✳ **K0814** Power wheelchair, group 1 standard, portable, captains chair, patient weight capacity up to and including 300 pounds Ⓑ Qp Qh 🦽   Y

*Capped rental*

✳ **K0815** Power wheelchair, group 1 standard, sling/solid seat and back, patient weight capacity up to and including 300 pounds Ⓑ Qp Qh 🦽   Y

*Capped rental*

✳ **K0816** Power wheelchair, group 1 standard, captains chair, patient weight capacity up to and including 300 pounds Ⓑ Qp Qh 🦽   Y

*Capped rental*

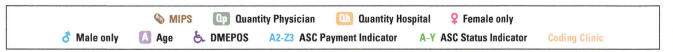

TEMPORARY CODES ASSIGNED TO DME REGIONAL CARRIERS    K0730 – K0816

✳ **K0820** Power wheelchair, group 2 standard, portable, sling/solid seat/back, patient weight capacity up to and including 300 pounds Ⓑ Qp Qh ♿ Y

*Capped rental*

✳ **K0821** Power wheelchair, group 2 standard, portable, captains chair, patient weight capacity up to and including 300 pounds Ⓑ Qp Qh ♿ Y

*Capped rental*

✳ **K0822** Power wheelchair, group 2 standard, sling/solid seat/back, patient weight capacity up to and including 300 pounds Ⓑ Qp Qh ♿ Y

*Capped rental*

✳ **K0823** Power wheelchair, group 2 standard, captains chair, patient weight capacity up to and including 300 pounds Ⓑ Qp Qh ♿ Y

*Capped rental*

✳ **K0824** Power wheelchair, group 2 heavy duty, sling/solid seat/back, patient weight capacity 301 to 450 pounds Ⓑ Qp Qh ♿ Y

*Capped rental*

✳ **K0825** Power wheelchair, group 2 heavy duty, captains chair, patient weight capacity 301 to 450 pounds Ⓑ Qp Qh ♿ Y

*Capped rental*

✳ **K0826** Power wheelchair, group 2 very heavy duty, sling/solid seat/back, patient weight capacity 451 to 600 pounds Ⓑ Qp Qh ♿ Y

*Capped rental*

✳ **K0827** Power wheelchair, group 2 very heavy duty, captains chair, patient weight capacity 451 to 600 pounds Ⓑ Qp Qh ♿ Y

*Capped rental*

✳ **K0828** Power wheelchair, group 2 extra heavy duty, sling/solid seat/back, patient weight capacity 601 pounds or more Ⓑ Qp Qh ♿ Y

*Capped rental*

✳ **K0829** Power wheelchair, group 2 extra heavy duty, captains chair, patient weight 601 pounds or more Ⓑ Qp Qh ♿ Y

*Capped rental*

✳ **K0830** Power wheelchair, group 2 standard, seat elevator, sling/solid seat/back, patient weight capacity up to and including 300 pounds Ⓑ Qp Qh Y

*Capped rental*

✳ **K0831** Power wheelchair, group 2 standard, seat elevator, captains chair, patient weight capacity up to and including 300 pounds Ⓑ Qp Qh Y

✳ **K0835** Power wheelchair, group 2 standard, single power option, sling/solid seat/back, patient weight capacity up to and including 300 pounds Ⓑ Qp Qh ♿ Y

*Capped rental*

✳ **K0836** Power wheelchair, group 2 standard, single power option, captains chair, patient weight capacity up to and including 300 pounds Ⓑ Qp Qh ♿ Y

*Capped rental*

✳ **K0837** Power wheelchair, group 2 heavy duty, single power option, sling/solid seat/back, patient weight capacity 301 to 450 pounds Ⓑ Qp Qh ♿ Y

*Capped rental*

✳ **K0838** Power wheelchair, group 2 heavy duty, single power option, captains chair, patient weight capacity 301 to 450 pounds Ⓑ Qp Qh ♿ Y

*Capped rental*

✳ **K0839** Power wheelchair, group 2 very heavy duty, single power option, sling/solid seat/back, patient weight capacity 451 to 600 pounds Ⓑ Qp Qh Y

*Capped rental*

✳ **K0840** Power wheelchair, group 2 extra heavy duty, single power option, sling/solid seat/back, patient weight capacity 601 pounds or more Ⓑ Qp Qh ♿ Y

*Capped rental*

✳ **K0841** Power wheelchair, group 2 standard, multiple power option, sling/solid seat/back, patient weight capacity up to and including 300 pounds Ⓑ Qp Qh ♿ Y

*Capped rental*

✳ **K0842** Power wheelchair, group 2 standard, multiple power option, captains chair, patient weight capacity up to and including 300 pounds Ⓑ Qp Qh ♿ Y

*Capped rental*

✳ **K0843** Power wheelchair, group 2 heavy duty, multiple power option, sling/solid seat/back, patient weight capacity 301 to 450 pounds Ⓑ Qp Qh ♿ Y

*Capped rental*

✳ **K0848** Power wheelchair, group 3 standard, sling/solid seat/back, patient weight capacity up to and including 300 pounds Ⓑ Qp Qh ♿ Y

*Capped rental*

---

▶ New    ⟳ Revised    ✔ Reinstated    ~~deleted~~ Deleted    ⃠ Not covered or valid by Medicare

✿ Special coverage instructions    ✳ Carrier discretion    Ⓑ Bill Part B MAC    Ⓓ Bill DME MAC

* **K0849** Power wheelchair, group 3 standard, captains chair, patient weight capacity up to and including 300 pounds ⑧ Qp Qh ♿ Y
*Capped rental*

* **K0850** Power wheelchair, group 3 heavy duty, sling/solid seat/back, patient weight capacity 301 to 450 pounds ⑧ Qp Qh ♿ Y
*Capped rental*

* **K0851** Power wheelchair, group 3 heavy duty, captains chair, patient weight capacity 301 to 450 pounds ⑧ Qp Qh ♿ Y
*Capped rental*

* **K0852** Power wheelchair, group 3 very heavy duty, sling/solid seat/back, patient weight capacity 451 to 600 pounds ⑧ Qp Qh ♿ Y
*Capped rental*

* **K0853** Power wheelchair, group 3 very heavy duty, captains chair, patient weight capacity 451 to 600 pounds ⑧ Qp Qh ♿ Y
*Capped rental*

* **K0854** Power wheelchair, group 3 extra heavy duty, sling/solid seat/back, patient weight capacity 601 pounds or more ⑧ Qp Qh ♿ Y
*Capped rental*

* **K0855** Power wheelchair, group 3 extra heavy duty, captains chair, patient weight capacity 601 pounds or more ⑧ Qp Qh ♿ Y
*Capped rental*

* **K0856** Power wheelchair, group 3 standard, single power option, sling/solid seat/back, patient weight capacity up to and including 300 pounds ⑧ Qp Qh ♿ Y
*Capped rental*

* **K0857** Power wheelchair, group 3 standard, single power option, captains chair, patient weight capacity up to and including 300 pounds ⑧ Qp Qh ♿ Y
*Capped rental*

* **K0858** Power wheelchair, group 3 heavy duty, single power option, sling/solid seat/back, patient weight 301 to 450 pounds ⑧ Qp Qh ♿ Y
*Capped rental*

* **K0859** Power wheelchair, group 3 heavy duty, single power option, captains chair, patient weight capacity 301 to 450 pounds ⑧ Qp Qh ♿ Y
*Capped rental*

* **K0860** Power wheelchair, group 3 very heavy duty, single power option, sling/solid seat/back, patient weight capacity 451 to 600 pounds ⑧ Qp Qh ♿ Y
*Capped rental*

* **K0861** Power wheelchair, group 3 standard, multiple power option, sling/solid seat/back, patient weight capacity up to and including 300 pounds ⑧ Qp Qh ♿ Y
*Capped rental*

* **K0862** Power wheelchair, group 3 heavy duty, multiple power option, sling/solid seat/back, patient weight capacity 301 to 450 pounds ⑧ Qp Qh ♿ Y
*Capped rental*

* **K0863** Power wheelchair, group 3 very heavy duty, multiple power option, sling/solid seat/back, patient weight capacity 451 to 600 pounds ⑧ Qp Qh ♿ Y
*Capped rental*

* **K0864** Power wheelchair, group 3 extra heavy duty, multiple power option, sling/solid seat/back, patient weight capacity 601 pounds or more ⑧ Qp Qh ♿ Y
*Capped rental*

* **K0868** Power wheelchair, group 4 standard, sling/solid seat/back, patient weight capacity up to and including 300 pounds ⑧ Qp Qh Y
*Capped rental*

* **K0869** Power wheelchair, group 4 standard, captains chair, patient weight capacity up to and including 300 pounds ⑧ Qp Qh Y
*Capped rental*

* **K0870** Power wheelchair, group 4 heavy duty, sling/solid seat/back, patient weight capacity 301 to 450 pounds ⑧ Qp Qh Y
*Capped rental*

* **K0871** Power wheelchair, group 4 very heavy duty, sling/solid seat/back, patient weight capacity 451 to 600 pounds ⑧ Qp Qh Y
*Capped rental*

* **K0877** Power wheelchair, group 4 standard, single power option, sling/solid seat/back, patient weight capacity up to and including 300 pounds ⑧ Qp Qh Y
*Capped rental*

* **K0878** Power wheelchair, group 4 standard, single power option, captains chair, patient weight capacity up to and including 300 pounds Ⓑ Qp Qh Y

  Capped rental

* **K0879** Power wheelchair, group 4 heavy duty, single power option, sling/solid seat/back, patient weight capacity 301 to 450 pounds Ⓑ Qp Qh Y

  Capped rental

* **K0880** Power wheelchair, group 4 very heavy duty, single power option, sling/solid seat/back, patient weight 451 to 600 pounds Ⓑ Qp Qh Y

  Capped rental

* **K0884** Power wheelchair, group 4 standard, multiple power option, sling/solid seat/back, patient weight capacity up to and including 300 pounds Ⓑ Qp Qh Y

  Capped rental

* **K0885** Power wheelchair, group 4 standard, multiple power option, captains chair, patient weight capacity up to and including 300 pounds Ⓑ Qp Qh Y

  Capped rental

* **K0886** Power wheelchair, group 4 heavy duty, multiple power option, sling/solid seat/back, patient weight capacity 301 to 450 pounds Ⓑ Qp Qh Y

  Capped rental

* **K0890** Power wheelchair, group 5 pediatric, single power option, sling/solid seat/back, patient weight capacity up to and including 125 pounds Ⓑ Qp Qh A Y

  Capped rental

* **K0891** Power wheelchair, group 5 pediatric, multiple power option, sling/solid seat/back, patient weight capacity up to and including 125 pounds Ⓑ Qp Qh A Y

  Capped rental

* **K0898** Power wheelchair, not otherwise classified Ⓑ Qp Qh Y

* **K0899** Power mobility device, not coded by DME PDAC or does not meet criteria Ⓑ Y

## Customized DME: Other than Wheelchair

⊙ **K0900** Customized durable medical equipment, other than wheelchair Ⓑ Qp Qh Y

## Miscellaneous

▶ * **K1001** Electronic positional obstructive sleep apnea treatment, with sensor, includes all components and accessories, any type Y

▶ ⊘ **K1002** Cranial electrotherapy stimulation (CES) system, includes all supplies and accessories, any type E1

▶ * **K1003** Whirlpool tub, walk-in, portable Y

▶ * **K1004** Low frequency ultrasonic diathermy treatment device for home use, includes all components and accessories Y

▶ * **K1005** Disposable collection and storage bag for breast milk, any size, any type, each Y

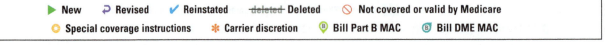

▶ New  ↩ Revised  ✔ Reinstated  ~~deleted~~ Deleted  ⊘ Not covered or valid by Medicare
⊙ Special coverage instructions  * Carrier discretion  Ⓑ Bill Part B MAC  Ⓑ Bill DME MAC

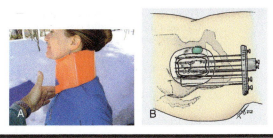

**Figure 19** (A) Flexible cervical collar. (B) Adjustable cervical collar.

## ORTHOTICS (L0100–L4999)

NOTE: DMEPOS fee schedule https://www.cms.gov/Medicare/Medicare-Fee-for-Service-Payment/DMEPOSFeeSched/DMEPOS-Fee-Schedule.html

### Cervical Orthotics

✳ **L0112** Cranial cervical orthosis, congenital torticollis type, with or without soft interface material, adjustable range of motion joint, custom fabricated ⑧ Qp Qh ♿ A

✳ **L0113** Cranial cervical orthosis, torticollis type, with or without joint, with or without soft interface material, prefabricated, includes fitting and adjustment ⑧ Qp Qh ♿ A

✳ **L0120** Cervical, flexible, non-adjustable, prefabricated, off-the-shelf (foam collar) ⑧ Qp Qh ♿ A

*Cervical orthoses including soft and rigid devices may be used as nonoperative management for cervical trauma*

✳ **L0130** Cervical, flexible, thermoplastic collar, molded to patient ⑧ Qp Qh ♿ A

✳ **L0140** Cervical, semi-rigid, adjustable (plastic collar) ⑧ Qp Qh ♿ A

✳ **L0150** Cervical, semi-rigid, adjustable molded chin cup (plastic collar with mandibular/occipital piece) ⑧ Qp Qh ♿ A

✳ **L0160** Cervical, semi-rigid, wire frame occipital/mandibular support, prefabricated, off-the-shelf ⑧ Qp Qh ♿ A

✳ **L0170** Cervical, collar, molded to patient model ⑧ Qp Qh ♿ A

✳ **L0172** Cervical, collar, semi-rigid thermoplastic foam, two-piece, prefabricated, off-the-shelf ⑧ Qp Qh ♿ A

✳ **L0174** Cervical, collar, semi-rigid, thermoplastic foam, two piece with thoracic extension, prefabricated, off-the-shelf ⑧ Qp Qh ♿ A

### Multiple Post Collar: Cervical

✳ **L0180** Cervical, multiple post collar, occipital/mandibular supports, adjustable ⑧ Qp Qh ♿ A

✳ **L0190** Cervical, multiple post collar, occipital/mandibular supports, adjustable cervical bars (SOMI, Guilford, Taylor types) ⑧ Qp Qh ♿ A

✳ **L0200** Cervical, multiple post collar, occipital/mandibular supports, adjustable cervical bars, and thoracic extension ⑧ Qp Qh ♿ A

### Thoracic Rib Belt

✳ **L0220** Thoracic, rib belt, custom fabricated ⑧ Qp Qh ♿ A

### Thoracic-Lumbar-Sacral Orthotics

✳ **L0450** TLSO, flexible, provides trunk support, upper thoracic region, produces intracavitary pressure to reduce load on the intervertebral disks with rigid stays or panel(s), includes shoulder straps and closures, prefabricated, off-the-shelf ⑧ Qp Qh ♿ A

*Used to immobilize specified area of spine, and is generally worn under clothing*

✳ **L0452** TLSO, flexible, provides trunk support, upper thoracic region, produces intracavitary pressure to reduce load on the intervertebral disks with rigid stays or panel(s), includes shoulder straps and closures, custom fabricated ⑧ Qp Qh ♿ A

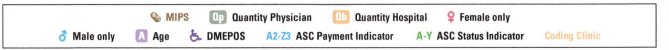

✎ MIPS   Qp Quantity Physician   Qh Quantity Hospital   ♀ Female only

♂ Male only   A Age   ♿ DMEPOS   A2-Z3 ASC Payment Indicator   A-Y ASC Status Indicator   Coding Clinic

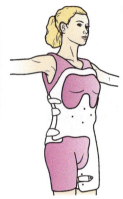

**Figure 20** Thoracic-lumbar-sacral-orthosis (TLSO).

✱ **L0454** TLSO flexible, provides trunk support, extends from sacrococcygeal junction to above T-9 vertebra, restricts gross trunk motion in the sagittal plane, produces intracavitary pressure to reduce load on the intervertebral disks with rigid stays or panel(s), includes shoulder straps and closures, prefabricated item that has been trimmed, bent, molded, assembled, or otherwise customized to fit a specific patient by an individual with expertise Ⓑ Qp Qh ⅄     A

*Used to immobilize specified areas of spine; and is generally designed to be worn under clothing; not specifically designed for patients in wheelchairs*

✱ **L0455** TLSO, flexible, provides trunk support, extends from sacrococcygeal junction to above T-9 vertebra, restricts gross trunk motion in the sagittal plane, produces intracavitary pressure to reduce load on the intervertebral disks with rigid stays or panel(s), includes shoulder straps and closures, prefabricated, off-the-shelf Ⓑ Qp Qh ⅄     A

✱ **L0456** TLSO, flexible, provides trunk support, thoracic region, rigid posterior panel and soft anterior apron, extends from the sacrococcygeal junction and terminates just inferior to the scapular spine, restricts gross trunk motion in the sagittal plane, produces intracavitary pressure to reduce load on the intervertebral disks, includes straps and closures, prefabricated item that has been trimmed, bent, molded, assembled, or otherwise customized to fit a specific patient by an individual with expertise Ⓑ Qp Qh ⅄     A

✱ **L0457** TLSO, flexible, provides trunk support, thoracic region, rigid posterior panel and soft anterior apron, extends from the sacrococcygeal junction and terminates just inferior to the scapular spine, restricts gross trunk motion in the sagittal plane, produces intracavitary pressure to reduce load on the intervertebral disks, includes straps and closures, prefabricated, off-the-shelf Ⓑ Qp Qh ⅄     A

✱ **L0458** TLSO, triplanar control, modular segmented spinal system, two rigid plastic shells, posterior extends from the sacrococcygeal junction and terminates just inferior to the scapular spine, anterior extends from the symphysis pubis to the xiphoid, soft liner, restricts gross trunk motion in the sagittal, coronal, and transverse planes, lateral strength is provided by overlapping plastic and stabilizing closures, includes straps and closures, prefabricated, includes fitting and adjustment Ⓑ Qp Qh ⅄     A

*To meet Medicare's definition of body jacket, orthosis has to have rigid plastic shell that circles trunk with overlapping edges and stabilizing closures, and entire circumference of shell must be made of same rigid material.*

\* **L0460** TLSO, triplanar control, modular segmented spinal system, two rigid plastic shells, posterior extends from the sacrococcygeal junction and terminates just inferior to the scapular spine, anterior extends from the symphysis pubis to the sternal notch, soft liner, restricts gross trunk motion in the sagittal, coronal, and transverse planes, lateral strength is provided by overlapping plastic and stabilizing closures, includes straps and closures, prefabricated item that has been trimmed, bent, molded, assembled, or otherwise customized to fit a specific patient by an individual with expertise Ⓑ Qp Qh ᴛ     A

\* **L0462** TLSO, triplanar control, modular segmented spinal system, three rigid plastic shells, posterior extends from the sacrococcygeal junction and terminates just inferior to the scapular spine, anterior extends from the symphysis pubis to the sternal notch, soft liner, restricts gross trunk motion in the sagittal, coronal, and transverse planes, lateral strength is provided by overlapping plastic and stabilizing closures, includes straps and closures, prefabricated, includes fitting and adjustment Ⓑ Qp Qh ᴛ     A

\* **L0464** TLSO, triplanar control, modular segmented spinal system, four rigid plastic shells, posterior extends from sacrococcygeal junction and terminates just inferior to scapular spine, anterior extends from symphysis pubis to the sternal notch, soft liner, restricts gross trunk motion in sagittal, coronal, and transverse planes, lateral strength is provided by overlapping plastic and stabilizing closures, includes straps and closures, prefabricated, includes fitting and adjustment Ⓑ Qp Qh ᴛ     A

\* **L0466** TLSO, sagittal control, rigid posterior frame and flexible soft anterior apron with straps, closures and padding, restricts gross trunk motion in sagittal plane, produces intracavitary pressure to reduce load on intervertebral disks, prefabricated item that has been trimmed, bent, molded, assembled, or otherwise customized to fit a specific patient by an individual with expertise Ⓑ Qp Qh ᴛ     A

\* **L0467** TLSO, sagittal control, rigid posterior frame and flexible soft anterior apron with straps, closures and padding, restricts gross trunk motion in sagittal plane, produces intracavitary pressure to reduce load on intervertebral disks, prefabricated, off-the-shelf Ⓑ Qp Qh ᴛ     A

\* **L0468** TLSO, sagittal-coronal control, rigid posterior frame and flexible soft anterior apron with straps, closures and padding, extends from sacrococcygeal junction over scapulae, lateral strength provided by pelvic, thoracic, and lateral frame pieces, restricts gross trunk motion in sagittal, and coronal planes, produces intracavitary pressure to reduce load on intervertebral disks, prefabricated item that has been trimmed, bent, molded, assembled, or otherwise customized to fit a specific patient by an individual with expertise Ⓑ Qp Qh ᴛ     A

\* **L0469** TLSO, sagittal-coronal control, rigid posterior frame and flexible soft anterior apron with straps, closures and padding, extends from sacrococcygeal junction over scapulae, lateral strength provided by pelvic, thoracic, and lateral frame pieces, restricts gross trunk motion in sagittal and coronal planes, produces intracavitary pressure to reduce load on intervertebral disks, prefabricated, off-the-shelf Ⓑ Qp Qh ᴛ     A

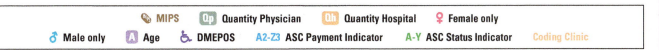

🐾 MIPS     Qp Quantity Physician     Qh Quantity Hospital     ♀ Female only
♂ Male only     Ⓐ Age     ᴛ DMEPOS     A2-Z3 ASC Payment Indicator     A-Y ASC Status Indicator     Coding Clinic

* **L0470** TLSO, triplanar control, rigid posterior frame and flexible soft anterior apron with straps, closures and padding, extends from sacrococcygeal junction to scapula, lateral strength provided by pelvic, thoracic, and lateral frame pieces, rotational strength provided by subclavicular extensions, restricts gross trunk motion in sagittal, coronal, and transverse planes, provides intracavitary pressure to reduce load on the intervertebral disks, includes fitting and shaping the frame, prefabricated, includes fitting and adjustment Ⓑ Qp Qh ♿   A

* **L0472** TLSO, triplanar control, hyperextension, rigid anterior and lateral frame extends from symphysis pubis to sternal notch with two anterior components (one pubic and one sternal), posterior and lateral pads with straps and closures, limits spinal flexion, restricts gross trunk motion in sagittal, coronal, and transverse planes, includes fitting and shaping the frame, prefabricated, includes fitting and adjustment Ⓑ Qp Qh ♿   A

* **L0480** TLSO, triplanar control, one piece rigid plastic shell without interface liner, with multiple straps and closures, posterior extends from sacrococcygeal junction and terminates just inferior to scapular spine, anterior extends from symphysis pubis to sternal notch, anterior or posterior opening, restricts gross trunk motion in sagittal, coronal, and transverse planes, includes a carved plaster or CAD-CAM model, custom fabricated Ⓑ Qp Qh ♿   A

* **L0482** TLSO, triplanar control, one piece rigid plastic shell with interface liner, multiple straps and closures, posterior extends from sacrococcygeal junction and terminates just inferior to scapular spine, anterior extends from symphysis pubis to sternal notch, anterior or posterior opening, restricts gross trunk motion in sagittal, coronal, and transverse planes, includes a carved plaster or CAD-CAM model, custom fabricated Ⓑ Qp Qh ♿   A

* **L0484** TLSO, triplanar control, two piece rigid plastic shell without interface liner, with multiple straps and closures, posterior extends from sacrococcygeal junction and terminates just inferior to scapular spine, anterior extends from symphysis pubis to sternal notch, lateral strength is enhanced by overlapping plastic, restricts gross trunk motion in the sagittal, coronal, and transverse planes, includes a carved plaster or CAD-CAM model, custom fabricated Ⓑ Qp Qh ♿   A

* **L0486** TLSO, triplanar control, two piece rigid plastic shell with interface liner, multiple straps and closures, posterior extends from sacrococcygeal junction and terminates just inferior to scapular spine, anterior extends from symphysis pubis to sternal notch, lateral strength is enhanced by overlapping plastic, restricts gross trunk motion in the sagittal, coronal, and transverse planes, includes a carved plaster or CAD-CAM model, custom fabricated Ⓑ Qp Qh ♿   A

* **L0488** TLSO, triplanar control, one piece rigid plastic shell with interface liner, multiple straps and closures, posterior extends from sacrococcygeal junction and terminates just inferior to scapular spine, anterior extends from symphysis pubis to sternal notch, anterior or posterior opening, restricts gross trunk motion in sagittal, coronal, and transverse planes, prefabricated, includes fitting and adjustment Ⓑ Qp Qh ♿   A

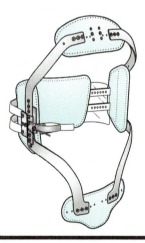

**Figure 21**  Thoracic-lumbar-sacral orthosis (TLSO) Jewett flexion control.

▶ **New**   ↻ **Revised**   ✔ **Reinstated**   ~~deleted~~ **Deleted**   ⊘ **Not covered or valid by Medicare**   ✺ **Special coverage instructions**   ✳ **Carrier discretion**   Ⓑ **Bill Part B MAC**   Ⓑ **Bill DME MAC**

**✳ L0490**   TLSO, sagittal-coronal control, one piece rigid plastic shell, with overlapping reinforced anterior, with multiple straps and closures, posterior extends from sacrococcygeal junction and terminates at or before the T-9 vertebra, anterior extends from symphysis pubis to xiphoid, anterior opening, restricts gross trunk motion in sagittal and coronal planes, prefabricated, includes fitting and adjustment Ⓑ Ⓠp Ⓠh ♿          A

**✳ L0491**   TLSO, sagittal-coronal control, modular segmented spinal system, two rigid plastic shells, posterior extends from the sacrococcygeal junction and terminates just inferior to the scapular spine, anterior extends from the symphysis pubis to the xiphoid, soft liner, restricts gross trunk motion in the sagittal and coronal planes, lateral strength is provided by overlapping plastic and stabilizing closures, includes straps and closures, prefabricated, includes fitting and adjustment Ⓑ Ⓠp Ⓠh ♿          A

**✳ L0492**   TLSO, sagittal-coronal control, modular segmented spinal system, three rigid plastic shells, posterior extends from the sacrococcygeal junction and terminates just inferior to the scapular spine, anterior extends from the symphysis pubis to the xiphoid, soft liner, restricts gross trunk motion in the sagittal and coronal planes, lateral strength is provided by overlapping plastic and stabilizing closures, includes straps and closures, prefabricated, includes fitting and adjustment Ⓑ Ⓠp Ⓠh ♿          A

## Sacroilliac Orthotics

**✳ L0621**   Sacroiliac orthosis, flexible, provides pelvic-sacral support, reduces motion about the sacroiliac joint, includes straps, closures, may include pendulous abdomen design, prefabricated, off-the-shelf Ⓑ Ⓠp Ⓠh ♿          A

**✳ L0622**   Sacroiliac orthosis, flexible, provides pelvic-sacral support, reduces motion about the sacroiliac joint, includes straps, closures, may include pendulous abdomen design, custom fabricated Ⓑ Ⓠp Ⓠh ♿          A

Type of custom-fabricated device for which impression of specific body part is made (e.g., by means of plaster cast, or CAD-CAM [computer-aided design] technology); impression then used to make specific patient model

**✳ L0623**   Sacroiliac orthosis, provides pelvic-sacral support, with rigid or semi-rigid panels over the sacrum and abdomen, reduces motion about the sacroiliac joint, includes straps, closures, may include pendulous abdomen design, prefabricated, off-the-shelf Ⓑ Ⓠp Ⓠh ♿          A

**✳ L0624**   Sacroiliac orthosis, provides pelvic-sacral support, with rigid or semi-rigid panels placed over the sacrum and abdomen, reduces motion about the sacroiliac joint, includes straps, closures, may include pendulous abdomen design, custom fabricated Ⓑ Ⓠp Ⓠh ♿          A

Custom fitted

## Lumbar Orthotics

**✳ L0625**   Lumbar orthosis, flexible, provides lumbar support, posterior extends from L-1 to below L-5 vertebra, produces intracavitary pressure to reduce load on the intervertebral discs, includes straps, closures, may include pendulous abdomen design, shoulder straps, stays, prefabricated, off-the-shelf Ⓑ Ⓠp Ⓠh ♿          A

**✳ L0626**   Lumbar orthosis, sagittal control, with rigid posterior panel(s), posterior extends from L-1 to below L-5 vertebra, produces intracavitary pressure to reduce load on the intervertebral discs, includes straps, closures, may include padding, stays, shoulder straps, pendulous abdomen design, prefabricated item that has been trimmed, bent, molded, assembled, or otherwise customized to fit a specific patient by an individual with expertise Ⓑ Ⓠp Ⓠh ♿          A

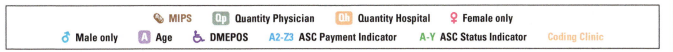

🪙 MIPS    Ⓠp Quantity Physician    Ⓠh Quantity Hospital    ♀ Female only

♂ Male only    Ⓐ Age    ♿ DMEPOS    A2-Z3 ASC Payment Indicator    A-Y ASC Status Indicator    Coding Clinic

✳ **L0627** Lumbar orthosis, sagittal control, with rigid anterior and posterior panels, posterior extends from L-1 to below L-5 vertebra, produces intracavitary pressure to reduce load on the intervertebral discs, includes straps, closures, may include padding, shoulder straps, pendulous abdomen design, prefabricated item that has been trimmed, bent, molded, assembled, or otherwise customized to fit a specific patient by an individual with expertise Ⓑ Qp Qh ♿ A

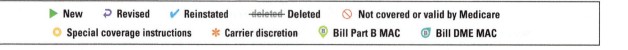

**Figure 22** Lumbar-sacral orthosis.

## Lumbar-Sacral Orthotics

✳ **L0628** Lumbar-sacral orthosis, flexible, provides lumbo-sacral support, posterior extends from sacrococcygeal junction to T-9 vertebra, produces intracavitary pressure to reduce load on the intervertebral discs, includes straps, closures, may include stays, shoulder straps, pendulous abdomen design, prefabricated, off-the-shelf Ⓑ Qp Qh ♿ A

✳ **L0629** Lumbar-sacral orthosis, flexible, provides lumbo-sacral support, posterior extends from sacrococcygeal junction to T-9 vertebra, produces intracavitary pressure to reduce load on the intervertebral discs, includes straps, closures, may include stays, shoulder straps, pendulous abdomen design, custom fabricated Ⓑ Qp Qh ♿ A

*Custom fitted*

✳ **L0630** Lumbar-sacral orthosis, sagittal control, with rigid posterior panel(s), posterior extends from sacrococcygeal junction to T-9 vertebra, produces intracavitary pressure to reduce load on the intervertebral discs, includes straps, closures, may include padding, stays, shoulder straps, pendulous abdomen design, prefabricated item that has been trimmed, bent, molded, assembled, or otherwise customized to fit a specific patient by an individual with expertise Ⓑ Qp Qh ♿ A

✳ **L0631** Lumbar-sacral orthosis, sagittal control, with rigid anterior and posterior panels, posterior extends from sacrococcygeal junction to T-9 vertebra, produces intracavitary pressure to reduce load on the intervertebral discs, includes straps, closures, may include padding, shoulder straps, pendulous abdomen design, prefabricated item that has been trimmed, bent, molded, assembled, or otherwise customized to fit a specific patient by an individual with expertise Ⓑ Qp Qh ♿ A

✳ **L0632** Lumbar-sacral orthosis, sagittal control, with rigid anterior and posterior panels, posterior extends from sacrococcygeal junction to T-9 vertebra, produces intracavitary pressure to reduce load on the intervertebral discs, includes straps, closures, may include padding, shoulder straps, pendulous abdomen design, custom fabricated Ⓑ Qp Qh ♿ A

*Custom fitted*

✳ **L0633** Lumbar-sacral orthosis, sagittal-coronal control, with rigid posterior frame/panel(s), posterior extends from sacrococcygeal junction to T-9 vertebra, lateral strength provided by rigid lateral frame/panels, produces intracavitary pressure to reduce load on intervertebral discs, includes straps, closures, may include padding, stays, shoulder straps, pendulous abdomen design, prefabricated item that has been trimmed, bent, molded, assembled, or otherwise customized to fit a specific patient by an individual with expertise Ⓑ Qp Qh ♿ A

---

▶ New   ↻ Revised   ✔ Reinstated   ~~deleted~~ Deleted   ⊘ Not covered or valid by Medicare
✺ Special coverage instructions   ✳ Carrier discretion   Ⓑ Bill Part B MAC   Ⓑ Bill DME MAC

✳ **L0634** Lumbar-sacral orthosis, sagittal-coronal control, with rigid posterior frame/panel(s), posterior extends from sacrococcygeal junction to T-9 vertebra, lateral strength provided by rigid lateral frame/panel(s), produces intracavitary pressure to reduce load on intervertebral discs, includes straps, closures, may include padding, stays, shoulder straps, pendulous abdomen design, custom fabricated Ⓑ Ⓠp Ⓠh ♿      A

Custom fitted

✳ **L0635** Lumbar-sacral orthosis, sagittal-coronal control, lumbar flexion, rigid posterior frame/panel(s), lateral articulating design to flex the lumbar spine, posterior extends from sacrococcygeal junction to T-9 vertebra, lateral strength provided by rigid lateral frame/panel(s), produces intracavitary pressure to reduce load on intervertebral discs, includes straps, closures, may include padding, anterior panel, pendulous abdomen design, prefabricated, includes fitting and adjustment Ⓑ Ⓠp Ⓠh ♿      A

✳ **L0636** Lumbar sacral orthosis, sagittal-coronal control, lumbar flexion, rigid posterior frame/panels, lateral articulating design to flex the lumbar spine, posterior extends from sacrococcygeal junction to T-9 vertebra, lateral strength provided by rigid lateral frame/panels, produces intracavitary pressure to reduce load on intervertebral discs, includes straps, closures, may include padding, anterior panel, pendulous abdomen design, custom fabricated Ⓑ Ⓠp Ⓠh ♿      A

Custom fitted

✳ **L0637** Lumbar-sacral orthosis, sagittal-coronal control, with rigid anterior and posterior frame/panels, posterior extends from sacrococcygeal junction to T-9 vertebra, lateral strength provided by rigid lateral frame/panels, produces intracavitary pressure to reduce load on intervertebral discs, includes straps, closures, may include padding, shoulder straps, pendulous abdomen design, prefabricated item that has been trimmed, bent, molded, assembled, or otherwise customized to fit a specific patient by an individual with expertise Ⓑ Ⓠp Ⓠh ♿      A

✳ **L0638** Lumbar-sacral orthosis, sagittal-coronal control, with rigid anterior and posterior frame/panels, posterior extends from sacrococcygeal junction to T-9 vertebra, lateral strength provided by rigid lateral frame/panels, produces intracavitary pressure to reduce load on intervertebral discs, includes straps, closures, may include padding, shoulder straps, pendulous abdomen design, custom fabricated Ⓑ Ⓠp Ⓠh ♿      A

✳ **L0639** Lumbar-sacral orthosis, sagittal-coronal control, rigid shell(s)/panel(s), posterior extends from sacrococcygeal junction to T-9 vertebra, anterior extends from symphysis pubis to xyphoid, produces intracavitary pressure to reduce load on the intervertebral discs, overall strength is provided by overlapping rigid material and stabilizing closures, includes straps, closures, may include soft interface, pendulous abdomen design, prefabricated item that has been trimmed, bent, molded, assembled, or otherwise customized to fit a specific patient by an individual with expertise Ⓑ Ⓠp Ⓠh ♿      A

Characterized by rigid plastic shell that encircles trunk with overlapping edges and stabilizing closures and provides high degree of immobility

✳ **L0640** Lumbar-sacral orthosis, sagittal-coronal control, rigid shell(s)/panel(s), posterior extends from sacrococcygeal junction to T-9 vertebra, anterior extends from symphysis pubis to xyphoid, produces intracavitary pressure to reduce load on the intervertebral discs, overall strength is provided by overlapping rigid material and stabilizing closures, includes straps, closures, may include soft interface, pendulous abdomen design, custom fabricated Ⓑ Ⓠp Ⓠh ♿      A

Custom fitted

## Lumbar Orthotics

✳ **L0641** Lumbar orthosis, sagittal control, with rigid posterior panel(s), posterior extends from L-1 to below L-5 vertebra, produces intracavitary pressure to reduce load on the intervertebral discs, includes straps, closures, may include padding, stays, shoulder straps, pendulous abdomen design, prefabricated, off-the-shelf Ⓑ Ⓠp Ⓠh ♿      A

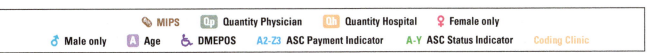

🏷 MIPS    Ⓠp **Quantity Physician**    Ⓠh **Quantity Hospital**    ♀ **Female only**

♂ **Male only**    Ⓐ **Age**    ♿ **DMEPOS**    A2-Z3 **ASC Payment Indicator**    A-Y **ASC Status Indicator**    Coding Clinic

✳ **L0642** Lumbar orthosis, sagittal control, with rigid anterior and posterior panels, posterior extends from L-1 to below L-5 vertebra, produces intracavitary pressure to reduce load on the intervertebral discs, includes straps, closures, may include padding, shoulder straps, pendulous abdomen design, prefabricated, off-the-shelf Ⓑ Qp Qh ⚬  A

## Lumbar-Sacral Orthotics

✳ **L0643** Lumbar-sacral orthosis, sagittal control, with rigid posterior panel(s), posterior extends from sacrococcygeal junction to T-9 vertebra, produces intracavitary pressure to reduce load on the intervertebral discs, includes straps, closures, may include padding, stays, shoulder straps, pendulous abdomen design, prefabricated, off-the-shelf Ⓑ Qp Qh ⚬  A

✳ **L0648** Lumbar-sacral orthosis, sagittal control, with rigid anterior and posterior panels, posterior extends from sacrococcygeal junction to T-9 vertebra, produces intracavitary pressure to reduce load on the intervertebral discs, includes straps, closures, may include padding, shoulder straps, pendulous abdomen design, prefabricated, off-the-shelf Ⓑ Qp Qh ⚬  A

✳ **L0649** Lumbar-sacral orthosis, sagittal-coronal control, with rigid posterior frame/panel(s), posterior extends from sacrococcygeal junction to T-9 vertebra, lateral strength provided by rigid lateral frame/panels, produces intracavitary pressure to reduce load on intervertebral discs, includes straps, closures, may include padding, stays, shoulder straps, pendulous abdomen design, prefabricated, off-the-shelf Ⓑ Qp Qh ⚬  A

✳ **L0650** Lumbar-sacral orthosis, sagittal-coronal control, with rigid anterior and posterior frame/panel(s), posterior extends from sacrococcygeal junction to T-9 vertebra, lateral strength provided by rigid lateral frame/panel(s), produces intracavitary pressure to reduce load on intervertebral discs, includes straps, closures, may include padding, shoulder straps, pendulous abdomen design, prefabricated, off-the-shelf Ⓑ Qp Qh ⚬  A

✳ **L0651** Lumbar-sacral orthosis, sagittal-coronal control, rigid shell(s)/panel(s), posterior extends from sacrococcygeal junction to T-9 vertebra, anterior extends from symphysis pubis to xyphoid, produces intracavitary pressure to reduce load on the intervertebral discs, overall strength is provided by overlapping rigid material and stabilizing closures, includes straps, closures, may include soft interface, pendulous abdomen design, prefabricated, off-the-shelf Ⓑ Qp Qh  A

## Cervical-Thoracic-Lumbar-Sacral

✳ **L0700** Cervical-thoracic-lumbar-sacral-orthoses (CTLSO), anterior-posterior-lateral control, molded to patient model (Minerva type) Ⓑ Qp Qh ⚬  A

✳ **L0710** CTLSO, anterior-posterior-lateral-control, molded to patient model, with interface material (Minerva type) Ⓑ Qp Qh ⚬  A

## HALO Procedure

✳ **L0810** HALO procedure, cervical halo incorporated into jacket vest Ⓑ Qp Qh ⚬  A

✳ **L0820** HALO procedure, cervical halo incorporated into plaster body jacket Ⓑ Qp Qh ⚬  A

✳ **L0830** HALO procedure, cervical halo incorporated into Milwaukee type orthosis Ⓑ Qp Qh  A

✳ **L0859** Addition to HALO procedure, magnetic resonance image compatible systems, rings and pins, any material Ⓑ Qp Qh ⚬  A

✳ **L0861** Addition to HALO procedure, replacement liner/interface material Ⓑ Qp Qh ⚬  A

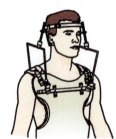

**Figure 23**  Halo device.

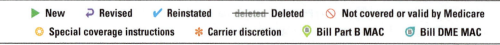

| ▶ New | ↻ Revised | ✔ Reinstated | ~~deleted~~ Deleted | ⦸ Not covered or valid by Medicare |
|---|---|---|---|---|
| ⊛ Special coverage instructions | ✳ Carrier discretion | Ⓑ Bill Part B MAC | Ⓑ Bill DME MAC | |

## Additions to Spinal Orthotics

**NOTE:** TLSO - Thoraci-lumbar-sacral orthoses/ Spinal orthoses may be prefabricated, prefitted, or custom fabricated. Conservative treatment for back pain may include the use of spinal orthoses.

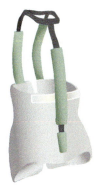

**Figure 24** Milwaukee CTLSO.

✳ **L0970**  TLSO, corset front Ⓑ Qp Qh ♿  A

✳ **L0972**  LSO, corset front Ⓑ Qp Qh ♿  A

✳ **L0974**  TLSO, full corset Ⓑ Qp Qh ♿  A

✳ **L0976**  LSO, full corset Ⓑ Qp Qh ♿  A

✳ **L0978**  Axillary crutch extension Ⓑ Qp Qh ♿  A

✳ **L0980**  Peroneal straps, prefabricated, off-the-shelf, pair Ⓑ Qp Qh ♿  A

✳ **L0982**  Stocking supporter grips, prefabricated, off-the-shelf, set of four (4) Ⓑ Qp Qh ♿  A

Convenience item

✳ **L0984**  Protective body sock, prefabricated, off-the-shelf, each Ⓑ Qp Qh ♿  A

Garment made of cloth or similar material that is worn under spinal orthosis and is not primarily medical in nature

✳ **L0999**  Addition to spinal orthosis, not otherwise specified Ⓑ  A

## Orthotic Devices: Scoliosis Procedures

**NOTE:** Orthotic care of scoliosis differs from other orthotic care in that the treatment is more dynamic in nature and uses ongoing continual modification of the orthosis to the patient's changing condition. This coding structure uses the proper names, or eponyms, of the procedures because they have historic and universal acceptance in the profession. It should be recognized that variations to the basic procedures described by the founders/ developers are accepted in various medical and orthotic practices throughout the country. All procedures include a model of patient when indicated.

✳ **L1000**  Cervical-thoracic-lumbar-sacral orthosis (CTLSO) (Milwaukee), inclusive of furnishing initial orthosis, including model Ⓑ Qp Qh ♿  A

✳ **L1001**  Cervical thoracic lumbar sacral orthosis, immobilizer, infant size, prefabricated, includes fitting and adjustment Ⓑ Qp Qh ♿  A

✳ **L1005**  Tension based scoliosis orthosis and accessory pads, includes fitting and adjustment Ⓑ Qp Qh ♿  A

✳ **L1010**  Addition to cervical-thoracic-lumbar-sacral orthosis (CTLSO) or scoliosis orthosis, axilla sling Ⓑ Qp Qh ♿  A

✳ **L1020**  Addition to CTLSO or scoliosis orthosis, kyphosis pad Ⓑ Qp Qh ♿  A

✳ **L1025**  Addition to CTLSO or scoliosis orthosis, kyphosis pad, floating Ⓑ Qp Qh ♿  A

✳ **L1030**  Addition to CTLSO or scoliosis orthosis, lumbar bolster pad Ⓑ Qp Qh ♿  A

✳ **L1040**  Addition to CTLSO or scoliosis orthosis, lumbar or lumbar rib pad Ⓑ Qp Qh ♿  A

✳ **L1050**  Addition to CTLSO or scoliosis orthosis, sternal pad Ⓑ Qp Qh ♿  A

✳ **L1060**  Addition to CTLSO or scoliosis orthosis, thoracic pad Ⓑ Qp Qh ♿  A

✳ **L1070**  Addition to CTLSO or scoliosis orthosis, trapezius sling Ⓑ Qp Qh ♿  A

✳ **L1080**  Addition to CTLSO or scoliosis orthosis, outrigger Ⓑ Qp Qh ♿  A

✳ **L1085**  Addition to CTLSO or scoliosis orthosis, outrigger, bilateral with vertical extensions Ⓑ Qp Qh ♿  A

✳ **L1090**  Addition to CTLSO or scoliosis orthosis, lumbar sling Ⓑ Qp Qh ♿  A

✳ **L1100**  Addition to CTLSO or scoliosis orthosis, ring flange, plastic or leather Ⓑ Qp Qh ♿  A

✳ **L1110**  Addition to CTLSO or scoliosis orthosis, ring flange, plastic or leather, molded to patient model Ⓑ Qp Qh ♿  A

✳ **L1120**  Addition to CTLSO, scoliosis orthosis, cover for upright, each Ⓑ Qp Qh ♿  A

---

| 🏷 MIPS | Qp Quantity Physician | Qh Quantity Hospital | ♀ Female only |
|---|---|---|---|
| ♂ Male only | Ⓐ Age | ♿ DMEPOS | A2-Z3 ASC Payment Indicator | A-Y ASC Status Indicator | Coding Clinic |

## Thoracic-Lumbar-Sacral (Low Profile)

✳ **L1200**  Thoracic-lumbar-sacral-orthosis (TLSO), inclusive of furnishing initial orthosis only Ⓑ Qp Qh ♿  A

✳ **L1210**  Addition to TLSO, (low profile), lateral thoracic extension Ⓑ Qp Qh ♿  A

✳ **L1220**  Addition to TLSO, (low profile), anterior thoracic extension Ⓑ Qp Qh ♿  A

✳ **L1230**  Addition to TLSO, (low profile), Milwaukee type superstructure Ⓑ Qp Qh ♿  A

✳ **L1240**  Addition to TLSO, (low profile), lumbar derotation pad Ⓑ Qp Qh ♿  A

✳ **L1250**  Addition to TLSO, (low profile), anterior ASIS pad Ⓑ Qp Qh ♿  A

✳ **L1260**  Addition to TLSO, (low profile), anterior thoracic derotation pad Ⓑ Qp Qh ♿  A

✳ **L1270**  Addition to TLSO, (low profile), abdominal pad Ⓑ Qp Qh ♿  A

✳ **L1280**  Addition to TLSO, (low profile), rib gusset (elastic), each Ⓑ Qp Qh ♿  A

✳ **L1290**  Addition to TLSO, (low profile), lateral trochanteric pad Ⓑ Qp Qh ♿  A

## Other Scoliosis Procedures

✳ **L1300**  Other scoliosis procedure, body jacket molded to patient model Ⓑ Qp Qh ♿  A

✳ **L1310**  Other scoliosis procedure, postoperative body jacket Ⓑ Qp Qh ♿  A

✳ **L1499**  Spinal orthosis, not otherwise specified Ⓑ Qp Qh  A

## Orthotic Devices: Lower Limb (L1600-L3649)

**NOTE:** the procedures in L1600-L2999 are considered as base or basic proceduresand may be modified by listing procedure from the Additions Sections and adding them to the base procedure.

### Hip: Flexible

✳ **L1600**  Hip orthosis, abduction control of hip joints, flexible, frejka type with cover, prefabricated item that has been trimmed, bent, molded, assembled, or otherwise customized to fit a specific patient by an individual with expertise Ⓑ Qp Qh ♿  A

✳ **L1610**  Hip orthosis, abduction control of hip joints, flexible, (frejka cover only), prefabricated item that has been trimmed, bent, molded, assembled, or otherwise customized to fit a specific patient by an individual with expertise Ⓑ Qp Qh ♿  A

✳ **L1620**  Hip orthosis, abduction control of hip joints, flexible, (Pavlik harness), prefabricated item that has been trimmed, bent, molded, assembled, or otherwise customized to fit a specific patient by an individual with expertise Ⓑ Qp Qh ♿  A

✳ **L1630**  Hip orthosis, abduction control of hip joints, semi-flexible (Von Rosen type), custom-fabricated Ⓑ Qp Qh ♿  A

✳ **L1640**  Hip orthosis, abduction control of hip joints, static, pelvic band or spreader bar, thigh cuffs, custom-fabricated Ⓑ Qp Qh ♿  A

✳ **L1650**  Hip orthosis, abduction control of hip joints, static, adjustable, (Ilfled type), prefabricated, includes fitting and adjustment Ⓑ Qp Qh ♿  A

✳ **L1652**  Hip orthosis, bilateral thigh cuffs with adjustable abductor spreader bar, adult size, prefabricated, includes fitting and adjustment, any type Ⓑ Qp Qh Ⓐ ♿  A

✳ **L1660**  Hip orthosis, abduction control of hip joints, static, plastic, prefabricated, includes fitting and adjustment Ⓑ Qp Qh ♿  A

✳ **L1680**  Hip orthosis, abduction control of hip joints, dynamic, pelvic control, adjustable hip motion control, thigh cuffs (Rancho hip action type), custom fabrication Ⓑ Qp Qh ♿  A

✳ **L1685**  Hip orthosis, abduction control of hip joint, postoperative hip abduction type, custom fabricated Ⓑ Qp Qh ♿  A

✳ **L1686**  Hip orthosis, abduction control of hip joint, postoperative hip abduction type, prefabricated, includes fitting and adjustment Ⓑ Qp Qh ♿  A

✳ **L1690**  Combination, bilateral, lumbo-sacral, hip, femur orthosis providing adduction and internal rotation control, prefabricated, includes fitting and adjustment Ⓑ Qp Qh  A

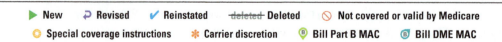

▶ New    ↩ Revised    ✔ Reinstated    ~~deleted~~ Deleted    ⊘ Not covered or valid by Medicare
⊙ Special coverage instructions    ✳ Carrier discretion    Ⓑ Bill Part B MAC    Ⓑ Bill DME MAC

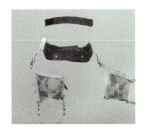

**Figure 25** Thoracic-hip-knee-ankle orthosis (THKAO).

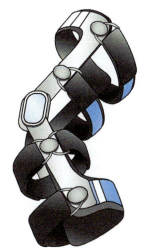

**Figure 27** Knee orthosis.

## Legg Perthes

* **L1700**   Legg-Perthes orthosis, (Toronto type), custom-fabricated Ⓑ Qp Qh ⓓ    A

* **L1710**   Legg-Perthes orthosis, (Newington type), custom-fabricated Ⓑ Qp Qh ⓓ    A

* **L1720**   Legg-Perthes orthosis, trilateral, (Tachdjian type), custom-fabricated Ⓑ Qp Qh ⓓ    A

* **L1730**   Legg-Perthes orthosis, (Scottish Rite type), custom-fabricated Ⓑ Qp Qh ⓓ A

* **L1755**   Legg-Perthes orthosis, (Patten bottom type), custom-fabricated Ⓑ Qp Qh ⓓ A

## Knee (KO)

* **L1810**   Knee orthosis, elastic with joints, prefabricated item that has been trimmed, bent, molded, assembled, or otherwise customized to fit a specific patient by an individual with expertise Ⓑ Qp Qh ⓓ    A

* **L1812**   Knee orthosis, elastic with joints, prefabricated, off-the-shelf Ⓑ Qp Qh ⓓ    A

* **L1820**   Knee orthosis, elastic with condylar pads and joints, with or without patellar control, prefabricated, includes fitting and adjustment Ⓑ Qp Qh ⓓ    A

* **L1830**   Knee orthosis, immobilizer, canvas longitudinal, prefabricated, off-the-shelf Ⓑ Qp Qh ⓓ    A

* **L1831**   Knee orthosis, locking knee joint(s), positional orthosis, prefabricated, includes fitting and adjustment Ⓑ Qp Qh ⓓ    A

* **L1832**   Knee orthosis, adjustable knee joints (unicentric or polycentric), positional orthosis, rigid support, prefabricated item that has been trimmed, bent, molded, assembled, or otherwise customized to fit a specific patient by an individual with expertise Ⓑ Qp Qh ⓓ    A

* **L1833**   Knee orthosis, adjustable knee joints (unicentric or polycentric), positional orthosis, rigid support, prefabricated, off-the-shelf Ⓑ Qp Qh ⓓ    A

* **L1834**   Knee orthosis, without knee joint, rigid, custom-fabricated Ⓑ Qp Qh ⓓ    A

* **L1836**   Knee orthosis, rigid, without joint(s), includes soft interface material, prefabricated, off-the-shelf Ⓑ Qp Qh ⓓ    A

* **L1840**   Knee orthosis, derotation, medial-lateral, anterior cruciate ligament, custom fabricated Ⓑ Qp Qh ⓓ    A

* **L1843**   Knee orthosis, single upright, thigh and calf, with adjustable flexion and extension joint (unicentric or polycentric), medial-lateral and rotation control, with or without varus/valgus adjustment, prefabricated item that has been trimmed, bent, molded, assembled, or otherwise customized to fit a specific patient by an individual with expertise Ⓑ Qp Qh ⓓ    A

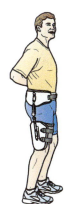

**Figure 26** Hip orthosis.

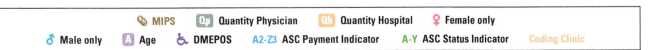

🏷 MIPS    Qp Quantity Physician    Qh Quantity Hospital    ♀ Female only    ♂ Male only    Ⓐ Age    ⓓ DMEPOS    A2-Z3 ASC Payment Indicator    A-Y ASC Status Indicator    Coding Clinic

* **L1844** Knee orthosis, single upright, thigh and calf, with adjustable flexion and extension joint (unicentric or polycentric), medial-lateral and rotation control, with or without varus/ valgus adjustment, custom fabricated Ⓑ Qp Qh ♿ A

* **L1845** Knee orthosis, double upright, thigh and calf, with adjustable flexion and extension joint (unicentric or polycentric), medial-lateral and rotation control, with or without varus/valgus adjustment, prefabricated item that has been trimmed, bent, molded, assembled, or otherwise customized to fit a specific patient by an individual with expertise Ⓑ Qp Qh ♿ A

* **L1846** Knee orthrosis, double upright, thigh and calf, with adjustable flexion and extension joint (unicentric or polycentric), medial-lateral and rotation control, with or without varus/ valgus adjustment, custom fabricated Ⓑ Qp Qh ♿ A

* **L1847** Knee orthosis, double upright with adjustable joint, with inflatable air support chamber(s), prefabricated item that has been trimmed, bent, molded, assembled, or otherwise customized to fit a specific patient by an individual with expertise Ⓑ Qp Qh ♿ A

* **L1848** Knee orthosis, double upright with adjustable joint, with inflatable air support chamber(s), prefabricated, off-the-shelf Ⓑ Qp Qh ♿ A

* **L1850** Knee orthosis, Swedish type, prefabricated, off-the-shelf Ⓑ Qp Qh ♿ A

* **L1851** Knee orthosis (KO), single upright, thigh and calf, with adjustable flexion and extension joint (unicentric or polycentric), medial-lateral and rotation control, with or without varus/valgus adjustment, prefabricated, off-the-shelf Qp Qh ♿ A

* **L1852** Knee orthosis (KO), double upright, thigh and calf, with adjustable flexion and extension joint (unicentric or polycentric), medial-lateral and rotation control, with or without varus/valgus adjustment, prefabricated, off-the-shelf Qp Qh ♿ A

* **L1860** Knee orthosis, modification of supracondylar prosthetic socket, custom fabricated (SK) Ⓑ Qp Qh ♿ A

## Ankle-Foot (AFO)

* **L1900** Ankle foot orthosis (AFO), spring wire, dorsiflexion assist calf band, custom-fabricated Ⓑ Qp Qh ♿ A

* **L1902** Ankle orthosis, ankle gauntlet or similiar, with or without joints, prefabricated, off-the-shelf Ⓑ Qp Qh ♿ A

* **L1904** Ankle orthosis, ankle gauntlet or similiar, with or without joints, custom fabricated Ⓑ Qp Qh ♿ A

* **L1906** Ankle foot orthosis, multiligamentus ankle support, prefabricated, off-the-shelf Ⓑ Qp Qh ♿ A

* **L1907** Ankle orthosis, supramalleolar with straps, with or without interface/pads, custom fabricated Ⓑ Qp Qh ♿ A

* **L1910** Ankle foot orthosis, posterior, single bar, clasp attachment to shoe counter, prefabricated, includes fitting and adjustment Ⓑ Qp Qh ♿ A

* **L1920** Ankle foot orthosis, single upright with static or adjustable stop (Phelps or Perlstein type), custom fabricated Ⓑ Qp Qh ♿ A

* **L1930** Ankle-foot orthosis, plastic or other material, prefabricated, includes fitting and adjustment Ⓑ Qp Qh ♿ A

* **L1932** AFO, rigid anterior tibial section, total carbon fiber or equal material, prefabricated, includes fitting and adjustment Ⓑ Qp Qh ♿ A

* **L1940** Ankle foot orthosis, plastic or other material, custom fabricated Ⓑ Qp Qh ♿ A

* **L1945** Ankle foot orthosis, plastic, rigid anterior tibial section (floor reaction), custom fabricated Ⓑ Qp Qh ♿ A

* **L1950** Ankle foot orthosis, spiral, (Institute of Rehabilitation Medicine type), plastic, custom fabricated Ⓑ Qp Qh ♿ A

* **L1951** Ankle foot orthosis, spiral, (Institute of Rehabilitative Medicine type), plastic or other material, prefabricated, includes fitting and adjustment Ⓑ Qp Qh ♿ A

* **L1960** Ankle foot orthosis, posterior solid ankle, plastic, custom fabricated Ⓑ Qp Qh ♿ A

* **L1970** Ankle foot orthosis, plastic, with ankle joint, custom fabricated Ⓑ Qp Qh ♿ A

* **L1971** Ankle foot orthosis, plastic or other material with ankle joint, prefabricated, includes fitting and adjustment Ⓑ Qp Qh ♿ A

---

▶ New  ↻ Revised  ✔ Reinstated  ~~deleted~~ Deleted  ⊘ Not covered or valid by Medicare

⊙ Special coverage instructions  * Carrier discretion  Ⓑ Bill Part B MAC  Ⓑ Bill DME MAC

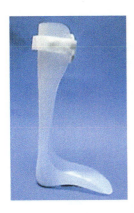

**Figure 28** Ankle-foot orthosis (AFO).

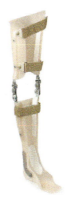

**Figure 29** Knee-ankle-foot orthosis (KAFO).

\* **L1980** Ankle foot orthosis, single upright free plantar dorsiflexion, solid stirrup, calf band/cuff (single bar 'BK' orthosis), custom fabricated Ⓑ Ⓠp Ⓠh 🚹    A

\* **L1990** Ankle foot orthosis, double upright free plantar dorsiflexion, solid stirrup, calf band/cuff (double bar 'BK' orthosis), custom fabricated Ⓑ Ⓠp Ⓠh 🚹    A

## Hip-Knee-Ankle-Foot (or Any Combination)

NOTE: L2000, L2020, and L2036 are base procedures to be used with any knee joint. L2010 and L2030 are to be used only with no knee joint.

\* **L2000** Knee ankle foot orthosis, single upright, free knee, free ankle, solid stirrup, thigh and calf bands/cuffs (single bar 'AK' orthosis), custom-fabricated Ⓑ Ⓠp Ⓠh 🚹    A

\* **L2005** Knee ankle foot orthosis, any material, single or double upright, stance control, automatic lock and swing phase release, any type activation; includes ankle joint, any type, custom fabricated Ⓑ Ⓠp Ⓠh 🚹    A

▶ \* **L2006** Knee ankle foot device, any material, single or double upright, swing and/or stance phase microprocessor control with adjustability, includes all components (e.g., sensors, batteries, charger), any type activation, with or without ankle joint(s), custom fabricated    A

\* **L2010** Knee ankle foot orthosis, single upright, free ankle, solid stirrup, thigh and calf bands/cuffs (single bar 'AK' orthosis), without knee joint, custom-fabricated Ⓑ Ⓠp Ⓠh 🚹    A

\* **L2020** Knee ankle foot orthosis, double upright, free knee, free ankle, solid stirrup, thigh and calf bands/cuffs (double bar 'AK' orthosis), custom fabricated Ⓑ Ⓠp Ⓠh 🚹    A

\* **L2030** Knee ankle foot orthosis, double upright, free ankle, solid stirrup, thigh and calf bands/cuffs (double bar 'AK' orthosis), without knee joint, custom fabricated Ⓑ Ⓠp Ⓠh 🚹    A

\* **L2034** Knee ankle foot orthosis, full plastic, single upright, with or without free motion knee, medial lateral rotation control, with or without free motion ankle, custom fabricated Ⓑ Ⓠp Ⓠh 🚹    A

\* **L2035** Knee ankle foot orthosis, full plastic, static (pediatric size), without free motion ankle, prefabricated, includes fitting and adjustment Ⓑ Ⓠp Ⓠh Ⓐ 🚹    A

\* **L2036** Knee ankle foot orthosis, full plastic, double upright, with or without free motion knee, with or without free motion ankle, custom fabricated Ⓑ Ⓠp Ⓠh 🚹    A

\* **L2037** Knee ankle foot orthosis, full plastic, single upright, with or without free motion knee, with or without free motion ankle, custom fabricated Ⓑ Ⓠp Ⓠh 🚹    A

\* **L2038** Knee ankle foot orthosis, full plastic, with or without free motion knee, multi-axis ankle, custom fabricated Ⓑ Ⓠp Ⓠh 🚹    A

## Torsion Control: Hip-Knee-Ankle-Foot (TLSO)

\* **L2040** Hip knee ankle foot orthosis, torsion control, bilateral rotation straps, pelvic band/belt, custom fabricated Ⓑ Ⓠp Ⓠh 🚹    A

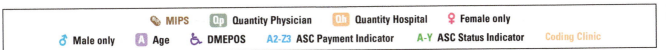

🖐 **MIPS**    Ⓠp **Quantity Physician**    Ⓠh **Quantity Hospital**    ♀ **Female only**

♂ **Male only**    Ⓐ **Age**    🚹 **DMEPOS**    **A2-Z3** **ASC Payment Indicator**    **A-Y** **ASC Status Indicator**    *Coding Clinic*

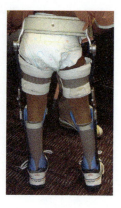

**Figure 30** Hip-knee-ankle-foot orthosis (HKAFO).

\* **L2050** Hip knee ankle foot orthosis, torsion control, bilateral torsion cables, hip joint, pelvic band/belt, custom fabricated Ⓑ Qp Qh ⚕ A

\* **L2060** Hip knee ankle foot orthosis, torsion control, bilateral torsion cables, ball bearing hip joint, pelvic band/belt, custom fabricated Ⓑ Qp Qh ⚕ A

\* **L2070** Hip knee ankle foot orthosis, torsion control, unilateral rotation straps, pelvic band/belt, custom fabricated Ⓑ Qp Qh A

\* **L2080** Hip knee ankle foot orthosis, torsion control, unilateral torsion cable, hip joint, pelvic band/belt, custom fabricated Ⓑ Qp Qh A

\* **L2090** Hip knee ankle foot orthosis, torsion control, unilateral torsion cable, ball bearing hip joint, pelvic band/belt, custom fabricated Ⓑ Qp Qh A

## Fracture Orthotics: Ankle-Foot and Knee-Ankle-Foot

\* **L2106** Ankle foot orthosis, fracture orthosis, tibial fracture cast orthosis, thermoplastic type casting material, custom fabricated Ⓑ Qp Qh ⚕ A

\* **L2108** Ankle foot orthosis, fracture orthosis, tibial fracture cast orthosis, custom fabricated Ⓑ Qp Qh ⚕ A

\* **L2112** Ankle foot orthosis, fracture orthosis, tibial fracture orthosis, soft, prefabricated, includes fitting and adjustment Ⓑ Qp Qh A

\* **L2114** Ankle foot orthosis, fracture orthosis, tibial fracture orthosis, semi-rigid, prefabricated, includes fitting and adjustment Ⓑ Qp Qh ⚕ A

\* **L2116** Ankle foot orthosis, fracture orthosis, tibial fracture orthosis, rigid, prefabricated, includes fitting and adjustment Ⓑ Qp Qh ⚕ A

\* **L2126** Knee ankle foot orthosis, fracture orthosis, femoral fracture cast orthosis, thermoplastic type casting material, custom fabricated Ⓑ Qp Qh ⚕ A

\* **L2128** Knee ankle foot orthosis, fracture orthosis, femoral fracture cast orthosis, custom fabricated Ⓑ Qp Qh ⚕ A

\* **L2132** KAFO, femoral fracture cast orthosis, soft, prefabricated, includes fitting and adjustment Ⓑ Qp Qh ⚕ A

\* **L2134** KAFO, femoral fracture cast orthosis, semi-rigid, prefabricated, includes fitting and adjustment Ⓑ Qp Qh ⚕ A

\* **L2136** KAFO, fracture orthosis, femoral fracture cast orthosis, rigid, prefabricated, includes fitting and adjustment Ⓑ Qp Qh A

## Additions to Fracture Orthotics

\* **L2180** Addition to lower extremity fracture orthosis, plastic shoe insert with ankle joints Ⓑ Qp Qh ⚕ A

\* **L2182** Addition to lower extremity fracture orthosis, drop lock knee joint Ⓑ Qp Qh A

\* **L2184** Addition to lower extremity fracture orthosis, limited motion knee joint Ⓑ Qp Qh A

\* **L2186** Addition to lower extremity fracture orthosis, adjustable motion knee joint, Lerman type Ⓑ Qp Qh A

\* **L2188** Addition to lower extremity fracture orthosis, quadrilateral brim Ⓑ Qp Qh A

\* **L2190** Addition to lower extremity fracture orthosis, waist belt Ⓑ Qp Qh A

\* **L2192** Addition to lower extremity fracture orthosis, hip joint, pelvic band, thigh flange, and pelvic belt Ⓑ Qp Qh ⚕ A

## Additions to Lower Extremity Orthotics

\* **L2200** Addition to lower extremity, limited ankle motion, each joint Ⓑ Qp Qh ⚕ A

\* **L2210** Addition to lower extremity, dorsiflexion assist (plantar flexion resist), each joint Ⓑ Qp Qh ⚕ A

\* **L2220** Addition to lower extremity, dorsiflexion and plantar flexion assist/resist, each joint Ⓑ Qp Qh ⚕ A

\* **L2230** Addition to lower extremity, split flat caliper stirrups and plate attachment Ⓑ Qp Qh ⚕ A

▶ New  ↻ Revised  ✔ Reinstated  ~~deleted~~ Deleted  ⊘ Not covered or valid by Medicare

⊙ Special coverage instructions  \* Carrier discretion  Ⓑ Bill Part B MAC  Ⓑ Bill DME MAC

* **L2232** Addition to lower extremity orthosis, rocker bottom for total contact ankle foot orthosis, for custom fabricated orthosis only Ⓑ Qp Qh ♿   A

* **L2240** Addition to lower extremity, round caliper and plate attachment Ⓑ Qp Qh ♿   A

* **L2250** Addition to lower extremity, foot plate, molded to patient model, stirrup attachment Ⓑ Qp Qh ♿   A

* **L2260** Addition to lower extremity, reinforced solid stirrup (Scott-Craig type) Ⓑ Qp Qh ♿   A

* **L2265** Addition to lower extremity, long tongue stirrup Ⓑ Qp Qh ♿   A

* **L2270** Addition to lower extremity, varus/valgus correction ('T') strap, padded/lined or malleolus pad Ⓑ Qp Qh ♿   A

* **L2275** Addition to lower extremity, varus/valgus correction, plastic modification, padded/lined Ⓑ Qp Qh ♿   A

* **L2280** Addition to lower extremity, molded inner boot Ⓑ Qp Qh ♿   A

* **L2300** Addition to lower extremity, abduction bar (bilateral hip involvement), jointed, adjustable Ⓑ Qp Qh ♿   A

* **L2310** Addition to lower extremity, abduction bar-straight Ⓑ Qp Qh ♿   A

* **L2320** Addition to lower extremity, non-molded lacer, for custom fabricated orthosis only Ⓑ Qp Qh ♿   A

* **L2330** Addition to lower extremity, lacer molded to patient model, for custom fabricated orthosis only Ⓑ Qp Qh ♿   A

  Used whether closure is lacer or Velcro

* **L2335** Addition to lower extremity, anterior swing band Ⓑ Qp Qh ♿   A

* **L2340** Addition to lower extremity, pre-tibial shell, molded to patient model Ⓑ Qp Qh ♿   A

* **L2350** Addition to lower extremity, prosthetic type, (BK) socket, molded to patient model, (used for 'PTB' and 'AFO' orthoses) Ⓑ Qp Qh ♿   A

* **L2360** Addition to lower extremity, extended steel shank Ⓑ Qp Qh ♿   A

* **L2370** Addition to lower extremity, Patten bottom Ⓑ Qp Qh ♿   A

* **L2375** Addition to lower extremity, torsion control, ankle joint and half solid stirrup Ⓑ Qp Qh ♿   A

* **L2380** Addition to lower extremity, torsion control, straight knee joint, each joint Ⓑ Qp Qh ♿   A

* **L2385** Addition to lower extremity, straight knee joint, heavy duty, each joint Ⓑ Qp ♿   A

* **L2387** Addition to lower extremity, polycentric knee joint, for custom fabricated knee ankle foot orthosis, each joint Ⓑ Qp ♿   A

* **L2390** Addition to lower extremity, offset knee joint, each joint Ⓑ Qp ♿   A

* **L2395** Addition to lower extremity, offset knee joint, heavy duty, each joint Ⓑ Qp ♿   A

* **L2397** Addition to lower extremity orthosis, suspension sleeve Ⓑ Qp ♿   A

## Additions to Straight Knee or Offset Knee Joints

* **L2405** Addition to knee joint, drop lock, each Ⓑ Qp ♿   A

* **L2415** Addition to knee lock with integrated release mechanism (bail, cable, or equal), any material, each joint Ⓑ Qp ♿   A

* **L2425** Addition to knee joint, disc or dial lock for adjustable knee flexion, each joint Ⓑ Qp ♿   A

* **L2430** Addition to knee joint, ratchet lock for active and progressive knee extension, each joint Ⓑ Qp ♿   A

* **L2492** Addition to knee joint, lift loop for drop lock ring Ⓑ Qp ♿   A

## Additions to Thigh/Weight Bearing Gluteal/Ischial Weight Bearing

* **L2500** Addition to lower extremity, thigh/weight bearing, gluteal/ischial weight bearing, ring Ⓑ Qp Qh ♿   A

* **L2510** Addition to lower extremity, thigh/weight bearing, quadri-lateral brim, molded to patient model Ⓑ Qp Qh ♿   A

* **L2520** Addition to lower extremity, thigh/weight bearing, quadri-lateral brim, custom fitted Ⓑ Qp Qh ♿   A

* **L2525** Addition to lower extremity, thigh/weight bearing, ischial containment/narrow M-L brim molded to patient model Ⓑ Qp Qh ♿   A

* **L2526** Addition to lower extremity, thigh/weight bearing, ischial containment/narrow M-L brim, custom fitted Ⓑ Qp Qh ♿   A

* **L2530** Addition to lower extremity, thigh-weight bearing, lacer, non-molded Ⓑ Qp Qh ♿   A

---

🖐 MIPS    Qp Quantity Physician    Qh Quantity Hospital    ♀ Female only    ♂ Male only    Ⓐ Age    ♿ DMEPOS    A2-Z3 ASC Payment Indicator    A-Y ASC Status Indicator    Coding Clinic

\* **L2540** Addition to lower extremity, thigh/ weight bearing, lacer, molded to patient model Ⓑ Qp Qh ♿     A

\* **L2550** Addition to lower extremity, thigh/ weight bearing, high roll cuff Ⓑ Qp Qh ♿     A

## Additions to Pelvic and Thoracic Control

\* **L2570** Addition to lower extremity, pelvic control, hip joint, Clevis type two position joint, each Ⓑ Qp Qh ♿     A

\* **L2580** Addition to lower extremity, pelvic control, pelvic sling Ⓑ Qp Qh ♿     A

\* **L2600** Addition to lower extremity, pelvic control, hip joint, Clevis type, or thrust bearing, free, each Ⓑ Qp Qh ♿     A

\* **L2610** Addition to lower extremity, pelvic control, hip joint, Clevis or thrust bearing, lock, each Ⓑ Qp Qh ♿     A

\* **L2620** Addition to lower extremity, pelvic control, hip joint, heavy duty, each Ⓑ Qp Qh ♿     A

\* **L2622** Addition to lower extremity, pelvic control, hip joint, adjustable flexion, each Ⓑ Qp Qh ♿     A

\* **L2624** Addition to lower extremity, pelvic control, hip joint, adjustable flexion, extension, abduction control, each Ⓑ Qp Qh ♿     A

\* **L2627** Addition to lower extremity, pelvic control, plastic, molded to patient model, reciprocating hip joint and cables Ⓑ Qp Qh ♿     A

\* **L2628** Addition to lower extremity, pelvic control, metal frame, reciprocating hip joint and cables Ⓑ Qp Qh ♿     A

\* **L2630** Addition to lower extremity, pelvic control, band and belt, unilateral Ⓑ Qp Qh ♿     A

\* **L2640** Addition to lower extremity, pelvic control, band and belt, bilateral Ⓑ Qp Qh ♿     A

\* **L2650** Addition to lower extremity, pelvic and thoracic control, gluteal pad, each Ⓑ Qp Qh ♿     A

\* **L2660** Addition to lower extremity, thoracic control, thoracic band Ⓑ Qp Qh ♿     A

\* **L2670** Addition to lower extremity, thoracic control, paraspinal uprights Ⓑ Qp Qh ♿     A

\* **L2680** Addition to lower extremity, thoracic control, lateral support uprights Ⓑ Qp Qh ♿     A

## General Additions

\* **L2750** Addition to lower extremity orthosis, plating chrome or nickel, per bar Ⓑ Qp ♿     A

\* **L2755** Addition to lower extremity orthosis, high strength, lightweight material, all hybrid lamination/prepreg composite, per segment, for custom fabricated orthosis only Ⓑ Qp ♿     A

\* **L2760** Addition to lower extremity orthosis, extension, per extension, per bar (for lineal adjustment for growth) Ⓑ Qp ♿     A

\* **L2768** Orthotic side bar disconnect device, per bar Ⓑ Qp ♿     A

\* **L2780** Addition to lower extremity orthosis, non-corrosive finish, per bar Ⓑ Qp ♿ A

\* **L2785** Addition to lower extremity orthosis, drop lock retainer, each Ⓑ Qp ♿     A

\* **L2795** Addition to lower extremity orthosis, knee control, full kneecap Ⓑ Qp Qh ♿     A

\* **L2800** Addition to lower extremity orthosis, knee control, knee cap, medial or lateral pull, for use with custom fabricated orthosis only Ⓑ Qp Qh ♿     A

\* **L2810** Addition to lower extremity orthosis, knee control, condylar pad Ⓑ Qp ♿ A

\* **L2820** Addition to lower extremity orthosis, soft interface for molded plastic, below knee section Ⓑ Qp Qh ♿     A

Only report if soft interface provided, either leather or other material

\* **L2830** Addition to lower extremity orthosis, soft interface for molded plastic, above knee section Ⓑ Qp Qh ♿     A

\* **L2840** Addition to lower extremity orthosis, tibial length sock, fracture or equal, each Ⓑ Qp ♿     A

\* **L2850** Addition to lower extremity orthosis, femoral length sock, fracture or equal, each Ⓑ Qp ♿     A

⊘ **L2861** Addition to lower extremity joint, knee or ankle, concentric adjustable torsion style mechanism for custom fabricated orthotics only, each Ⓑ Qp Qh     E1

\* **L2999** Lower extremity orthoses, not otherwise specified Ⓑ     A

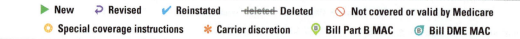

▶ New    ↻ Revised    ✔ Reinstated    ~~deleted~~ Deleted    ⊘ Not covered or valid by Medicare

🟡 Special coverage instructions    \* Carrier discretion    Ⓑ Bill Part B MAC    Ⓑ Bill DME MAC

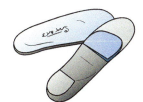

**Figure 31** Foot inserts.

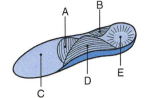

**Figure 32** Arch support.

## Foot (Orthopedic Shoes) (L3000-L3649)

### Inserts

✿ **L3000** Foot, insert, removable, molded to patient model, 'UCB' type, Berkeley shell, each Ⓑ Qp Qh   A

  If both feet casted and supplied with an orthosis, bill L3000-LT and L3000-RT

  *IOM: 100-02, 15, 290*

✿ **L3001** Foot, insert, removable, molded to patient model, Spenco, each Ⓑ Qp Qh   A

  *IOM: 100-02, 15, 290*

✿ **L3002** Foot, insert, removable, molded to patient model, Plastazote or equal, each Ⓑ Qp Qh   A

  *IOM: 100-02, 15, 290*

✿ **L3003** Foot, insert, removable, molded to patient model, silicone gel, each Ⓑ Qp Qh   A

  *IOM: 100-02, 15, 290*

✿ **L3010** Foot, insert, removable, molded to patient model, longitudinal arch support, each Ⓑ Qp Qh   A

  *IOM: 100-02, 15, 290*

✿ **L3020** Foot, insert, removable, molded to patient model, longitudinal/metatarsal support, each Ⓑ Qp Qh   A

  *IOM: 100-02, 15, 290*

✿ **L3030** Foot, insert, removable, formed to patient foot, each Ⓑ Qp Qh   A

  *IOM: 100-02, 15, 290*

∗ **L3031** Foot, insert/plate, removable, addition to lower extremity orthosis, high strength, lightweight material, all hybrid lamination/prepreg composite, each Ⓑ Qp Qh   A

### Arch Support, Removable, Premolded

✿ **L3040** Foot, arch support, removable, premolded, longitudinal, each Ⓑ Qp Qh   A

  *IOM: 100-02, 15, 290*

✿ **L3050** Foot, arch support, removable, premolded, metatarsal, each Ⓑ Qp Qh   A

  *IOM: 100-02, 15, 290*

✿ **L3060** Foot, arch support, removable, premolded, longitudinal/metatarsal, each Ⓑ Qp Qh   A

  *IOM: 100-02, 15, 290*

### Arch Support, Non-removable, Attached to Shoe

✿ **L3070** Foot, arch support, non-removable attached to shoe, longitudinal, each Ⓑ Qp Qh   A

  *IOM: 100-02, 15, 290*

✿ **L3080** Foot, arch support, non-removable attached to shoe, metatarsal, each Ⓑ Qp Qh   A

  *IOM: 100-02, 15, 290*

✿ **L3090** Foot, arch support, non-removable attached to shoe, longitudinal/metatarsal, each Ⓑ Qp Qh   A

  *IOM: 100-02, 15, 290*

✿ **L3100** Hallus-valgus night dynamic splint, prefabricated, off-the-shelf Ⓑ Qp Qh   A

  *IOM: 100-02, 15, 290*

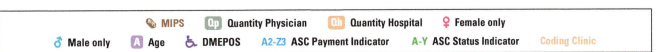

**Figure 33** Hallux valgus splint.

🖐 MIPS   Qp Quantity Physician   Qh Quantity Hospital   ♀ Female only

♂ Male only   Ⓐ Age   & DMEPOS   A2-Z3 ASC Payment Indicator   A-Y ASC Status Indicator   Coding Clinic

## Abduction and Rotation Bars

⚙ **L3140** Foot, abduction rotation bar, including shoes Ⓑ Qp Qh ♿     A

*IOM: 100-02, 15, 290*

⚙ **L3150** Foot, abduction rotation bar, without shoes Ⓑ Qp Qh ♿     A

*IOM: 100-02, 15, 290*

✱ **L3160** Foot, adjustable shoe-styled positioning device Ⓑ Qp Qh     A

⚙ **L3170** Foot, plastic, silicone or equal, heel stabilizer, prefabricated, off-the-shelf, each Ⓑ Qp Qh ♿     A

*IOM: 100-02, 15, 290*

## Orthopedic Footwear

⚙ **L3201** Orthopedic shoe, oxford with supinator or pronator, infant Ⓑ Ⓐ     A

*IOM: 100-02, 15, 290*

⚙ **L3202** Orthopedic shoe, oxford with supinator or pronator, child Ⓑ Ⓐ     A

*IOM: 100-02, 15, 290*

⚙ **L3203** Orthopedic shoe, oxford with supinator or pronator, junior Ⓑ Ⓐ     A

*IOM: 100-02, 15, 290*

⚙ **L3204** Orthopedic shoe, hightop with supinator or pronator, infant Ⓑ Ⓐ     A

*IOM: 100-02, 15, 290*

⚙ **L3206** Orthopedic shoe, hightop with supinator or pronator, child Ⓑ Ⓐ     A

*IOM: 100-02, 15, 290*

⚙ **L3207** Orthopedic shoe, hightop with supinator or pronator, junior Ⓑ Ⓐ     A

*IOM: 100-02, 15, 290*

⚙ **L3208** Surgical boot, infant, each Ⓑ Ⓐ     A

*IOM: 100-02, 15, 100*

⚙ **L3209** Surgical boot, each, child Ⓑ Ⓐ     A

*IOM: 100-02, 15, 100*

⚙ **L3211** Surgical boot, each, junior Ⓑ Ⓐ     A

*IOM: 100-02, 15, 100*

⚙ **L3212** Benesch boot, pair, infant Ⓑ Ⓐ     A

*IOM: 100-02, 15, 100*

⚙ **L3213** Benesch boot, pair, child Ⓑ Ⓐ     A

*IOM: 100-02, 15, 100*

⚙ **L3214** Benesch boot, pair, junior Ⓑ Ⓐ     A

*IOM: 100-02, 15, 100*

⊘ **L3215** Orthopedic footwear, ladies shoe, oxford, each Ⓑ Qp Qh ♀     E1

*Medicare Statute 1862a8*

⊘ **L3216** Orthopedic footwear, ladies shoe, depth inlay, each Ⓑ Qp Qh ♀     E1

*Medicare Statute 1862a8*

⊘ **L3217** Orthopedic footwear, ladies shoe, hightop, depth inlay, each Ⓑ Qp Qh ♀     E1

*Medicare Statute 1862a8*

⊘ **L3219** Orthopedic footwear, mens shoe, oxford, each Ⓑ Qp Qh ♂     E1

*Medicare Statute 1862a8*

⊘ **L3221** Orthopedic footwear, mens shoe, depth inlay, each Ⓑ Qp Qh ♂     E1

*Medicare Statute 1862a8*

⊘ **L3222** Orthopedic footwear, mens shoe, hightop, depth inlay, each Ⓑ Qp Qh ♂     E1

*Medicare Statute 1862a8*

⚙ **L3224** Orthopedic footwear, ladies shoe, oxford, used as an integral part of a brace (orthosis) Ⓑ Qp Qh ♀ ♿     A

*IOM: 100-02, 15, 290*

⚙ **L3225** Orthopedic footwear, mens shoe, oxford, used as an integral part of a brace (orthosis) Ⓑ Qp Qh ♂ ♿     A

*IOM: 100-02, 15, 290*

⚙ **L3230** Orthopedic footwear, custom shoe, depth inlay, each Ⓑ Qp Qh     A

*IOM: 100-02, 15, 290*

⚙ **L3250** Orthopedic footwear, custom molded shoe, removable inner mold, prosthetic shoe, each Ⓑ Qp Qh     A

*IOM: 100-02, 15, 290*

⚙ **L3251** Foot, shoe molded to patient model, silicone shoe, each Ⓑ Qp Qh     A

*IOM: 100-02, 15, 290*

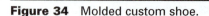

**Figure 34**   Molded custom shoe.

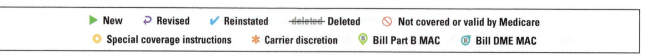

▶ New    ↻ Revised    ✔ Reinstated    ~~deleted~~ Deleted    ⊘ Not covered or valid by Medicare
⚙ Special coverage instructions    ✱ Carrier discretion    Ⓑ Bill Part B MAC    Ⓑ Bill DME MAC

**L3252** Foot, shoe molded to patient model, Plastazote (or similar), custom fabricated, each Ⓑ Qp Qh A
*IOM: 100-02, 15, 290*

**L3253** Foot, molded shoe Plastazote (or similar), custom fitted, each Ⓑ Qp Qh A
*IOM: 100-02, 15, 290*

**L3254** Non-standard size or width Ⓑ A
*IOM: 100-02, 15, 290*

**L3255** Non-standard size or length Ⓑ A
*IOM: 100-02, 15, 290*

**L3257** Orthopedic footwear, additional charge for split size Ⓑ A
*IOM: 100-02, 15, 290*

**L3260** Surgical boot/shoe, each Ⓑ E1
*IOM: 100-02, 15, 100*

* **L3265** Plastazote sandal, each Ⓑ A

## Shoe Lifts

**L3300** Lift, elevation, heel, tapered to metatarsals, per inch Ⓑ Qp ♿ A
*IOM: 100-02, 15, 290*

**L3310** Lift, elevation, heel and sole, Neoprene, per inch Ⓑ Qp ♿ A
*IOM: 100-02, 15, 290*

**L3320** Lift, elevation, heel and sole, cork, per inch Ⓑ Qp A
*IOM: 100-02, 15, 290*

**L3330** Lift, elevation, metal extension (skate) Ⓑ Qp Qh ♿ A
*IOM: 100-02, 15, 290*

**L3332** Lift, elevation, inside shoe, tapered, up to one-half inch Ⓑ Qp Qh ♿ A
*IOM: 100-02, 15, 290*

**L3334** Lift, elevation, heel, per inch Ⓑ Qp ♿ A
*IOM: 100-02, 15, 290*

## Shoe Wedges

**L3340** Heel wedge, SACH Ⓑ Qp Qh ♿ A
*IOM: 100-02, 15, 290*

**L3350** Heel wedge Ⓑ Qp Qh ♿ A
*IOM: 100-02, 15, 290*

**L3360** Sole wedge, outside sole Ⓑ Qp Qh ♿ A
*IOM: 100-02, 15, 290*

**L3370** Sole wedge, between sole Ⓑ Qp Qh ♿ A
*IOM: 100-02, 15, 290*

**L3380** Clubfoot wedge Ⓑ Qp Qh ♿ A
*IOM: 100-02, 15, 290*

**L3390** Outflare wedge Ⓑ Qp Qh ♿ A
*IOM: 100-02, 15, 290*

**L3400** Metatarsal bar wedge, rocker Ⓑ Qp Qh ♿ A
*IOM: 100-02, 15, 290*

**L3410** Metatarsal bar wedge, between sole Ⓑ Qp Qh ♿ A
*IOM: 100-02, 15, 290*

**L3420** Full sole and heel wedge, between sole Ⓑ Qp Qh ♿ A
*IOM: 100-02, 15, 290*

## Shoe Heels

**L3430** Heel, counter, plastic reinforced Ⓑ Qp Qh ♿ A
*IOM: 100-02, 15, 290*

**L3440** Heel, counter, leather reinforced Ⓑ Qp Qh ♿ A
*IOM: 100-02, 15, 290*

**L3450** Heel, SACH cushion type Ⓑ Qp Qh ♿ A
*IOM: 100-02, 15, 290*

**L3455** Heel, new leather, standard Ⓑ Qp Qh ♿ A
*IOM: 100-02, 15, 290*

**L3460** Heel, new rubber, standard Ⓑ Qp Qh ♿ A
*IOM: 100-02, 15, 290*

**L3465** Heel, Thomas with wedge Ⓑ Qp Qh ♿ A
*IOM: 100-02, 15, 290*

**L3470** Heel, Thomas extended to ball Ⓑ Qp Qh ♿ A
*IOM: 100-02, 15, 290*

**L3480** Heel, pad and depression for spur Ⓑ Qp Qh ♿ A
*IOM: 100-02, 15, 290*

**L3485** Heel, pad, removable for spur Ⓑ Qp Qh A
*IOM: 100-02, 15, 290*

## Orthopedic Shoe Additions: Other

**L3500** Orthopedic shoe addition, insole, leather Ⓑ Qp Qh ♿ A
*IOM: 100-02, 15, 290*

⊛ **L3510** Orthopedic shoe addition, insole, rubber Ⓑ Qp Qh ♿ A

*IOM: 100-02, 15, 290*

⊛ **L3520** Orthopedic shoe addition, insole, felt covered with leather Ⓑ Qp Qh ♿ A

*IOM: 100-02, 15, 290*

⊛ **L3530** Orthopedic shoe addition, sole, half Ⓑ Qp Qh ♿ A

*IOM: 100-02, 15, 290*

⊛ **L3540** Orthopedic shoe addition, sole, full Ⓑ Qp Qh ♿ A

*IOM: 100-02, 15, 290*

⊛ **L3550** Orthopedic shoe addition, toe tap standard Ⓑ Qp Qh ♿ A

*IOM: 100-02, 15, 290*

⊛ **L3560** Orthopedic shoe addition, toe tap, horseshoe Ⓑ Qp Qh ♿ A

*IOM: 100-02, 15, 290*

⊛ **L3570** Orthopedic shoe addition, special extension to instep (leather with eyelets) Ⓑ Qp Qh ♿ A

*IOM: 100-02, 15, 290*

⊛ **L3580** Orthopedic shoe addition, convert instep to Velcro closure Ⓑ Qp Qh ♿ A

*IOM: 100-02, 15, 290*

⊛ **L3590** Orthopedic shoe addition, convert firm shoe counter to soft counter Ⓑ Qp Qh ♿ A

*IOM: 100-02, 15, 290*

⊛ **L3595** Orthopedic shoe addition, March bar Ⓑ Qp Qh ♿ A

*IOM: 100-02, 15, 290*

## Transfer or Replacement

⊛ **L3600** Transfer of an orthosis from one shoe to another, caliper plate, existing Ⓑ Qp Qh ♿ A

*IOM: 100-02, 15, 290*

⊛ **L3610** Transfer of an orthosis from one shoe to another, caliper plate, new Ⓑ Qp Qh ♿ A

*IOM: 100-02, 15, 290*

⊛ **L3620** Transfer of an orthosis from one shoe to another, solid stirrup, existing Ⓑ Qp Qh ♿ A

*IOM: 100-02, 15, 290*

⊛ **L3630** Transfer of an orthosis from one shoe to another, solid stirrup, new Ⓑ Qp Qh ♿ A

*IOM: 100-02, 15, 290*

⊛ **L3640** Transfer of an orthosis from one shoe to another, Dennis Browne splint (Riveton), both shoes Ⓑ Qp Qh ♿ A

*IOM: 100-02, 15, 290*

⊛ **L3649** Orthopedic shoe, modification, addition or transfer, not otherwise specified Ⓑ A

*IOM: 100-02, 15, 290*

## Orthotic Devices: Upper Limb

**NOTE:** The procedures in this section are considered as base or basic procedures and may be modified by listing procedures from the Additions section and adding them to the base procedure.

### Shoulder

⁎ **L3650** Shoulder orthosis, figure of eight design abduction restrainer, prefabricated, off-the-shelf Ⓑ Qp Qh A

⁎ **L3660** Shoulder orthosis, figure of eight design abduction restrainer, canvas and webbing, prefabricated, off-the-shelf Ⓑ Qp Qh A

⁎ **L3670** Shoulder orthosis, acromio/clavicular (canvas and webbing type), prefabricated, off-the-shelf Ⓑ Qp Qh A

⁎ **L3671** Shoulder orthosis, shoulder joint design, without joints, may include soft interface, straps, custom fabricated, includes fitting and adjustment Ⓑ Qp Qh ♿ A

⁎ **L3674** Shoulder orthosis, abduction positioning (airplane design), thoracic component and support bar, with or without nontorsion joint/turnbuckle, may include soft interface, straps, custom fabricated, includes fitting and adjustment Ⓑ Qp Qh ♿ A

⁎ **L3675** Shoulder orthosis, vest type abduction restrainer, canvas webbing type or equal, prefabricated, off-the-shelf Ⓑ Qp Qh ♿ A

⊛ **L3677** Shoulder orthosis, shoulder joint design, without joints, may include soft interface, straps, prefabricated item that has been trimmed, bent, molded, assembled, or otherwise customized to fit a specific patient by an individual with expertise Ⓑ Qp Qh A

⁎ **L3678** Shoulder orthosis, shoulder joint design, without joints, may include soft interface, straps, prefabricated, off-the-shelf Ⓑ Qp Qh A

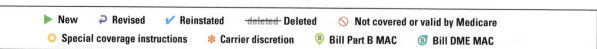

▶ New　⟳ Revised　✔ Reinstated　deleted Deleted　⊘ Not covered or valid by Medicare
⊛ Special coverage instructions　⁎ Carrier discretion　Ⓑ Bill Part B MAC　Ⓑ Bill DME MAC

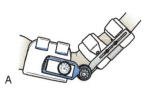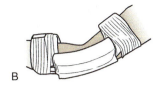

**Figure 35** Elbow orthoses.

## Elbow

❋ **L3702** Elbow orthosis, without joints, may include soft interface, straps, custom fabricated, includes fitting and adjustment Ⓑ Ⓠp Ⓠh ♿     A

❋ **L3710** Elbow orthosis, elastic with metal joints, prefabricated, off-the-shelf Ⓑ Ⓠp Ⓠh ♿     A

❋ **L3720** Elbow orthosis, double upright with forearm/arm cuffs, free motion, custom fabricated Ⓑ Ⓠp Ⓠh ♿     A

❋ **L3730** Elbow orthosis, double upright with forearm/arm cuffs, extension/flexion assist, custom fabricated Ⓑ Ⓠp Ⓠh ♿     A

❋ **L3740** Elbow orthosis, double upright with forearm/arm cuffs, adjustable position lock with active control, custom fabricated Ⓑ Ⓠp Ⓠh ♿     A

❋ **L3760** Elbow orthosis (EO), with adjustable position locking joint(s), prefabricated, item that has been trimmed, bent, molded, assembled, or otherwise customized to fit a specific patient by an individual with expertise Ⓑ Ⓠp Ⓠh ♿     A

❋ **L3761** Elbow orthosis (EO), with adjustable position locking joint(s), prefabricated, off-the-shelf     A

❋ **L3762** Elbow orthosis, rigid, without joints, includes soft interface material, prefabricated, off-the-shelf Ⓑ Ⓠp Ⓠh ♿     A

❋ **L3763** Elbow wrist hand orthosis, rigid, without joints, may include soft interface, straps, custom fabricated, includes fitting and adjustment Ⓑ Ⓠp Ⓠh ♿     A

❋ **L3764** Elbow wrist hand orthosis, includes one or more nontorsion joints, elastic bands, turnbuckles, may include soft interface, straps, custom fabricated, includes fitting and adjustment Ⓑ Ⓠp Ⓠh ♿     A

❋ **L3765** Elbow wrist hand finger orthosis, rigid, without joints, may include soft interface, straps, custom fabricated, includes fitting and adjustment Ⓑ Ⓠp Ⓠh ♿     A

❋ **L3766** Elbow wrist hand finger orthosis, includes one or more nontorsion joints, elastic bands, turnbuckles, may include soft interface, straps, custom fabricated, includes fitting and adjustment Ⓑ Ⓠp Ⓠh ♿     A

## Wrist-Hand-Finger Orthosis (WHFO)

❋ **L3806** Wrist hand finger orthosis, includes one or more nontorsion joint(s), turnbuckles, elastic bands/springs, may include soft interface material, straps, custom fabricated, includes fitting and adjustment Ⓑ Ⓠp Ⓠh ♿     A

❋ **L3807** Wrist hand finger orthosis, without joint(s), prefabricated item that has been trimmed, bent, molded, assembled, or otherwise customized to fit a specific patient by an individual with expertise Ⓑ Ⓠp Ⓠh ♿     A

❋ **L3808** Wrist hand finger orthosis, rigid without joints, may include soft interface material; straps, custom fabricated, includes fitting and adjustment Ⓑ Ⓠp Ⓠh ♿     A

❋ **L3809** Wrist hand finger orthosis, without joint(s), prefabricated, off-the-shelf, any type Ⓑ Ⓠp Ⓠh ♿     A

🚫 **L3891** Addition to upper extremity joint, wrist or elbow, concentric adjustable torsion style mechanism for custom fabricated orthotics only, each Ⓑ Ⓠp Ⓠh     E1

❋ **L3900** Wrist hand finger orthosis, dynamic flexor hinge, reciprocal wrist extension/flexion, finger flexion/extension, wrist or finger driven, custom fabricated Ⓑ Ⓠp Ⓠh ♿     A

❋ **L3901** Wrist hand finger orthosis, dynamic flexor hinge, reciprocal wrist extension/flexion, finger flexion/extension, cable driven, custom fabricated Ⓑ Ⓠp Ⓠh ♿     A

❋ **L3904** Wrist hand finger orthosis, external powered, electric, custom fabricated Ⓑ Ⓠp Ⓠh ♿     A

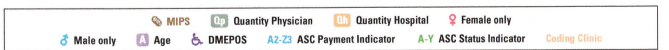

🐾 **MIPS**    Ⓠp **Quantity Physician**    Ⓠh **Quantity Hospital**    ♀ **Female only**

♂ **Male only**    Ⓐ **Age**    ♿ **DMEPOS**    **A2-Z3 ASC Payment Indicator**    **A-Y ASC Status Indicator**    Coding Clinic

## Other Upper Extremity Orthotics

* **L3905** Wrist hand orthosis, includes one or more nontorsion joints, elastic bands, turnbuckles, may include soft interface, straps, custom fabricated, includes fitting and adjustment Ⓑ Qp Qh ⓓ    A

* **L3906** Wrist hand orthosis, without joints, may include soft interface, straps, custom fabricated, includes fitting and adjustment Ⓑ Qp Qh ⓓ    A

* **L3908** Wrist hand orthosis, wrist extension control cock-up, non-molded, prefabricated, off-the-shelf Ⓑ Qp Qh ⓓ    A

* **L3912** Hand finger orthosis (HFO), flexion glove with elastic finger control, prefabricated, off-the-shelf Ⓑ Qp Qh ⓓ    A

* **L3913** Hand finger orthosis, without joints, may include soft interface, straps, custom fabricated, includes fitting and adjustment Ⓑ Qp Qh ⓓ    A

* **L3915** Wrist hand orthosis, includes one or more nontorsion joint(s), elastic bands, turnbuckles, may include soft interface, straps, prefabricated item that has been trimmed, bent, molded, assembled, or otherwise customized to fit a specific patient by an individual with expertise Ⓑ Qp Qh ⓓ    A

* **L3916** Wrist hand orthosis, includes one or more nontorsion joint(s), elastic bands, turnbuckles, may include soft interface, straps, prefabricated, off-the-shelf Ⓑ Qp Qh ⓓ    A

* **L3917** Hand orthosis, metacarpal fracture orthosis, prefabricated item that has been trimmed, bent, molded, assembled, or otherwise customized to fit a specific patient by an individual with expertise Ⓑ Qp Qh ⓓ    A

* **L3918** Hand orthosis, metacarpal fracture orthosis, prefabricated, off-the-shelf Ⓑ Qp Qh ⓓ    A

* **L3919** Hand orthosis, without joints, may include soft interface, straps, custom fabricated, includes fitting and adjustment Ⓑ Qp Qh ⓓ    A

* **L3921** Hand finger orthosis, includes one or more nontorsion joints, elastic bands, turnbuckles, may include soft interface, straps, custom fabricated, includes fitting and adjustment Ⓑ Qp Qh ⓓ    A

* **L3923** Hand finger orthosis, without joints, may include soft interface, straps, prefabricated item that has been trimmed, bent, molded, assembled, or otherwise customized to fit a specific patient by an individual with expertise Ⓑ Qp Qh    A

* **L3924** Hand finger orthosis, without joints, may include soft interface, straps, prefabricated, off-the-shelf Ⓑ Qp Qh ⓓ    A

* **L3925** Finger orthosis, proximal interphalangeal (PIP)/distal interphalangeal (DIP), non torsion joint/spring, extension/flexion, may include soft interface material, prefabricated, off-the-shelf Ⓑ Qp Qh ⓓ    A

* **L3927** Finger orthosis, proximal interphalangeal (PIP)/distal interphalangeal (DIP), without joint/spring, extension/flexion (e.g., static or ring type), may include soft interface material, prefabricated, off-the-shelf Ⓑ Qp Qh ⓓ    A

* **L3929** Hand finger orthosis, includes one or more nontorsion joint(s), turnbuckles, elastic bands/springs, may include soft interface material, straps, prefabricated item that has been trimmed, bent, molded, assembled, or otherwise customized to fit a specific patient by an individual with expertise Ⓑ Qp Qh ⓓ    A

* **L3930** Hand finger orthosis, includes one or more nontorsion joint(s), turnbuckles, elastic bands/springs, may include soft interface material, straps, prefabricated, off-the-shelf Ⓑ Qp Qh ⓓ    A

* **L3931** Wrist hand finger orthosis, includes one or more nontorsion joint(s), turnbuckles, elastic bands/springs, may include soft interface material, straps, prefabricated, includes fitting and adjustment Ⓑ Qp Qh ⓓ    A

* **L3933** Finger orthosis, without joints, may include soft interface, custom fabricated, includes fitting and adjustment Ⓑ Qp Qh ⓓ    A

* **L3935** Finger orthosis, nontorsion joint, may include soft interface, custom fabricated, includes fitting and adjustment Ⓑ Qp Qh ⓓ    A

* **L3956** Addition of joint to upper extremity orthosis, any material, per joint Ⓑ Qp ⓓ    A

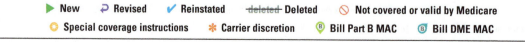

▶ New    ↺ Revised    ✔ Reinstated    ~~deleted~~ Deleted    ⊘ Not covered or valid by Medicare
🌕 Special coverage instructions    * Carrier discretion    Ⓑ Bill Part B MAC    Ⓑ Bill DME MAC

## Shoulder-Elbow-Wrist-Hand Orthotics (SEWHO) (L3960-L3973)

✳ **L3960** Shoulder elbow wrist hand orthosis, abduction positioning, airplane design, prefabricated, includes fitting and adjustment Ⓑ Qp Qh ♿    A

✳ **L3961** Shoulder elbow wrist hand orthosis, shoulder cap design, without joints, may include soft interface, straps, custom fabricated, includes fitting and adjustment Ⓑ Qp Qh ♿    A

✳ **L3962** Shoulder elbow wrist hand orthosis, abduction positioning, Erb's palsy design, prefabricated, includes fitting and adjustment Ⓑ Qp Qh ♿    A

✳ **L3967** Shoulder elbow wrist hand orthosis, abduction positioning (airplane design), thoracic component and support bar, without joints, may include soft interface, straps, custom fabricated, includes fitting and adjustment Ⓑ Qp Qh ♿    A

✳ **L3971** Shoulder elbow wrist hand orthosis, shoulder cap design, includes one or more nontorsion joints, elastic bands, turnbuckles, may include soft interface, straps, custom fabricated, includes fitting and adjustment Ⓑ Qp Qh ♿    A

✳ **L3973** Shoulder elbow wrist hand orthosis, abduction positioning (airplane design), thoracic component and support bar, includes one or more nontorsion joints, elastic bands, turnbuckles, may include soft interface, straps, custom fabricated, includes fitting and adjustment Ⓑ Qp Qh ♿    A

## Shoulder-Elbow-Wrist-Hand-Finger Orthotics

✳ **L3975** Shoulder elbow wrist hand finger orthosis, shoulder cap design, without joints, may include soft interface, straps, custom fabricated, includes fitting and adjustment Ⓑ Qp Qh ♿    A

✳ **L3976** Shoulder elbow wrist hand finger orthosis, abduction positioning (airplane design), thoracic component and support bar, without joints, may include soft interface, straps, custom fabricated, includes fitting and adjustment Ⓑ Qp Qh ♿    A

✳ **L3977** Shoulder elbow wrist hand finger orthosis, shoulder cap design, includes one or more nontorsion joints, elastic bands, turnbuckles, may include soft interface, straps, custom fabricated, includes fitting and adjustment Ⓑ Qp Qh ♿    A

✳ **L3978** Shoulder elbow wrist hand finger orthosis, abduction positioning (airplane design), thoracic component and support bar, includes one or more nontorsion joints, elastic bands, turnbuckles, may include soft interface, straps, custom fabricated, includes fitting and adjustment Ⓑ Qp Qh ♿    A

## Fracture Orthotics

✳ **L3980** Upper extremity fracture orthosis, humeral, prefabricated, includes fitting and adjustment Ⓑ Qp Qh ♿    A

✳ **L3981** Upper extremity fracture orthosis, humeral, prefabricated, includes shoulder cap design, with or without joints, forearm section, may include soft interface, straps, includes fitting and adjustments Ⓑ Qp Qh ♿    A

✳ **L3982** Upper extremity fracture orthosis, radius/ulnar, prefabricated, includes fitting and adjustment Ⓑ Qp Qh ♿    A

✳ **L3984** Upper extremity fracture orthosis, wrist, prefabricated, includes fitting and adjustment Ⓑ Qp Qh ♿    A

✳ **L3995** Addition to upper extremity orthosis, sock, fracture or equal, each Ⓑ Qp ♿    A

✳ **L3999** Upper limb orthosis, not otherwise specified Ⓑ    A

## Repairs

✳ **L4000** Replace girdle for spinal orthosis (CTLSO or SO) Ⓑ Qp Qh ♿    A

✳ **L4002** Replacement strap, any orthosis, includes all components, any length, any type Ⓑ Qp ♿    A

✳ **L4010** Replace trilateral socket brim Ⓑ Qp Qh ♿    A

✳ **L4020** Replace quadrilateral socket brim, molded to patient model Ⓑ Qp Qh ♿    A

✳ **L4030** Replace quadrilateral socket brim, custom fitted Ⓑ Qp Qh ♿    A

✳ **L4040** Replace molded thigh lacer, for custom fabricated orthosis only Ⓑ Qp Qh ♿    A

✳ **L4045** Replace non-molded thigh lacer, for custom fabricated orthosis only Ⓑ Qp Qh ♿    A

✳ **L4050** Replace molded calf lacer, for custom fabricated orthosis only Ⓑ Qp Qh ♿    A

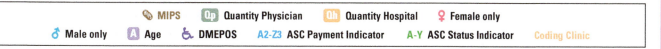

🖐 MIPS    Qp Quantity Physician    Qh Quantity Hospital    ♀ Female only

♂ Male only    Ⓐ Age    ♿ DMEPOS    A2-Z3 ASC Payment Indicator    A-Y ASC Status Indicator    Coding Clinic

\* **L4055** Replace non-molded calf lacer, for custom fabricated orthosis only Ⓑ 📗Qp 📙Qh ♿     A

\* **L4060** Replace high roll cuff Ⓑ 📗Qp 📙Qh ♿     A

\* **L4070** Replace proximal and distal upright for KAFO Ⓑ 📗Qp 📙Qh ♿     A

\* **L4080** Replace metal bands KAFO, proximal thigh 📗Qp 📙Qh ♿     A

\* **L4090** Replace metal bands KAFO-AFO, calf or distal thigh Ⓑ 📗Qp ♿     A

\* **L4100** Replace leather cuff KAFO, proximal thigh Ⓑ 📗Qp 📙Qh ♿     A

\* **L4110** Replace leather cuff KAFO-AFO, calf or distal thigh Ⓑ 📗Qp ♿     A

\* **L4130** Replace pretibial shell Ⓑ 📗Qp 📙Qh ♿     A

⊙ **L4205** Repair of orthotic device, labor component, per 15 minutes Ⓑ 📗Qp     A

    *IOM: 100-02, 15, 110.2*

⊙ **L4210** Repair of orthotic device, repair or replace minor parts Ⓑ 📗Qp 📙Qh     A

    *IOM: 100-02, 15, 110.2; 100-02, 15, 120*

## Ancillary Orthotic Services

\* **L4350** Ankle control orthosis, stirrup style, rigid, includes any type interface (e.g., pneumatic, gel), prefabricated, off-the-shelf Ⓑ 📗Qp 📙Qh ♿     A

\* **L4360** Walking boot, pneumatic and/or vacuum, with or without joints, with or without interface material, prefabricated item that has been trimmed, bent, molded, assembled, or otherwise customized to fit a specific patient by an individual with expertise Ⓑ 📗Qp 📙Qh ♿     A

    *Noncovered when walking boots used primarily to relieve pressure, especially on sole of foot, or are used for patients with foot ulcers*

\* **L4361** Walking boot, pneumatic and/or vacuum, with or without joints, with or without interface material, prefabricated, off-the-shelf Ⓑ 📗Qp 📙Qh ♿     A

\* **L4370** Pneumatic full leg splint, prefabricated, off-the-shelf Ⓑ 📗Qp 📙Qh ♿     A

\* **L4386** Walking boot, non-pneumatic, with or without joints, with or without interface material, prefabricated item that has been trimmed, bent, molded, assembled, or otherwise customized to fit a specific patient by an individual with expertise Ⓑ 📗Qp 📙Qh ♿     A

\* **L4387** Walking boot, non-pneumatic, with or without joints, with or without interface material, prefabricated, off-the-shelf Ⓑ 📗Qp 📙Qh ♿     A

\* **L4392** Replacement, soft interface material, static AFO Ⓑ 📗Qp 📙Qh ♿     A

\* **L4394** Replace soft interface material, foot drop splint Ⓑ 📗Qp 📙Qh ♿     A

\* **L4396** Static or dynamic ankle foot orthosis, including soft interface material, adjustable for fit, for positioning, may be used for minimal ambulation, prefabricated item that has been trimmed, bent, molded, assembled, or otherwise customized to fit a specific patient by an individual with expertise Ⓑ 📗Qp 📙Qh ♿     A

\* **L4397** Static or dynamic ankle foot orthosis, including soft interface material, adjustable for fit, for positioning, may be used for minimal ambulation, prefabricated, off-the-shelf Ⓑ 📗Qp 📙Qh ♿     A

\* **L4398** Foot drop splint, recumbent positioning device, prefabricated, off-the-shelf Ⓑ 📗Qp 📙Qh ♿     A

\* **L4631** Ankle foot orthosis, walking boot type, varus/valgus correction, rocker bottom, anterior tibial shell, soft interface, custom arch support, plastic or other material, includes straps and closures, custom fabricated Ⓑ 📗Qp 📙Qh ♿     A

---

▶ New    ⮌ Revised    ✔ Reinstated    ~~deleted~~ Deleted    ⊘ Not covered or valid by Medicare

⊙ Special coverage instructions    \* Carrier discretion    Ⓑ Bill Part B MAC    Ⓑ Bill DME MAC

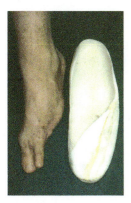

**Figure 36** Partial foot.

## PROSTHETICS (L5000-L9999)

### Lower Limb (L5000-L5999)

NOTE: The procedures in this section are considered as base or basic procedures and may be modified by listing items/procedures or special materials from the Additions section and adding them to the base procedure.

### Partial Foot

✿ **L5000** Partial foot, shoe insert with longitudinal arch, toe filler ⑧ 【Qp】【Qh】 &   A

    *IOM: 100-02, 15, 290*

✿ **L5010** Partial foot, molded socket, ankle height, with toe filler ⑧ 【Qp】【Qh】 &   A

    *IOM: 100-02, 15, 290*

✿ **L5020** Partial foot, molded socket, tibial tubercle height, with toe filler ⑧ 【Qp】【Qh】 &   A

    *IOM: 100-02, 15, 290*

### Ankle

✳ **L5050** Ankle, Symes, molded socket, SACH foot ⑧ 【Qp】【Qh】 &   A

✳ **L5060** Ankle, Symes, metal frame, molded leather socket, articulated ankle/foot ⑧ 【Qp】【Qh】 &   A

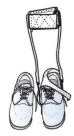

**Figure 37** Ankle Symes.

### Below Knee

✳ **L5100** Below knee, molded socket, shin, SACH foot ⑧ 【Qp】【Qh】 &   A

✳ **L5105** Below knee, plastic socket, joints and thigh lacer, SACH foot ⑧ 【Qp】【Qh】 &   A

### Knee Disarticulation

✳ **L5150** Knee disarticulation (or through knee), molded socket, external knee joints, shin, SACH foot ⑧ 【Qp】【Qh】 &   A

✳ **L5160** Knee disarticulation (or through knee), molded socket, bent knee configuration, external knee joints, shin, SACH foot ⑧ 【Qp】【Qh】 &   A

### Above Knee

✳ **L5200** Above knee, molded socket, single axis constant friction knee, shin, SACH foot ⑧ 【Qp】【Qh】 &   A

✳ **L5210** Above knee, short prosthesis, no knee joint ('stubbies'), with foot blocks, no ankle joints, each ⑧ 【Qp】【Qh】 &   A

✳ **L5220** Above knee, short prosthesis, no knee joint ('stubbies'), with articulated ankle/foot, dynamically aligned, each ⑧ 【Qp】【Qh】 &   A

✳ **L5230** Above knee, for proximal femoral focal deficiency, constant friction knee, shin, SACH foot ⑧ 【Qp】【Qh】 &   A

### Hip Disarticulation

✳ **L5250** Hip disarticulation, Canadian type; molded socket, hip joint, single axis constant friction knee, shin, SACH foot ⑧ 【Qp】【Qh】 &   A

✳ **L5270** Hip disarticulation, tilt table type; molded socket, locking hip joint, single axis constant friction knee, shin, SACH foot ⑧ 【Qp】【Qh】 &   A

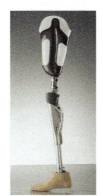

**Figure 38** Above knee.

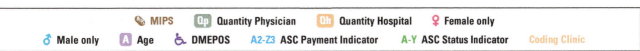

🐾 MIPS   【Qp】 Quantity Physician   【Qh】 Quantity Hospital   ♀ Female only

♂ Male only   Ⓐ Age   & DMEPOS   A2-Z3 ASC Payment Indicator   A-Y ASC Status Indicator   Coding Clinic

## Hemipelvectomy

* **L5280** Hemipelvectomy, Canadian type; molded socket, hip joint, single axis constant friction knee, shin, SACH foot Ⓑ Qp Qh ⛑     A

## Endoskeletal

* **L5301** Below knee, molded socket, shin, SACH foot, endoskeletal system Ⓑ Qp Qh ⛑   A

* **L5312** Knee disarticulation (or through knee), molded socket, single axis knee, pylon, sach foot, endoskeletal system Ⓑ Qp Qh ⛑   A

* **L5321** Above knee, molded socket, open end, SACH foot, endoskeletal system, single axis knee Ⓑ Qp Qh ⛑   A

* **L5331** Hip disarticulation, Canadian type, molded socket, endoskeletal system, hip joint, single axis knee, SACH foot Ⓑ Qp Qh ⛑   A

* **L5341** Hemipelvectomy, Canadian type, molded socket, endoskeletal system, hip joint, single axis knee, SACH foot Ⓑ Qp Qh ⛑   A

## Immediate Postsurgical or Early Fitting Procedures

* **L5400** Immediate post surgical or early fitting, application of initial rigid dressing, including fitting, alignment, suspension, and one cast change, below knee Ⓑ Qp Qh ⛑   A

* **L5410** Immediate post surgical or early fitting, application of initial rigid dressing, including fitting, alignment and suspension, below knee, each additional cast change and realignment Ⓑ Qp Qh ⛑   A

* **L5420** Immediate post surgical or early fitting, application of initial rigid dressing, including fitting, alignment and suspension and one cast change 'AK' or knee disarticulation Ⓑ Qp Qh ⛑   A

* **L5430** Immediate postsurgical or early fitting, application of initial rigid dressing, including fitting, alignment, and suspension, 'AK' or knee disarticulation, each additional cast change and realignment Ⓑ Qp Qh ⛑   A

* **L5450** Immediate post surgical or early fitting, application of non-weight bearing rigid dressing, below knee Ⓑ Qp Qh ⛑   A

* **L5460** Immediate post surgical or early fitting, application of non-weight bearing rigid dressing, above knee Ⓑ Qp Qh ⛑   A

## Initial Prosthesis

* **L5500** Initial, below knee 'PTB' type socket, non-alignable system, pylon, no cover, SACH foot, plaster socket, direct formed Ⓑ Qp Qh ⛑   A

* **L5505** Initial, above knee-knee disarticulation, ischial level socket, non-alignable system, pylon, no cover, SACH foot, plaster socket, direct formed Ⓑ Qp Qh ⛑   A

## Preparatory Prosthesis

* **L5510** Preparatory, below knee 'PTB' type socket, non-alignable system, pylon, no cover, SACH foot, plaster socket, molded to model Ⓑ Qp Qh ⛑   A

* **L5520** Preparatory, below knee 'PTB' type socket, non-alignable system, pylon, no cover, SACH foot, thermoplastic or equal, direct formed Ⓑ Qp Qh ⛑   A

* **L5530** Preparatory, below knee 'PTB' type socket, non-alignable system, pylon, no cover, SACH foot, thermoplastic or equal, molded to model Ⓑ Qp Qh ⛑   A

* **L5535** Preparatory, below knee 'PTB' type socket, non-alignable system, no cover, SACH foot, prefabricated, adjustable open end socket Ⓑ Qp Qh ⛑   A

* **L5540** Preparatory, below knee 'PTB' type socket, non-alignable system, pylon, no cover, SACH foot, laminated socket, molded to model Qp Qh ⛑   A

* **L5560** Preparatory, above knee - knee disarticulation, ischial level socket, non-alignable system, pylon, no cover, SACH foot, plaster socket, molded to model Ⓑ Qp Qh ⛑   A

* **L5570** Preparatory, above knee - knee disarticulation, ischial level socket, non-alignable system, pylon, no cover, SACH foot, thermoplastic or equal, direct formed Ⓑ Qp Qh ⛑   A

* **L5580** Preparatory, above knee - knee disarticulation, ischial level socket, non-alignable system, pylon, no cover, SACH foot, thermoplastic or equal, molded to model Ⓑ Qp Qh ⛑   A

* **L5585** Preparatory, above knee - knee disarticulation, ischial level socket, non-alignable system, pylon, no cover, SACH foot, prefabricated adjustable open end socket Ⓑ Qp Qh ⛑   A

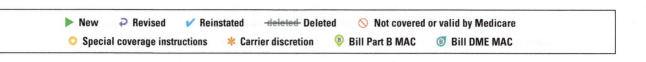

▶ New   ↻ Revised   ✔ Reinstated   deleted Deleted   ⊘ Not covered or valid by Medicare   ○ Special coverage instructions   * Carrier discretion   Ⓑ Bill Part B MAC   Ⓓ Bill DME MAC

* **L5590** Preparatory, above knee - knee disarticulation, ischial level socket, non-alignable system, pylon, no cover, SACH foot, laminated socket, molded to model Ⓑ Ⓠp Ⓠh    A

* **L5595** Preparatory, hip disarticulation-hemipelvectomy, pylon, no cover, SACH foot, thermoplastic or equal, molded to patient model Ⓑ Ⓠp Ⓠh    A

* **L5600** Preparatory, hip disarticulation-hemipelvectomy, pylon, no cover, SACH foot, laminated socket, molded to patient model Ⓑ Ⓠp Ⓠh    A

## Additions to Lower Extremity

* **L5610** Addition to lower extremity, endoskeletal system, above knee, hydracadence system Ⓑ Ⓠp Ⓠh    A

* **L5611** Addition to lower extremity, endoskeletal system, above knee-knee disarticulation, 4 bar linkage, with friction swing phase control Ⓑ Ⓠp Ⓠh    A

* **L5613** Addition to lower extremity, endoskeletal system, above knee-knee disarticulation, 4 bar linkage, with hydraulic swing phase control Ⓑ Ⓠp Ⓠh    A

* **L5614** Addition to lower extremity, exoskeletal system, above knee-knee disarticulation, 4 bar linkage, with pneumatic swing phase control Ⓑ Ⓠp Ⓠh    A

* **L5616** Addition to lower extremity, endoskeletal system, above knee, universal multiplex system, friction swing phase control Ⓑ Ⓠp Ⓠh    A

* **L5617** Addition to lower extremity, quick change self-aligning unit, above knee or below knee, each Ⓑ Ⓠp Ⓠh    A

## Additions to Test Sockets

* **L5618** Addition to lower extremity, test socket, Symes Ⓑ Ⓠp    A

* **L5620** Addition to lower extremity, test socket, below knee Ⓑ Ⓠp    A

* **L5622** Addition to lower extremity, test socket, knee disarticulation Ⓑ Ⓠp    A

* **L5624** Addition to lower extremity, test socket, above knee Ⓑ Ⓠp    A

* **L5626** Addition to lower extremity, test socket, hip disarticulation Ⓑ Ⓠp    A

* **L5628** Addition to lower extremity, test socket, hemipelvectomy Ⓑ Ⓠp Ⓠh    A

## Additions to Socket Variations

* **L5629** Addition to lower extremity, below knee, acrylic socket Ⓑ Ⓠp Ⓠh    A

* **L5630** Addition to lower extremity, Symes type, expandable wall socket Ⓑ Ⓠp Ⓠh    A

* **L5631** Addition to lower extremity, above knee or knee disarticulation, acrylic socket Ⓑ Ⓠp Ⓠh    A

* **L5632** Addition to lower extremity, Symes type, 'PTB' brim design socket Ⓑ Ⓠp Ⓠh    A

* **L5634** Addition to lower extremity, Symes type, posterior opening (Canadian) socket Ⓑ Ⓠp Ⓠh    A

* **L5636** Addition to lower extremity, Symes type, medial opening socket Ⓑ Ⓠp Ⓠh    A

* **L5637** Addition to lower extremity, below knee, total contact Ⓑ Ⓠp Ⓠh    A

* **L5638** Addition to lower extremity, below knee, leather socket Ⓑ Ⓠp Ⓠh    A

* **L5639** Addition to lower extremity, below knee, wood socket Ⓑ Ⓠp Ⓠh    A

* **L5640** Addition to lower extremity, knee disarticulation, leather socket Ⓑ Ⓠp Ⓠh    A

* **L5642** Addition to lower extremity, above knee, leather socket Ⓑ Ⓠp Ⓠh    A

* **L5643** Addition to lower extremity, hip disarticulation, flexible inner socket, external frame Ⓑ Ⓠp Ⓠh    A

* **L5644** Addition to lower extremity, above knee, wood socket Ⓑ Ⓠp Ⓠh    A

* **L5645** Addition to lower extremity, below knee, flexible inner socket, external frame Ⓑ Ⓠp Ⓠh    A

* **L5646** Addition to lower extremity, below knee, air, fluid, gel or equal, cushion socket Ⓑ Ⓠp Ⓠh    A

* **L5647** Addition to lower extremity, below knee, suction socket Ⓑ Ⓠp Ⓠh    A

* **L5648** Addition to lower extremity, above knee, air, fluid, gel or equal, cushion socket Ⓑ Ⓠp Ⓠh    A

* **L5649** Addition to lower extremity, ischial containment/narrow M-L socket Ⓑ Ⓠp Ⓠh    A

* **L5650** Additions to lower extremity, total contact, above knee or knee disarticulation socket Ⓑ Ⓠp Ⓠh    A

---

🖐 MIPS    Ⓠp Quantity Physician    Ⓠh Quantity Hospital    ♀ Female only

♂ Male only    Ⓐ Age    & DMEPOS    A2-Z3 ASC Payment Indicator    A-Y ASC Status Indicator    Coding Clinic

\* **L5651** Addition to lower extremity, above knee, flexible inner socket, external frame Ⓑ ⒬ᵖ ⒬ʰ ♿     A

\* **L5652** Addition to lower extremity, suction suspension, above knee or knee disarticulation socket Ⓑ ⒬ᵖ ⒬ʰ ♿     A

\* **L5653** Addition to lower extremity, knee disarticulation, expandable wall socket Ⓑ ⒬ᵖ ⒬ʰ ♿     A

## Additions to Socket Insert and Suspension

\* **L5654** Addition to lower extremity, socket insert, Symes, (Kemblo, Pelite, Aliplast, Plastazote or equal) ⒬ᵖ ⒬ʰ ♿     A

\* **L5655** Addition to lower extremity, socket insert, below knee (Kemblo, Pelite, Aliplast, Plastazote or equal) Ⓑ ⒬ᵖ ⒬ʰ ♿     A

\* **L5656** Addition to lower extremity, socket insert, knee disarticulation (Kemblo, Pelite, Aliplast, Plastazote or equal) Ⓑ ⒬ᵖ ⒬ʰ ♿     A

\* **L5658** Addition to lower extremity, socket insert, above knee (Kemblo, Pelite, Aliplast, Plastazote or equal) Ⓑ ⒬ᵖ ⒬ʰ ♿     A

\* **L5661** Addition to lower extremity, socket insert, multi-durometer Symes Ⓑ ⒬ᵖ ⒬ʰ ♿     A

\* **L5665** Addition to lower extremity, socket insert, multi-durometer, below knee Ⓑ ⒬ᵖ ⒬ʰ ♿     A

\* **L5666** Addition to lower extremity, below knee, cuff suspension Ⓑ ⒬ᵖ ⒬ʰ ♿     A

\* **L5668** Addition to lower extremity, below knee, molded distal cushion Ⓑ ⒬ᵖ ⒬ʰ ♿     A

\* **L5670** Addition to lower extremity, below knee, molded supracondylar suspension ('PTS' or similar) Ⓑ ⒬ᵖ ⒬ʰ ♿     A

\* **L5671** Addition to lower extremity, below knee/above knee suspension locking mechanism (shuttle, lanyard or equal), excludes socket insert Ⓑ ⒬ᵖ ⒬ʰ ♿     A

\* **L5672** Addition to lower extremity, below knee, removable medial brim suspension Ⓑ ⒬ᵖ ⒬ʰ ♿     A

\* **L5673** Addition to lower extremity, below knee/above knee, custom fabricated from existing mold or prefabricated, socket insert, silicone gel, elastomeric or equal, for use with locking mechanism Ⓑ ⒬ᵖ ♿     A

\* **L5676** Additions to lower extremity, below knee, knee joints, single axis, pair Ⓑ ⒬ᵖ ⒬ʰ ♿     A

\* **L5677** Additions to lower extremity, below knee, knee joints, polycentric, pair Ⓑ ⒬ᵖ ⒬ʰ ♿     A

\* **L5678** Additions to lower extremity, below knee, joint covers, pair Ⓑ ⒬ᵖ ⒬ʰ ♿     A

\* **L5679** Addition to lower extremity, below knee/above knee, custom fabricated from existing mold or prefabricated, socket insert, silicone gel, elastomeric or equal, not for use with locking mechanism Ⓑ ⒬ᵖ     A

\* **L5680** Addition to lower extremity, below knee, thigh lacer, non-molded Ⓑ ⒬ᵖ ⒬ʰ     A

\* **L5681** Addition to lower extremity, below knee/above knee, custom fabricated socket insert for congenital or atypical traumatic amputee, silicone gel, elastomeric or equal, for use with or without locking mechanism, initial only (for other than initial, use code L5673 or L5679) Ⓑ ⒬ᵖ ⒬ʰ     A

\* **L5682** Addition to lower extremity, below knee, thigh lacer, gluteal/ischial, molded Ⓑ ⒬ᵖ ⒬ʰ     A

\* **L5683** Addition to lower extremity, below knee/above knee, custom fabricated socket insert for other than congenital or atypical traumatic amputee, silicone gel, elastomeric, or equal, for use with or without locking mechanism, initial only (for other than initial, use code L5673 or L5679) Ⓑ ⒬ᵖ ⒬ʰ     A

\* **L5684** Addition to lower extremity, below knee, fork strap Ⓑ ⒬ᵖ ⒬ʰ ♿     A

\* **L5685** Addition to lower extremity prosthesis, below knee, suspension/sealing sleeve, with or without valve, any material, each Ⓑ ⒬ᵖ ♿     A

\* **L5686** Addition to lower extremity, below knee, back check (extension control) Ⓑ ⒬ᵖ ⒬ʰ     A

\* **L5688** Addition to lower extremity, below knee, waist belt, webbing Ⓑ ⒬ᵖ ⒬ʰ ♿     A

\* **L5690** Addition to lower extremity, below knee, waist belt, padded and lined Ⓑ ⒬ᵖ ⒬ʰ ♿     A

\* **L5692** Addition to lower extremity, above knee, pelvic control belt, light Ⓑ ⒬ᵖ ⒬ʰ ♿     A

\* **L5694** Addition to lower extremity, above knee, pelvic control belt, padded and lined Ⓑ ⒬ᵖ ⒬ʰ ♿     A

---

▶ New    ↻ Revised    ✔ Reinstated    ~~deleted~~ Deleted    ⊘ Not covered or valid by Medicare

⊛ Special coverage instructions    \* Carrier discretion    Ⓑ Bill Part B MAC    Ⓑ Bill DME MAC

* **L5695** Addition to lower extremity, above knee, pelvic control, sleeve suspension, neoprene or equal, each 🅑 Qp Qh ♿   A

* **L5696** Addition to lower extremity, above knee or knee disarticulation, pelvic joint 🅑 Qp Qh ♿   A

* **L5697** Addition to lower extremity, above knee or knee disarticulation, pelvic band 🅑 Qp Qh ♿   A

* **L5698** Addition to lower extremity, above knee or knee disarticulation, Silesian bandage 🅑 Qp Qh ♿   A

* **L5699** All lower extremity prostheses, shoulder harness 🅑 Qp Qh ♿   A

## Replacement Sockets

* **L5700** Replacement, socket, below knee, molded to patient model 🅑 Qp Qh ♿   A

* **L5701** Replacement, socket, above knee/knee disarticulation, including attachment plate, molded to patient model 🅑 Qp Qh ♿   A

* **L5702** Replacement, socket, hip disarticulation, including hip joint, molded to patient model 🅑 Qp Qh ♿   A

* **L5703** Ankle, Symes, molded to patient model, socket without solid ankle cushion heel (SACH) foot, replacement only 🅑 Qp Qh ♿   A

## Protective Covers

* **L5704** Custom shaped protective cover, below knee 🅑 Qp Qh ♿   A

* **L5705** Custom shaped protective cover, above knee 🅑 Qp Qh ♿   A

* **L5706** Custom shaped protective cover, knee disarticulation 🅑 Qp Qh ♿   A

* **L5707** Custom shaped protective cover, hip disarticulation 🅑 Qp Qh ♿   A

## Additions to Exoskeletal–Knee-Shin System

* **L5710** Addition, exoskeletal knee-shin system, single axis, manual lock 🅑 Qp Qh ♿   A

* **L5711** Additions exoskeletal knee-shin system, single axis, manual lock, ultra-light material 🅑 Qp Qh ♿   A

* **L5712** Addition, exoskeletal knee-shin system, single axis, friction swing and stance phase control (safety knee) 🅑 Qp Qh ♿   A

* **L5714** Addition, exoskeletal knee-shin system, single axis, variable friction swing phase control 🅑 Qp Qh ♿   A

* **L5716** Addition, exoskeletal knee-shin system, polycentric, mechanical stance phase lock 🅑 Qp Qh ♿   A

* **L5718** Addition, exoskeletal knee-shin system, polycentric, friction swing and stance phase control 🅑 Qp Qh ♿   A

* **L5722** Addition, exoskeletal knee-shin system, single axis, pneumatic swing, friction stance phase control 🅑 Qp Qh ♿   A

* **L5724** Addition, exoskeletal knee-shin system, single axis, fluid swing phase control 🅑 Qp Qh ♿   A

* **L5726** Addition, exoskeletal knee-shin system, single axis, external joints, fluid swing phase control 🅑 Qp Qh ♿   A

* **L5728** Addition, exoskeletal knee-shin system, single axis, fluid swing and stance phase control 🅑 Qp Qh ♿   A

* **L5780** Addition, exoskeletal knee-shin system, single axis, pneumatic/hydra pneumatic swing phase control 🅑 Qp Qh ♿   A

## Vacuum Pumps

* **L5781** Addition to lower limb prosthesis, vacuum pump, residual limb volume management and moisture evacuation system 🅑 Qp Qh ♿   A

* **L5782** Addition to lower limb prosthesis, vacuum pump, residual limb volume management and moisture evacuation system, heavy duty 🅑 Qp Qh ♿   A

## Component Modification

* **L5785** Addition, exoskeletal system, below knee, ultra-light material (titanium, carbon fiber, or equal) 🅑 Qp Qh ♿   A

* **L5790** Addition, exoskeletal system, above knee, ultra-light material (titanium, carbon fiber, or equal) 🅑 Qp Qh ♿   A

* **L5795** Addition, exoskeletal system, hip disarticulation, ultra-light material (titanium, carbon fiber, or equal) 🅑 Qp Qh ♿   A

## Endoskeletal

* **L5810** Addition, endoskeletal knee-shin system, single axis, manual lock 🅑 Qp Qh ♿   A

* **L5811** Addition, endoskeletal knee-shin system, single axis, manual lock, ultralight material 🅑 Qp Qh ♿   A

🖐 MIPS   Qp Quantity Physician   Qh Quantity Hospital   ♀ Female only
♂ Male only   🅐 Age   ♿ DMEPOS   A2-Z3 ASC Payment Indicator   A-Y ASC Status Indicator   Coding Clinic

PROSTHETICS   L5695 – L5811

365

* **L5812** Addition, endoskeletal knee-shin system, single axis, friction swing and stance phase control (safety knee) Ⓑ Qp Qh   A

* **L5814** Addition, endoskeletal knee-shin system, polycentric, hydraulic swing phase control, mechanical stance phase lock Ⓑ Qp Qh   A

* **L5816** Addition, endoskeletal knee-shin system, polycentric, mechanical stance phase lock Ⓑ Qp Qh   A

* **L5818** Addition, endoskeletal knee-shin system, polycentric, friction swing, and stance phase control Ⓑ Qp Qh   A

* **L5822** Addition, endoskeletal knee-shin system, single axis, pneumatic swing, friction stance phase control Ⓑ Qp Qh   A

* **L5824** Addition, endoskeletal knee-shin system, single axis, fluid swing phase control Ⓑ Qp Qh   A

* **L5826** Addition, endoskeletal knee-shin system, single axis, hydraulic swing phase control, with miniature high activity frame Ⓑ Qp Qh   A

* **L5828** Addition, endoskeletal knee-shin system, single axis, fluid swing and stance phase control Ⓑ Qp Qh   A

* **L5830** Addition, endoskeletal knee-shin system, single axis, pneumatic/swing phase control Ⓑ Qp Qh   A

* **L5840** Addition, endoskeletal knee/shin system, 4-bar linkage or multiaxial, pneumatic swing phase control Ⓑ Qp Qh   A

* **L5845** Addition, endoskeletal, knee-shin system, stance flexion feature, adjustable Ⓑ Qp Qh   A

* **L5848** Addition to endoskeletal, knee-shin system, fluid stance extension, dampening feature, with or without adjustability Ⓑ Qp Qh   A

* **L5850** Addition, endoskeletal system, above knee or hip disarticulation, knee extension assist Ⓑ Qp Qh   A

* **L5855** Addition, endoskeletal system, hip disarticulation, mechanical hip extension assist Ⓑ Qp Qh   A

* **L5856** Addition to lower extremity prosthesis, endoskeletal knee-shin system, microprocessor control feature, swing and stance phase; includes electronic sensor(s), any type Ⓑ Qp Qh   A

* **L5857** Addition to lower extremity prosthesis, endoskeletal knee-shin system, microprocessor control feature, swing phase only; includes electronic sensor(s), any type Ⓑ Qp Qh   A

* **L5858** Addition to lower extremity prosthesis, endoskeletal knee shin system, microprocessor control feature, stance phase only, includes electronic sensor(s), any type Ⓑ Qp Qh   A

* **L5859** Addition to lower extremity prosthesis, endoskeletal knee-shin system, powered and programmable flexion/extension assist control, includes any type motor(s) Ⓑ Qp Qh   A

* **L5910** Addition, endoskeletal system, below knee, alignable system Ⓑ Qp Qh   A

* **L5920** Addition, endoskeletal system, above knee or hip disarticulation, alignable system Ⓑ Qp Qh   A

* **L5925** Addition, endoskeletal system, above knee, knee disarticulation or hip disarticulation, manual lock Ⓑ Qp Qh   A

* **L5930** Addition, endoskeletal system, high activity knee control frame Ⓑ Qp Qh   A

* **L5940** Addition, endoskeletal system, below knee, ultra-light material (titanium, carbon fiber or equal) Ⓑ Qp Qh   A

* **L5950** Addition, endoskeletal system, above knee, ultra-light material (titanium, carbon fiber or equal) Ⓑ Qp Qh   A

* **L5960** Addition, endoskeletal system, hip disarticulation, ultra-light material (titanium, carbon fiber, or equal) Ⓑ Qp Qh   A

* **L5961** Addition, endoskeletal system, polycentric hip joint, pneumatic or hydraulic control, rotation control, with or without flexion, and/or extension control Ⓑ Qp Qh   A

* **L5962** Addition, endoskeletal system, below knee, flexible protective outer surface covering system Ⓑ Qp Qh   A

* **L5964** Addition, endoskeletal system, above knee, flexible protective outer surface covering system Ⓑ Qp Qh   A

* **L5966** Addition, endoskeletal system, hip disarticulation, flexible protective outer surface covering system Ⓑ Qp Qh   A

---

▶ New    ↻ Revised    ✔ Reinstated    deleted Deleted    ⊘ Not covered or valid by Medicare

✿ Special coverage instructions    ✱ Carrier discretion    Ⓑ Bill Part B MAC    Ⓓ Bill DME MAC

## PROSTHETICS

### Additions to Ankle and/or Foot

* **L5968** Addition to lower limb prosthesis, multiaxial ankle with swing phase active dorsiflexion feature Ⓑ Qp Qh ♿    A

* **L5969** Addition, endoskeletal ankle-foot or ankle system, power assist, includes any type motor(s) Ⓑ Qp Qh    A

* **L5970** All lower extremity prostheses, foot, external keel, SACH foot Ⓑ Qp Qh ♿    A

* **L5971** All lower extremity prosthesis, solid ankle cushion keel (SACH) foot, replacement only Ⓑ Qp Qh ♿    A

* **L5972** All lower extremity prostheses (foot, flexible keel) Ⓑ Qp Qh ♿    A

* **L5973** Endoskeletal ankle foot system, microprocessor controlled feature, dorsiflexion and/or plantar flexion control, includes power source Ⓑ Qh ♿    A

* **L5974** All lower extremity prostheses, foot, single axis ankle/foot Ⓑ Qp Qh ♿    A

* **L5975** All lower extremity prostheses, combination single axis ankle and flexible keel foot Ⓑ Qp Qh ♿    A

* **L5976** All lower extremity prostheses, energy storing foot (Seattle Carbon Copy II or equal) Ⓑ Qp Qh ♿    A

* **L5978** All lower extremity prostheses, foot, multiaxial ankle/foot Ⓑ Qp Qh ♿    A

* **L5979** All lower extremity prostheses, multiaxial ankle, dynamic response foot, one piece system Ⓑ Qp Qh ♿    A

* **L5980** All lower extremity prostheses, flex foot system Ⓑ Qp Qh ♿    A

* **L5981** All lower extremity prostheses, flexwalk system or equal Ⓑ Qp Qh ♿    A

* **L5982** All exoskeletal lower extremity prostheses, axial rotation unit Ⓑ Qp Qh ♿    A

* **L5984** All endoskeletal lower extremity prostheses, axial rotation unit, with or without adjustability Ⓑ Qp Qh ♿    A

* **L5985** All endoskeletal lower extremity prostheses, dynamic prosthetic pylon Ⓑ Qp Qh ♿    A

* **L5986** All lower extremity prostheses, multiaxial rotation unit ('MCP' or equal) Ⓑ Qp Qh ♿    A

* **L5987** All lower extremity prostheses, shank foot system with vertical loading pylon Ⓑ Qp Qh ♿    A

* **L5988** Addition to lower limb prosthesis, vertical shock reducing pylon feature Ⓑ Qp Qh ♿    A

* **L5990** Addition to lower extremity prosthesis, user adjustable heel height Ⓑ Qp Qh ♿    A

* **L5999** Lower extremity prosthesis, not otherwise specified Ⓑ    A

### Upper Limb (L6000-L7600)

**NOTE:** The procedures in L6000-L6599 are considered as base or basic procedures and may be modified by listing procedures from the additions sections. The base procedures include only standard friction wrist and control cable system unless otherwise specified.

### Partial Hand

* **L6000** Partial hand, thumb remaining Ⓑ Qp Qh ♿    A

* **L6010** Partial hand, little and/or ring finger remaining Ⓑ Qp Qh ♿    A

* **L6020** Partial hand, no finger remaining Ⓑ Qp Qh ♿    A

* **L6026** Transcarpal/metacarpal or partial hand disarticulation prosthesis, external power, self-suspended, inner socket with removable forearm section, electrodes and cables, two batteries, charger, myoelectric control of terminal device, excludes terminal device(s) Ⓑ Qp Qh ♿    A

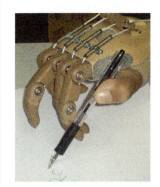

**Figure 39** Partial hand.

— PROSTHETICS L5968 – L6026

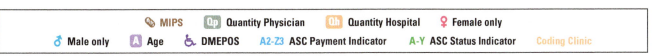

🐾 MIPS   Qp Quantity Physician   Qh Quantity Hospital   ♀ Female only   ♂ Male only   A Age   ♿ DMEPOS   A2-Z3 ASC Payment Indicator   A-Y ASC Status Indicator   Coding Clinic

## Wrist Disarticulation

  ✱ **L6050**   Wrist disarticulation, molded socket, flexible elbow hinges, triceps pad Ⓑ Qp Qh ♿   A

  ✱ **L6055**   Wrist disarticulation, molded socket with expandable interface, flexible elbow hinges, triceps pad Ⓑ Qp Qh ♿   A

## Below Elbow

  ✱ **L6100**   Below elbow, molded socket, flexible elbow hinge, triceps pad Ⓑ Qp Qh ♿   A

  ✱ **L6110**   Below elbow, molded socket, (Muenster or Northwestern suspension types) Ⓑ Qp Qh ♿   A

  ✱ **L6120**   Below elbow, molded double wall split socket, step-up hinges, half cuff Ⓑ Qp Qh ♿   A

  ✱ **L6130**   Below elbow, molded double wall split socket, stump activated locking hinge, half cuff Ⓑ Qp Qh ♿   A

## Elbow Disarticulation

  ✱ **L6200**   Elbow disarticulation, molded socket, outside locking hinge, forearm Ⓑ Qp Qh ♿   A

  ✱ **L6205**   Elbow disarticulation, molded socket with expandable interface, outside locking hinges, forearm Ⓑ Qp Qh ♿   A

## Above Elbow

  ✱ **L6250**   Above elbow, molded double wall socket, internal locking elbow, forearm Ⓑ Qp Qh ♿   A

## Shoulder Disarticulation

  ✱ **L6300**   Shoulder disarticulation, molded socket, shoulder bulkhead, humeral section, internal locking elbow, forearm Ⓑ Qp Qh ♿   A

  ✱ **L6310**   Shoulder disarticulation, passive restoration (complete prosthesis) Ⓑ Qp Qh ♿   A

  ✱ **L6320**   Shoulder disarticulation, passive restoration (shoulder cap only) Ⓑ Qp Qh ♿   A

## Interscapular Thoracic

  ✱ **L6350**   Interscapular thoracic, molded socket, shoulder bulkhead, humeral section, internal locking elbow, forearm Ⓑ Qp Qh ♿   A

  ✱ **L6360**   Interscapular thoracic, passive restoration (complete prosthesis) Ⓑ Qp Qh ♿   A

  ✱ **L6370**   Interscapular thoracic, passive restoration (shoulder cap only) Ⓑ Qp Qh ♿   A

## Immediate and Early Postsurgical Procedures

  ✱ **L6380**   Immediate post surgical or early fitting, application of initial rigid dressing, including fitting alignment and suspension of components, and one cast change, wrist disarticulation or below elbow Ⓑ Qp Qh ♿   A

  ✱ **L6382**   Immediate post surgical or early fitting, application of initial rigid dressing including fitting alignment and suspension of components, and one cast change, elbow disarticulation or above elbow Ⓑ Qp Qh ♿   A

  ✱ **L6384**   Immediate post surgical or early fitting, application of initial rigid dressing including fitting alignment and suspension of components, and one cast change, shoulder disarticulation or interscapular thoracic Ⓑ Qp Qh ♿ A

  ✱ **L6386**   Immediate post surgical or early fitting, each additional cast change and realignment Ⓑ Qp Qh ♿   A

  ✱ **L6388**   Immediate post surgical or early fitting, application of rigid dressing only Ⓑ Qp Qh ♿   A

## Molded Socket

  ✱ **L6400**   Below elbow, molded socket, endoskeletal system, including soft prosthetic tissue shaping Ⓑ Qp Qh ♿   A

  ✱ **L6450**   Elbow disarticulation, molded socket, endoskeletal system, including soft prosthetic tissue shaping Ⓑ Qp Qh ♿   A

  ✱ **L6500**   Above elbow, molded socket, endoskeletal system, including soft prosthetic tissue shaping Ⓑ Qp Qh ♿   A

  ✱ **L6550**   Shoulder disarticulation, molded socket, endoskeletal system, including soft prosthetic tissue shaping Ⓑ Qp Qh ♿   A

  ✱ **L6570**   Interscapular thoracic, molded socket, endoskeletal system, including soft prosthetic tissue shaping Ⓑ Qp Qh ♿   A

---

▶ New    ↻ Revised    ✔ Reinstated    ~~deleted~~ Deleted    ⊘ Not covered or valid by Medicare

⊛ Special coverage instructions    ✱ Carrier discretion    Ⓑ Bill Part B MAC    Ⓑ Bill DME MAC

## Preparatory Prosthetic

**\* L6580** Preparatory, wrist disarticulation or below elbow, single wall plastic socket, friction wrist, flexible elbow hinges, figure of eight harness, humeral cuff, Bowden cable control, USMC or equal pylon, no cover, molded to patient model Ⓑ Ⓠp Ⓠh ♿   A

**\* L6582** Preparatory, wrist disarticulation or below elbow, single wall socket, friction wrist, flexible elbow hinges, figure of eight harness, humeral cuff, Bowden cable control, USMC or equal pylon, no cover, direct formed Ⓑ Ⓠp Ⓠh ♿   A

**\* L6584** Preparatory, elbow disarticulation or above elbow, single wall plastic socket, friction wrist, locking elbow, figure of eight harness, fair lead cable control, USMC or equal pylon, no cover, molded to patient model Ⓑ Ⓠp Ⓠh ♿   A

**\* L6586** Preparatory, elbow disarticulation or above elbow, single wall socket, friction wrist, locking elbow, figure of eight harness, fair lead cable control, USMC or equal pylon, no cover, direct formed Ⓑ Ⓠp Ⓠh ♿   A

**\* L6588** Preparatory, shoulder disarticulation or interscapular thoracic, single wall plastic socket, shoulder joint, locking elbow, friction wrist, chest strap, fair lead cable control, USMC or equal pylon, no cover, molded to patient model Ⓑ Ⓠp Ⓠh ♿   A

**\* L6590** Preparatory, shoulder disarticulation or interscapular thoracic, single wall socket, shoulder joint, locking elbow, friction wrist, chest strap, fair lead cable control, USMC or equal pylon, no cover, direct formed Ⓑ Ⓠp Ⓠh ♿   A

## Additions to Upper Limb

**NOTE:** The following procedures/modifications/components may be added to other base procedures. The items in this section should reflect the additional complexity of each modification procedure, in addition to base procedure, at the time of the original order.

**\* L6600** Upper extremity additions, polycentric hinge, pair Ⓑ Ⓠp Ⓠh ♿   A

**\* L6605** Upper extremity additions, single pivot hinge, pair Ⓑ Ⓠp Ⓠh ♿   A

**\* L6610** Upper extremity additions, flexible metal hinge, pair Ⓑ Ⓠp Ⓠh ♿   A

**\* L6611** Addition to upper extremity prosthesis, external powered, additional switch, any type Ⓑ Ⓠp Ⓠh ♿   A

**\* L6615** Upper extremity addition, disconnect locking wrist unit Ⓑ Ⓠp Ⓠh ♿   A

**\* L6616** Upper extremity addition, additional disconnect insert for locking wrist unit, each Ⓑ Ⓠp Ⓠh ♿   A

**\* L6620** Upper extremity addition, flexion/extension wrist unit, with or without friction Ⓑ Ⓠp Ⓠh ♿   A

**\* L6621** Upper extremity prosthesis addition, flexion/extension wrist with or without friction, for use with external powered terminal device Ⓑ Ⓠp Ⓠh ♿   A

**\* L6623** Upper extremity addition, spring assisted rotational wrist unit with latch release Ⓑ Ⓠp Ⓠh ♿   A

**\* L6624** Upper extremity addition, flexion/extension and rotation wrist unit Ⓑ Ⓠp Ⓠh ♿   A

**\* L6625** Upper extremity addition, rotation wrist unit with cable lock Ⓑ Ⓠp Ⓠh ♿   A

**\* L6628** Upper extremity addition, quick disconnect hook adapter, Otto Bock or equal Ⓑ Ⓠp Ⓠh ♿   A

**\* L6629** Upper extremity addition, quick disconnect lamination collar with coupling piece, Otto Bock or equal Ⓑ Ⓠp Ⓠh ♿   A

**\* L6630** Upper extremity addition, stainless steel, any wrist Ⓑ Ⓠp Ⓠh ♿   A

**\* L6632** Upper extremity addition, latex suspension sleeve, each Ⓑ Ⓠp ♿   A

**\* L6635** Upper extremity addition, lift assist for elbow Ⓑ Ⓠp Ⓠh ♿   A

**\* L6637** Upper extremity addition, nudge control elbow lock Ⓑ Ⓠp Ⓠh ♿   A

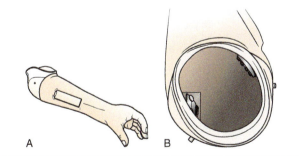

**Figure 40** Upper extremity addition.

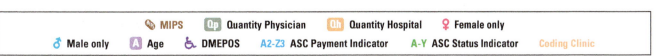

🪶 MIPS    Ⓠp Quantity Physician    Ⓠh Quantity Hospital    ♀ Female only

♂ Male only    Ⓐ Age    ♿ DMEPOS    A2-Z3 ASC Payment Indicator    A-Y ASC Status Indicator    Coding Clinic

* **L6638** Upper extremity addition to prosthesis, electric locking feature, only for use with manually powered elbow Ⓑ Qp Qh ♿    A

* **L6640** Upper extremity additions, shoulder abduction joint, pair Ⓑ Qp Qh ♿    A

* **L6641** Upper extremity addition, excursion amplifier, pulley type Ⓑ Qp Qh ♿    A

* **L6642** Upper extremity addition, excursion amplifier, lever type Ⓑ Qp Qh ♿    A

* **L6645** Upper extremity addition, shoulder flexion-abduction joint, each Ⓑ Qp Qh ♿    A

* **L6646** Upper extremity addition, shoulder joint, multipositional locking, flexion, adjustable abduction friction control, for use with body powered or external powered system Ⓑ Qp Qh ♿    A

* **L6647** Upper extremity addition, shoulder lock mechanism, body powered actuator Ⓑ Qp Qh ♿    A

* **L6648** Upper extremity addition, shoulder lock mechanism, external powered actuator Ⓑ Qp Qh ♿    A

* **L6650** Upper extremity addition, shoulder universal joint, each Ⓑ Qp Qh ♿    A

* **L6655** Upper extremity addition, standard control cable, extra Ⓑ Qp ♿    A

* **L6660** Upper extremity addition, heavy duty control cable Ⓑ Qp ♿    A

* **L6665** Upper extremity addition, Teflon, or equal, cable lining Ⓑ Qp ♿    A

* **L6670** Upper extremity addition, hook to hand, cable adapter Ⓑ Qp Qh ♿    A

* **L6672** Upper extremity addition, harness, chest or shoulder, saddle type Ⓑ Qp Qh ♿    A

* **L6675** Upper extremity addition, harness, (e.g., figure of eight type), single cable design Ⓑ Qp Qh ♿    A

* **L6676** Upper extremity addition, harness, (e.g., figure of eight type), dual cable design Ⓑ Qp Qh ♿    A

* **L6677** Upper extremity addition, harness, triple control, simultaneous operation of terminal device and elbow Ⓑ Qp Qh ♿    A

* **L6680** Upper extremity addition, test socket, wrist disarticulation or below elbow Ⓑ Qp ♿    A

* **L6682** Upper extremity addition, test socket, elbow disarticulation or above elbow Ⓑ Qp ♿    A

* **L6684** Upper extremity addition, test socket, shoulder disarticulation or interscapular thoracic Ⓑ Qp ♿    A

* **L6686** Upper extremity addition, suction socket Ⓑ Qp Qh ♿    A

* **L6687** Upper extremity addition, frame type socket, below elbow or wrist disarticulation Ⓑ Qp Qh ♿    A

* **L6688** Upper extremity addition, frame type socket, above elbow or elbow disarticulation Ⓑ Qp Qh ♿    A

* **L6689** Upper extremity addition, frame type socket, shoulder disarticulation Ⓑ Qp Qh ♿    A

* **L6690** Upper extremity addition, frame type socket, interscapular-thoracic Ⓑ Qp Qh ♿    A

* **L6691** Upper extremity addition, removable insert, each Ⓑ Qp ♿    A

* **L6692** Upper extremity addition, silicone gel insert or equal, each Ⓑ Qp ♿    A

* **L6693** Upper extremity addition, locking elbow, forearm counterbalance Ⓑ Qp Qh ♿    A

* **L6694** Addition to upper extremity prosthesis, below elbow/above elbow, custom fabricated from existing mold or prefabricated, socket insert, silicone gel, elastomeric or equal, for use with locking mechanism Ⓑ Qp Qh ♿    A

* **L6695** Addition to upper extremity prosthesis, below elbow/above elbow, custom fabricated from existing mold or prefabricated, socket insert, silicone gel, elastomeric or equal, not for use with locking mechanism Ⓑ Qp Qh ♿    A

* **L6696** Addition to upper extremity prosthesis, below elbow/above elbow, custom fabricated socket insert for congenital or atypical traumatic amputee, silicone gel, elastomeric or equal, for use with or without locking mechanism, initial only (for other than initial, use code L6694 or L6695) Ⓑ Qp Qh ♿    A

* **L6697** Addition to upper extremity prosthesis, below elbow/above elbow, custom fabricated socket insert for other than congenital or atypical traumatic amputee, silicone gel, elastomeric or equal, for use with or without locking mechanism, initial only (for other than initial, use code L6694 or L6695) Ⓑ Qp Qh ♿    A

* **L6698** Addition to upper extremity prosthesis, below elbow/above elbow, lock mechanism, excludes socket insert Ⓑ Qp Qh ♿    A

---

▶ New   ↻ Revised   ✔ Reinstated   ~~deleted~~ Deleted   ⊘ Not covered or valid by Medicare
✪ Special coverage instructions   ✳ Carrier discretion   Ⓑ Bill Part B MAC   Ⓓ Bill DME MAC

## Terminal Devices (L6703-L6882)

✳ **L6703**  Terminal device, passive hand/mitt, any material, any size Ⓑ Qp Qh ♿     A

✳ **L6704**  Terminal device, sport/recreational/work attachment, any material, any size Ⓑ Qp Qh ♿     A

✳ **L6706**  Terminal device, hook, mechanical, voluntary opening, any material, any size, lined or unlined Ⓑ Qp Qh ♿     A

✳ **L6707**  Terminal device, hook, mechanical, voluntary closing, any material, any size, lined or unlined Ⓑ Qp Qh ♿     A

✳ **L6708**  Terminal device, hand, mechanical, voluntary opening, any material, any size Ⓑ Qp Qh ♿     A

✳ **L6709**  Terminal device, hand, mechanical, voluntary closing, any material, any size Ⓑ Qp Qh ♿     A

✳ **L6711**  Terminal device, hook, mechanical, voluntary opening, any material, any size, lined or unlined, pediatric Ⓑ Qp Qh A ♿     A

✳ **L6712**  Terminal device, hook, mechanical, voluntary closing, any material, any size, lined or unlined, pediatric Ⓑ Qp Qh A ♿     A

✳ **L6713**  Terminal device, hand, mechanical, voluntary opening, any material, any size, pediatric Ⓑ Qp Qh A ♿     A

✳ **L6714**  Terminal device, hand, mechanical, voluntary closing, any material, any size, pediatric Ⓑ Qp Qh A ♿     A

✳ **L6715**  Terminal device, multiple articulating digit, includes motor(s), initial issue or replacement Ⓑ Qp Qh ♿     A

✳ **L6721**  Terminal device, hook or hand, heavy duty, mechanical, voluntary opening, any material, any size, lined or unlined Ⓑ Qp Qh ♿     A

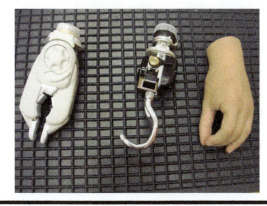

**Figure 41**   Terminal devices, hand and hook.

✳ **L6722**  Terminal device, hook or hand, heavy duty, mechanical, voluntary closing, any material, any size, lined or unlined Ⓑ Qp Qh ♿     A

❂ **L6805**  Addition to terminal device, modifier wrist unit Ⓑ Qp Qh ♿     A

    *IOM: 100-02, 15, 120; 100-04, 3, 10.4*

❂ **L6810**  Addition to terminal device, precision pinch device Ⓑ Qp Qh ♿     A

    *IOM: 100-02, 15, 120; 100-04, 3, 10.4*

✳ **L6880**  Electric hand, switch or myoelectric controlled, independently articulating digits, any grasp pattern or combination of grasp patterns, includes motor(s) Ⓑ Qp Qh ♿     A

✳ **L6881**  Automatic grasp feature, addition to upper limb electric prosthetic terminal device Ⓑ Qp Qh ♿     A

❂ **L6882**  Microprocessor control feature, addition to upper limb prosthetic terminal device Ⓑ Qp Qh ♿     A

    *IOM: 100-02, 15, 120; 100-04, 3, 10.4*

## Replacement Sockets

✳ **L6883**  Replacement socket, below elbow/wrist disarticulation, molded to patient model, for use with or without external power Ⓑ Qp Qh ♿     A

✳ **L6884**  Replacement socket, above elbow/elbow disarticulation, molded to patient model, for use with or without external power Ⓑ Qp Qh ♿     A

✳ **L6885**  Replacement socket, shoulder disarticulation/interscapular thoracic, molded to patient model, for use with or without external power Ⓑ Qp Qh ♿     A

## Hand Restoration

✳ **L6890**  Addition to upper extremity prosthesis, glove for terminal device, any material, prefabricated, includes fitting and adjustment Ⓑ Qp Qh ♿     A

✳ **L6895**  Addition to upper extremity prosthesis, glove for terminal device, any material, custom fabricated Ⓑ Qp Qh ♿     A

✳ **L6900**  Hand restoration (casts, shading and measurements included), partial hand, with glove, thumb or one finger remaining Ⓑ Qp Qh ♿     A

✳ **L6905**  Hand restoration (casts, shading and measurements included), partial hand, with glove, multiple fingers remaining Ⓑ Qp Qh ♿     A

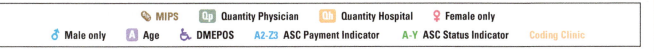

🔖 MIPS    Qp Quantity Physician    Qh Quantity Hospital    ♀ Female only    ♂ Male only    A Age    ♿ DMEPOS    A2-Z3 ASC Payment Indicator    A-Y ASC Status Indicator    Coding Clinic

**\* L6910** Hand restoration (casts, shading and measurements included), partial hand, with glove, no fingers remaining Ⓑ 🟢Qp 🟠Qh ♿    A

**\* L6915** Hand restoration (shading, and measurements included), replacement glove for above Ⓑ 🟢Qp 🟠Qh ♿    A

## External Power

**\* L6920** Wrist disarticulation, external power, self-suspended inner socket, removable forearm shell, Otto Bock or equal switch, cables, two batteries and one charger, switch control of terminal device Ⓑ 🟢Qp 🟠Qh ♿    A

**\* L6925** Wrist disarticulation, external power, self-suspended inner socket, removable forearm shell, Otto Bock or equal electrodes, cables, two batteries and one charger, myoelectronic control of terminal device Ⓑ 🟢Qp 🟠Qh ♿    A

**\* L6930** Below elbow, external power, self-suspended inner socket, removable forearm shell, Otto Bock or equal switch, cables, two batteries and one charger, switch control of terminal device Ⓑ 🟢Qp 🟠Qh ♿    A

**\* L6935** Below elbow, external power, self-suspended inner socket, removable forearm shell, Otto Bock or equal electrodes, cables, two batteries and one charger, myoelectronic control of terminal device Ⓑ 🟢Qp 🟠Qh ♿    A

**\* L6940** Elbow disarticulation, external power, molded inner socket, removable humeral shell, outside locking hinges, forearm, Otto Bock or equal switch, cables, two batteries and one charger, switch control of terminal device Ⓑ 🟢Qp 🟠Qh ♿    A

**\* L6945** Elbow disarticulation, external power, molded inner socket, removable humeral shell, outside locking hinges, forearm, Otto Bock or equal electrodes, cables, two batteries and one charger, myoelectronic control of terminal device Ⓑ 🟢Qp 🟠Qh ♿    A

**\* L6950** Above elbow, external power, molded inner socket, removable humeral shell, internal locking elbow, forearm, Otto Bock or equal switch, cables, two batteries and one charger, switch control of terminal device Ⓑ 🟢Qp 🟠Qh ♿    A

**\* L6955** Above elbow, external power, molded inner socket, removable humeral shell, internal locking elbow, forearm, Otto Bock or equal electrodes, cables, two batteries and one charger, myoelectronic control of terminal device Ⓑ 🟢Qp 🟠Qh ♿    A

**\* L6960** Shoulder disarticulation, external power, molded inner socket, removable shoulder shell, shoulder bulkhead, humeral section, mechanical elbow, forearm, Otto Bock or equal switch, cables, two batteries and one charger, switch control of terminal device Ⓑ 🟢Qp 🟠Qh ♿    A

**\* L6965** Shoulder disarticulation, external power, molded inner socket, removable shoulder shell, shoulder bulkhead, humeral section, mechanical elbow, forearm, Otto Bock or equal electrodes, cables, two batteries and one charger, myoelectronic control of terminal device Ⓑ 🟢Qp 🟠Qh ♿    A

**\* L6970** Interscapular-thoracic, external power, molded inner socket, removable shoulder shell, shoulder bulkhead, humeral section, mechanical elbow, forearm, Otto Bock or equal switch, cables, two batteries and one charger, switch control of terminal device Ⓑ 🟢Qp 🟠Qh ♿    A

**\* L6975** Interscapular-thoracic, external power, molded inner socket, removable shoulder shell, shoulder bulkhead, humeral section, mechanical elbow, forearm, Otto Bock or equal electrodes, cables, two batteries and one charger, myoelectronic control of terminal device Ⓑ 🟢Qp 🟠Qh ♿    A

## Additions to Electronic Hand or Hook

**\* L7007** Electric hand, switch or myoelectric controlled, adult Ⓑ 🟢Qp 🟠Qh 🟣A ♿    A

**\* L7008** Electric hand, switch or myoelectric controlled, pediatric Ⓑ 🟢Qp 🟠Qh 🟣A ♿    A

**\* L7009** Electric hook, switch or myoelectric controlled, adult Ⓑ 🟢Qp 🟠Qh 🟣A ♿    A

**\* L7040** Prehensile actuator, switch controlled Ⓑ 🟢Qp 🟠Qh ♿    A

**\* L7045** Electric hook, switch or myoelectric controlled, pediatric Ⓑ 🟢Qp 🟠Qh 🟣A ♿    A

---

▶ New    ↻ Revised    ✔ Reinstated    ~~deleted~~ Deleted    ⊘ Not covered or valid by Medicare
⊙ Special coverage instructions    \* Carrier discretion    Ⓑ Bill Part B MAC    Ⓑ Bill DME MAC

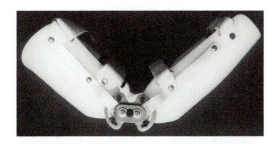

**Figure 42** Electronic elbow.

## Additions to Electronic Elbow

* **L7170** Electronic elbow, Hosmer or equal, switch controlled ⓑ 🅠p 🅠h 🔧    A

* **L7180** Electronic elbow, microprocessor sequential control of elbow and terminal device ⓑ 🅠p 🅠h ♿    A

* **L7181** Electronic elbow, microprocessor simultaneous control of elbow and terminal device ⓑ 🅠p 🅠h ♿    A

* **L7185** Electronic elbow, adolescent, Variety Village or equal, switch controlled ⓑ 🅠p 🅠h 🔧    A

* **L7186** Electronic elbow, child, Variety Village or equal, switch controlled ⓑ 🅠p 🅠h Ⓐ ♿    A

* **L7190** Electronic elbow, adolescent, Variety Village or equal, myoelectronically controlled ⓑ 🅠p 🅠h ♿    A

* **L7191** Electronic elbow, child, Variety Village or equal, myoelectronically controlled ⓑ 🅠p 🅠h Ⓐ ♿    A

## Wrist

* **L7259** Electronic wrist rotator, any type ⓑ 🅠p 🅠h 🔧    A

## Battery Components

* **L7360** Six volt battery, each ⓑ 🅠p 🔧    A

* **L7362** Battery charger, six volt, each ⓑ 🅠p 🅠h ♿    A

* **L7364** Twelve volt battery, each ⓑ 🅠p 🔧    A

* **L7366** Battery charger, twelve volt, each ⓑ 🅠p 🅠h ♿    A

* **L7367** Lithium ion battery, rechargeable, replacement ⓑ 🅠p 🔧    A

* **L7368** Lithium ion battery charger, replacement only ⓑ 🅠p 🅠h ♿    A

## Additions

* **L7400** Addition to upper extremity prosthesis, below elbow/wrist disarticulation, ultralight material (titanium, carbon fiber or equal) ⓑ 🅠p 🅠h 🔧    A

* **L7401** Addition to upper extremity prosthesis, above elbow disarticulation, ultralight material (titanium, carbon fiber or equal) ⓑ 🅠p 🅠h 🔧    A

* **L7402** Addition to upper extremity prosthesis, shoulder disarticulation/interscapular thoracic, ultralight material (titanium, carbon fiber or equal) ⓑ 🅠p 🅠h 🔧    A

* **L7403** Addition to upper extremity prosthesis, below elbow/wrist disarticulation, acrylic material ⓑ 🅠p 🅠h 🔧    A

* **L7404** Addition to upper extremity prosthesis, above elbow disarticulation, acrylic material ⓑ 🅠p 🅠h 🔧    A

* **L7405** Addition to upper extremity prosthesis, shoulder disarticulation/interscapular thoracic, acrylic material ⓑ 🅠p 🅠h 🔧    A

## Other/Repair

* **L7499** Upper extremity prosthesis, not otherwise specified ⓑ    A

✪ **L7510** Repair of prosthetic device, repair or replace minor parts 🅟 ⓑ 🅠p 🅠h    A

*IOM: 100-02, 15, 110.2; 100-02, 15, 120; 100-04, 32, 100*

* **L7520** Repair prosthetic device, labor component, per 15 minutes 🅟 ⓑ    A

⊘ **L7600** Prosthetic donning sleeve, any material, each ⓑ    E1

*Medicare Statute 1862(1)(a)*

## General

### Prosthetic Socket Insert

* **L7700** Gasket or seal, for use with prosthetic socket insert, any type, each    A

### Penile Prosthetics

⊘ **L7900** Male vacuum erection system ⓑ 🅠p 🅠h ♂    E1

*Medicare Statute 1834a*

⊘ **L7902** Tension ring, for vacuum erection device, any type, replacement only, each ⓑ 🅠p 🅠h    E1

*Medicare Statute 1834a*

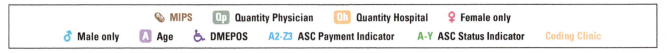

🐌 MIPS   🅠p Quantity Physician   🅠h Quantity Hospital   ♀ Female only   ♂ Male only   Ⓐ Age   🔧 DMEPOS   A2-Z3 ASC Payment Indicator   A-Y ASC Status Indicator   Coding Clinic

## Breast Prosthetics

⚙ **L8000** Breast prosthesis, mastectomy bra, without integrated breast prosthesis form, any size, any type Ⓑ Qp ♀ ⚕  A

*IOM: 100-02, 15, 120*

⚙ **L8001** Breast prosthesis, mastectomy bra, with integrated breast prosthesis form, unilateral, any size, any type Ⓑ Qp ♀ ⚕  A

*IOM: 100-02, 15, 120*

⚙ **L8002** Breast prosthesis, mastectomy bra, with integrated breast prosthesis form, bilateral, any size, any type Ⓑ Qp ♀ ⚕  A

*IOM: 100-02, 15, 120*

⚙ **L8010** Breast prosthesis, mastectomy sleeve Ⓑ ♀  A

*IOM: 100-02, 15, 120*

⚙ **L8015** External breast prosthesis garment, with mastectomy form, post mastectomy Ⓑ Qp ♀ ⚕  A

*IOM: 100-02, 15, 120*

⚙ **L8020** Breast prosthesis, mastectomy form Ⓑ Qp ♀ ⚕  A

*IOM: 100-02, 15, 120*

⚙ **L8030** Breast prosthesis, silicone or equal, without integral adhesive Ⓑ Qp Qh ♀ ⚕  A

*IOM: 100-02, 15, 120*

⚙ **L8031** Breast prosthesis, silicone or equal, with integral adhesive Ⓑ Qp Qh ⚕  A

*IOM: 100-02, 15, 120*

↻ ✱ **L8032** Nipple prosthesis, prefabricated, reusable, any type, each Ⓑ Qp Qh ⚕  A

▶ ✱ **L8033** Nipple prosthesis, custom fabricated, reusable, any material, any type, each  A

⚙ **L8035** Custom breast prosthesis, post mastectomy, molded to patient model Ⓑ Qp Qh ♀ ⚕  A

*IOM: 100-02, 15, 120*

✱ **L8039** Breast prosthesis, not otherwise specified Ⓑ Qp Qh ♀  A

## Nasal, Orbital, Auricular Prostherics

✱ **L8040** Nasal prosthesis, provided by a non-physician Ⓑ Qp Qh ⚕  A

✱ **L8041** Midfacial prosthesis, provided by a non-physician Ⓑ Qp Qh ⚕  A

✱ **L8042** Orbital prosthesis, provided by a non-physician Ⓑ Qp Qh ⚕  A

✱ **L8043** Upper facial prosthesis, provided by a non-physician Ⓑ Qp Qh ⚕  A

✱ **L8044** Hemi-facial prosthesis, provided by a non-physician Ⓑ Qp Qh ⚕  A

✱ **L8045** Auricular prosthesis, provided by a non-physician Ⓑ Qp Qh ⚕  A

✱ **L8046** Partial facial prosthesis, provided by a non-physician Ⓑ Qp Qh ⚕  A

✱ **L8047** Nasal septal prosthesis, provided by a non-physician Ⓑ Qp Qh ⚕  A

✱ **L8048** Unspecified maxillofacial prosthesis, by report, provided by a non-physician Ⓑ Qp Qh  A

✱ **L8049** Repair or modification of maxillofacial prosthesis, labor component, 15 minute increments, provided by a non-physician Ⓑ Qp  A

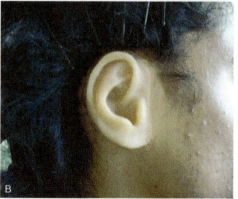
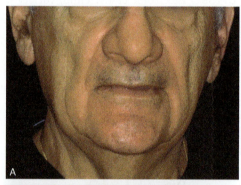

**Figure 44** (A) Nasal prosthesis, (B) Auricular prosthesis.

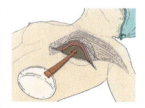

**Figure 43** Implant breast prosthesis.

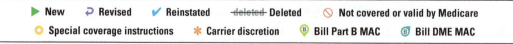

▶ New  ↻ Revised  ✔ Reinstated  ~~deleted~~ Deleted  ⊘ Not covered or valid by Medicare
⚙ Special coverage instructions  ✱ Carrier discretion  Ⓑ Bill Part B MAC  Ⓑ Bill DME MAC

## Trusses

⚙ **L8300**  Truss, single with standard pad Ⓑ Qp Qh ♿  A

*IOM: 100-02, 15, 120; 100-03, 4, 280.11; 100-03, 4, 280.12; 100-04, 4, 240*

⚙ **L8310**  Truss, double with standard pads Ⓑ Qp Qh  A

*IOM: 100-02, 15, 120; 100-03, 4, 280.11; 100-03, 4, 280.12; 100-04, 4, 240*

⚙ **L8320**  Truss, addition to standard pad, water pad Ⓑ Qp Qh ♿  A

*IOM: 100-02, 15, 120; 100-03, 4, 280.11; 100-03, 4, 280.12; 100-04, 4, 240*

⚙ **L8330**  Truss, addition to standard pad, scrotal pad Ⓑ Qp Qh ♂ ♿  A

*IOM: 100-02, 15, 120; 100-03, 4, 280.11; 100-03, 4, 280.12; 100-04, 4, 240*

## Prosthetic Socks

⚙ **L8400**  Prosthetic sheath, below knee, each Ⓑ Qp ♿  A

*IOM: 100-02, 15, 200*

⚙ **L8410**  Prosthetic sheath, above knee, each Ⓑ Qp  A

*IOM: 100-02, 15, 200*

⚙ **L8415**  Prosthetic sheath, upper limb, each Ⓑ Qp ♿  A

*IOM: 100-02, 15, 200*

✳ **L8417**  Prosthetic sheath/sock, including a gel cushion layer, below knee or above knee, each Ⓖ Qp ♿  A

⚙ **L8420**  Prosthetic sock, multiple ply, below knee, each Ⓑ Qp ♿  A

*IOM: 100-02, 15, 200*

⚙ **L8430**  Prosthetic sock, multiple ply, above knee, each Ⓑ Qp ♿  A

*IOM: 100-02, 15, 200*

⚙ **L8435**  Prosthetic sock, multiple ply, upper limb, each Ⓑ Qp ♿  A

*IOM: 100-02, 15, 200*

⚙ **L8440**  Prosthetic shrinker, below knee, each Ⓖ Qp ♿  A

*IOM: 100-02, 15, 200*

⚙ **L8460**  Prosthetic shrinker, above knee, each Ⓑ Qp ♿  A

*IOM: 100-02, 15, 200*

⚙ **L8465**  Prosthetic shrinker, upper limb, each Qp ♿  A

*IOM: 100-02, 15, 200*

⚙ **L8470**  Prosthetic sock, single ply, fitting, below knee, each Ⓑ Qp ♿  A

*IOM: 100-02, 15, 200*

⚙ **L8480**  Prosthetic sock, single ply, fitting, above knee, each Ⓑ Qp ♿  A

*IOM: 100-02, 15, 200*

⚙ **L8485**  Prosthetic sock, single ply, fitting, upper limb, each Ⓑ Qp ♿  A

*IOM: 100-02, 15, 200*

## Unlisted

✳ **L8499**  Unlisted procedure for miscellaneous prosthetic services Ⓥ Ⓑ  A

## Prosthetic Implants (L8500-L9900)

## Larynx, Tracheoesophageal

⚙ **L8500**  Artificial larynx, any type Ⓖ Qp Qh ♿  A

*IOM: 100-02, 15, 120; 100-03, 1, 50.2; 100-04, 4, 240*

⚙ **L8501**  Tracheostomy speaking valve Ⓖ Qp Qh  A

*IOM: 100-03, 1, 50.4*

✳ **L8505**  Artificial larynx replacement battery/accessory, any type Ⓑ  A

✳ **L8507**  Tracheo-esophageal voice prosthesis, patient inserted, any type, each Ⓖ Qp Qh ♿  A

✳ **L8509**  Tracheo-esophageal voice prosthesis, inserted by a licensed health care provider, any type Ⓥ Ⓖ Qp Qh ♿  A

⚙ **L8510**  Voice amplifier Ⓖ Qp Qh ♿  A

*IOM: 100-03, 1, 50.2*

✳ **L8511**  Insert for indwelling tracheoesophageal prosthesis, with or without valve, replacement only, each Ⓥ Ⓑ Qp Qh  A

✳ **L8512**  Gelatin capsules or equivalent, for use with tracheoesophageal voice prosthesis, replacement only, per 10 Ⓥ Ⓖ ♿  A

✳ **L8513**  Cleaning device used with tracheoesophageal voice prosthesis, pipet, brush, or equal, replacement only, each Ⓥ Ⓖ ♿  A

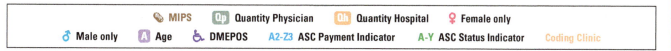

✳ **L8514** Tracheoesophageal puncture dilator, replacement only, each Ⓑ Ⓓ Qp Qh 🦽     A

✳ **L8515** Gelatin capsule, application device for use with tracheoesophageal voice prosthesis, each Ⓑ Ⓓ Qp Qh 🦽    A

## Breast

⚙ **L8600** Implantable breast prosthesis, silicone or equal Ⓑ Qp Qh ♀ 🦽    N1   N

*IOM: 100-02, 15, 120; 100-3, 2, 140.2*

## Bulking Agents

⚙ **L8603** Injectable bulking agent, collagen implant, urinary tract, 2.5 ml syringe, includes shipping and necessary supplies Ⓑ 🦽    N1   N

Bill on paper, acquisition cost invoice required

*IOM: 100-03, 4, 280.1*

✳ **L8604** Injectable bulking agent, dextranomer/hyaluronic acid copolymer implant, urinary tract, 1 ml, includes shipping and necessary supplies ⦿ Qp Qh   N1   N

✳ **L8605** Injectable bulking agent, dextranomer/hyaluronic acid copolymer implant, anal canal, 1 ml, includes shipping and necessary supplies Ⓑ Qp Qh 🦽   N1   N

⚙ **L8606** Injectable bulking agent, synthetic implant, urinary tract, 1 ml syringe, includes shipping and necessary supplies Ⓑ Qp Qh 🦽    N1   N

Bill on paper, acquisition cost invoice required

*IOM: 100-03, 4, 280.1*

⚙ **L8607** Injectable bulking agent for vocal cord medialization, 0.1 ml, includes shipping and necessary supplies Ⓑ Qp Qh 🦽    N1   N

*IOM: 100-03, 4, 280.1*

## Eye and Ear

✳ **L8608** Miscellaneous external component, supply or accessory for use with the Argus II retinal prosthesis system    N

✳ **L8609** Artificial cornea Ⓑ Qp Qh 🦽   N1   N

⚙ **L8610** Ocular implant Ⓑ Qp Qh 🦽   N1   N

*IOM: 100-02, 15, 120*

⚙ **L8612** Aqueous shunt Ⓑ Qp Qh 🦽   N1   N

*IOM: 100-02, 15, 120*

*Cross Reference Q0074*

⚙ **L8613** Ossicula implant ⦿ Qp Qh 🦽   N1   N

*IOM: 100-02, 15, 120*

⚙ **L8614** Cochlear device, includes all internal and external components Ⓑ Qp Qh 🦽    N1   N

*IOM: 100-02, 15, 120; 100-03, 1, 50.3*

⚙ **L8615** Headset/headpiece for use with cochlear implant device, replacement Ⓑ Qp Qh 🦽    A

*IOM: 100-03, 1, 50.3*

⚙ **L8616** Microphone for use with cochlear implant device, replacement Ⓑ Qp Qh 🦽    A

*IOM: 100-03, 1, 50.3*

⚙ **L8617** Transmitting coil for use with cochlear implant device, replacement Ⓑ Qp Qh 🦽    A

*IOM: 100-03, 1, 50.3*

⚙ **L8618** Transmitter cable for use with cochlear implant device or auditory osseointegrated device, replacement Ⓑ Qp Qh 🦽    A

*IOM: 100-03, 1, 50.3*

⚙ **L8619** Cochlear implant, external speech processor and controller, integrated system, replacement Ⓓ Qp Qh 🦽    A

*IOM: 100-03, 1, 50.3*

✳ **L8621** Zinc air battery for use with cochlear implant device and auditory osseointegrated sound processors, replacement, each Ⓑ Qp Qh 🦽    A

✳ **L8622** Alkaline battery for use with cochlear implant device, any size, replacement, each Ⓑ Qp Qh 🦽    A

✳ **L8623** Lithium ion battery for use with cochlear implant device speech processor, other than ear level, replacement, each Ⓓ 🦽    A

✳ **L8624** Lithium ion battery for use with cochlear implant or auditory osseointegrated device speech processor, ear level, replacement, each Ⓓ 🦽    A

⚙ **L8625** External recharging system for battery for use with cochlear implant or auditory osseointegrated device, replacement only, each    A

*IOM: 103-03, PART 1, 50.3*

⚙ **L8627** Cochlear implant, external speech processor, component, replacement Ⓑ Qp Qh 🦽    A

*IOM: 103-03, PART 1, 50.3*

⚙ **L8628** Cochlear implant, external controller component, replacement Ⓑ Qp Qh 🦽    A

*IOM: 103-03, PART 1, 50.3*

---

▶ New    ⟳ Revised    ✔ Reinstated    ~~deleted~~ Deleted    ⊘ Not covered or valid by Medicare

⚙ Special coverage instructions    ✳ Carrier discretion    Ⓑ Bill Part B MAC    Ⓓ Bill DME MAC

○ **L8629** Transmitting coil and cable, integrated, for use with cochlear implant device, replacement ⊕ Qp Qh ♿      A

*IOM: 103-03, PART 1, 50.3*

## Hand and Foot

○ **L8630** Metacarpophalangeal joint implant Ⓑ ♿      N1   N

*IOM: 100-02, 15, 120*

○ **L8631** Metacarpal phalangeal joint replacement, two or more pieces, metal (e.g., stainless steel or cobalt chrome), ceramic-like material (e.g., pyrocarbon), for surgical implantation (all sizes, includes entire system) Ⓑ Qp Qh ♿    N1   N

*IOM: 100-02, 15, 120*

○ **L8641** Metatarsal joint implant Ⓑ Qp Qh ♿     N1   N

*IOM: 100-02, 15, 120*

○ **L8642** Hallux implant ⊕ Qp Qh ♿    N1   N

May be billed by ambulatory surgical center or surgeon

*IOM: 100-02, 15, 120*

*Cross Reference Q0073*

○ **L8658** Interphalangeal joint spacer, silicone or equal, each Ⓑ Qp Qh ♿    N1   N

*IOM: 100-02, 15, 120*

○ **L8659** Interphalangeal finger joint replacement, 2 or more pieces, metal (e.g., stainless steel or cobalt chrome), ceramic-like material (e.g., pyrocarbon) for surgical implantation, any size Ⓑ Qp Qh ♿    N1   N

*IOM: 100-02, 15, 120*

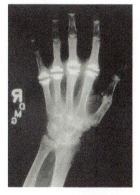

**Figure 45** Metacarpophalangeal implant.

## Vascular

○ **L8670** Vascular graft material, synthetic, implant Ⓑ Qp Qh ♿        N1   N

*IOM: 100-02, 15, 120*

## Neurostimulator

○ **L8679** Implantable neurostimulator, pulse generator, any type Ⓑ Qp Qh ♿   N1   N

*IOM: 100-03, 4, 280.4*

⊘ **L8680** Implantable neurostimulator electrode, each Ⓑ Qh         E1

Related CPT codes: 43647, 63650, 63655, 64553, 64555, 64560, 64561, 64565, 64573, 64575, 64577, 64580, 64581.

○ **L8681** Patient programmer (external) for use with implantable programmable neurostimulator pulse generator, replacement only Ⓑ Qp Qh     A

*IOM: 100-03, 4, 280.4*

○ **L8682** Implantable neurostimulator radiofrequency receiver Ⓑ Qp Qh ♿    N1   N

*IOM: 100-03, 4, 280.4*

○ **L8683** Radiofrequency transmitter (external) for use with implantable neurostimulator radiofrequency receiver Ⓑ Qp Qh ♿   A

*IOM: 100-03, 4, 280.4*

○ **L8684** Radiofrequency transmitter (external) for use with implantable sacral root neurostimulator receiver for bowel and bladder management, replacement Ⓑ Qp Qh ♿   A

*IOM: 100-03, 4, 280.4*

⊘ **L8685** Implantable neurostimulator pulse generator, single array, rechargeable, includes extension Ⓑ Qp Qh    E1

Related CPT codes: 61885, 64590, 63685.

⊘ **L8686** Implantable neurostimulator pulse generator, single array, non-rechargeable, includes extension Ⓑ Qp Qh    E1

Related CPT codes: 61885, 64590, 63685.

⊘ **L8687** Implantable neurostimulator pulse generator, dual array, rechargeable, includes extension Ⓑ Qp Qh    E1

Related CPT codes: 64590, 63685, 61886.

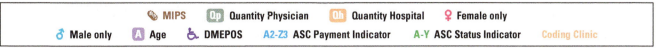

🖐 **MIPS**    Qp **Quantity Physician**    Qh **Quantity Hospital**    ♀ **Female only**

♂ **Male only**    Ⓐ **Age**    ♿ **DMEPOS**    A2-Z3 **ASC Payment Indicator**    A-Y **ASC Status Indicator**    **Coding Clinic**

⃠ **L8688**  Implantable neurostimulator pulse generator, dual array, non-rechargeable, includes extension Ⓑ **Qp** **Qh**     E1

Related CPT codes: 61885, 64590, 63685.

✿ **L8689**  External recharging system for battery (internal) for use with implantable neurostimulator, replacement only Ⓑ **Qp** **Qh** ♿     A

*IOM: 100-03, 4, 280.4*

## Miscellaneous Orthotic and Prosthetic Components, Services, and Supplies

✻ **L8690**  Auditory osseointegrated device, includes all internal and external components Ⓑ **Qp** **Qh** ♿     N1  N

Related CPT codes: 69714, 69715, 69717, 69718.

✻ **L8691**  Auditory osseointegrated device, external sound processor, excludes transducer/actuator, replacement only, each Ⓑ **Qp** **Qh** ♿     A

⃠ **L8692**  Auditory osseointegrated device, external sound processor, used without osseointegration, body worn, includes headband or other means of external attachment Ⓑ **Qp** **Qh**     E1

*Medicare Statute 1862(a)(7)*

✻ **L8693**  Auditory osseointegrated device abutment, any length, replacement only Ⓑ **Qp** **Qh** ♿     A

✻ **L8694**  Auditory osseointegrated device, transducer/actuator, replacement only, each     A

✿ **L8695**  External recharging system for battery (external) for use with implantable neurostimulator, replacement only Ⓑ **Qp** **Qh** ♿     A

*IOM: 100-03, 4, 280.4*

✿ **L8696**  Antenna (external) for use with implantable diaphragmatic/phrenic nerve stimulation device, replacement, each Ⓑ **Qp** **Qh** ♿     A

✿ **L8698**  Miscellaneous component, supply or accessory for use with total artificial heart system Ⓑ     A

✻ **L8699**  Prosthetic implant, not otherwise specified Ⓑ     N1  N

✻ **L8701**  Powered upper extremity range of motion assist device, elbow, wrist, hand with single or double upright(s), includes microprocessor, sensors, all components and accessories, custom fabricated Ⓑ     A

✻ **L8702**  Powered upper extremity range of motion assist device, elbow, wrist, hand, finger, single or double upright(s), includes microprocessor, sensors, all components and accessories, custom fabricated Ⓑ     A

✻ **L9900**  Orthotic and prosthetic supply, accessory, and/or service component of another HCPCS "L" code Ⓑ Ⓑ     N1  N

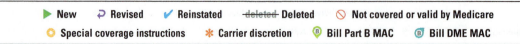

▶ New    ↻ Revised    ✔ Reinstated    ~~deleted~~ Deleted    ⃠ Not covered or valid by Medicare
✿ Special coverage instructions    ✻ Carrier discretion    Ⓑ Bill Part B MAC    Ⓑ Bill DME MAC

## OTHER MEDICAL SERVICES (M0000-M0301)

⊘ **M0075** Cellular therapy Ⓑ E1

⊘ **M0076** Prolotherapy Ⓟ E1

Prolotherapy stimulates production of new ligament tissue. Not covered by Medicare.

⊘ **M0100** Intragastric hypothermia using gastric freezing Ⓑ E1

⊘ **M0300** IV chelation therapy (chemical endarterectomy) Ⓑ E1

⊘ **M0301** Fabric wrapping of abdominal aneurysm Ⓟ E1

Treatment for abdominal aneurysms that involves wrapping aneurysms with cellophane or fascia lata. Fabric wrapping of abdominal aneurysms is not a covered Medicare procedure.

~~M1000~~ ~~Pain screened as moderate to severe~~ ✖

~~M1001~~ ~~Plan of care to address moderate to severe pain documented on or before the date of the second visit with a clinician~~ ✖

~~M1002~~ ~~Plan of care for moderate to severe pain not documented on or before the date of the second visit with a clinician, reason not given~~ ✖

✱ **M1003** TB screening performed and results interpreted within twelve months prior to initiation of first-time biologic disease modifying anti-rheumatic drug therapy for RA Ⓟ M

✱ **M1004** Documentation of medical reason for not screening for TB or interpreting results (i.e., patient positive for TB and documentation of past treatment; patient who has recently completed a course of anti-TB therapy) Ⓑ M

✱ **M1005** TB screening not performed or results not interpreted, reason not given Ⓑ M

✱ **M1006** Disease activity not assessed, reason not given Ⓑ M

✱ **M1007** >=50% of total number of a patient's outpatient RA encounters assessed Ⓑ M

✱ **M1008** <50% of total number of a patient's outpatient RA encounters assessed Ⓑ M

↪ ✱ **M1009** Discharge/discontinuation of the episode of care documented in the medical record Ⓟ M

↪ ✱ **M1010** Discharge/discontinuation of the episode of care documented in the medical record Ⓑ M

↪ ✱ **M1011** Discharge/discontinuation of the episode of care documented in the medical record Ⓑ M

↪ ✱ **M1012** Discharge/discontinuation of the episode of care documented in the medical record Ⓑ M

↪ ✱ **M1013** Discharge/discontinuation of the episode of care documented in the medical record Ⓑ M

↪ ✱ **M1014** Discharge/discontinuation of the episode of care documented in the medical record Ⓑ M

↪ ✱ **M1015** Discharge/discontinuation of the episode of care documented in the medical record Ⓟ M

✱ **M1016** Female patients unable to bear children Ⓑ M

✱ **M1017** Patient admitted to palliative care services Ⓑ M

✱ **M1018** Patients with an active diagnosis or history of cancer (except basal cell and squamous cell skin carcinoma), patients who are heavy tobacco smokers, lung cancer screening patients Ⓑ M

✱ **M1019** Adolescent patients 12 to 17 years of age with major depression or dysthymia who reached remission at twelve months as demonstrated by a twelve month (+/-60 days) PHQ-9 or PHQ-9m score of less than five Ⓑ M

✱ **M1020** Adolescent patients 12 to 17 years of age with major depression or dysthymia who did not reach remission at twelve months as demonstrated by a twelve month (+/-60 days) PHQ-9 or PHQ-9m score of less than 5. Either PHQ-9 or PHQ-9m score was not assessed or is greater than or equal to 5 Ⓑ M

✱ **M1021** Patient had only urgent care visits during the performance period Ⓑ M

✱ **M1022** Patients who were in hospice at any time during the performance period Ⓑ M

✱ **M1023** Adolescent patients 12 to 17 years of age with major depression or dysthymia who reached remission at six months as demonstrated by a six month (+/-60 days) PHQ-9 or PHQ-9m score of less than five Ⓟ M

| 🐾 MIPS | 🆀ᵖ Quantity Physician | 🆀ʰ Quantity Hospital | ♀ Female only |
| ♂ Male only | Ⓐ Age | DMEPOS | A2-Z3 ASC Payment Indicator | A-Y ASC Status Indicator | Coding Clinic |

* **M1024** Adolescent patients 12 to 17 years of age with major depression or dysthymia who did not reach remission at six months as demonstrated by a six month (+/-60 days) PHQ-9 or PHQ-9m score of less than five. Either PHQ-9 or PHQ-9m score was not assessed or is greater than or equal to five Ⓑ M

* **M1025** Patients who were in hospice at any time during the performance period Ⓑ M

* **M1026** Patients who were in hospice at any time during the performance period Ⓑ M

* **M1027** Imaging of the head (CT or MRI) was obtained Ⓑ M

* **M1028** Documentation of patients with primary headache diagnosis and imaging other than CT or MRI obtained Ⓑ M

* **M1029** Imaging of the head (CT or MRI) was not obtained, reason not given Ⓑ M

~~M1030~~ ~~Patients with clinical indications for imaging of the head~~ ✖

* **M1031** Patients with no clinical indications for imaging of the head Ⓑ M

* **M1032** Adults currently taking pharmacotherapy for OUD Ⓑ M

* **M1033** Pharmacotherapy for OUD initiated after June 30th of performance period Ⓑ M

* **M1034** Adults who have at least 180 days of continuous pharmacotherapy with a medication prescribed for OUD without a gap of more than seven days Ⓑ M

* **M1035** Adults who are deliberately phased out of medication assisted treatment (MAT) prior to 180 days of continuous treatment Ⓑ M

* **M1036** Adults who have not had at least 180 days of continuous pharmacotherapy with a medication prescribed for oud without a gap of more than seven days Ⓑ M

* **M1037** Patients with a diagnosis of lumbar spine region cancer at the time of the procedure Ⓑ M

* **M1038** Patients with a diagnosis of lumbar spine region fracture at the time of the procedure Ⓑ M

* **M1039** Patients with a diagnosis of lumbar spine region infection at the time of the procedure Ⓑ M

* **M1040** Patients with a diagnosis of lumbar idiopathic or congenital scoliosis Ⓑ M

* **M1041** Patient had cancer, fracture or infection related to the lumbar spine or patient had idiopathic or congenital scoliosis Ⓑ M

~~M1042~~ ~~Functional status measurement with score was obtained utilizing the Oswestry Disability Index (ODI version 2.1a) patient reported outcome tool within three months preoperatively and at one year (9 to 15 months) postoperatively~~ ✖

↻ * **M1043** Functional status was not measured by the Oswestry Disability Index (ODI version 2.1a) at one year (9 to 15 months) postoperatively Ⓑ M

~~M1044~~ ~~Functional status was measured by the Oswestry Disability Index (ODI version 2.1a) patient reported outcome tool within three months preoperatively and at one year (9 to 15 months) postoperatively~~ ✖

↻ * **M1045** Functional status measured by the Oxford Knee Score (OKS) at one year (9 to 15 months) postoperatively was greater than or equal to 37 Ⓑ M

↻ * **M1046** Functional status the Oxford Knee Score (OKS) at one year (9 to 15 months) postoperatively was less than 37 Ⓑ M

~~M1047~~ ~~Functional status was measured by the Oxford Knee Score (OKS) patient reported outcome tool within three months preoperatively and at one year (9 to 15 months) postoperatively~~ ✖

~~M1048~~ ~~Functional status measurement with score was obtained utilizing the Oswestry Disability Index (ODI version 2.1a) patient reported outcome tool within three months preoperatively and at three months (6 to 20 weeks) postoperatively~~ ✖

↻ * **M1049** Functional status was not measured by the Oswestry Disability Index (ODI version 2.1a) at three months (6 to 20 weeks) postoperatively Ⓑ M

~~M1050~~ ~~Functional status was measured by the Oswestry Disability Index (ODI version 2.1a) patient reported outcome tool within three months preoperatively and at three months (6 to 20 weeks) postoperatively~~ ✖

▶ New   ↻ Revised   ✔ Reinstated   ~~deleted~~ Deleted   ⊘ Not covered or valid by Medicare
○ Special coverage instructions   * Carrier discretion   Ⓑ Bill Part B MAC   Ⓑ Bill DME MAC

\* **M1051** Patient had cancer, fracture or infection related to the lumbar spine or patient had idiopathic or congenital scoliosis Ⓑ M

↻ \* **M1052** Leg pain was not measured by the Visual Analog Scale (VAS) at one year (9 to 15 months) postoperatively Ⓑ M

~~**M1053** Leg pain was measured by the visual analog scale (VAS) within three months preoperatively and at one year (9 to 15 months) postoperatively~~ ✖

\* **M1054** Patient had only urgent care visits during the performance period Ⓑ M

\* **M1055** Aspirin or another antiplatelet therapy used Ⓑ M

\* **M1056** Prescribed anticoagulant medication during the performance period, history of GI bleeding, history of intracranial bleeding, bleeding disorder and specific provider documented reasons: allergy to aspirin or anti-platelets, use of non-steroidal anti-inflammatory agents, drug-drug interaction, uncontrolled hypertension >180/110 mmhg or gastroesophageal reflux disease Ⓑ M

\* **M1057** Aspirin or another antiplatelet therapy not used, reason not given Ⓑ M

\* **M1058** Patient was a permanent nursing home resident at any time during the performance period Ⓑ M

\* **M1059** Patient was in hospice or receiving palliative care at any time during the performance period Ⓑ M

\* **M1060** Patient died prior to the end of the performance period Ⓑ M

\* **M1061** Patient pregnancy Ⓑ M

\* **M1062** Patient immunocompromised Ⓑ M

\* **M1063** Patients receiving high doses of immunosuppressive therapy Ⓑ M

\* **M1064** Shingrix vaccine documented as administered or previously received Ⓑ M

\* **M1065** Shingrix vaccine was not administered for reasons documented by clinician (e.g., patient administered vaccine other than shingrix, patient allergy or other medical reasons, patient declined or other patient reasons, vaccine not available or other system reasons) Ⓑ M

\* **M1066** Shingrix vaccine not documented as administered, reason not given Ⓑ M

\* **M1067** Hospice services for patient provided any time during the measurement period Ⓑ M

\* **M1068** Adults who are not ambulatory Ⓑ M

\* **M1069** Patient screened for future fall risk Ⓑ M

\* **M1070** Patient not screened for future fall risk, reason not given Ⓑ M

\* **M1071** Patient had any additional spine procedures performed on the same date as the lumbar discectomy/laminotomy Ⓑ M

▶ \* **M1106** The start of an episode of care documented in the medical record M

▶ \* **M1107** Documentation stating patient has a diagnosis of a degenerative neurological condition such as ALS, MS, or Parkinson's diagnosed at any time before or during the episode of care M

▶ \* **M1108** Ongoing care not indicated, patient seen only 1-2 visits (e.g., home program only, referred to another provider or facility, consultation only) M

▶ \* **M1109** Ongoing care not indicated, patient discharged after only 1-2 visits due to specific medical events, documented in the medical record that make the treatment episode impossible such as the patient becomes hospitalized or scheduled for surgery or hospitalized M

▶ \* **M1110** Ongoing care not indicated, patient self-discharged early and seen only 1-2 visits (e.g., financial or insurance reasons, transportation problems, or reason unknown) M

▶ \* **M1111** The start of an episode of care documented in the medical record M

▶ \* **M1112** Documentation stating patient has a diagnosis of a degenerative neurological condition such as ALS, MS, or Parkinson's diagnosed at any time before or during the episode of care M

▶ \* **M1113** Ongoing care not indicated, patient seen only 1-2 visits (e.g., home program only, referred to another provider or facility, consultation only) M

▶ \* **M1114** Ongoing care not indicated, patient discharged after only 1-2 visits due to specific medical events, documented in the medical record that make the treatment episode impossible such as the patient becomes hospitalized or scheduled for surgery or hospitalized M

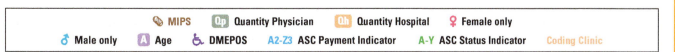

🔖 MIPS   Ⓠₚ Quantity Physician   Ⓠₕ Quantity Hospital   ♀ Female only

♂ Male only   Ⓐ Age   ♿ DMEPOS   A2-Z3 ASC Payment Indicator   A-Y ASC Status Indicator   Coding Clinic

▶ ✳ **M1115** Ongoing care not indicated, patient self-discharged early and seen only 1-2 visits (e.g., financial or insurance reasons, transportation problems, or reason unknown) M

▶ ✳ **M1116** The start of an episode of care documented in the medical record M

▶ ✳ **M1117** Documentation stating patient has a diagnosis of a degenerative neurological condition such as ALS, MS, or Parkinson's diagnosed at any time before or during the episode of care M

▶ ✳ **M1118** Ongoing care not indicated, patient seen only 1-2 visits (e.g., home program only, referred to another provider or facility, consultation only) M

▶ ✳ **M1119** Ongoing care not indicated, patient discharged after only 1-2 visits due to specific medical events, documented in the medical record that make the treatment episode impossible such as the patient becomes hospitalized or scheduled for surgery or hospitalized M

▶ ✳ **M1120** Ongoing care not indicated, patient self-discharged early and seen only 1-2 visits (e.g., financial or insurance reasons, transportation problems, or reason unknown) M

▶ ✳ **M1121** The start of an episode of care documented in the medical record M

▶ ✳ **M1122** Documentation stating patient has a diagnosis of a degenerative neurological condition such as ALS, MS, or Parkinson's diagnosed at any time before or during the episode of care M

▶ ✳ **M1123** Ongoing care not indicated, patient seen only 1-2 visits (e.g., home program only, referred to another provider or facility, consultation only) M

▶ ✳ **M1124** Ongoing care not indicated, patient discharged after only 1-2 visits due to specific medical events, documented in the medical record that make the treatment episode impossible such as the patient becomes hospitalized or scheduled for surgery M

▶ ✳ **M1125** Ongoing care not indicated, patient self-discharged early and seen only 1-2 visits (e.g., financial or insurance reasons, transportation problems, or reason unknown) M

▶ ✳ **M1126** The start of an episode of care documented in the medical record M

▶ ✳ **M1127** Documentation stating patient has a diagnosis of a degenerative neurological condition such as ALS, MS, or Parkinson's diagnosed at any time before or during the episode of care M

▶ ✳ **M1128** Ongoing care not indicated, patient seen only 1-2 visits (e.g., home program only, referred to another provider or facility, consultation only) M

▶ ✳ **M1129** Ongoing care not indicated, patient discharged after only 1-2 visits due to specific medical events, documented in the medical record that make the treatment episode impossible such as the patient becomes hospitalized or scheduled for surgery M

▶ ✳ **M1130** Ongoing care not indicated, patient self-discharged early and seen only 1-2 visits (e.g., financial or insurance reasons, transportation problems, or reason unknown) M

▶ ✳ **M1131** Documentation stating patient has a diagnosis of a degenerative neurological condition such as ALS, MS, or Parkinson's diagnosed at any time before or during the episode of care M

▶ ✳ **M1132** Ongoing care not indicated, patient seen only 1-2 visits (e.g., home program only, referred to another provider or facility, consultation only) M

▶ ✳ **M1133** Ongoing care not indicated, patient discharged after only 1-2 visits due to specific medical events, documented in the medical record that make the treatment episode impossible such as the patient becomes hospitalized or scheduled for surgery M

▶ ✳ **M1134** Ongoing care not indicated, patient self-discharged early and seen only 1-2 visits (e.g., financial or insurance reasons, transportation problems, or reason unknown) M

▶ ✳ **M1135** The start of an episode of care documented in the medical record M

▶ ✳ **M1136** The start of an episode of care documented in the medical record M

▶ ✳ **M1137** Documentation stating patient has a diagnosis of a degenerative neurological condition such as ALS, MS, or Parkinson's diagnosed at any time before or during the episode of care M

▶ ✳ **M1138** Ongoing care not indicated, patient seen only 1-2 visits (e.g., home program only, referred to another provider or facility, consultation only) M

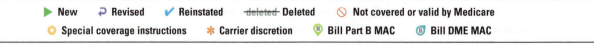

▶ New    ↩ Revised    ✔ Reinstated    ~~deleted~~ Deleted    ⊘ Not covered or valid by Medicare
✿ Special coverage instructions    ✳ Carrier discretion    Ⓑ Bill Part B MAC    Ⓓ Bill DME MAC

▶ ✳ **M1139** Ongoing care not indicated, patient self-discharged early and seen only 1-2 visits (e.g., financial or insurance reasons, transportation problems, or reason unknown)　M

▶ ✳ **M1140** Ongoing care not indicated, patient discharged after only 1-2 visits due to specific medical events, documented in the medical record that make the treatment episode impossible such as the patient becomes hospitalized or scheduled for surgery for surgery or hospitalized　M

▶ ✳ **M1141** Functional status was not measured by the Oxford Knee Score (OKS) at one year (9 to 15 months) postoperatively　M

▶ ✳ **M1142** Emergent cases　M

▶ ✳ **M1143** Initiated episode of rehabilitation therapy, medical, or chiropractic care for neck impairment　M

▶ ✳ **M1144** Ongoing care not indicated, patient seen only 1-2 visits (e.g., home program only, referred to another provider or facility, consultation only)　M

# LABORATORY SERVICES (P0000-P9999)

## Chemistry and Toxicology Tests

⚙ **P2028** Cephalin floculation, blood ⑧ Qp Qh     A

This code appears on a CMS list of codes that represent obsolete and unreliable tests and procedures. Verify before reporting.

*IOM: 100-03, 4, 300.1*

⚙ **P2029** Congo red, blood ⑧ Qp Qh     A

This code appears on a CMS list of codes that represent obsolete and unreliable tests and procedures. Verify before reporting.

*IOM: 100-03, 4, 300.1*

⊘ **P2031** Hair analysis (excluding arsenic) ⑧    E1

*IOM: 100-03, 4, 300.1*

⚙ **P2033** Thymol turbidity, blood ⑧ Qp Qh     A

This code appears on a CMS list of codes that represent obsolete and unreliable tests and procedures. Verify before reporting.

*IOM: 100-03, 4, 300.1*

⚙ **P2038** Mucoprotein, blood (seromucoid) (medical necessity procedure) ⑧ Qp Qh     A

This code appears on a CMS list of codes that represent obsolete and unreliable tests and procedures. Verify before reporting.

*IOM: 100-03, 4, 300.1*

## Pathology Screening Tests

⚙ **P3000** Screening Papanicolaou smear, cervical or vaginal, up to three smears, by technician under physician supervision ⑧ Qp Qh ♀     A

Co-insurance and deductible waived

Assign for Pap smear ordered for screening purposes only, conventional method, performed by technician

*IOM: 100-03, 3, 190.2,*

*Laboratory Certification: Cytology*

⚙ **P3001** Screening Papanicolaou smear, cervical or vaginal, up to three smears, requiring interpretation by physician ⑧ Qp Qh ♀     B

Co-insurance and deductible waived

Report professional component for Pap smears requiring physician interpretation. There are CPT codes assigned for diagnostic Paps, such as, 88141; HCPCS are for screening Paps.

*IOM: 100-03, 3, 190.2*

*Laboratory Certification: Cytology*

## Microbiology Tests

⊘ **P7001** Culture, bacterial, urine; quantitative, sensitivity study ⑧    E1

*Cross Reference CPT*

*Laboratory Certification: Bacteriology*

## Miscellaneous Pathology

⚙ **P9010** Blood (whole), for transfusion, per unit ⑧ Qp Qh     R

Blood furnished on an outpatient basis, subject to Medicare Part B blood deductible; applicable to first 3 pints of whole blood or equivalent units of packed red cells in calendar year

*IOM: 100-01, 3, 20.5; 100-02, 1, 10*

⚙ **P9011** Blood, split unit ⑧ Qp Qh     R

Reports all splitting activities of any blood component

*IOM: 100-01, 3, 20.5; 100-02, 1, 10*

⚙ **P9012** Cryoprecipitate, each unit ⑧ Qp Qh    R

*IOM: 100-01, 3, 20.5; 100-02, 1, 10*

⚙ **P9016** Red blood cells, leukocytes reduced, each unit ⑧ Qp Qh     R

*IOM: 100-01, 3, 20.5; 100-02, 1, 10*

⚙ **P9017** Fresh frozen plasma (single donor), frozen within 8 hours of collection, each unit ⑧ Qp Qh     R

*IOM: 100-01, 3, 20.5; 100-02, 1, 10*

⚙ **P9019** Platelets, each unit ⑧ Qp Qh    R

*IOM: 100-01, 3, 20.5; 100-02, 1, 10*

⚙ **P9020** Platelet rich plasma, each unit ⑧ Qp Qh     R

*IOM: 100-01, 3, 20.5; 100-02, 1, 10*

⚙ **P9021** Red blood cells, each unit ⑧ Qp Qh   R

*IOM: 100-01, 3, 20.5; 100-02, 1, 10*

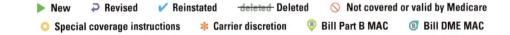

▶ New    ↻ Revised    ✔ Reinstated    ~~deleted~~ Deleted    ⊘ Not covered or valid by Medicare
⚙ Special coverage instructions    ✱ Carrier discretion    ⑧ Bill Part B MAC    ⑩ Bill DME MAC

⚙ **P9022** Red blood cells, washed, each unit Ⓑ Qp Qh     R

*IOM: 100-01, 3, 20.5; 100-02, 1, 10*

⚙ **P9023** Plasma, pooled multiple donor, solvent/detergent treated, frozen, each unit Ⓑ Qp Qh     R

*IOM: 100-01, 3, 20.5; 100-02, 1, 10*

⚙ **P9031** Platelets, leukocytes reduced, each unit Ⓑ Qp Qh     R

*IOM: 100-01, 3, 20.5; 100-02, 1, 10*

⚙ **P9032** Platelets, irradiated, each unit Ⓑ Qp Qh     R

*IOM: 100-01, 3, 20.5; 100-02, 1, 10*

⚙ **P9033** Platelets, leukocytes reduced, irradiated, each unit Ⓑ Qp Qh     R

*IOM: 100-01, 3, 20.5; 100-02, 1, 10*

⚙ **P9034** Platelets, pheresis, each unit Ⓑ Qp Qh     R

*IOM: 100-01, 3, 20.5; 100-02, 1, 10*

⚙ **P9035** Platelets, pheresis, leukocytes reduced, each unit Ⓑ Qp Qh     R

*IOM: 100-01, 3, 20.5; 100-02, 1, 10*

⚙ **P9036** Platelets, pheresis, irradiated, each unit Ⓑ Qp Qh     R

*IOM: 100-01, 3, 20.5; 100-02, 1, 10*

⚙ **P9037** Platelets, pheresis, leukocytes reduced, irradiated, each unit Ⓑ Qp Qh     R

*IOM: 100-01, 3, 20.5; 100-02, 1, 10*

⚙ **P9038** Red blood cells, irradiated, each unit Ⓑ Qp Qh     R

*IOM: 100-01, 3, 20.5; 100-02, 1, 10*

⚙ **P9039** Red blood cells, deglycerolized, each unit Ⓑ Qp Qh     R

*IOM: 100-01, 3, 20.5; 100-02, 1, 10*

⚙ **P9040** Red blood cells, leukocytes reduced, irradiated, each unit Ⓑ Qp Qh     R

*IOM: 100-01, 3, 20.5; 100-02, 1, 10*

✳ **P9041** Infusion, albumin (human), 5%, 50 ml Ⓑ Qp Qh     K2 K

⚙ **P9043** Infusion, plasma protein fraction (human), 5%, 50 ml Ⓑ Qp Qh     R

*IOM: 100-01, 3, 20.5; 100-02, 1, 10*

⚙ **P9044** Plasma, cryoprecipitate reduced, each unit Ⓑ Qp Qh     R

*IOM: 100-01, 3, 20.5; 100-02, 1, 10*

✳ **P9045** Infusion, albumin (human), 5%, 250 ml Ⓑ Qp Qh     K2 K

✳ **P9046** Infusion, albumin (human), 25%, 20 ml Ⓑ Qp Qh     K2 K

✳ **P9047** Infusion, albumin (human), 25%, 50 ml Qp Qh     K2 K

✳ **P9048** Infusion, plasma protein fraction (human), 5%, 250 ml Ⓑ Qp Qh     R

✳ **P9050** Granulocytes, pheresis, each unit Ⓑ Qp Qh     E2

⚙ **P9051** Whole blood or red blood cells, leukocytes reduced, CMV-negative, each unit Ⓑ Qp Qh     R

*Medicare Statute 1833(t)*

⚙ **P9052** Platelets, HLA-matched leukocytes reduced, apheresis/pheresis, each unit Ⓑ Qp Qh     R

*Medicare Statute 1833(t)*

⚙ **P9053** Platelets, pheresis, leukocytes reduced, CMV-negative, irradiated, each unit Ⓑ Qp Qh     R

Freezing and thawing are reported separately, see Transmittal 1487 (Hospital outpatient)

*Medicare Statute 1833(t)*

⚙ **P9054** Whole blood or red blood cells, leukocytes reduced, frozen, deglycerol, washed, each unit Ⓑ Qp Qh     R

*Medicare Statute 1833(t)*

⚙ **P9055** Platelets, leukocytes reduced, CMV-negative, apheresis/pheresis, each unit Ⓑ Qp Qh     R

*Medicare Statute 1833(t)*

⚙ **P9056** Whole blood, leukocytes reduced, irradiated, each unit Ⓑ Qp Qh     R

*Medicare Statute 1833(t)*

⚙ **P9057** Red blood cells, frozen/deglycerolized/washed, leukocytes reduced, irradiated, each unit Ⓑ Qp Qh     R

*Medicare Statute 1833(t)*

⚙ **P9058** Red blood cells, leukocytes reduced, CMV-negative, irradiated, each unit Ⓑ Qp Qh     R

*Medicare Statute 1833(t)*

⚙ **P9059** Fresh frozen plasma between 8-24 hours of collection, each unit Ⓑ Qp Qh     R

*Medicare Statute 1833(t)*

⚙ **P9060** Fresh frozen plasma, donor retested, each unit Ⓑ Qp Qh     R

*Medicare Statute 1833(t)*

⚙ **P9070** Plasma, pooled multiple donor, pathogen reduced, frozen, each unit Ⓑ Qp Qh     R

*Medicare Statute 1833(T)*

---

| 🐾 MIPS | Qp Quantity Physician | Qh Quantity Hospital | ♀ Female only |
|---|---|---|---|
| ♂ Male only | Ⓐ Age | ♿ DMEPOS | A2-Z3 ASC Payment Indicator    A-Y ASC Status Indicator    Coding Clinic |

⚙ **P9071**  Plasma (single donor), pathogen reduced, frozen, each unit 🅑 Qp Qh  **R**

*IOM: 100-01, 3, 20.5; 100-02, 1, 10*

*Medicare Statute 1833T*

⚙ **P9073**  Platelets, pheresis, pathogen-reduced, each unit  **R**

*IOM: 100-01, 3, 20.5; 100-02, 1, 10*

*Medicare Statute 1833T*

▶ ✳ **P9099**  Blood component or product not otherwise classified  **E2**

⚙ **P9100**  Pathogen(s) test for platelets  **S**

*IOM: 100-03, 4, 300.1*

## Travel Allowance for Specimen Collection

⚙ **P9603**  Travel allowance one way in connection with medically necessary laboratory specimen collection drawn from home bound or nursing home bound patient; prorated miles actually traveled 🅑 Qp Qh  **A**

Fee for clinical laboratory travel (P9603) is $1.025 per mile for CY2015.

*IOM: 100-04, 16, 60*

⚙ **P9604**  Travel allowance one way in connection with medically necessary laboratory specimen collection drawn from home bound or nursing home bound patient; prorated trip charge 🅑 Qp Qh  **A**

For CY2010, the fee for clinical laboratory travel is $10.30 per flat rate trip for CY2015.

*IOM: 100-04, 16, 60*

## Catheterization for Specimen Collection

⚙ **P9612**  Catheterization for collection of specimen, single patient, all places of service 🅑 Qp Qh  **A**

NCCI edits indicate that when 51701 is comprehensive or is a Column 1 code, P9612 cannot be reported. When the catheter insertion is a component of another procedure, do not report straight catheterization separately.

*IOM: 100-04, 16, 60*

*Coding Clinic: 2007, Q3, P7*

⚙ **P9615**  Catheterization for collection of specimen(s) (multiple patients) 🅑 Qp Qh  **N**

*IOM: 100-04, 16, 60*

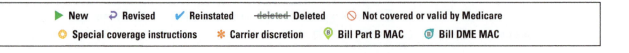

▶ New   ↻ Revised   ✔ Reinstated   ~~deleted~~ Deleted   ⊘ Not covered or valid by Medicare
⚙ Special coverage instructions   ✳ Carrier discretion   🅑 Bill Part B MAC   🅑 Bill DME MAC

## TEMPORARY CODES ASSIGNED BY CMS
## (Q0000-Q9999)

### Cardiokymography

⚙ **Q0035** Cardiokymography Ⓑ Qp Qh    Q1

Report modifier 26 if professional component only

*IOM: 100-03, 1, 20.24*

### Infusion Therapy

⚙ **Q0081** Infusion therapy, using other than chemotherapeutic drugs, per visit Ⓥ Qh    B

IV piggyback only assigned one time per patient encounter per day. Report for hydration or the intravenous administration of antibiotics, antiemetics, or analgesics. Bill on paper. Requires a report.

*IOM: 100-03, 4, 280.14*

Coding Clinic: 2004, Q2, P11; Q1, P5, 8; 2002, Q2, P10; Q1, P7

### Chemotherapy Administration

✳ **Q0083** Chemotherapy administration by other than infusion technique only (e.g., subcutaneous, intramuscular, push), per visit Ⓥ Qh    B

Coding Clinic: 2002, Q1, P7

⚙ **Q0084** Chemotherapy administration by infusion technique only, per visit Ⓥ Qh    B

*IOM: 100-03, 4, 280.14*

Coding Clinic: 2004, Q2, P11; 2002, Q1, P7

✳ **Q0085** Chemotherapy administration by both infusion technique and other technique(s) (e.g., subcutaneous, intramuscular, push), per visit Ⓥ Qh    B

Coding Clinic: 2002, Q1, P7

### Smear Preparation

⚙ **Q0091** Screening Papanicolaou smear; obtaining, preparing and conveyance of cervical or vaginal smear to laboratory Ⓑ Qp Qh ♀    S

Medicare does not cover comprehensive preventive medicine services; however, services described by G0101 and Q0091 (only for Medicare patients) are covered. Includes the services necessary to procure and transport the specimen to the laboratory.

*IOM: 100-03, 3, 190.2*

Coding Clinic: 2002, Q4, P8

### Portable X-ray Setup

⚙ **Q0092** Set-up portable x-ray equipment Ⓑ    N

*IOM: 100-04, 13, 90*

### Miscellaneous Lab Services

✳ **Q0111** Wet mounts, including preparations of vaginal, cervical or skin specimens Ⓑ Qp Qh    A

*Laboratory Certification: Bacteriology, Mycology, Parasitology*

✳ **Q0112** All potassium hydroxide (KOH) preparations Ⓑ Qp Qh    A

*Laboratory Certification: Mycology*

✳ **Q0113** Pinworm examinations Ⓑ Qp Qh    A

*Laboratory Certification: Parasitology*

✳ **Q0114** Fern test Ⓑ Qp Qh ♀    A

*Laboratory Certification: Routine chemistry*

✳ **Q0115** Post-coital direct, qualitative examinations of vaginal or cervical mucous Ⓑ Qp Qh ♀    A

*Laboratory Certification: Hematology*

### Drugs

✳ **Q0138** Injection, ferumoxytol, for treatment of iron deficiency anemia, 1 mg (non-ESRD use) Ⓥ Qp Qh    K2 K

Feraheme is FDA approved for chronic kidney disease.

*Other: Feraheme*

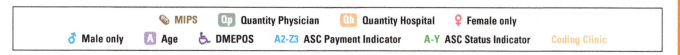

🐾 MIPS    Qp Quantity Physician    Qh Quantity Hospital    ♀ Female only    ♂ Male only    A Age    ♿ DMEPOS    A2-Z3 ASC Payment Indicator    A-Y ASC Status Indicator    Coding Clinic

**387**

TEMPORARY CODES ASSIGNED BY CMS    Q0035 — Q0138

* **Q0139** Injection, ferumoxytol, for treatment of iron deficiency anemia, 1 mg (for ESRD on dialysis) ⑧ Qp Qh  K2 K

*Other: Feraheme*

⊘ **Q0144** Azithromycin dihydrate, oral, capsules/powder, 1 gm ⑧ ⑥ Qp Qh  E1

*Other: Zithromax, Zmax*

* **Q0161** Chlorpromazine hydrochloride, 5 mg, oral, FDA approved prescription anti-emetic, for use as a complete therapeutic substitute for an IV anti-emetic at the time of chemotherapy treatment, not to exceed a 48 hour dosage regimen ⑧ Qp Qh  N1 N

⊛ **Q0162** Ondansetron 1 mg, oral, FDA-approved prescription anti-emetic, for use as a complete therapeutic substitute for an iv anti-emetic at the time of chemotherapy treatment, not to exceed a 48 hour dosage regimen ⑧ Qp Qh  N1 N

*Other: Zofran*

*Medicare Statute 4557*

Coding Clinic: 2012, Q1, P9

⊛ **Q0163** Diphenhydramine hydrochloride, 50 mg, oral, FDA approved prescription anti-emetic, for use as a complete therapeutic substitute for an IV anti-emetic at time of chemotherapy treatment not to exceed a 48 hour dosage regimen ⑧ Qp Qh  N1 N

*Other: Alercap, Alertab, Allergy Relief Medicine, Allermax, Anti-Hist, Antihistamine, Banophen, Complete Allergy Medication, Complete Allergy medicine, Diphedryl, Diphenhist, Diphenhydramine, Dormin Sleep Aid, Genahist, Geridryl, Good Sense Antihistamine Allergy Relief, Good Sense Nighttime Sleep Aid, Mediphedryl, Night Time Sleep Aid, Nytol Quickcaps, Nytol Quickgels maximum strength, Quality Choice Sleep Aid, Quality Choice Rest Simply, Rapidpaq Dicopanol, Rite Aid Allergy, Serabrina La France, Siladryl Allergy, Silphen, Simply Sleep, Sleep Tabs, Sleepinal, Sominex, Twilite, Valu-Dryl Allergy*

*Medicare Statute 4557*

Coding Clinic: 2012, Q2, P10

⊛ **Q0164** Prochlorperazine maleate, 5 mg, oral, FDA approved prescription anti-emetic, for use as a complete therapeutic substitute for an IV anti-emetic at the time of chemotherapy treatment, not to exceed a 48 hour dosage regimen ⑧ Qp Qh  N1 N

*Other: Compazine*

*Medicare Statute 4557*

Coding Clinic: 2012, Q2, P10

⊛ **Q0166** Granisetron hydrochloride, 1 mg, oral, FDA approved prescription anti-emetic, for use as a complete therapeutic substitute for an IV anti-emetic at the time of chemotherapy treatment, not to exceed a 24 hour dosage regimen ⑧ Qp Qh  N1 N

*Other: Kytril*

*Medicare Statute 4557*

Coding Clinic: 2012, Q2, P10

⊛ **Q0167** Dronabinol, 2.5 mg, oral, FDA approved prescription anti-emetic, for use as a complete therapeutic substitute for an IV anti-emetic at the time of chemotherapy treatment, not to exceed a 48 hour dosage regimen ⑧ Qp Qh  N1 N

*Other: Marinol*

*Medicare Statute 4557*

Coding Clinic: 2012, Q2, P10

⊛ **Q0169** Promethazine hydrochloride, 12.5 mg, oral, FDA approved prescription anti-emetic, for use as a complete therapeutic substitute for an IV anti-emetic at the time of chemotherapy treatment, not to exceed a 48 hour dosage regimen ⑧ Qp Qh  N1 N

*Other: Anergan, Chlorpromazine, Hydroxyzine Pamoate, Phenazine, Phenergan, Prorex, Prothazine, V-Gan*

*Medicare Statute 4557*

Coding Clinic: 2012, Q2, P10

⊛ **Q0173** Trimethobenzamide hydrochloride, 250 mg, oral, FDA approved prescription anti-emetic, for use as a complete therapeutic substitute for an IV anti-emetic at the time of chemotherapy treatment, not to exceed a 48 hour dosage regimen ⑧ Qp Qh  N1 N

*Other: Arrestin, Ticon, Tigan, Tiject*

*Medicare Statute 4557*

Coding Clinic: 2012, Q2, P10

---

| ▶ New | ↩ Revised | ✔ Reinstated | deleted Deleted | ⊘ Not covered or valid by Medicare |
|---|---|---|---|---|
| ⊛ Special coverage instructions | | * Carrier discretion | ⑧ Bill Part B MAC | ⑥ Bill DME MAC |

◉ **Q0174**   Thiethylperazine maleate, 10 mg, oral, FDA approved prescription anti-emetic, for use as a complete therapeutic substitute for an IV anti-emetic at the time of chemotherapy treatment, not to exceed a 48 hour dosage regimen ⓑ 〔Qp〕 〔Qh〕                            E2

*Other: Torecan*

*Medicare Statute 4557*

**Coding Clinic: 2012, Q2, P10**

◉ **Q0175**   Perphenazine, 4 mg, oral, FDA approved prescription anti-emetic, for use as a complete therapeutic substitute for an IV anti-emetic at the time of chemotherapy treatment, not to exceed a 48 hour dosage regimen ⓑ 〔Qp〕 〔Qh〕                       N1  N

*Medicare Statute 4557*

**Coding Clinic: 2012, Q2, P10**

◉ **Q0177**   Hydroxyzine pamoate, 25 mg, oral, FDA approved prescription anti-emetic, for use as a complete therapeutic substitute for an IV anti-emetic at the time of chemotherapy treatment, not to exceed a 48 hour dosage regimen ⓑ 〔Qp〕 〔Qh〕                       N1  N

*Other: Vistaril*

*Medicare Statute 4557*

**Coding Clinic: 2012, Q2, P10**

◉ **Q0180**   Dolasetron mesylate, 100 mg, oral, FDA approved prescription anti-emetic, for use as a complete therapeutic substitute for an IV anti-emetic at the time of chemotherapy treatment, not to exceed a 24 hour dosage regimen ⓑ 〔Qp〕 〔Qh〕                       N1  N

*Other: Anzemet*

*Medicare Statute 4557*

**Coding Clinic: 2012, Q2, P10**

◉ **Q0181**   Unspecified oral dosage form, FDA approved prescription anti-emetic, for use as a complete therapeutic substitute for a IV anti-emetic at the time of chemotherapy treatment, not to exceed a 48 hour dosage regimen ⓑ                       N1  N

*Medicare Statute 4557*

**Coding Clinic: 2012, Q2, P10**

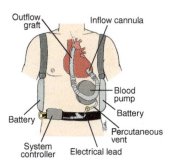

**Figure 46**   Ventricular assist device.

## Ventricular Assist Devices

◉ **Q0477**   Power module patient cable for use with electric or electric/pneumatic ventricular assist device, replacement only ⓑ                                                A

◉ **Q0478**   Power adapter for use with electric or electric/pneumatic ventricular assist device, vehicle type ⓑ 〔Qp〕 〔Qh〕 ♿                A

CMS has determined the reasonable useful lifetime is one year. Add modifier RA to claims to report when battery is replaced because it was lost, stolen, or irreparably damaged.

◉ **Q0479**   Power module for use with electric or electric/pneumatic ventricular assist device, replacemment only ⓑ 〔Qp〕 〔Qh〕 ♿                A

CMS has determined the reasonable useful lifetime is one year. Add modifier RA in cases where the battery is being replaced because it was lost, stolen, or irreparably damaged.

◉ **Q0480**   Driver for use with pneumatic ventricular assist device, replacement only ⓥ 〔Qp〕 〔Qh〕 ♿                A

◉ **Q0481**   Microprocessor control unit for use with electric ventricular assist device, replacement only ⓑ 〔Qp〕 〔Qh〕 ♿                A

◉ **Q0482**   Microprocessor control unit for use with electric/pneumatic combination ventricular assist device, replacement only ⓑ 〔Qp〕 〔Qh〕 ♿                A

◉ **Q0483**   Monitor/display module for use with electric ventricular assist device, replacement only ⓑ 〔Qp〕 〔Qh〕 ♿                A

◉ **Q0484**   Monitor/display module for use with electric or electric/pneumatic ventricular assist device, replacement only ⓑ 〔Qp〕 〔Qh〕 ♿                A

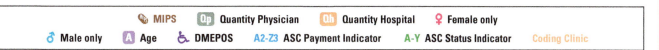

◎ **Q0485** Monitor control cable for use with electric ventricular assist device, replacement only ⑧ Qp Qh ♿   A

◎ **Q0486** Monitor control cable for use with electric/pneumatic ventricular assist device, replacement only ⑧ Qp Qh ♿   A

◎ **Q0487** Leads (pneumatic/electrical) for use with any type electric/pneumatic ventricular assist device, replacement only ⑧ Qp Qh ♿   A

◎ **Q0488** Power pack base for use with electric ventricular assist device, replacement only ⑧ Qp Qh   A

◎ **Q0489** Power pack base for use with electric/pneumatic ventricular assist device, replacement only ⑨ Qp Qh ♿   A

◎ **Q0490** Emergency power source for use with electric ventricular assist device, replacement only ⑧ Qp Qh ♿   A

◎ **Q0491** Emergency power source for use with electric/pneumatic ventricular assist device, replacement only ⑧ Qp Qh ♿   A

◎ **Q0492** Emergency power supply cable for use with electric ventricular assist device, replacement only ⑧ Qp Qh ♿   A

◎ **Q0493** Emergency power supply cable for use with electric/pneumatic ventricular assist device, replacement only ⑧ Qp Qh ♿   A

◎ **Q0494** Emergency hand pump for use with electric or electric/pneumatic ventricular assist device, replacement only ⑧ Qp Qh ♿   A

◎ **Q0495** Battery/power pack charger for use with electric or electric/pneumatic ventricular assist device, replacement only ⑧ Qp Qh ♿   A

◎ **Q0496** Battery, other than lithium-ion, for use with electric or electric/pneumatic ventricular assist device, replacement only ⑧ ♿   A

Reasonable useful lifetime is 6 months (CR3931).

◎ **Q0497** Battery clips for use with electric or electric/pneumatic ventricular assist device, replacement only ⑧ Qp Qh ♿   A

◎ **Q0498** Holster for use with electric or electric/pneumatic ventricular assist device, replacement only ⑧ Qp Qh ♿   A

◎ **Q0499** Belt/vest/bag for use to carry external peripheral components of any type ventricular assist device, replacement only ⑧ Qp Qh ♿   A

◎ **Q0500** Filters for use with electric or electric/pneumatic ventricular assist device, replacement only ⑧ ♿   A

◎ **Q0501** Shower cover for use with electric or electric/pneumatic ventricular assist device, replacement only ⑧ Qp Qh ♿   A

◎ **Q0502** Mobility cart for pneumatic ventricular assist device, replacement only ⑧ Qp Qh ♿   A

◎ **Q0503** Battery for pneumatic ventricular assist device, replacement only, each ⑧ Qp Qh ♿   A

Reasonable useful lifetime is 6 months (CR3931).

◎ **Q0504** Power adapter for pneumatic ventricular assist device, replacement only, vehicle type ⑧ Qp Qh ♿   A

◎ **Q0506** Battery, lithium-ion, for use with electric or electric/pneumatic, ventricular assist device, replacement only ⑧ Qp Qh ♿   A

Reasonable useful lifetime is 12 months. Add -RA for replacement if lost, stolen, or irreparable damage.

◎ **Q0507** Miscellaneous supply or accessory for use with an external ventricular assist device ⑧ Qp Qh   A

◎ **Q0508** Miscellaneous supply or accessory for use with an implanted ventricular assist device ⑧ Qp Qh   A

◎ **Q0509** Miscellaneous supply or accessory for use with any implanted ventricular assist device for which payment was not made under Medicare Part A ⑧ Qp Qh   A

## Pharmacy: Supply and Dispensing Fee

◎ **Q0510** Pharmacy supply fee for initial immunosuppressive drug(s), first month following transplant ⑧ Qp Qh   B

◎ **Q0511** Pharmacy supply fee for oral anti-cancer, oral anti-emetic or immunosuppressive drug(s); for the first prescription in a 30-day period ⑧ Qp Qh   B

◎ **Q0512** Pharmacy supply fee for oral anti-cancer, oral anti-emetic or immunosuppressive drug(s); for a subsequent prescription in a 30-day period ⑧ Qp Qh   B

---

▶ New    ↵ Revised    ✔ Reinstated    ~~deleted~~ Deleted    ⊘ Not covered or valid by Medicare

◎ Special coverage instructions    ✷ Carrier discretion    ⑧ Bill Part B MAC    ⑨ Bill DME MAC

**390**

⊙ **Q0513**  Pharmacy dispensing fee for inhalation drug(s); per 30 days Ⓑ Qp Qh          B

⊙ **Q0514**  Pharmacy dispensing fee for inhalation drug(s); per 90 days Ⓑ Qp Qh          B

## Sermorelin Acetate

⊙ **Q0515**  Injection, sermorelin acetate, 1 microgram Ⓑ Qp Qh          E2

*IOM: 100-02, 15, 50*

## New Technology: Intraocular Lens

⊙ **Q1004**  New technology intraocular lens category 4 as defined in Federal Register notice Ⓑ Qp Qh          E1

⊙ **Q1005**  New technology intraocular lens category 5 as defined in Federal Register notice Ⓑ Qp Qh          E1

## Solutions and Drugs

⊙ **Q2004**  Irrigation solution for treatment of bladder calculi, for example renacidin, per 500 ml Ⓑ Qp Qh          N1 N

*IOM: 100-02, 15, 50*

*Medicare Statute 1861S2B*

⊙ **Q2009**  Injection, fosphenytoin, 50 mg phenytoin equivalent Ⓑ Qp Qh          K2 K

*IOM: 100-02, 15, 50*

*Medicare Statute 1861S2B*

⊙ **Q2017**  Injection, teniposide, 50 mg Ⓑ Qp Qh          K2 K

*IOM: 100-02, 15, 50*

*Medicare Statute 1861S2B*

⊙ **Q2026**  Injection, radiesse, 0.1 ml Ⓑ Qp Qh  E2

*Coding Clinic: 2010, Q3, P8*

⊙ **Q2028**  Injection, sculptra, 0.5 mg Ⓑ Qp Qh  E2

⊙ **Q2034**  Influenza virus vaccine, split virus, for intramuscular use (Agriflu) Sipuleucel-t, minimum of 50 million autologous CD54+ cells activated with PAP-GM-CSF, including leukapheresis and all other preparatory procedures, per infusion Ⓑ Qp Qh          L1 L

*IOM: 100-02, 15, 50*

⊙ **Q2035**  Influenza virus vaccine, split virus, when administered to individuals 3 years of age and older, for intramuscular use (Afluria) Ⓑ Qp Qh Ⓐ          L1 L

Preventive service; no deductible

*IOM: 100-02, 15, 50*

Coding Clinic: 2011, Q1, P7; 2010, Q4, P8-9

⊙ **Q2036**  Influenza virus vaccine, split virus, when administered to individuals 3 years of age and older, for intramuscular use (Flulaval) Ⓑ Qp Qh Ⓐ          L1 L

Preventive service; no deductible

*IOM: 100-02, 15, 50*

Coding Clinic: 2011, Q1, P7; 2010, Q4, P8-9

⊙ **Q2037**  Influenza virus vaccine, split virus, when administered to individuals3 years of age and older, for intramuscular use (Fluvirin) Ⓑ Qp Qh Ⓐ          L1 L

Preventive service; no deductible

*IOM: 100-02, 15, 50*

Coding Clinic: 2011, Q1, P7; 2010, Q4, P8-9

⊙ **Q2038**  Influenza virus vaccine, split virus, when administered to individuals 3 years of age or older, for intramuscular use (Fluzone) Ⓑ Qp Qh Ⓐ          L1 L

Preventive service; no deductible

*IOM: 100-02, 15, 50*

Coding Clinic: 2011, Q1, P7; 2010, Q4, P8-9

⊙ **Q2039**  Influenza virus vaccine, not otherwise specified Ⓑ Qp Qh Ⓐ          L1 L

Preventive service; no deductible

*IOM: 100-02, 15, 50*

Coding Clinic: 2011, Q1, P7; 2010, Q4, P8-9

⊙ **Q2041**  Axicabtagene ciloleucel, up to 200 million autologous anti-CD 19 CAR-positive viable T cells, including leukapheresis and dose preparation procedures, per therapeutic dose Ⓑ          G

⊙ **Q2042**  Tisagenlecleucel, up to 600 million CAR-positive viable T cells, including leukapheresis and dose preparation procedures, per therapeutic dose Ⓑ          G

🐾 MIPS    Qp Quantity Physician    Qh Quantity Hospital    ♀ Female only    ♂ Male only    Ⓐ Age    ♿ DMEPOS    A2-Z3 ASC Payment Indicator    A-Y ASC Status Indicator    Coding Clinic

⊛ **Q2043** Sipuleucel-T, minimum of 50 million autologous CD54+ cells activated with PAP-GM-CSF, including leukapheresis and all other preparatory procedures, per infusion ⑧ Qp Qh    K2 K

*Other: Provenge*

Coding Clinic: 2012, Q2, P7; Q1, P7, 9; 2011, Q3, P9

✳ **Q2049** Injection, doxorubicin hydrochloride, liposomal, imported lipodox, 10 mg ⑧ ⑧ Qp Qh    K2 K

Coding Clinic: 2012, Q3, P10

⊛ **Q2050** Injection, doxorubicin hydrochloride, liposomal, not otherwise specified, 10 mg ⑧ ⑧ Qp Qh    K2 K

*Other: Doxil*

*IOM: 100-02, 15, 50*

⊛ **Q2052** Services, supplies and accessories used in the home under the Medicare intravenous immune globulin (IVIG) demonstration ⑧ Qp Qh    E1

Coding Clinic: 2014, Q2, P6

## Brachytherapy Radioelements

⊛ **Q3001** Radioelements for brachytherapy, any type, each ⑧    B

*IOM: 100-04, 12, 70; 100-04, 13, 20*

## Telehealth

✳ **Q3014** Telehealth originating site facility fee ⑧ Qp Qh    A

Effective January of each year, the fee for telehealth services is increased by the Medicare Economic Index (MEI). The telehealth originating facility site fee (HCPCS code Q3014) for 2011 was 80 percent of the lesser of the actual charge or $24.10.

## Drugs

⊛ **Q3027** Injection, interferon beta-1a, 1 mcg for intramuscular use ⑧ Qp Qh    K2 K

*Other: Avonex*

*IOM: 100-02, 15, 50*

⊘ **Q3028** Injection, interferon beta-1a, 1 mcg for subcutaneous use ⑧ Qp Qh    E1

## Skin Test

⊛ **Q3031** Collagen skin test ⑧ Qp Qh    N1 N

*IOM: 100-03, 4, 280.1*

## Supplies: Cast

Q4001-Q4051: Payment on a reasonable charge basis is required for splints, casts by regulations contained in 42 CFR 405.501.

✳ **Q4001** Casting supplies, body cast adult, with or without head, plaster ⑧ Qp Qh A ♿    B

✳ **Q4002** Cast supplies, body cast adult, with or without head, fiberglass ⑧ Qp Qh A ♿    B

✳ **Q4003** Cast supplies, shoulder cast, adult (11 years +), plaster ⑧ Qp Qh A ♿ B

✳ **Q4004** Cast supplies, shoulder cast, adult (11 years +), fiberglass ⑧ Qp Qh A ♿    B

✳ **Q4005** Cast supplies, long arm cast, adult (11 years +), plaster ⑧ A ♿    B

✳ **Q4006** Cast supplies, long arm cast, adult (11 years +), fiberglass ⑧ A ♿    B

✳ **Q4007** Cast supplies, long arm cast, pediatric (0-10 years), plaster ⑧ A ♿    B

✳ **Q4008** Cast supplies, long arm cast, pediatric (0-10 years), fiberglass ⑧ A ♿    B

✳ **Q4009** Cast supplies, short arm cast, adult (11 years +), plaster ⑧ A ♿    B

✳ **Q4010** Cast supplies, short arm cast, adult (11 years +), fiberglass ⑧ A ♿    B

✳ **Q4011** Cast supplies, short arm cast, pediatric (0-10 years), plaster ⑧ A ♿    B

✳ **Q4012** Cast supplies, short arm cast, pediatric (0-10 years), fiberglass ⑧ A ♿    B

✳ **Q4013** Cast supplies, gauntlet cast (includes lower forearm and hand), adult (11 years +), plaster ⑧ A ♿    B

✳ **Q4014** Cast supplies, gauntlet cast (includes lower forearm and hand), adult (11 years +), fiberglass ⑧ A ♿    B

✳ **Q4015** Cast supplies, gauntlet cast (includes lower forearm and hand), pediatric (0-10 years), plaster ⑧ A ♿    B

✳ **Q4016** Cast supplies, gauntlet cast (includes lower forearm and hand), pediatric (0-10 years), fiberglass ⑧ A ♿    B

✳ **Q4017** Cast supplies, long arm splint, adult (11 years +), plaster ⑧ A ♿    B

| ▶ New | ↩ Revised | ✔ Reinstated | ~~deleted~~ Deleted | ⊘ Not covered or valid by Medicare |
|---|---|---|---|---|
| ⊛ Special coverage instructions | | ✳ Carrier discretion | ⑧ Bill Part B MAC | ⑧ Bill DME MAC |

❋ **Q4018** Cast supplies, long arm splint, adult (11 years +), fiberglass 🔵 Ⓐ ♿    B

❋ **Q4019** Cast supplies, long arm splint, pediatric (0-10 years), plaster Ⓑ Ⓐ ♿    B

❋ **Q4020** Cast supplies, long arm splint, pediatric (0-10 years), fiberglass Ⓑ Ⓐ ♿    B

❋ **Q4021** Cast supplies, short arm splint, adult (11 years +), plaster 🔵 Ⓐ ♿    B

❋ **Q4022** Cast supplies, short arm splint, adult (11 years +), fiberglass Ⓑ Ⓐ ♿    B

❋ **Q4023** Cast supplies, short arm splint, pediatric (0-10 years), plaster Ⓑ Ⓐ ♿ B

❋ **Q4024** Cast supplies, short arm splint, pediatric (0-10 years), fiberglass Ⓑ Ⓐ ♿    B

❋ **Q4025** Cast supplies, hip spica (one or both legs), adult (11 years +), plaster Ⓑ Qp Qh Ⓐ ♿    B

❋ **Q4026** Cast supplies, hip spica (one or both legs), adult (11 years +), fiberglass Ⓑ Qp Qh Ⓐ ♿    B

❋ **Q4027** Cast supplies, hip spica (one or both legs), pediatric (0-10 years), plaster Ⓑ Qp Qh Ⓐ ♿    B

❋ **Q4028** Cast supplies, hip spica (one or both legs), pediatric (0-10 years), fiberglass Ⓑ Qp Qh Ⓐ ♿    B

❋ **Q4029** Cast supplies, long leg cast, adult (11 years +), plaster 🔵 Ⓐ ♿    B

❋ **Q4030** Cast supplies, long leg cast, adult (11 years +), fiberglass Ⓑ Ⓐ ♿    B

❋ **Q4031** Cast supplies, long leg cast, pediatric (0-10 years), plaster Ⓑ Ⓐ ♿    B

❋ **Q4032** Cast supplies, long leg cast, pediatric (0-10 years), fiberglass Ⓑ Ⓐ ♿    B

❋ **Q4033** Cast supplies, long leg cylinder cast, adult (11 years +), plaster 🔵 Ⓐ ♿    B

❋ **Q4034** Cast supplies, long leg cylinder cast, adult (11 years +), fiberglass Ⓑ Ⓐ ♿ B

❋ **Q4035** Cast supplies, long leg cylinder cast, pediatric (0-10 years), plaster Ⓑ Ⓐ ♿    B

❋ **Q4036** Cast supplies, long leg cylinder cast, pediatric (0-10 years), fiberglass Ⓑ Ⓐ ♿    B

❋ **Q4037** Cast supplies, short leg cast, adult (11 years +), plaster Ⓑ Ⓐ ♿    B

❋ **Q4038** Cast supplies, short leg cast, adult (11 years +), fiberglass Ⓑ Ⓐ ♿    B

❋ **Q4039** Cast supplies, short leg cast, pediatric (0-10 years), plaster Ⓑ Ⓐ ♿    B

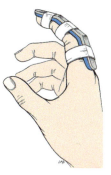

**Figure 47**    Finger splint.

❋ **Q4040** Cast supplies, short leg cast, pediatric (0-10 years), fiberglass Ⓑ Ⓐ ♿    B

❋ **Q4041** Cast supplies, long leg splint, adult (11 years +), plaster Ⓑ Ⓐ ♿    B

❋ **Q4042** Cast supplies, long leg splint, adult (11 years +), fiberglass 🔵 Ⓐ ♿    B

❋ **Q4043** Cast supplies, long leg splint, pediatric (0-10 years), plaster 🔵 Ⓐ ♿    B

❋ **Q4044** Cast supplies, long leg splint, pediatric (0-10 years), fiberglass Ⓑ Ⓐ ♿    B

❋ **Q4045** Cast supplies, short leg splint, adult (11 years +), plaster Ⓑ Ⓐ ♿    B

❋ **Q4046** Cast supplies, short leg splint, adult (11 years +), fiberglass Ⓑ Ⓐ ♿    B

❋ **Q4047** Cast supplies, short leg splint, pediatric (0-10 years), plaster Ⓑ Ⓐ ♿    B

❋ **Q4048** Cast supplies, short leg splint, pediatric (0-10 years), fiberglass Ⓑ Ⓐ ♿    B

❋ **Q4049** Finger splint, static 🔵 ♿    B

❋ **Q4050** Cast supplies, for unlisted types and materials of casts Ⓑ    B

❋ **Q4051** Splint supplies, miscellaneous (includes thermoplastics, strapping, fasteners, padding and other supplies) 🔵    B

## Drugs

❋ **Q4074** Iloprost, inhalation solution, FDA-approved final product, non-compounded, administered through DME, unit dose form, up to 20 micrograms 🔵 Ⓑ Qp Qh    Y

*Other: Ventavis*

⊙ **Q4081** Injection, epoetin alfa, 100 units (for ESRD on dialysis) Ⓑ Qp Qh    N

*Other: Epogen, Procrit*

❋ **Q4082** Drug or biological, not otherwise classified, Part B drug competitive acquisition program (CAP) 🔵    B

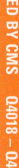

---

🔖 **MIPS**    Qp **Quantity Physician**    Qh **Quantity Hospital**    ♀ **Female only**

♂ **Male only**    Ⓐ **Age**    ♿ **DMEPOS**    A2-Z3 **ASC Payment Indicator**    A-Y **ASC Status Indicator**    **Coding Clinic**

## Skin Substitutes

✳ **Q4100** Skin substitute, not otherwise specified Ⓑ N1 N

    Coding Clinic: 2018, Q2, P3; 2012, Q2, P7

✳ **Q4101** Apligraf, per square centimeter Ⓑ Qp Qh N1 N

    Coding Clinic: 2012, Q2, P7; 2011, Q1, P9

✳ **Q4102** Oasis Wound Matrix, per square centimeter Ⓑ Qp Qh N1 N

    Coding Clinic: 2012, Q3, P8; Q2, P7; 2011, Q1, P9

✳ **Q4103** Oasis Burn Matrix, per square centimeter Ⓑ Qp Qh N1 N

    Coding Clinic: 2012, Q2, P7; 2011, Q1, P9

✳ **Q4104** Integra Bilayer Matrix Wound Dressing (BMWD), per square centimeter Ⓑ Qp Qh N1 N

    Coding Clinic: 2012, Q2, P7; 2011, Q1, P9; 2010, Q2, P8

✳ **Q4105** Integra Dermal Regeneration Template (DRT) or integra omnigraft dermal regeneration matrix, per square centimeter Ⓑ Qp Qh N1 N

    Coding Clinic: 2012, Q2, P7; 2011, Q1, P9; 2010, Q2, P8

✳ **Q4106** Dermagraft, per square centimeter Ⓑ Qp Qh N1 N

    Coding Clinic: 2012, Q2, P7; 2011, Q1, P9

✳ **Q4107** Graftjacket, per square centimeter Ⓑ Qp Qh N1 N

    Coding Clinic: 2012, Q2, P7; 2011, Q1, P9

✳ **Q4108** Integra Matrix, per square centimeter Ⓑ Qp Qh N1 N

    Coding Clinic: 2012, Q2, P7; 2011, Q1, P9; 2010, Q2, P8

✳ **Q4110** Primatrix, per square centimeter Ⓑ Qp Qh N1 N

    Coding Clinic: 2012, Q2, P7; 2011, Q1, P9

✳ **Q4111** GammaGraft, per square centimeter Ⓑ Qp Qh N1 N

    Coding Clinic: 2012, Q2, P7; 2011, Q1, P9

✳ **Q4112** Cymetra, injectable, 1 cc Ⓑ Qp Qh N1 N

    Coding Clinic: 2012, Q2, P7; 2011, Q1, P9

✳ **Q4113** GraftJacket Xpress, injectable, 1 cc Ⓑ Qp Qh N1 N

    Coding Clinic: 2012, Q2, P7; 2011, Q1, P9

✳ **Q4114** Integra Flowable Wound Matrix, injectable, 1 cc Ⓑ Qp Qh N1 N

    Coding Clinic: 2012, Q2, P7; 2010, Q2, P8

✳ **Q4115** Alloskin, per square centimeter Ⓑ Qp Qh N1 N

    Coding Clinic: 2012, Q2, P7; 2011, Q1, P9

✳ **Q4116** Alloderm, per square centimeter Ⓑ Qp Qh N1 N

    Coding Clinic: 2012, Q2, P7; 2011, Q1, P9

✳ **Q4117** Hyalomatrix, per square centimeter Ⓑ Qp Qh N1 N

    *IOM: 100-02, 15, 50*

✳ **Q4118** Matristem micromatrix, 1 mg Ⓑ Qp Qh N1 N

    Coding Clinic: 2013, Q4, P2; 2012, Q2, P7; 2011, Q1, P6

✳ **Q4121** Theraskin, per square centimeter Ⓑ Qp Qh N1 N

    Coding Clinic: 2012, Q2, P7; 2011, Q1, P6

↻ ✳ **Q4122** Dermacell, Dermacell AWM or Dermacell AWM Porous, per square centimeter Ⓑ Qp Qh N1 N

    Coding Clinic: 2012, Q2, P7; Q1, P8

✳ **Q4123** AlloSkin RT, per square centimeter Ⓑ Qp Qh N1 N

✳ **Q4124** Oasis Ultra Tri-layer Wound Matrix, per square centimeter Ⓑ Qp Qh N1 N

    Coding Clinic: 2012, Q2, P7; Q1, P9

✳ **Q4125** Arthroflex, per square centimeter Ⓑ Qp Qh N1 N

✳ **Q4126** Memoderm, dermaspan, tranzgraft or integuply, per square centimeter Ⓑ Qp Qh N1 N

✳ **Q4127** Talymed, per square centimeter Ⓑ Qp Qh N1 N

✳ **Q4128** FlexHD, Allopatch HD, or Matrix HD, per square centimeter Ⓑ Qp Qh N1 N

✳ **Q4130** Strattice TM, per square centimeter Ⓑ Qp Qh N1 N

    Coding Clinic: 2012, Q2, P7

✳ **Q4132** Grafix core and GrafixPL core, per square centimeter Ⓑ Qp Qh N1 N

✳ **Q4133** Grafix prime, GrafixPL prime, stravix and stravixpl, per square centimeter Ⓑ Qp Qh N1 N

✳ **Q4134** Hmatrix, per square centimeter Ⓑ Qp Qh N1 N

✳ **Q4135** Mediskin, per square centimeter Ⓑ Qp Qh N1 N

✳ **Q4136** Ez-derm, per square centimeter Ⓑ Qp Qh N1 N

✳ **Q4137** Amnioexcel, amnioexcel plus or biodexcel, per square centimeter Ⓑ Qp Qh N1 N

✳ **Q4138** Biodfence dryflex, per square centimeter Ⓑ Qp Qh N1 N

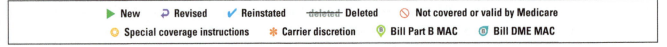

▶ New    ↻ Revised    ✔ Reinstated    ~~deleted~~ Deleted    ⊘ Not covered or valid by Medicare

✪ Special coverage instructions    ✳ Carrier discretion    Ⓑ Bill Part B MAC    Ⓑ Bill DME MAC

* **Q4139** Amniomatrix or biodmatrix, injectable, 1 cc Ⓥ Qp Qh   N1 N

* **Q4140** Biodfence, per square centimeter Ⓑ Qp Qh   N1 N

* **Q4141** Alloskin ac, per square centimeter Ⓑ Qp Qh   N1 N

* **Q4142** XCM biologic tissue matrix, per square centimeter Ⓥ Qp Qh   N1 N

* **Q4143** Repriza, per square centimeter Ⓑ Qp Qh   N1 N

* **Q4145** Epifix, injectable, 1 mg Ⓑ Qp Qh   N1 N

* **Q4146** Tensix, per square centimeter Ⓥ Qp Qh   N1 N

* **Q4147** Architect, architect PX, or architect FX, extracellular matrix, per square centimeter Ⓥ Qp Qh   N1 N

* **Q4148** Neox cord 1K, Neox cord RT, or Clarix cord 1K, per square centimeter Ⓑ Qp Qh   N1 N

* **Q4149** Excellagen, 0.1 cc Ⓥ Qp Qh   N1 N

* **Q4150** AlloWrap DS or dry, per square centimeter Ⓥ Qp Qh   N1 N

* **Q4151** Amnioband or guardian, per square centimeter Ⓥ Qp Qh   N1 N

* **Q4152** DermaPure, per square centimeter Ⓑ Qp Qh   N1 N

* **Q4153** Dermavest and Plurivest, per square centimeter Ⓥ Qp Qh   N1 N

* **Q4154** Biovance, per square centimeter Ⓥ Qp Qh   N1 N

* **Q4155** Neoxflo or clarixflo, 1 mg Ⓑ Qp Qh   N1 N

* **Q4156** Neox 100 or Clarix 100, per square centimeter Ⓥ Qp Qh   N1 N

* **Q4157** Revitalon, per square centimeter Ⓥ Qp Qh   N1 N

* **Q4158** Kerecis Omega3, per square centimeter Ⓥ Qp Qh   N1 N

* **Q4159** Affinity, per square centimeter Ⓥ Qp Qh   N1 N

* **Q4160** Nushield, per square centimeter Ⓥ Qp Qh   N1 N

* **Q4161** Bio-ConneKt Wound Matrix, per square centimeter Ⓑ Qp Qh   N1 N

* **Q4162** Woundex flow, BioSkin flow 0.5 cc Ⓑ Qp Qh   N1 N

* **Q4163** Woundex, BioSkin per square centimeter Ⓥ Qp Qh   N1 N

* **Q4164** Helicoll, per square centimeter Ⓥ Qp Qh   N1 N

� * **Q4165** Keramatrix or kerasorb, per square centimeter Ⓑ Qp Qh   N1 N

* **Q4166** Cytal, per square centimeter Ⓑ Qp Qh   N1 N
Coding Clinic: 2017, Q1, P10

* **Q4167** TruSkin, per square centimeter Ⓥ Qp Qh   N1 N
Coding Clinic: 2017, Q1, P10

* **Q4168** AmnioBand, 1 mg Ⓑ Qp Qh   N1 N
Coding Clinic: 2017, Q1, P10

* **Q4169** Artacent wound, per square centimeter Ⓑ Qp Qh   N1 N
Coding Clinic: 2017, Q1, P10

* **Q4170** Cygnus, per square centimeter Ⓥ Qp Qh   N1 N
Coding Clinic: 2017, Q1, P10

* **Q4171** Interfyl, 1 mg Ⓑ Qp Qh   N1 N
Coding Clinic: 2017, Q1, P10

* **Q4173** PalinGen or PalinGen XPlus, per square centimeter Ⓥ Qp Qh   N1 N
Coding Clinic: 2017, Q1, P10

* **Q4174** PalinGen or ProMatrX, 0.36 mg per 0.25 cc Ⓑ Qp Qh   N1 N
Coding Clinic: 2017, Q1, P10

* **Q4175** Miroderm, per square centimeter Ⓑ Qp Qh   N1 N
Coding Clinic: 2017, Q1, P10

* **Q4176** Neopatch, per square centimeter Ⓑ   N1 N

* **Q4177** Floweramnioflo, 0.1 cc Ⓑ   N1 N

* **Q4178** Floweramniopatch, per square centimeter Ⓑ   N1 N

* **Q4179** Flowerderm, per square centimeter Ⓑ   N1 N

* **Q4180** Revita, per square centimeter Ⓑ   N1 N

* **Q4181** Amnio wound, per square centimeter Ⓑ   N1 N

* **Q4182** Transcyte, per square centimeter Ⓑ   N1 N

* **Q4183** Surgigraft, per square centimeter Ⓑ   N

↺ * **Q4184** Cellesta or cellesta duo, per square centimeter Ⓑ   N

* **Q4185** Cellesta flowable amnion (25 mg per cc); per 0.5 cc Ⓑ   N

* **Q4186** Epifix, per square centimeter Ⓑ   N

* **Q4187** Epicord, per square centimeter Ⓑ   N

* **Q4188** Amnioarmor, per square centimeter Ⓑ   N

* **Q4189** Artacent ac, 1 mg Ⓑ   N

* **Q4190** Artacent ac, per square centimeter Ⓑ   N

| 🐾 MIPS | Qp Quantity Physician | Qh Quantity Hospital | ♀ Female only |
| ♂ Male only | Ⓐ Age | ♿ DMEPOS | A2-Z3 ASC Payment Indicator | A-Y ASC Status Indicator | Coding Clinic |

\* **Q4191** Restorigin, per square centimeter Ⓑ N

\* **Q4192** Restorigin, 1 cc Ⓑ N

\* **Q4193** Coll-e-derm, per square centimeter Ⓑ N

\* **Q4194** Novachor, per square centimeter Ⓑ N

\* **Q4195** Puraply, per square centimeter Ⓑ G

\* **Q4196** Puraply am, per square centimeter Ⓑ G

\* **Q4197** Puraply xt, per square centimeter Ⓑ N

\* **Q4198** Genesis amniotic membrane, per square centimeter Ⓑ N

\* **Q4200** Skin te, per square centimeter Ⓑ N

\* **Q4201** Matrion, per square centimeter Ⓑ N

\* **Q4202** Keroxx (2.5g/cc), 1cc Ⓑ N

\* **Q4203** Derma-gide, per square centimeter Ⓑ N

\* **Q4204** Xwrap, per square centimeter Ⓑ N

▶ \* **Q4205** Membrane graft or membrane wrap, per square centimeter

▶ \* **Q4206** Fluid flow or fluid Gf, 1 cc N

▶ \* **Q4208** Novafix, per square cenitmeter N

▶ \* **Q4209** Surgraft, per square centimeter N

▶ \* **Q4210** Axolotl graft or axolotl dualgraft, per square centimeter N

▶ \* **Q4211** Amnion bio or axobiomembrane, per square centimeter N

▶ \* **Q4212** Allogen, per cc N

▶ \* **Q4213** Ascent, 0.5 mg N

▶ \* **Q4214** Cellesta cord, per square centimeter N

▶ \* **Q4215** Axolotl ambient or axolotl cryo, 0.1 mg N

▶ \* **Q4216** Artacent cord, per square centimeter N

▶ \* **Q4217** Woundfix, BioWound, Woundfix Plus, BioWound Plus, Woundfix Xplus or BioWound Xplus, per square centimeter N

▶ \* **Q4218** Surgicord, per square centimeter N

▶ \* **Q4219** Surgigraft-dual, per square centimeter N

▶ \* **Q4220** BellaCell HD or Surederm, per square centimeter N

▶ \* **Q4221** Amniowrap2, per square centimeter N

▶ \* **Q4222** Progenamatrix, per square centimeter N

▶ \* **Q4226** MyOwn skin, includes harvesting and preparation procedures, per square centimeter N

## Hospice Care

✸ **Q5001** Hospice or home health care provided in patient's home/residence Ⓑ B

✸ **Q5002** Hospice or home health care provided in assisted living facility Ⓑ B

✸ **Q5003** Hospice care provided in nursing long term care facility (LTC) or non-skilled nursing facility (NF) Ⓑ B

✸ **Q5004** Hospice care provided in skilled nursing facility (SNF) Ⓑ B

✸ **Q5005** Hospice care provided in inpatient hospital Ⓑ B

✸ **Q5006** Hospice care provided in inpatient hospice facility Ⓑ B

Hospice care provided in an inpatient hospice facility. These are residential facilities, which are places for patients to live while receiving routine home care or continuous home care. These hospice residential facilities are not certified by Medicare or Medicaid for provision of General Inpatient (GIP) or respite care, and regulations at 42 CFR 418.202(e) do not allow provision of GIP or respite care at hospice residential facilities.

✸ **Q5007** Hospice care provided in long term care facility Ⓑ B

✸ **Q5008** Hospice care provided in inpatient psychiatric facility Ⓑ B

✸ **Q5009** Hospice or home health care provided in place not otherwise specified (NOS) Ⓑ B

✸ **Q5010** Hospice home care provided in a hospice facility Ⓑ B

## Biosimilar Drugs

✸ **Q5101** Injection, filgrastim-sndz, biosimilar, (zarxio), 1 microgram Ⓑ Ⓑ Qp Qh K2 G

*Other: Zarxio*

✸ **Q5103** Injection, infliximab-dyyb, biosimilar, (inflectra), 10 mg Ⓑ Ⓑ G

*Other: Remicade, Inflectra, Renflexis*

✸ **Q5104** Injection, infliximab-abda, biosimilar, (renflexis), 10 mgn Ⓑ Ⓑ K2 G

*Other: Remicade*

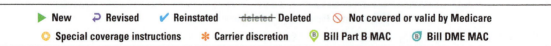

▶ New ↻ Revised ✔ Reinstated ~~deleted~~ Deleted ⊘ Not covered or valid by Medicare
✸ Special coverage instructions \* Carrier discretion Ⓑ Bill Part B MAC Ⓑ Bill DME MAC

↻ ✿ **Q5105** Injection, epoetin alfa-epbx, biosimilar, (retacrit) (for ESRD on dialysis), 100 units Ⓑ Ⓑ    K2 G

*Other: Retacrit*

↻ ✿ **Q5106** Injection, epoetin alfa-epbx, biosimilar, (retacrit) (for non-ESRD use), 1000 units Ⓑ Ⓑ    G

*Other: Retacrit*

✿ **Q5107** Injection, bevacizumab-awwb, biosimilar, (mvasi), 10 mg Ⓑ Ⓑ    E2

*Other: Avastin*

✿ **Q5108** Injection, pegfilgrastim-jmdb, biosimilar, (fulphila), 0.5 mg Ⓑ Ⓑ    K

*Other: Neulasta*

✿ **Q5109** Injection, infliximab-qbtx, biosimilar, (ixifi), 10 mg Ⓑ Ⓑ    E2

*Other: Remicade, Inflectra, Renflexis*

✿ **Q5110** Injection, filgrastim-aafi, biosimilar, (nivestym), 1 microgram Ⓑ Ⓑ    K

*Other: Nivestym*

▶ ✳ **Q5112** Injection, trastuzumab-dttb, biosimilar, (ontruzant), 10 mg    E2

▶ ✳ **Q5113** Injection, trastuzumab-pkrb, biosimilar, (herzuma), 10 mg    E2

▶ ✳ **Q5114** Injection, trastuzumab-dkst, biosimilar, (ogivri), 10 mg    E2

▶ ✿ **Q5115** Injection, rituximab-abbs, biosimilar, (truxima), 10 mg    E2

▶ ✳ **Q5116** Injection, trastuzumab-qyyp, biosimilar, (trazimera), 10 mg    E2

▶ ✳ **Q5117** Injection, trastuzumab-anns, biosimilar, (kanjinti), 10 mg    K2 G

▶ ✳ **Q5118** Injection, bevacizumab-bvzr, biosimilar, (zirabev), 10 mg    E2

## Contrast Agents

✳ **Q9950** Injection, sulfur hexafluoride lipid microspheres, per ml Ⓑ Qp Qh    N1 N

*Other: Lumason*

✿ **Q9951** Low osmolar contrast material, 400 or greater mg/ml iodine concentration, per ml Ⓑ Qp Qh    N1 N

*IOM: 100-04, 12, 70; 100-04, 13, 20; 100-04, 13, 90*

Coding Clinic: 2012, Q3, P8

✿ **Q9953** Injection, iron-based magnetic resonance contrast agent, per ml Ⓑ Qp Qh    N1 N

*IOM: 100-04, 12, 70; 100-04, 13, 20; 100-04, 13, 90*

Coding Clinic: 2012, Q3, P8

✿ **Q9954** Oral magnetic resonance contrast agent, per 100 ml Ⓑ Qp Qh    N1 N

*IOM: 100-04, 12, 70; 100-04, 13, 20; 100-04, 13, 90*

Coding Clinic: 2012, Q3, P8

✳ **Q9955** Injection, perflexane lipid microspheres, per ml Ⓑ Qp Qh    N1 N

Coding Clinic: 2012, Q3, P8

✳ **Q9956** Injection, octafluoropropane microspheres, per ml Ⓑ Qp Qh    N1 N

*Other: Optison*

Coding Clinic: 2012, Q3, P8

✳ **Q9957** Injection, perflutren lipid microspheres, per ml Ⓑ Qp Qh    N1 N

*Other: Definity*

Coding Clinic: 2012, Q3, P8

✿ **Q9958** High osmolar contrast material, up to 149 mg/ml iodine concentration, per ml Ⓑ Qp Qh    N1 N

*Other: Conray 30, Cysto-Conray II, Cystografin*

*IOM: 100-04, 12, 70; 100-04, 13, 20; 100-04, 13, 90*

Coding Clinic: 2012, Q3, P8; 2007, Q1, P6

✿ **Q9959** High osmolar contrast material, 150-199 mg/ml iodine concentration, per ml Ⓑ Qp Qh    N1 N

*IOM: 100-04, 12, 70; 100-04, 13, 20; 100-04, 13, 90*

Coding Clinic: 2012, Q3, P8; 2007, Q1, P6

✿ **Q9960** High osmolar contrast material, 200-249 mg/ml iodine concentration, per ml Ⓑ Qp Qh    N1 N

*Other: Conray 43*

*IOM: 100-04, 12, 70; 100-04, 13, 20; 100-04, 13, 90*

Coding Clinic: 2012, Q3, P8; 2007, Q1, P6

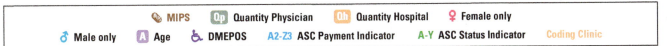

🖐 **MIPS**    Qp **Quantity Physician**    Qh **Quantity Hospital**    ♀ **Female only**
♂ **Male only**    Ⓐ **Age**    ♿ **DMEPOS**    A2-Z3 **ASC Payment Indicator**    A-Y **ASC Status Indicator**    **Coding Clinic**

⚙ **Q9961** High osmolar contrast material, 250-299 mg/mliodine concentration, per ml Ⓑ Qp Qh    N1   N

*Other: Conray, Cholografin Meglumine*

IOM: 100-04, 12, 70; 100-04, 13, 20; 100-04, 13, 90

Coding Clinic: 2012, Q3, P8; 2007, Q1, P6

⚙ **Q9962** High osmolar contrast material, 300-349 mg/ml iodine concentration, per ml Ⓑ Qp Qh    N1   N

IOM: 100-04, 12, 70; 100-04, 13, 20; 100-04, 13, 90

Coding Clinic: 2012, Q3, P8; 2007, Q1, P6

⚙ **Q9963** High osmolar contrast material, 350-399 mg/ml iodine concentration, per ml Ⓑ Qp Qh    N1   N

*Other: Gastrografin, MD-76R, MD Gastroview, Sinografin*

IOM: 100-04, 12, 70; 100-04, 13, 20; 100-04, 13, 90

Coding Clinic: 2012, Q3, P8; 2007, Q1, P6

⚙ **Q9964** High osmolar contrast material, 400 or greater mg/ml iodine concentration, per ml Ⓑ Qp Qh   N1   N

IOM: 100-04, 12, 70; 100-04, 13, 20; 100-04, 13, 90

Coding Clinic: 2012, Q3, P8; 2007, Q1, P6

⚙ **Q9965** Low osmolar contrast material, 100-199 mg/ml iodine concentration, per ml Ⓑ    N1   N

*Other: Omnipaque*

IOM: 100-04, 12, 70; 100-04, 13, 20; 100-04, 13, 90

Coding Clinic: 2012, Q3, P8

⚙ **Q9966** Low osmolar contrast material, 200-299 mg/ml iodine concentration, per ml Ⓑ Qp Qh    N1   N

*Other: Isovue, Omnipaque, Optiray, Ultravist 240, Visipaque*

IOM: 100-04, 12, 70; 100-04, 13, 20; 100-04, 13, 90

Coding Clinic: 2012, Q3, P8

⚙ **Q9967** Low osmolar contrast material, 300-399 mg/ml iodine concentration, per ml Ⓑ Qp Qh    N1   N

*Other: Hexabrix 320, Isovue, Omnipaque, Optiray, Oxilan, Ultravist, Vispaque*

IOM: 100-04, 12, 70; 100-04, 13, 20; 100-04, 13, 90

Coding Clinic: 2012, Q3, P8

✳ **Q9968** Injection, non-radioactive, non-contrast, visualization adjunct (e.g., Methylene Blue, Isosulfan Blue), 1 mg Ⓑ    K2   K

⚙ **Q9969** Tc-99m from non-highly enriched uranium source, full cost recovery add-on, per study dose Ⓑ Qp Qh    K

## Radiopharmaceuticals

⚙ **Q9982** Flutemetamol F18, diagnostic, per study dose, up to 5 millicuries Ⓑ Qp Qh    K2   G

*Other: Vizamyl*

⚙ **Q9983** Florbetaben F18, diagnostic, per study dose, up to 8.1 millicuries Ⓑ Qp Qh    K2   G

*Other: Neuraceq*

✳ **Q9991** Injection, buprenorphine extended-release (sublocade), less than or equal to 100 mg Ⓑ Ⓓ    G

*Other: Subutex, Buprenex, Belbuca, Probuphine, Butrans*

✳ **Q9992** Injection, buprenorphine extended-release (sublocade), greater than 100 mg Ⓑ Ⓓ    G

*Other: Subutex, Buprenex, Belbuca, Probuphine, Butrans*

▶ New   ↻ Revised   ✔ Reinstated   ~~deleted~~ Deleted   ⊘ Not covered or valid by Medicare

⚙ Special coverage instructions   ✳ Carrier discretion   Ⓑ Bill Part B MAC   Ⓓ Bill DME MAC

# DIAGNOSTIC RADIOLOGY SERVICES
## (R0000-R9999)

## Transportation/Setup of Portable Equipment

○ **R0070** Transportation of portable x-ray equipment and personnel to home or nursing home, per trip to facility or location, one patient seen ⑧ Qp Qh  B

CMS Transmittal B03-049; specific instructions to contractors on pricing

*IOM: 100-04, 13, 90; 100-04, 13, 90.3*

○ **R0075** Transportation of portable x-ray equipment and personnel to home or nursing home, per trip to facility or location, more than one patient seen ⑧ Qp Qh  B

This code would not apply to the x-ray equipment if stored at the location where the x-ray was performed (e.g., a nursing home).

*IOM: 100-04, 13, 90; 100-04, 13, 90.3*

○ **R0076** Transportation of portable ECG to facility or location, per patient ⑧ Qp Qh  B

EKG procedure code 93000 or 93005 must be submitted on same claim as transportation code. Bundled status on physician fee schedule

*IOM: 100-01, 5, 90.2; 100-02, 15, 80; 100-03, 1, 20.15; 100-04, 13, 90; 100-04, 16, 10; 100-04, 16, 110.4*

---

🔾 MIPS  Qp Quantity Physician  Qh Quantity Hospital  ♀ Female only
♂ Male only  Ⓐ Age  ♿ DMEPOS  A2-Z3 ASC Payment Indicator  A-Y ASC Status Indicator  Coding Clinic

## TEMPORARY NATIONAL CODES ESTABLISHED BY PRIVATE PAYERS (S0000-S9999)

**NOTE:** Medicare and other federal payers do not recognize "S" codes; however, S codes may be useful for claims to some private insurers.

### Non-Medicare Drugs

⊘ **S0012** Butorphanol tartrate, nasal spray, 25 mg

⊘ **S0014** Tacrine hydrochloride, 10 mg

⊘ **S0017** Injection, aminocaproic acid, 5 grams

⊘ **S0020** Injection, bupivacaine hydrochloride, 30 ml

⊘ **S0021** Injection, cefoperazone sodium, 1 gram

⊘ **S0023** Injection, cimetidine hydrochloride, 300 mg

⊘ **S0028** Injection, famotidine, 20 mg

⊘ **S0030** Injection, metronidazole, 500 mg

⊘ **S0032** Injection, nafcillin sodium, 2 grams

⊘ **S0034** Injection, ofloxacin, 400 mg

⊘ **S0039** Injection, sulfamethoxazole and trimethoprim, 10 ml

⊘ **S0040** Injection, ticarcillin disodium and clavulanate potassium, 3.1 grams

⊘ **S0073** Injection, aztreonam, 500 mg

⊘ **S0074** Injection, cefotetan disodium, 500 mg

⊘ **S0077** Injection, clindamycin phosphate, 300 mg

⊘ **S0078** Injection, fosphenytoin sodium, 750 mg

⊘ **S0080** Injection, pentamidine isethionate, 300 mg

⊘ **S0081** Injection, piperacillin sodium, 500 mg

⊘ **S0088** Imatinib, 100 mg

⊘ **S0090** Sildenafil citrate, 25 mg Ⓐ

⊘ **S0091** Granisetron hydrochloride, 1 mg (for circumstances falling under the Medicare Statute, use Q0166)

⊘ **S0092** Injection, hydromorphone hydrochloride, 250 mg (loading dose for infusion pump)

⊘ **S0093** Injection, morphine sulfate, 500 mg (loading dose for infusion pump)

⊘ **S0104** Zidovudine, oral, 100 mg

⊘ **S0106** Bupropion HCl sustained release tablet, 150 mg, per bottle of 60 tablets

⊘ **S0108** Mercaptopurine, oral, 50 mg

⊘ **S0109** Methadone, oral, 5 mg

⊘ **S0117** Tretinoin, topical, 5 grams

⊘ **S0119** Ondansetron, oral, 4 mg (for circumstances falling under the Medicare statute, use HCPCS Q code)

⊘ **S0122** Injection, menotropins, 75 IU

⊘ **S0126** Injection, follitropin alfa, 75 IU

⊘ **S0128** Injection, follitropin beta, 75 IU

⊘ **S0132** Injection, ganirelix acetate, 250 mcg

⊘ **S0136** Clozapine, 25 mg

⊘ **S0137** Didanosine (DDI), 25 mg

⊘ **S0138** Finasteride, 5 mg

⊘ **S0139** Minoxidil, 10 mg

⊘ **S0140** Saquinavir, 200 mg

⊘ **S0142** Colistimethate sodium, inhalation solution administered through DME, concentrated form, per mg

⊘ **S0145** Injection, pegylated interferon alfa-2a, 180 mcg per ml

⊘ **S0148** Injection, pegylated interferon ALFA-2b, 10 mcg

⊘ **S0155** Sterile dilutant for epoprostenol, 50 ml

⊘ **S0156** Exemestane, 25 mg

⊘ **S0157** Becaplermin gel 0.01%, 0.5 gm

⊘ **S0160** Dextroamphetamine sulfate, 5 mg

⊘ **S0164** Injection, pantoprazole sodium, 40 mg

⊘ **S0166** Injection, olanzapine, 2.5 mg

⊘ **S0169** Calcitrol, 0.25 microgram

⊘ **S0170** Anastrozole, oral, 1 mg

⊘ **S0171** Injection, bumetanide, 0.5 mg

⊘ **S0172** Chlorambucil, oral, 2 mg

⊘ **S0174** Dolasetron mesylate, oral 50 mg (for circumstances falling under the Medicare Statute, use Q0180)

⊘ **S0175** Flutamide, oral, 125 mg

⊘ **S0176** Hydroxyurea, oral, 500 mg

⊘ **S0177** Levamisole hydrochloride, oral, 50 mg

⊘ **S0178** Lomustine, oral, 10 mg

⊘ **S0179** Megestrol acetate, oral, 20 mg

⊘ **S0182** Procarbazine hydrochloride, oral, 50 mg

⊘ **S0183** Prochlorperazine maleate, oral, 5 mg (for circumstances falling under the Medicare Statute, use Q0164)

⊘ **S0187** Tamoxifen citrate, oral, 10 mg

---

▶ New    ↻ Revised    ✔ Reinstated    ~~deleted~~ Deleted    ⊘ Not covered or valid by Medicare

⊕ Special coverage instructions    ✳ Carrier discretion    Ⓑ Bill Part B MAC    Ⓓ Bill DME MAC

⊘ **S0189**   Testosterone pellet, 75 mg

⊘ **S0190**   Mifepristone, oral, 200 mg

⊘ **S0191**   Misoprostol, oral 200 mcg

⊘ **S0194**   Dialysis/stress vitamin supplement, oral, 100 capsules

⊘ **S0197**   Prenatal vitamins, 30-day supply ♀

## Provider Services

⊘ **S0199**   Medically induced abortion by oral ingestion of medication including all associated services and supplies (e.g., patient counseling, office visits, confirmation of pregnancy by HCG, ultrasound to confirm duration of pregnancy, ultrasound to confirm completion of abortion) except drugs ♀

🐾 ⊘ **S0201**   Partial hospitalization services, less than 24 hours, per diem

⊘ **S0207**   Paramedic intercept, non-hospital-based ALS service (non-voluntary), non-transport

⊘ **S0208**   Paramedic intercept, hospital-based ALS service (non-voluntary), non-transport

⊘ **S0209**   Wheelchair van, mileage, per mile

⊘ **S0215**   Non-emergency transportation; mileage per mile

⊘ **S0220**   Medical conference by a physician with interdisciplinary team of health professionals or representatives of community agencies to coordinate activities of patient care (patient is present); approximately 30 minutes

⊘ **S0221**   Medical conference by a physician with interdisciplinary team of health professionals or representatives of community agencies to coordinate activities of patient care (patient is present); approximately 60 minutes

⊘ **S0250**   Comprehensive geriatric assessment and treatment planning performed by assessment team 🅐

⊘ **S0255**   Hospice referral visit (advising patient and family of care options) performed by nurse, social worker, or other designated staff

⊘ **S0257**   Counseling and discussion regarding advance directives or end of life care planning and decisions, with patient and/or surrogate (list separately in addition to code for appropriate evaluation and management service)

⊘ **S0260**   History and physical (outpatient or office) related to surgical procedure (list separately in addition to code for appropriate evaluation and management service)

⊘ **S0265**   Genetic counseling, under physician supervision, each 15 minutes

⊘ **S0270**   Physician management of patient home care, standard monthly case rate (per 30 days)

⊘ **S0271**   Physician management of patient home care, hospice monthly case rate (per 30 days)

⊘ **S0272**   Physician management of patient home care, episodic care monthly case rate (per 30 days)

⊘ **S0273**   Physician visit at member's home, outside of a capitation arrangement

⊘ **S0274**   Nurse practitioner visit at member's home, outside of a capitation arrangement

⊘ **S0280**   Medical home program, comprehensive care coordination and planning, initial plan

⊘ **S0281**   Medical home program, comprehensive care coordination and planning, maintenance of plan

⊘ **S0285**   Colonoscopy consultation performed prior to a screening colonoscopy procedure

⊘ **S0302**   Completed Early Periodic Screening Diagnosis and Treatment (EPSDT) service (list in addition to code for appropriate evaluation and management service) 🅐

⊘ **S0310**   Hospitalist services (list separately in addition to code for appropriate evaluation and management service)

⊘ **S0311**   Comprehensive management and care coordination for advanced illness, per calendar month

⊘ **S0315**   Disease management program; initial assessment and initiation of the program

⊘ **S0316**   Disease management program; follow-up/reassessment

⊘ **S0317**   Disease management program; per diem

⊘ **S0320**   Telephone calls by a registered nurse to a disease management program member for monitoring purposes; per month

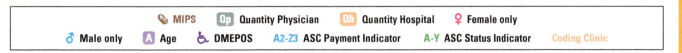

🐾 MIPS   Qp Quantity Physician   Qh Quantity Hospital   ♀ Female only   ♂ Male only   🅐 Age   ♿ DMEPOS   A2-Z3 ASC Payment Indicator   A-Y ASC Status Indicator   Coding Clinic

⊘ **S0340** Lifestyle modification program for management of coronary artery disease, including all supportive services; first quarter/stage

⊘ **S0341** Lifestyle modification program for management of coronary artery disease, including all supportive services; second or third quarter/stage

⊘ **S0342** Lifestyle modification program for management of coronary artery disease, including all supportive services; fourth quarter/stage

⊘ **S0353** Treatment planning and care coordination management for cancer, initial treatment

⊘ **S0354** Treatment planning and care coordination management for cancer, established patient with a change of regimen

⊘ **S0390** Routine foot care; removal and/or trimming of corns, calluses and/or nails and preventive maintenance in specific medical conditions (e.g., diabetes), per visit

⊘ **S0395** Impression casting of a foot performed by a practitioner other than the manufacturer of the orthotic

⊘ **S0400** Global fee for extracorporeal shock wave lithotripsy treatment of kidney stone(s)

## Vision Supplies

⊘ **S0500** Disposable contact lens, per lens

⊘ **S0504** Single vision prescription lens (safety, athletic, or sunglass), per lens

⊘ **S0506** Bifocal vision prescription lens (safety, athletic, or sunglass), per lens

⊘ **S0508** Trifocal vision prescription lens (safety, athletic, or sunglass), per lens

⊘ **S0510** Non-prescription lens (safety, athletic, or sunglass), per lens

⊘ **S0512** Daily wear specialty contact lens, per lens

⊘ **S0514** Color contact lens, per lens

⊘ **S0515** Scleral lens, liquid bandage device, per lens

⊘ **S0516** Safety eyeglass frames

⊘ **S0518** Sunglasses frames

⊘ **S0580** Polycarbonate lens (list this code in addition to the basic code for the lens)

⊘ **S0581** Nonstandard lens (list this code in addition to the basic code for the lens)

⊘ **S0590** Integral lens service, miscellaneous services reported separately

⊘ **S0592** Comprehensive contact lens evaluation

⊘ **S0595** Dispensing new spectacle lenses for patient supplied frame

⊘ **S0596** Phakic intraocular lens for correction of refractive error

## Screening and Examinations

⊘ **S0601** Screening proctoscopy

⊘ **S0610** Annual gynecological examination, new patient ♀

⊘ **S0612** Annual gynecological examination, established patient ♀

⊘ **S0613** Annual gynecological examination; clinical breast examination without pelvic evaluation ♀

⊘ **S0618** Audiometry for hearing aid evaluation to determine the level and degree of hearing loss

⊘ **S0620** Routine ophthalmological examination including refraction; new patient

Many non-Medicare vision plans may require code for routine encounter, no complaints

⊘ **S0621** Routine ophthalmological examination including refraction; established patient

Many non-Medicare vision plans may require code for routine encounter, no complaints

⊘ **S0622** Physical exam for college, new or established patient (list separately) in addition to appropriate evaluation and management code Ⓐ

## Provider Services and Supplies

⊘ **S0630** Removal of sutures; by a physician other than the physician who originally closed the wound

⊘ **S0800** Laser in situ keratomileusis (LASIK)

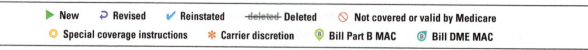

▶ New    ↻ Revised    ✔ Reinstated    ~~deleted~~ Deleted    ⊘ Not covered or valid by Medicare
Ⓞ Special coverage instructions    ✱ Carrier discretion    Ⓑ Bill Part B MAC    Ⓓ Bill DME MAC

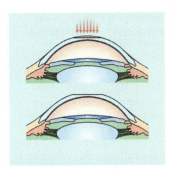

**Figure 48**
Phototherapeutic keratectomy (PRK).

⊘ **S0810** Photorefractive keratectomy (PRK)

⊘ **S0812** Phototherapeutic keratectomy (PTK)

⊘ **S1001** Deluxe item, patient aware (list in addition to code for basic item)

⊘ **S1002** Customized item (list in addition to code for basic item)

⊘ **S1015** IV tubing extension set

⊘ **S1016** Non-PVC (polyvinyl chloride) intravenous administration set, for use with drugs that are not stable in PVC (e.g., paclitaxel)

⊘ **S1030** Continuous noninvasive glucose monitoring device, purchase (for physician interpretation of data, use CPT code)

⊘ **S1031** Continuous noninvasive glucose monitoring device, rental, including sensor, sensor replacement, and download to monitor (for physician interpretation of data, use CPT code)

⊘ **S1034** Artificial pancreas device system (e.g., low glucose suspend (LGS) feature) including continuous glucose monitor, blood glucose device, insulin pump and computer algorithm that communicates with all of the devices

⊘ **S1035** Sensor; invasive (e.g., subcutaneous), disposable, for use with artificial pancreas device system

⊘ **S1036** Transmitter; external, for use with artificial pancreas device system

⊘ **S1037** Receiver (monitor); external, for use with artificial pancreas device system

⊘ **S1040** Cranial remolding orthosis, pediatric, rigid, with soft interface material, custom fabricated, includes fitting and adjustment(s) Ⓐ

~~S1090~~ ~~Mometasone furoate sinus implant, 370 micrograms~~ ✖

⊘ **S2053** Transplantation of small intestine and liver allografts

⊘ **S2054** Transplantation of multivisceral organs

⊘ **S2055** Harvesting of donor multivisceral organs, with preparation and maintenance of allografts; from cadaver donor

⊘ **S2060** Lobar lung transplantation

⊘ **S2061** Donor lobectomy (lung) for transplantation, living donor

⊘ **S2065** Simultaneous pancreas kidney transplantation

⊘ **S2066** Breast reconstruction with gluteal artery perforator (GAP) flap, including harvesting of the flap, microvascular transfer, closure of donor site and shaping the flap into a breast, unilateral ♀

⊘ **S2067** Breast reconstruction of a single breast with "stacked" deep inferior epigastric perforator (DIEP) flap(s) and/or gluteal artery perforator (GAP) flap(s), including harvesting of the flap(s), microvascular transfer, closure of donor site(s) and shaping the flap into a breast, unilateral ♀

⊘ **S2068** Breast reconstruction with deep inferior epigastric perforator (DIEP) flap, or superficial inferior epigastric artery (SIEA) flap, including harvesting of the flap, microvascular transfer, closure of donor site and shaping the flap into a breast, unilateral ♀

⊘ **S2070** Cystourethroscopy, with ureteroscopy and/or pyeloscopy; with endoscopic laser treatment of ureteral calculi (includes ureteral catheterization)

⊘ **S2079** Laparoscopic esophagomyotomy (Heller type)

⊘ **S2080** Laser-assisted uvulopalatoplasty (LAUP)

⊘ **S2083** Adjustment of gastric band diameter via subcutaneous port by injection or aspiration of saline

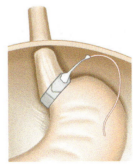

**Figure 49** Gastric band.

| | | | | |
|---|---|---|---|---|
| ⚙ MIPS | Ⓠp Quantity Physician | Ⓠh Quantity Hospital | ♀ Female only | |
| ♂ Male only | Ⓐ Age | ♿ DMEPOS | A2-Z3 ASC Payment Indicator | A-Y ASC Status Indicator | Coding Clinic |

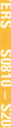

⊘ **S2095** Transcatheter occlusion or embolization for tumor destruction, percutaneous, any method, using yttrium-90 microspheres

⊘ **S2102** Islet cell tissue transplant from pancreas; allogeneic

⊘ **S2103** Adrenal tissue transplant to brain

⊘ **S2107** Adoptive immunotherapy i.e. development of specific anti-tumor reactivity (e.g., tumor-infiltrating lymphocyte therapy) per course of treatment

⊘ **S2112** Arthroscopy, knee, surgical for harvesting of cartilage (chondrocyte cells)

⊘ **S2115** Osteotomy, periacetabular, with internal fixation

⊘ **S2117** Arthroereisis, subtalar

⊘ **S2118** Metal-on-metal total hip resurfacing, including acetabular and femoral components

⊘ **S2120** Low density lipoprotein (LDL) apheresis using heparin-induced extracorporeal LDL precipitation

⊘ **S2140** Cord blood harvesting for transplantation, allogeneic

⊘ **S2142** Cord blood-derived stem cell transplantation, allogeneic

⊘ **S2150** Bone marrow or blood-derived stem cells (peripheral or umbilical), allogeneic or autologous, harvesting, transplantation, and related complications; including: pheresis and cell preparation/storage; marrow ablative therapy; drugs, supplies, hospitalization with outpatient follow-up; medical/surgical, diagnostic, emergency, and rehabilitative services; and the number of days of pre- and post-transplant care in the global definition

⊘ **S2152** Solid organ(s), complete or segmental, single organ or combination of organs; deceased or living donor(s), procurement, transplantation, and related complications; including: drugs; supplies; hospitalization with outpatient follow-up; medical/surgical, diagnostic, emergency, and rehabilitative services, and the number of days of pre- and post-transplant care in the global definition

⊘ **S2202** Echosclerotherapy

⊘ **S2205** Minimally invasive direct coronary artery bypass surgery involving mini-thoracotomy or mini-sternotomy surgery, performed under direct vision; using arterial graft(s), single coronary arterial graft

⊘ **S2206** Minimally invasive direct coronary artery bypass surgery involving mini-thoracotomy or mini-sternotomy surgery, performed under direct vision; using arterial graft(s), two coronary arterial grafts

⊘ **S2207** Minimally invasive direct coronary artery bypass surgery involving mini-thoracotomy or mini-sternotomy surgery, performed under direct vision; using venous graft only, single coronary venous graft

⊘ **S2208** Minimally invasive direct coronary artery bypass surgery involving mini-thoracotomy or mini-sternotomy surgery, performed under direct vision; using single arterial and venous graft(s), single venous graft

⊘ **S2209** Minimally invasive direct coronary artery bypass surgery involving mini-thoracotomy or mini-sternotomy surgery, performed under direct vision; using two arterial grafts and single venous graft

⊘ **S2225** Myringotomy, laser-assisted

⊘ **S2230** Implantation of magnetic component of semi-implantable hearing device on ossicles in middle ear

⊘ **S2235** Implantation of auditory brain stem implant

⊘ **S2260** Induced abortion, 17 to 24 weeks ♀

⊘ **S2265** Induced abortion, 25 to 28 weeks ♀

⊘ **S2266** Induced abortion, 29 to 31 weeks ♀

⊘ **S2267** Induced abortion, 32 weeks or greater ♀

⊘ **S2300** Arthroscopy, shoulder, surgical; with thermally-induced capsulorrhaphy

⊘ **S2325** Hip core decompression

Coding Clinic: 2017, Q3, P1

⊘ **S2340** Chemodenervation of abductor muscle(s) of vocal cord

⊘ **S2341** Chemodenervation of adductor muscle(s) of vocal cord

⊘ **S2342** Nasal endoscopy for post-operative debridement following functional endoscopic sinus surgery, nasal and/or sinus cavity(s), unilateral or bilateral

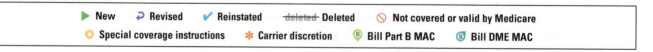

▶ New   ↩ Revised   ✔ Reinstated   ~~deleted~~ Deleted   ⊘ Not covered or valid by Medicare
⊕ Special coverage instructions   ✳ Carrier discretion   Ⓑ Bill Part B MAC   Ⓓ Bill DME MAC

⊘ **S2348** Decompression procedure, percutaneous, of nucleus pulpous of intervertebral disc, using radiofrequency energy, single or multiple levels, lumbar

⊘ **S2350** Diskectomy, anterior, with decompression of spinal cord and/or nerve root(s), including osteophytectomy; lumbar, single interspace

⊘ **S2351** Diskectomy, anterior, with decompression of spinal cord and/or nerve root(s) including osteophytectomy; lumbar, each additional interspace (list separately in addition to code for primary procedure)

⊘ **S2400** Repair, congenital diaphragmatic hernia in the fetus using temporary tracheal occlusion, procedure performed in utero ♀ **A**

⊘ **S2401** Repair, urinary tract obstruction in the fetus, procedure performed in utero ♀ **A**

⊘ **S2402** Repair, congenital cystic adenomatoid malformation in the fetus, procedure performed in utero ♀ **A**

⊘ **S2403** Repair, extralobar pulmonary sequestration in the fetus, procedure performed in utero ♀ **A**

⊘ **S2404** Repair, myelomeningocele in the fetus, procedure performed in utero ♀ **A**

⊘ **S2405** Repair of sacrococcygeal teratoma in the fetus, procedure performed in utero ♀ **A**

⊘ **S2409** Repair, congenital malformation of fetus, procedure performed in utero, not otherwise classified ♀ **A**

⊘ **S2411** Fetoscopic laser therapy for treatment of twin-to-twin transfusion syndrome **A**

⊘ **S2900** Surgical techniques requiring use of robotic surgical system (list separately in addition to code for primary procedure)

*Coding Clinic: 2010, Q2, P6*

⊘ **S3000** Diabetic indicator; retinal eye exam, dilated, bilateral

⊘ **S3005** Performance measurement, evaluation of patient self assessment, depression

⊘ **S3600** STAT laboratory request (situations other than S3601)

⊘ **S3601** Emergency STAT laboratory charge for patient who is homebound or residing in a nursing facility

✿ **S3620** Newborn metabolic screening panel, includes test kit, postage and the laboratory tests specified by the state for inclusion in this panel (e.g., galactose; hemoglobin, electrophoresis; hydroxyprogesterone, 17-D; phenylalanine (PKU); and thyroxine, total) **A**

⊘ **S3630** Eosinophil count, blood, direct

⊘ **S3645** HIV-1 antibody testing of oral mucosal transudate

⊘ **S3650** Saliva test, hormone level; during menopause ♀

⊘ **S3652** Saliva test, hormone level; to assess preterm labor risk ♀

⊘ **S3655** Antisperm antibodies test (immunobead) ♀

⊘ **S3708** Gastrointestinal fat absorption study

⊘ **S3722** Dose optimization by area under the curve (AUC) analysis, for infusional 5-fluorouracil

## Genetic Testing

⊘ **S3800** Genetic testing for amyotrophic lateral sclerosis (ALS)

⊘ **S3840** DNA analysis for germline mutations of the RET proto-oncogene for susceptibility to multiple endocrine neoplasia type 2

⊘ **S3841** Genetic testing for retinoblastoma

⊘ **S3842** Genetic testing for von Hippel-Lindau disease

⊘ **S3844** DNA analysis of the connexin 26 gene (GJB2) for susceptibility to congenital, profound deafness

⊘ **S3845** Genetic testing for alpha-thalassemia

⊘ **S3846** Genetic testing for hemoglobin E beta-thalassemia

⊘ **S3849** Genetic testing for Niemann-Pick disease

⊘ **S3850** Genetic testing for sickle cell anemia

⊘ **S3852** DNA analysis for APOE epilson 4 allele for susceptibility to Alzheimer's disease

⊘ **S3853** Genetic testing for myotonic muscular dystrophy

⊘ **S3854** Gene expression profiling panel for use in the management of breast cancer treatment ♀

⊘ **S3861** Genetic testing, sodium channel, voltage-gated, type V, alpha subunit (SCN5A) and variants for suspected Brugada syndrome

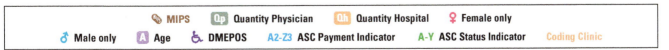

🏷 MIPS    **Qp** Quantity Physician    **Qh** Quantity Hospital    ♀ Female only    ♂ Male only    **A** Age    ♿ DMEPOS    **A2-Z3** ASC Payment Indicator    **A-Y** ASC Status Indicator    Coding Clinic

⊘ **S3865** Comprehensive gene sequence analysis for hypertrophic cardiomyopathy

⊘ **S3866** Genetic analysis for a specific gene mutation for hypertrophic cardiomyopathy (HCM) in an individual with a known HCM mutation in the family

⊘ **S3870** Comparative genomic hybridization (CGH) microarray testing for developmental delay, autism spectrum disorder and/or intellectual disability

## Other Tests

⊘ **S3900** Surface electromyography (EMG)

⊘ **S3902** Ballistrocardiogram

⊘ **S3904** Masters two step

Bill on paper. Requires a report.

## Obstetric and Fertility Services

⊘ **S4005** Interim labor facility global (labor occurring but not resulting in delivery) ♀

⊘ **S4011** In vitro fertilization; including but not limited to identification and incubation of mature oocytes, fertilization with sperm, incubation of embryo(s), and subsequent visualization for determination of development ♀

⊘ **S4013** Complete cycle, gamete intrafallopian transfer (GIFT), case rate ♀

⊘ **S4014** Complete cycle, zygote intrafallopian transfer (ZIFT), case rate ♀

⊘ **S4015** Complete in vitro fertilization cycle, not otherwise specified, case rate ♀

⊘ **S4016** Frozen in vitro fertilization cycle, case rate ♀

⊘ **S4017** Incomplete cycle, treatment cancelled prior to stimulation, case rate ♀

⊘ **S4018** Frozen embryo transfer procedure cancelled before transfer, case rate ♀

⊘ **S4020** In vitro fertilization procedure cancelled before aspiration, case rate ♀

⊘ **S4021** In vitro fertilization procedure cancelled after aspiration, case rate ♀

⊘ **S4022** Assisted oocyte fertilization, case rate ♀

⊘ **S4023** Donor egg cycle, incomplete, case rate ♀

⊘ **S4025** Donor services for in vitro fertilization (sperm or embryo), case rate

⊘ **S4026** Procurement of donor sperm from sperm bank ♂

⊘ **S4027** Storage of previously frozen embryos ♀

⊘ **S4028** Microsurgical epididymal sperm aspiration (MESA) ♂

⊘ **S4030** Sperm procurement and cryopreservation services; initial visit ♂

⊘ **S4031** Sperm procurement and cryopreservation services; subsequent visit ♂

⊘ **S4035** Stimulated intrauterine insemination (IUI), case rate ♀

⊘ **S4037** Cryopreserved embryo transfer, case rate ♀

⊘ **S4040** Monitoring and storage of cryopreserved embryos, per 30 days ♀

⊘ **S4042** Management of ovulation induction (interpretation of diagnostic tests and studies, non-face-to-face medical management of the patient), per cycle ♀

⊘ **S4981** Insertion of levonorgestrel-releasing intrauterine system ♀

⊘ **S4989** Contraceptive intrauterine device (e.g., Progestasert IUD), including implants and supplies ♀

## Therapeutic Substances and Medications

⊘ **S4990** Nicotine patches, legend

⊘ **S4991** Nicotine patches, non-legend

⊘ **S4993** Contraceptive pills for birth control ♀

Only billed by Family Planning Clinics

⊘ **S4995** Smoking cessation gum

⊘ **S5000** Prescription drug, generic

⊘ **S5001** Prescription drug, brand name

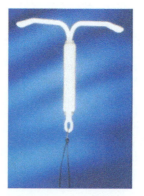

**Figure 50**  IUD.

▶ New   ↻ Revised   ✔ Reinstated   ~~deleted~~ Deleted   ⊘ Not covered or valid by Medicare

◉ Special coverage instructions   ✳ Carrier discretion   ⑧ Bill Part B MAC   ⑧ Bill DME MAC

⊘ **S5010** 5% dextrose and 0.45% normal saline, 1000 ml

⊘ **S5012** 5% dextrose with potassium chloride, 1000 ml

⊘ **S5013** 5% dextrose/0.45% normal saline with potassium chloride and magnesium sulfate, 1000 ml

⊘ **S5014** 5% dextrose/0.45% normal saline with potassium chloride and magnesium sulfate, 1500 ml

## Home Care Services

⊘ **S5035** Home infusion therapy, routine service of infusion device (e.g., pump maintenance)

⊘ **S5036** Home infusion therapy, repair of infusion device (e.g., pump repair)

⊘ **S5100** Day care services, adult; per 15 minutes [A]

⊘ **S5101** Day care services, adult; per half day [A]

⊘ **S5102** Day care services, adult; per diem [A]

⊘ **S5105** Day care services, center-based; services not included in program fee, per diem

⊘ **S5108** Home care training to home care client, per 15 minutes

⊘ **S5109** Home care training to home care client, per session

⊘ **S5110** Home care training, family; per 15 minutes

⊘ **S5111** Home care training, family; per session

⊘ **S5115** Home care training, non-family; per 15 minutes

⊘ **S5116** Home care training, non-family; per session

⊘ **S5120** Chore services; per 15 minutes

⊘ **S5121** Chore services; per diem

⊘ **S5125** Attendant care services; per 15 minutes

⊘ **S5126** Attendant care services; per diem

⊘ **S5130** Homemaker service, NOS; per 15 minutes

⊘ **S5131** Homemaker service, NOS; per diem

⊘ **S5135** Companion care, adult (e.g., IADL/ADL); per 15 minutes [A]

⊘ **S5136** Companion care, adult (e.g., IADL/ADL); per diem [A]

⊘ **S5140** Foster care, adult; per diem [A]

⊘ **S5141** Foster care, adult; per month [A]

⊘ **S5145** Foster care, therapeutic, child; per diem [A]

⊘ **S5146** Foster care, therapeutic, child; per month [A]

⊘ **S5150** Unskilled respite care, not hospice; per 15 minutes

⊘ **S5151** Unskilled respite care, not hospice; per diem

⊘ **S5160** Emergency response system; installation and testing

⊘ **S5161** Emergency response system; service fee, per month (excludes installation and testing)

⊘ **S5162** Emergency response system; purchase only

⊘ **S5165** Home modifications; per service

⊘ **S5170** Home delivered meals, including preparation; per meal

⊘ **S5175** Laundry service, external, professional; per order

⊘ **S5180** Home health respiratory therapy, initial evaluation

⊘ **S5181** Home health respiratory therapy, NOS, per diem

⊘ **S5185** Medication reminder service, non-face-to-face; per month

⊘ **S5190** Wellness assessment, performed by non-physician

⊘ **S5199** Personal care item, NOS, each

## Home Infusion Therapy

⊘ **S5497** Home infusion therapy, catheter care/maintenance, not otherwise classified; includes administrative services, professional pharmacy services, care coordination, and all necessary supplies and equipment (drugs and nursing visits coded separately), per diem

⊘ **S5498** Home infusion therapy, catheter care/maintenance, simple (single lumen), includes administrative services, professional pharmacy services, care coordination and all necessary supplies and equipment, (drugs and nursing visits coded separately), per diem

⊘ **S5501** Home infusion therapy, catheter care/maintenance, complex (more than one lumen), includes administrative services, professional pharmacy services, care coordination, and all necessary supplies and equipment (drugs and nursing visits coded separately), per diem

| 🐾 MIPS | Qp Quantity Physician | Qh Quantity Hospital | ♀ Female only |
| ♂ Male only | A Age | ♿ DMEPOS | A2-Z3 ASC Payment Indicator | A-Y ASC Status Indicator | Coding Clinic |

⊘ **S5502**    Home infusion therapy, catheter care/maintenance, implanted access device, includes administrative services, professional pharmacy services, care coordination, and all necessary supplies and equipment, (drugs and nursing visits coded separately), per diem (use this code for interim maintenance of vascular access not currently in use)

⊘ **S5517**    Home infusion therapy, all supplies necessary for restoration of catheter patency or declotting

⊘ **S5518**    Home infusion therapy, all supplies necessary for catheter repair

⊘ **S5520**    Home infusion therapy, all supplies (including catheter) necessary for a peripherally inserted central venous catheter (PICC) line insertion

*Bill on paper. Requires a report.*

⊘ **S5521**    Home infusion therapy, all supplies (including catheter) necessary for a midline catheter insertion

⊘ **S5522**    Home infusion therapy, insertion of peripherally inserted central venous catheter (PICC), nursing services only (no supplies or catheter included)

⊘ **S5523**    Home infusion therapy, insertion of midline central venous catheter, nursing services only (no supplies or catheter included)

## Insulin Services

⊘ **S5550**    Insulin, rapid onset, 5 units

⊘ **S5551**    Insulin, most rapid onset (Lispro or Aspart); 5 units

⊘ **S5552**    Insulin, intermediate acting (NPH or Lente); 5 units

⊘ **S5553**    Insulin, long acting; 5 units

⊘ **S5560**    Insulin delivery device, reusable pen; 1.5 ml size

⊘ **S5561**    Insulin delivery device, reusable pen; 3 ml size

⊘ **S5565**    Insulin cartridge for use in insulin delivery device other than pump; 150 units

⊘ **S5566**    Insulin cartridge for use in insulin delivery device other than pump; 300 units

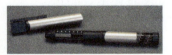

**Figure 51**  Nova pen.

⊘ **S5570**    Insulin delivery device, disposable pen (including insulin); 1.5 ml size

⊘ **S5571**    Insulin delivery device, disposable pen (including insulin); 3 ml size

## Imaging

⊘ **S8030**    Scleral application of tantalum ring(s) for localization of lesions for proton beam therapy

⊘ **S8035**    Magnetic source imaging

⊘ **S8037**    Magnetic resonance cholangiopancreatography (MRCP)

⊘ **S8040**    Topographic brain mapping

⊘ **S8042**    Magnetic resonance imaging (MRI), low-field

⊘ **S8055**    Ultrasound guidance for multifetal pregnancy reduction(s), technical component (only to be used when the physician doing the reduction procedure does not perform the ultrasound, guidance is included in the CPT code for multifetal pregnancy reduction - 59866) ♀

⊘ **S8080**    Scintimammography (radioimmunoscintigraphy of the breast), unilateral, including supply of radiopharmaceutical ♀

⊘ **S8085**    Fluorine-18 fluorodeoxyglucose (F-18 FDG) imaging using dual-head coincidence detection system (non-dedicated PET scan)

⊘ **S8092**    Electron beam computed tomography (also known as ultrafast CT, cine CT)

## Assistive Breathing Supplies

⊘ **S8096**    Portable peak flow meter

⊘ **S8097**    Asthma kit (including but not limited to portable peak expiratory flow meter, instructional video, brochure, and/or spacer)

⊘ **S8100**    Holding chamber or spacer for use with an inhaler or nebulizer; without mask

⊘ **S8101**    Holding chamber or spacer for use with an inhaler or nebulizer; with mask

⊘ **S8110**    Peak expiratory flow rate (physician services)

⊘ **S8120**    Oxygen contents, gaseous, 1 unit equals 1 cubic foot

⊘ **S8121**    Oxygen contents, liquid, 1 unit equals 1 pound

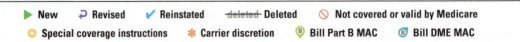

▶ New    ⟲ Revised    ✔ Reinstated    ~~deleted~~ Deleted    ⊘ Not covered or valid by Medicare
⊛ Special coverage instructions    ✳ Carrier discretion    Ⓑ Bill Part B MAC    Ⓓ Bill DME MAC

**408**

⊘ **S8130**   Interferential current stimulator, 2 channel

⊘ **S8131**   Interferential current stimulator, 4 channel

⊘ **S8185**   Flutter device

⊘ **S8186**   Swivel adapter

⊘ **S8189**   Tracheostomy supply, not otherwise classified

⊘ **S8210**   Mucus trap

## Miscellaneous Supplies and Services

⊘ **S8265**   Haberman feeder for cleft lip/palate

⊘ **S8270**   Enuresis alarm, using auditory buzzer and/or vibration device

⊘ **S8301**   Infection control supplies, not otherwise specified

⊘ **S8415**   Supplies for home delivery of infant Ⓐ

⊘ **S8420**   Gradient pressure aid (sleeve and glove combination), custom made

⊘ **S8421**   Gradient pressure aid (sleeve and glove combination), ready made

⊘ **S8422**   Gradient pressure aid (sleeve), custom made, medium weight

⊘ **S8423**   Gradient pressure aid (sleeve), custom made, heavy weight

⊘ **S8424**   Gradient pressure aid (sleeve), ready made

⊘ **S8425**   Gradient pressure aid (glove), custom made, medium weight

⊘ **S8426**   Gradient pressure aid (glove), custom made, heavy weight

⊘ **S8427**   Gradient pressure aid (glove), ready made

⊘ **S8428**   Gradient pressure aid (gauntlet), ready made

⊘ **S8429**   Gradient pressure exterior wrap

⊘ **S8430**   Padding for compression bandage, roll

⊘ **S8431**   Compression bandage, roll

⊘ **S8450**   Splint, prefabricated, digit (specify digit by use of modifier)

⊘ **S8451**   Splint, prefabricated, wrist or ankle

⊘ **S8452**   Splint, prefabricated, elbow

⊘ **S8460**   Camisole, post-mastectomy

⊘ **S8490**   Insulin syringes (100 syringes, any size)

⊘ **S8930**   Electrical stimulation of auricular acupuncture points; each 15 minutes of personal one-on-one contact with the patient

⊘ **S8940**   Equestrian/Hippotherapy, per session

⊘ **S8948**   Application of a modality (requiring constant provider attendance) to one or more areas; low-level laser; each 15 minutes

⊘ **S8950**   Complex lymphedema therapy, each 15 minutes

⊘ **S8990**   Physical or manipulative therapy performed for maintenance rather than restoration

⊘ **S8999**   Resuscitation bag (for use by patient on artificial respiration during power failure or other catastrophic event)

⊘ **S9001**   Home uterine monitor with or without associated nursing services ♀

⊘ **S9007**   Ultrafiltration monitor

⊘ **S9024**   Paranasal sinus ultrasound

⊘ **S9025**   Omnicardiogram/cardiointegram

⊘ **S9034**   Extracorporeal shockwave lithotripsy for gall stones (if performed with ERCP, use 43265)

⊘ **S9055**   Procuren or other growth factor preparation to promote wound healing

⊘ **S9056**   Coma stimulation per diem

⊘ **S9061**   Home administration of aerosolized drug therapy (e.g., pentamidine); administrative services, professional pharmacy services, care coordination, all necessary supplies and equipment (drugs and nursing visits coded separately), per diem

⊘ **S9083**   Global fee urgent care centers

⊘ **S9088**   Services provided in an urgent care center (list in addition to code for service)

⊘ **S9090**   Vertebral axial decompression, per session

⊘ **S9097**   Home visit for wound care

⊘ **S9098**   Home visit, phototherapy services (e.g., Bili-Lite), including equipment rental, nursing services, blood draw, supplies, and other services, per diem

⊘ **S9110**   Telemonitoring of patient in their home, including all necessary equipment; computer system, connections, and software; maintenance; patient education and support; per month

⊘ **S9117**   Back school, per visit

⊘ **S9122**   Home health aide or certified nurse assistant, providing care in the home; per hour

⚕ MIPS   Ⓠⱼ Quantity Physician   Ⓠₕ Quantity Hospital   ♀ Female only
♂ Male only   Ⓐ Age   ♿ DMEPOS   A2-Z3 ASC Payment Indicator   A-Y ASC Status Indicator   Coding Clinic

TEMPORARY NATIONAL CODES ESTABLISHED BY PRIVATE PAYERS   S8130 – S9122

⊘ **S9123** Nursing care, in the home; by registered nurse, per hour (use for general nursing care only, not to be used when CPT codes 99500-99602 can be used)

⊘ **S9124** Nursing care, in the home; by licensed practical nurse, per hour

⊘ **S9125** Respite care, in the home, per diem

⊘ **S9126** Hospice care, in the home, per diem

⊘ **S9127** Social work visit, in the home, per diem

⊘ **S9128** Speech therapy, in the home, per diem

⊘ **S9129** Occupational therapy, in the home, per diem

⊘ **S9131** Physical therapy; in the home, per diem

⊘ **S9140** Diabetic management program, follow-up visit to non-MD provider

⊘ **S9141** Diabetic management program, follow-up visit to MD provider

⊘ **S9145** Insulin pump initiation, instruction in initial use of pump (pump not included)

⊘ **S9150** Evaluation by ocularist

⊘ **S9152** Speech therapy, re-evaluation

## Home Management of Pregnancy

⊘ **S9208** Home management of preterm labor, including administrative services, professional pharmacy services, care coordination, and all necessary supplies or equipment (drugs and nursing visits coded separately), per diem (do not use this code with any home infusion per diem code) ♀

⊘ **S9209** Home management of preterm premature rupture of membranes (PPROM), including administrative services, professional pharmacy services, care coordination, and all necessary supplies or equipment (drugs and nursing visits coded separately), per diem (do not use this code with any home infusion per diem code) ♀

⊘ **S9211** Home management of gestational hypertension, includes administrative services, professional pharmacy services, care coordination, and all necessary supplies and equipment (drugs and nursing visits coded separately); per diem (do not use this code with any home infusion per diem code) ♀

⊘ **S9212** Home management of postpartum hypertension, includes administrative services, professional pharmacy services, care coordination, and all necessary supplies and equipment (drugs and nursing visits coded separately), per diem (do not use this code with any home infusion per diem code) ♀

⊘ **S9213** Home management of preeclampsia, includes administrative services, professional pharmacy services, care coordination, and all necessary supplies and equipment (drugs and nursing services coded separately); per diem (do not use this code with any home infusion per diem code) ♀

⊘ **S9214** Home management of gestational diabetes, includes administrative services, professional pharmacy services, care coordination, and all necessary supplies and equipment (drugs and nursing visits coded separately); per diem (do not use this code with any home infusion per diem code) ♀

## Home Infusion Therapy

⊘ **S9325** Home infusion therapy, pain management infusion; administrative services, professional pharmacy services, care coordination, and all necessary supplies and equipment, (drugs and nursing visits coded separately), per diem (do not use this code with S9326, S9327 or S9328)

⊘ **S9326** Home infusion therapy, continuous (twenty-four hours or more) pain management infusion; administrative services, professional pharmacy services, care coordination, and all necessary supplies and equipment (drugs and nursing visits coded separately), per diem

⊘ **S9327** Home infusion therapy, intermittent (less than twenty-four hours) pain management infusion; administrative services, professional pharmacy services, care coordination, and all necessary supplies and equipment (drugs and nursing visits coded separately), per diem

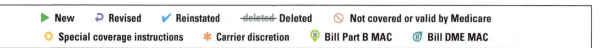

▶ New    ⟲ Revised    ✔ Reinstated    ~~deleted~~ Deleted    ⊘ Not covered or valid by Medicare

⊙ Special coverage instructions    ✳ Carrier discretion    Ⓑ Bill Part B MAC    Ⓓ Bill DME MAC

⊘ **S9328** Home infusion therapy, implanted pump pain management infusion; administrative services, professional pharmacy services, care coordination, and all necessary supplies and equipment (drugs and nursing visits coded separately), per diem

⊘ **S9329** Home infusion therapy, chemotherapy infusion; administrative services, professional pharmacy services, care coordination, and all necessary supplies and equipment (drugs and nursing visits coded separately), per diem (do not use this code with S9330 or S9331)

⊘ **S9330** Home infusion therapy, continuous (twenty-four hours or more) chemotherapy infusion; administrative services, professional pharmacy services, care coordination, and all necessary supplies and equipment (drugs and nursing visits coded separately), per diem

⊘ **S9331** Home infusion therapy, intermittent (less than twenty-four hours) chemotherapy infusion; administrative services, professional pharmacy services, care coordination, and all necessary supplies and equipment (drugs and nursing visits coded separately), per diem

⊘ **S9335** Home therapy, hemodialysis; administrative services, professional pharmacy services, care coordination, and all necessary supplies and equipment (drugs and nursing services coded separately), per diem

⊘ **S9336** Home infusion therapy, continuous anticoagulant infusion therapy (e.g., heparin), administrative services, professional pharmacy services, care coordination, and all necessary supplies and equipment (drugs and nursing visits coded separately), per diem

⊘ **S9338** Home infusion therapy, immunotherapy, administrative services, professional pharmacy services, care coordination, and all necessary supplies and equipment (drug and nursing visits coded separately), per diem

⊘ **S9339** Home therapy; peritoneal dialysis, administrative services, professional pharmacy services, care coordination and all necessary supplies and equipment (drugs and nursing visits coded separately), per diem

⊘ **S9340** Home therapy; enteral nutrition; administrative services, professional pharmacy services, care coordination, and all necessary supplies and equipment (enteral formula and nursing visits coded separately), per diem

⊘ **S9341** Home therapy; enteral nutrition via gravity; administrative services, professional pharmacy services, care coordination, and all necessary supplies and equipment (enteral formula and nursing visits coded separately), per diem

⊘ **S9342** Home therapy; enteral nutrition via pump; administrative services, professional pharmacy services, care coordination, and all necessary supplies and equipment (enteral formula and nursing visits coded separately), per diem

⊘ **S9343** Home therapy; enteral nutrition via bolus; administrative services, professional pharmacy services, care coordination, and all necessary supplies and equipment (enteral formula and nursing visits coded separately), per diem

⊘ **S9345** Home infusion therapy, anti-hemophilic agent infusion therapy (e.g., Factor VIII); administrative services, professional pharmacy services, care coordination, and all necessary supplies and equipment (drugs and nursing visits coded separately), per diem

⊘ **S9346** Home infusion therapy, alpha-1-proteinase inhibitor (e.g., Prolastin); administrative services, professional pharmacy services, care coordination, and all necessary supplies and equipment (drugs and nursing visits coded separately), per diem

⊘ **S9347** Home infusion therapy, uninterrupted, long-term, controlled rate intravenous or subcutaneous infusion therapy (e.g., Epoprostenol); administrative services, professional pharmacy services, care coordination, and all necessary supplies and equipment (drugs and nursing visits coded separately), per diem

⊘ **S9348** Home infusion therapy, sympathomimetic/inotropic agent infusion therapy (e.g., Dobutamine); administrative services, professional pharmacy services, care coordination, all necessary supplies and equipment (drugs and nursing visits coded separately), per diem

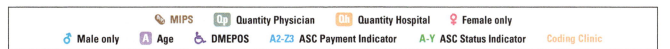

🖐 MIPS    📋 Quantity Physician    📋 Quantity Hospital    ♀ Female only

♂ Male only    A Age    ♿ DMEPOS    A2-Z3 ASC Payment Indicator    A-Y ASC Status Indicator    Coding Clinic

⊘ **S9349** Home infusion therapy, tocolytic infusion therapy; administrative services, professional pharmacy services, care coordination, and all necessary supplies and equipment (drugs and nursing visits coded separately), per diem

⊘ **S9351** Home infusion therapy, continuous or intermittent anti-emetic infusion therapy; administrative services, professional pharmacy services, care coordination, and all necessary supplies and equipment (drugs and visits coded separately), per diem

⊘ **S9353** Home infusion therapy, continuous insulin infusion therapy; administrative services, professional pharmacy services, care coordination, and all necessary supplies and equipment (drugs and nursing visits coded separately), per diem

⊘ **S9355** Home infusion therapy, chelation therapy; administrative services, professional pharmacy services, care coordination, and all necessary supplies and equipment (drugs and nursing visits coded separately), per diem

⊘ **S9357** Home infusion therapy, enzyme replacement intravenous therapy (e.g., Imiglucerase); administrative services, professional pharmacy services, care coordination, and all necessary supplies and equipment (drugs and nursing visits coded separately), per diem

⊘ **S9359** Home infusion therapy, anti-tumor necrosis factor intravenous therapy (e.g., Infliximab); administrative services, professional pharmacy services, care coordination, and all necessary supplies and equipment (drugs and nursing visits coded separately), per diem

⊘ **S9361** Home infusion therapy, diuretic intravenous therapy; administrative services, professional pharmacy services, care coordination, and all necessary supplies and equipment (drugs and nursing visits coded separately), per diem

⊘ **S9363** Home infusion therapy, anti-spasmotic therapy; administrative services, professional pharmacy services, care coordination, and all necessary supplies and equipment (drugs and nursing visits coded separately), per diem

⊘ **S9364** Home infusion therapy, total parenteral nutrition (TPN); administrative services, professional pharmacy services, care coordination, and all necessary supplies and equipment including standard TPN formula (lipids, specialty amino acid formulas, drugs other than in standard formula, and nursing visits coded separately) per diem (do not use with home infusion codes S9365-S9368 using daily volume scales)

⊘ **S9365** Home infusion therapy, total parenteral nutrition (TPN); one liter per day, administrative services, professional pharmacy services, care coordination, and all necessary supplies and equipment including standard TPN formula (lipids, specialty amino acid formulas, drugs other than in standard formula and nursing visits coded separately), per diem

⊘ **S9366** Home infusion therapy, total parenteral nutrition (TPN); more than one liter but no more than two liters per day, administrative services, professional pharmacy services, care coordination, and all necessary supplies and equipment including standard TPN formula (lipids, specialty amino acid formulas, drugs other than in standard formula and nursing visits coded separately), per diem

⊘ **S9367** Home infusion therapy, total parenteral nutrition (TPN); more than two liters but no more than three liters per day, administrative services, professional pharmacy services, care coordination, and all necessary supplies and equipment including standard TPN formula (lipids, specialty amino acid formulas, drugs other than in standard formula and nursing visits coded separately), per diem

⊘ **S9368** Home infusion therapy, total parenteral nutrition (TPN); more than three liters per day, administrative services, professional pharmacy services, care coordination, and all necessary supplies and equipment (including standard TPN formula; lipids, specialty amino acid formulas, drugs other than in standard formula and nursing visits coded separately), per diem

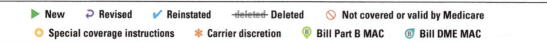

▶ New    ↩ Revised    ✔ Reinstated    ~~deleted~~ Deleted    ⊘ Not covered or valid by Medicare
⊕ Special coverage instructions    ✱ Carrier discretion    Ⓑ Bill Part B MAC    Ⓓ Bill DME MAC

⊘ **S9370** Home therapy, intermittent anti-emetic injection therapy; administrative services, professional pharmacy services, care coordination, and all necessary supplies and equipment (drugs and nursing visits coded separately), per diem

⊘ **S9372** Home therapy; intermittent anticoagulant injection therapy (e.g., heparin); administrative services, professional pharmacy services, care coordination, and all necessary supplies and equipment (drugs and nursing visits coded separately), per diem (do not use this code for flushing of infusion devices with heparin to maintain patency)

⊘ **S9373** Home infusion therapy, hydration therapy; administrative services, professional pharmacy services, care coordination, and all necessary supplies and equipment (drugs and nursing visits coded separately), per diem (do not use with hydration therapy codes S9374-S9377 using daily volume scales)

⊘ **S9374** Home infusion therapy, hydration therapy; one liter per day, administrative services, professional pharmacy services, care coordination, and all necessary supplies and equipment (drugs and nursing visits coded separately), per diem

⊘ **S9375** Home infusion therapy, hydration therapy; more than one liter but no more than two liters per day, administrative services, professional pharmacy services, care coordination, and all necessary supplies and equipment (drugs and nursing visits coded separately), per diem

⊘ **S9376** Home infusion therapy, hydration therapy; more than two liters but no more than three liters per day, administrative services, professional pharmacy services, care coordination, and all necessary supplies and equipment (drugs and nursing visits coded separately), per diem

⊘ **S9377** Home infusion therapy, hydration therapy; more than three liters per day, administrative services, professional pharmacy services, care coordination, and all necessary supplies (drugs and nursing visits coded separately), per diem

⊘ **S9379** Home infusion therapy, infusion therapy, not otherwise classified; administrative services, professional pharmacy services, care coordination, and all necessary supplies and equipment (drugs and nursing visits coded separately), per diem

## Miscellaneous Supplies and Services

⊘ **S9381** Delivery or service to high risk areas requiring escort or extra protection, per visit

⊘ **S9401** Anticoagulation clinic, inclusive of all services except laboratory tests, per session

⊘ **S9430** Pharmacy compounding and dispensing services

⊘ **S9433** Medical food nutritionally complete, administered orally, providing 100% of nutritional intake

⊘ **S9434** Modified solid food supplements for inborn errors of metabolism

⊘ **S9435** Medical foods for inborn errors of metabolism

⊘ **S9436** Childbirth preparation/Lamaze classes, non-physician provider, per session ♀

⊘ **S9437** Childbirth refresher classes, non-physician provider, per session ♀

⊘ **S9438** Cesarean birth classes, non-physician provider, per session ♀

⊘ **S9439** VBAC (vaginal birth after cesarean) classes, non-physician provider, per session ♀

⊘ **S9441** Asthma education, non-physician provider, per session

⊘ **S9442** Birthing classes, non-physician provider, per session ♀

⊘ **S9443** Lactation classes, non-physician provider, per session ♀

⊘ **S9444** Parenting classes, non-physician provider, per session

⊘ **S9445** Patient education, not otherwise classified, non-physician provider, individual, per session

⊘ **S9446** Patient education, not otherwise classified, non-physician provider, group, per session

⊘ **S9447** Infant safety (including CPR) classes, non-physician provider, per session

⊘ **S9449** Weight management classes, non-physician provider, per session

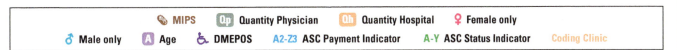

🕹 MIPS    Qp Quantity Physician    Qh Quantity Hospital    ♀ Female only
♂ Male only    A Age    ♿ DMEPOS    A2-Z3 ASC Payment Indicator    A-Y ASC Status Indicator    Coding Clinic

⊘ **S9451** Exercise classes, non-physician provider, per session

⊘ **S9452** Nutrition classes, non-physician provider, per session

⊘ **S9453** Smoking cessation classes, non-physician provider, per session

⊘ **S9454** Stress management classes, non-physician provider, per session

⊘ **S9455** Diabetic management program, group session

⊘ **S9460** Diabetic management program, nurse visit

⊘ **S9465** Diabetic management program, dietitian visit

⊘ **S9470** Nutritional counseling, dietitian visit

⊘ **S9472** Cardiac rehabilitation program, non-physician provider, per diem

⊘ **S9473** Pulmonary rehabilitation program, non-physician provider, per diem

⊘ **S9474** Enterostomal therapy by a registered nurse certified in enterostomal therapy, per diem

⊘ **S9475** Ambulatory setting substance abuse treatment or detoxification services, per diem

⊘ **S9476** Vestibular rehabilitation program, non-physician provider, per diem

⊘ **S9480** Intensive outpatient psychiatric services, per diem

⊘ **S9482** Family stabilization services, per 15 minutes

⊘ **S9484** Crisis intervention mental health services, per hour

⊘ **S9485** Crisis intervention mental health services, per diem

## Home Therapy Services

⊘ **S9490** Home infusion therapy, corticosteroid infusion; administrative services, professional pharmacy services, care coordination, and all necessary supplies and equipment (drugs and nursing visits coded separately), per diem

⊘ **S9494** Home infusion therapy, antibiotic, antiviral, or antifungal therapy; administrative services, professional pharmacy services, care coordination, and all necessary supplies and equipment (drugs and nursing visits coded separately) per diem (do not use this code with home infusion codes for hourly dosing schedules S9497-S9504)

⊘ **S9497** Home infusion therapy, antibiotic, antiviral, or antifungal therapy; once every 3 hours; administrative services, professional pharmacy services, care coordination, and all necessary supplies and equipment (drugs and nursing visits coded separately), per diem

⊘ **S9500** Home infusion therapy, antibiotic, antiviral, or antifungal therapy; once every 24 hours; administrative services, professional pharmacy services, care coordination, and all necessary supplies and equipment (drugs and nursing visits coded separately), per diem

⊘ **S9501** Home infusion therapy, antibiotic, antiviral, or antifungal therapy; once every 12 hours; administrative services, professional pharmacy services, care coordination, and all necessary supplies and equipment (drugs and nursing visits coded separately), per diem

⊘ **S9502** Home infusion therapy, antibiotic, antiviral, or antifungal therapy; once every 8 hours, administrative services, professional pharmacy services, care coordination, and all necessary supplies and equipment (drugs and nursing visits coded separately), per diem

⊘ **S9503** Home infusion therapy, antibiotic, antiviral, or antifungal; once every 6 hours; administrative services, professional pharmacy services, care coordination, and all necessary supplies and equipment (drugs and nursing visits coded separately), per diem

⊘ **S9504** Home infusion therapy, antibiotic, antiviral, or antifungal; once every 4 hours; administrative services, professional pharmacy services, care coordination, and all necessary supplies and equipment (drugs and nursing visits coded separately), per diem

⊘ **S9529** Routine venipuncture for collection of specimen(s), single home bound, nursing home, or skilled nursing facility patient

⊘ **S9537** Home therapy; hematopoietic hormone injection therapy (e.g., erythropoietin, G-CSF, GM-CSF); administrative services, professional pharmacy services, care coordination, and all necessary supplies and equipment (drugs and nursing visits coded separately), per diem

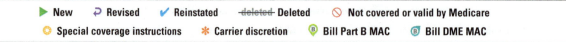

▶ New    ↻ Revised    ✔ Reinstated    ~~deleted~~ Deleted    ⊘ Not covered or valid by Medicare

🟡 Special coverage instructions    ✳ Carrier discretion    Ⓑ Bill Part B MAC    Ⓑ Bill DME MAC

⊘ **S9538** Home transfusion of blood product(s); administrative services, professional pharmacy services, care coordination, and all necessary supplies and equipment (blood products, drugs, and nursing visits coded separately), per diem

⊘ **S9542** Home injectable therapy; not otherwise classified, including administrative services, professional pharmacy services, care coordination, and all necessary supplies and equipment (drugs and nursing visits coded separately), per diem

⊘ **S9558** Home injectable therapy; growth hormone, including administrative services, professional pharmacy services, care coordination, and all necessary supplies and equipment (drugs and nursing visits coded separately), per diem

⊘ **S9559** Home injectable therapy; interferon, including administrative services, professional pharmacy services, care coordination, and all necessary supplies and equipment (drugs and nursing visits coded separately), per diem

⊘ **S9560** Home injectable therapy; hormonal therapy (e.g., Leuprolide, Goserelin), including administrative services, professional pharmacy services, care coordination, and all necessary supplies and equipment (drugs and nursing visits coded separately), per diem

⊘ **S9562** Home injectable therapy, palivizumab, including administrative services, professional pharmacy services, care coordination, and all necessary supplies and equipment (drugs and nursing visits coded separately), per diem

⊘ **S9590** Home therapy, irrigation therapy (e.g., sterile irrigation of an organ or anatomical cavity); including administrative services, professional pharmacy services, care coordination, and all necessary supplies and equipment (drugs and nursing visits coded separately), per diem

⊘ **S9810** Home therapy; professional pharmacy services for provision of infusion, specialty drug administration, and/or disease state management, not otherwise classified, per hour (do not use this code with any per diem code)

## Other Services and Fees

⊘ **S9900** Services by journal-listed Christian Science Practitioner for the purpose of healing, per diem

⊘ **S9901** Services by a journal-listed Christian Science nurse, per hour

⊘ **S9960** Ambulance service, conventional air service, nonemergency transport, one way (fixed wing)

⊘ **S9961** Ambulance service, conventional air service, nonemergency transport, one way (rotary wing)

⊘ **S9970** Health club membership, annual

⊘ **S9975** Transplant related lodging, meals and transportation, per diem

⊘ **S9976** Lodging, per diem, not otherwise classified

⊘ **S9977** Meals, per diem, not otherwise specified

⊘ **S9981** Medical records copying fee, administrative

⊘ **S9982** Medical records copying fee, per page

⊘ **S9986** Not medically necessary service (patient is aware that service not medically necessary)

⊘ **S9988** Services provided as part of a Phase I clinical trial

⊘ **S9989** Services provided outside of the United States of America (list in addition to code(s) for services(s))

⊘ **S9990** Services provided as part of a Phase II clinical trial

⊘ **S9991** Services provided as part of a Phase III clinical trial

⊘ **S9992** Transportation costs to and from trial location and local transportation costs (e.g., fares for taxicab or bus) for clinical trial participant and one caregiver/companion

⊘ **S9994** Lodging costs (e.g., hotel charges) for clinical trial participant and one caregiver/companion

⊘ **S9996** Meals for clinical trial participant and one caregiver/companion

⊘ **S9999** Sales tax

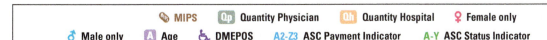

## TEMPORARY NATIONAL CODES ESTABLISHED BY MEDICAID (T1000-T9999)

### Not Valid For Medicare

⊘ **T1000** Private duty/independent nursing service(s) - licensed, up to 15 minutes

⊘ **T1001** Nursing assessment/evaluation

⊘ **T1002** RN services, up to 15 minutes

⊘ **T1003** LPN/LVN services, up to 15 minutes

⊘ **T1004** Services of a qualified nursing aide, up to 15 minutes

⊘ **T1005** Respite care services, up to 15 minutes

⊘ **T1006** Alcohol and/or substance abuse services, family/couple counseling

⊘ **T1007** Alcohol and/or substance abuse services, treatment plan development and/or modification

⊘ **T1009** Child sitting services for children of the individual receiving alcohol and/or substance abuse services A

⊘ **T1010** Meals for individuals receiving alcohol and/or substance abuse services (when meals not included in the program)

⊘ **T1012** Alcohol and/or substance abuse services, skills development

⊘ **T1013** Sign language or oral interpretive services, per 15 minutes

⊘ **T1014** Telehealth transmission, per minute, professional services bill separately

⊘ **T1015** Clinic visit/encounter, all-inclusive

⊘ **T1016** Case Management, each 15 minutes

⊘ **T1017** Targeted Case Management, each 15 minutes

⊘ **T1018** School-based individualized education program (IEP) services, bundled

⊘ **T1019** Personal care services, per 15 minutes, not for an inpatient or resident of a hospital, nursing facility, ICF/MR or IMD, part of the individualized plan of treatment (code may not be used to identify services provided by home health aide or certified nurse assistant)

⊘ **T1020** Personal care services, per diem, not for an inpatient or resident of a hospital, nursing facility, ICF/MR or IMD, part of the individualized plan of treatment (code may not be used to identify services provided by home health aide or certified nurse assistant)

⊘ **T1021** Home health aide or certified nurse assistant, per visit

⊘ **T1022** Contracted home health agency services, all services provided under contract, per day

⊘ **T1023** Screening to determine the appropriateness of consideration of an individual for participation in a specified program, project or treatment protocol, per encounter

⊘ **T1024** Evaluation and treatment by an integrated, specialty team contracted to provide coordinated care to multiple or severely handicapped children, per encounter A

⊘ **T1025** Intensive, extended multidisciplinary services provided in a clinic setting to children with complex medical, physical, mental and psychosocial impairments, per diem A

⊘ **T1026** Intensive, extended multidisciplinary services provided in a clinic setting to children with complex medical, physical, medical and psychosocial impairments, per hour A

⊘ **T1027** Family training and counseling for child development, per 15 minutes A

⊘ **T1028** Assessment of home, physical and family environment, to determine suitability to meet patient's medical needs

⊘ **T1029** Comprehensive environmental lead investigation, not including laboratory analysis, per dwelling

⊘ **T1030** Nursing care, in the home, by registered nurse, per diem

⊘ **T1031** Nursing care, in the home, by licensed practical nurse, per diem

⊘ **T1040** Medicaid certified community behavioral health clinic services, per diem

⊘ **T1041** Medicaid certified community behavioral health clinic services, per month

⊘ **T1502** Administration of oral, intramuscular and/or subcutaneous medication by health care agency/professional, per visit

⊘ **T1503** Administration of medication, other than oral and/or injectable, by a health care agency/professional, per visit

⊘ **T1505** Electronic medication compliance management device, includes all components and accessories, not otherwise classified

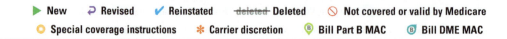

▶ New    ⮌ Revised    ✔ Reinstated    ~~deleted~~ Deleted    ⊘ Not covered or valid by Medicare
✪ Special coverage instructions    ✱ Carrier discretion    Ⓑ Bill Part B MAC    Ⓑ Bill DME MAC

○ **T1999** Miscellaneous therapeutic items and supplies, retail purchases, not otherwise classified; identify product in "remarks"

○ **T2001** Non-emergency transportation; patient attendant/escort

○ **T2002** Non-emergency transportation; per diem

○ **T2003** Non-emergency transportation; encounter/trip

○ **T2004** Non-emergency transport; commercial carrier, multi-pass

○ **T2005** Non-emergency transportation: stretcher van

○ **T2007** Transportation waiting time, air ambulance and non-emergency vehicle, one-half (1/2) hour increments

○ **T2010** Preadmission screening and resident review (PASRR) level I identification screening, per screen

○ **T2011** Preadmission screening and resident review (PASRR) level II evaluation, per evaluation

○ **T2012** Habilitation, educational, waiver; per diem

○ **T2013** Habilitation, educational, waiver; per hour

○ **T2014** Habilitation, prevocational, waiver; per diem

○ **T2015** Habilitation, prevocational, waiver; per hour

○ **T2016** Habilitation, residential, waiver; per diem

○ **T2017** Habilitation, residential, waiver; 15 minutes

○ **T2018** Habilitation, supported employment, waiver; per diem

○ **T2019** Habilitation, supported employment, waiver; per 15 minutes

○ **T2020** Day habilitation, waiver; per diem

○ **T2021** Day habilitation, waiver; per 15 minutes

○ **T2022** Case management, per month

○ **T2023** Targeted case management; per month

○ **T2024** Service assessment/plan of care development, waiver

○ **T2025** Waiver services; not otherwise specified (NOS)

○ **T2026** Specialized childcare, waiver; per diem

○ **T2027** Specialized childcare, waiver; per 15 minutes

○ **T2028** Specialized supply, not otherwise specified, waiver

○ **T2029** Specialized medical equipment, not otherwise specified, waiver

○ **T2030** Assisted living, waiver; per month

○ **T2031** Assisted living; waiver, per diem

○ **T2032** Residential care, not otherwise specified (NOS), waiver; per month

○ **T2033** Residential care, not otherwise specified (NOS), waiver; per diem

○ **T2034** Crisis intervention, waiver; per diem

○ **T2035** Utility services to support medical equipment and assistive technology/devices, waiver

○ **T2036** Therapeutic camping, overnight, waiver; each session

○ **T2037** Therapeutic camping, day, waiver; each session

○ **T2038** Community transition, waiver; per service

○ **T2039** Vehicle modifications, waiver; per service

○ **T2040** Financial management, self-directed, waiver; per 15 minutes

○ **T2041** Supports brokerage, self-directed, waiver; per 15 minutes

○ **T2042** Hospice routine home care; per diem

○ **T2043** Hospice continuous home care; per hour

○ **T2044** Hospice inpatient respite care; per diem

○ **T2045** Hospice general inpatient care; per diem

○ **T2046** Hospice long term care, room and board only; per diem

○ **T2048** Behavioral health; long-term care residential (non-acute care in a residential treatment program where stay is typically longer than 30 days), with room and board, per diem

○ **T2049** Non-emergency transportation; stretcher van, mileage; per mile

○ **T2101** Human breast milk processing, storage and distribution only ♀

○ **T4521** Adult sized disposable incontinence product, brief/diaper, small, each 🅐
*IOM: 100-03, 4, 280.1*

○ **T4522** Adult sized disposable incontinence product, brief/diaper, medium, each 🅐
*IOM: 100-03, 4, 280.1*

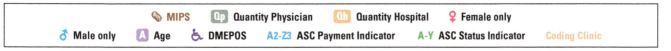

🅜 MIPS    🆀🅟 Quantity Physician    🆀🅷 Quantity Hospital    ♀ Female only    ♂ Male only    🅐 Age    ♿ DMEPOS    A2-Z3 ASC Payment Indicator    A-Y ASC Status Indicator    Coding Clinic

⊘ **T4523** Adult sized disposable incontinence product, brief/diaper, large, each Ⓐ

*IOM: 100-03, 4, 280.1*

⊘ **T4524** Adult sized disposable incontinence product, brief/diaper, extra large, each Ⓐ

*IOM: 100-03, 4, 280.1*

⊘ **T4525** Adult sized disposable incontinence product, protective underwear/pull-on, small size, each Ⓐ

*IOM: 100-03, 4, 280.1*

⊘ **T4526** Adult sized disposable incontinence product, protective underwear/pull-on, medium size, each Ⓐ

*IOM: 100-03, 4, 280.1*

⊘ **T4527** Adult sized disposable incontinence product, protective underwear/pull-on, large size, each Ⓐ

*IOM: 100-03, 4, 280.1*

⊘ **T4528** Adult sized disposable incontinence product, protective underwear/pull-on, extra large size, each Ⓐ

*IOM: 100-03, 4, 280.1*

⊘ **T4529** Pediatric sized disposable incontinence product, brief/diaper, small/medium size, each Ⓐ

*IOM: 100-03, 4, 280.1*

⊘ **T4530** Pediatric sized disposable incontinence product, brief/diaper, large size, each Ⓐ

*IOM: 100-03, 4, 280.1*

⊘ **T4531** Pediatric sized disposable incontinence product, protective underwear/pull-on, small/medium size, each Ⓐ

*IOM: 100-03, 4, 280.1*

⊘ **T4532** Pediatric sized disposable incontinence product, protective underwear/pull-on, large size, each Ⓐ

*IOM: 100-03, 4, 280.1*

⊘ **T4533** Youth sized disposable incontinence product, brief/diaper, each Ⓐ

*IOM: 100-03, 4, 280.1*

⊘ **T4534** Youth sized disposable incontinence product, protective underwear/pull-on, each Ⓐ

*IOM: 100-03, 4, 280.1*

⊘ **T4535** Disposable liner/shield/guard/pad/ undergarment, for incontinence, each

*IOM: 100-03, 4, 280.1*

⊘ **T4536** Incontinence product, protective underwear/pull-on, reusable, any size, each

*IOM: 100-03, 4, 280.1*

⊘ **T4537** Incontinence product, protective underpad, reusable, bed size, each

*IOM: 100-03, 4, 280.1*

⊘ **T4538** Diaper service, reusable diaper, each diaper

*IOM: 100-03, 4, 280.1*

⊘ **T4539** Incontinence product, diaper/brief, reusable, any size, each

*IOM: 100-03, 4, 280.1*

⊘ **T4540** Incontinence product, protective underpad, reusable, chair size, each

*IOM: 100-03, 4, 280.1*

⊘ **T4541** Incontinence product, disposable underpad, large, each

⊘ **T4542** Incontinence product, disposable underpad, small size, each

⊘ **T4543** Adult sized disposable incontinence product, protective brief/diaper, above extra large, each Ⓐ

*IOM: 100-03, 4, 280.1*

⊘ **T4544** Adult sized disposable incontinence product, protective underwear/pull-on, above extra large, each Ⓐ

*IOM: 100-03, 4, 280.1*

⊘ **T4545** Incontinence product, disposable, penile wrap, each ♂

⊘ **T5001** Positioning seat for persons with special orthopedic needs, supply, not otherwise specified

⊘ **T5999** Supply, not otherwise specified

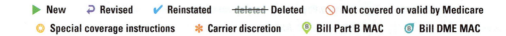

▶ New    ↺ Revised    ✔ Reinstated    ~~deleted~~ Deleted    ⊘ Not covered or valid by Medicare
   ⊙ Special coverage instructions    ✳ Carrier discretion    Ⓑ Bill Part B MAC    Ⓑ Bill DME MAC

## VISION SERVICES (V0000-V2999)

### Frames

✿ **V2020** Frames, purchases Ⓑ 〔Qp〕〔Qh〕 ♿ A

Includes cost of frame/replacement and dispensing fee. One unit of service represents one pair of eyeglass frames.

*IOM: 100-02, 15, 120*

⊘ **V2025** Deluxe frame Ⓑ 〔Qp〕〔Qh〕 E1

Not a benefit. Billing deluxe frames- submit V2020 on one line; V2025 on second line.

*IOM: 100-04, 1, 30.3.5*

If a CPT procedure code for supply of spectacles or a permanent prosthesis is reported, recode with the specific lens type listed below.

### Single Vision Lenses

✳ **V2100** Sphere, single vision, plano to plus or minus 4.00, per lens Ⓑ 〔Qp〕〔Qh〕 ♿ A

✳ **V2101** Sphere, single vision, plus or minus 4.12 to plus or minus 7.00d, per lens Ⓑ 〔Qp〕〔Qh〕 ♿ A

✳ **V2102** Sphere, single vision, plus or minus 7.12 to plus or minus 20.00d, per lens Ⓑ 〔Qp〕〔Qh〕 ♿ A

✳ **V2103** Spherocylinder, single vision, plano to plus or minus 4.00d sphere, .12 to 2.00d cylinder, per lens Ⓑ 〔Qp〕〔Qh〕 ♿ A

✳ **V2104** Spherocylinder, single vision, plano to plus or minus 4.00d sphere, 2.12 to 4.00d cylinder, per lens Ⓑ 〔Qp〕〔Qh〕 ♿ A

✳ **V2105** Spherocylinder, single vision, plano to plus or minus 4.00d sphere, 4.25 to 6.00d cylinder, per lens Ⓑ 〔Qp〕〔Qh〕 ♿ A

✳ **V2106** Spherocylinder, single vision, plano to plus or minus 4.00d sphere, over 6.00d cylinder, per lens Ⓑ 〔Qp〕〔Qh〕 ♿ A

✳ **V2107** Spherocylinder, single vision, plus or minus 4.25 to plus or minus 7.00 sphere, .12 to 2.00d cylinder, per lens Ⓑ 〔Qp〕〔Qh〕 ♿ A

✳ **V2108** Spherocylinder, single vision, plus or minus 4.25d to plus or minus 7.00d sphere, 2.12 to 4.00d cylinder, per lens Ⓑ 〔Qp〕〔Qh〕 ♿ A

✳ **V2109** Spherocylinder, single vision, plus or minus 4.25 to plus or minus 7.00d sphere, 4.25 to 6.00d cylinder, per lens Ⓑ 〔Qp〕〔Qh〕 ♿ A

✳ **V2110** Sperocylinder, single vision, plus or minus 4.25 to 7.00d sphere, over 6.00d cylinder, per lens Ⓑ 〔Qp〕〔Qh〕 ♿ A

✳ **V2111** Spherocylinder, single vision, plus or minus 7.25 to plus or minus 12.00d sphere, .25 to 2.25d cylinder, per lens Ⓑ 〔Qp〕〔Qh〕 ♿ A

✳ **V2112** Spherocylinder, single vision, plus or minus 7.25 to plus or minus 12.00d sphere, 2.25d to 4.00d cylinder, per lens Ⓑ 〔Qp〕〔Qh〕 ♿ A

✳ **V2113** Spherocylinder, single vision, plus or minus 7.25 to plus or minus 12.00d sphere, 4.25 to 6.00d cylinder, per lens Ⓑ 〔Qp〕〔Qh〕 ♿ A

✳ **V2114** Spherocylinder, single vision, sphere over plus or minus 12.00d, per lens Ⓑ 〔Qp〕〔Qh〕 ♿ A

✳ **V2115** Lenticular, (myodisc), per lens, single vision Ⓑ 〔Qp〕〔Qh〕 ♿ A

✳ **V2118** Aniseikonic lens, single vision Ⓑ 〔Qp〕〔Qh〕 A

✿ **V2121** Lenticular lens, per lens, single Ⓑ 〔Qp〕〔Qh〕 ♿ A

*IOM: 100-02, 15, 120; 100-04, 3, 10.4*

✳ **V2199** Not otherwise classified, single vision lens Ⓑ 〔Qp〕〔Qh〕 A

Bill on paper. Requires report of type of single vision lens and optical lab invoice.

### Bifocal Lenses

✳ **V2200** Sphere, bifocal, plano to plus or minus 4.00d, per lens Ⓑ 〔Qp〕〔Qh〕 ♿ A

✳ **V2201** Sphere, bifocal, plus or minus 4.12 to plus or minus 7.00d, per lens Ⓑ 〔Qp〕〔Qh〕 ♿ A

✳ **V2202** Sphere, bifocal, plus or minus 7.12 to plus or minus 20.00d, per lens Ⓑ 〔Qp〕〔Qh〕 ♿ A

✳ **V2203** Spherocylinder, bifocal, plano to plus or minus 4.00d sphere, .12 to 2.00d cylinder, per lens Ⓑ 〔Qp〕〔Qh〕 A

✳ **V2204** Spherocylinder, bifocal, plano to plus or minus 4.00d sphere, 2.12 to 4.00d cylinder, per lens Ⓑ 〔Qp〕〔Qh〕 ♿ A

✳ **V2205** Spherocylinder, bifocal, plano to plus or minus 4.00d sphere, 4.25 to 6.00d cylinder, per lens Ⓑ 〔Qp〕〔Qh〕 ♿ A

✳ **V2206** Spherocylinder, bifocal, plano to plus or minus 4.00d sphere, over 6.00d cylinder, per lens Ⓑ 〔Qp〕〔Qh〕 ♿ A

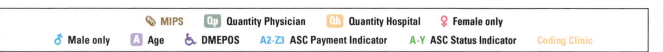

🔖 MIPS　〔Qp〕 Quantity Physician　〔Qh〕 Quantity Hospital　♀ Female only
♂ Male only　Ⓐ Age　♿ DMEPOS　A2-Z3 ASC Payment Indicator　A-Y ASC Status Indicator　Coding Clinic

\* **V2207** Spherocylinder, bifocal, plus or minus 4.25 to plus or minus 7.00d sphere, .12 to 2.00d cylinder, per lens Ⓑ Qp Qh ♿ A

\* **V2208** Spherocylinder, bifocal, plus or minus 4.25 to plus or minus 7.00d sphere, 2.12 to 4.00d cylinder, per lens Ⓑ Qp Qh ♿ A

\* **V2209** Spherocylinder, bifocal, plus or minus 4.25 to plus or minus 7.00d sphere, 4.25 to 6.00d cylinder, per lens Ⓑ Qp Qh ♿ A

\* **V2210** Spherocylinder, bifocal, plus or minus 4.25 to plus or minus 7.00d sphere, over 6.00d cylinder, per lens Ⓑ Qp Qh ♿ A

\* **V2211** Spherocylinder, bifocal, plus or minus 7.25 to plus or minus 12.00d sphere, .25 to 2.25d cylinder, per lens Ⓑ Qp Qh ♿ A

\* **V2212** Spherocylinder, bifocal, plus or minus 7.25 to plus or minus 12.00d sphere, 2.25 to 4.00d cylinder, per lens Ⓑ Qp Qh ♿ A

\* **V2213** Spherocylinder, bifocal, plus or minus 7.25 to plus or minus 12.00d sphere, 4.25 to 6.00d cylinder, per lens Ⓑ Qp Qh ♿ A

\* **V2214** Spherocylinder, bifocal, sphere over plus or minus 12.00d, per lens Ⓑ Qp Qh ♿ A

\* **V2215** Lenticular (myodisc), per lens, bifocal Ⓑ Qp Qh ♿ A

\* **V2218** Aniseikonic, per lens, bifocal Ⓑ Qp Qh ♿ A

\* **V2219** Bifocal seg width over 28 mm Ⓑ Qp Qh ♿ A

\* **V2220** Bifocal add over 3.25d Qp Qh ♿ A

⊛ **V2221** Lenticular lens, per lens, bifocal Ⓑ Qp Qh ♿ A

*IOM: 100-02, 15, 120; 100-04, 3, 10.4*

\* **V2299** Specialty bifocal (by report) Ⓑ Qp Qh A

Bill on paper. Requires report of type of specialty bifocal lens and optical lab invoice.

## Trifocal Lenses

\* **V2300** Sphere, trifocal, plano to plus or minus 4.00d, per lens Ⓑ Qp Qh ♿ A

\* **V2301** Sphere, trifocal, plus or minus 4.12 to plus or minus 7.00d per lens Ⓑ Qp Qh ♿ A

\* **V2302** Sphere, trifocal, plus or minus 7.12 to plus or minus 20.00, per lens Ⓑ Qp Qh ♿ A

\* **V2303** Spherocylinder, trifocal, plano to plus or minus 4.00d sphere, .12 to 2.00d cylinder, per lens Ⓑ Qp Qh ♿ A

\* **V2304** Spherocylinder, trifocal, plano to plus or minus 4.00d sphere, 2.25-4.00d cylinder, per lens Ⓑ Qp Qh ♿ A

\* **V2305** Spherocylinder, trifocal, plano to plus or minus 4.00d sphere, 4.25 to 6.00 cylinder, per lens Ⓑ Qp Qh ♿ A

\* **V2306** Spherocylinder, trifocal, plano to plus or minus 4.00d sphere, over 6.00d cylinder, per lens Ⓑ Qp Qh ♿ A

\* **V2307** Spherocylinder, trifocal, plus or minus 4.25 to plus or minus 7.00d sphere, .12 to 2.00d cylinder, per lens Ⓑ Qp Qh ♿ A

\* **V2308** Spherocylinder, trifocal, plus or minus 4.25 to plus or minus 7.00d sphere, 2.12 to 4.00d cylinder, per lens Ⓑ Qp Qh ♿ A

\* **V2309** Spherocylinder, trifocal, plus or minus 4.25 to plus or minus 7.00d sphere, 4.25 to 6.00d cylinder, per lens Ⓑ Qp Qh ♿ A

\* **V2310** Spherocylinder, trifocal, plus or minus 4.25 to plus or minus 7.00d sphere, over 6.00d cylinder, per lens Ⓑ Qp Qh ♿ A

\* **V2311** Spherocylinder, trifocal, plus or minus 7.25 to plus or minus 12.00d sphere, .25 to 2.25d cylinder, per lens Ⓑ Qp Qh ♿ A

\* **V2312** Spherocylinder, trifocal, plus or minus 7.25 to plus or minus 12.00d sphere, 2.25 to 4.00d cylinder, per lens Ⓑ Qp Qh ♿ A

\* **V2313** Spherocylinder, trifocal, plus or minus 7.25 to plus or minus 12.00d sphere, 4.25 to 6.00d cylinder, per lens Ⓑ Qp Qh ♿ A

\* **V2314** Spherocylinder, trifocal, sphere over plus or minus 12.00d, per lens Ⓑ Qp Qh ♿ A

\* **V2315** Lenticular, (myodisc), per lens, trifocal Ⓑ Qp Qh ♿ A

\* **V2318** Aniseikonic lens, trifocal Ⓑ Qp Qh ♿ A

\* **V2319** Trifocal seg width over 28 mm Ⓑ Qp Qh ♿ A

\* **V2320** Trifocal add over 3.25d Ⓑ Qp Qh ♿ A

▶ New  ↻ Revised  ✔ Reinstated  ~~deleted~~ Deleted  ⊘ Not covered or valid by Medicare

⊛ Special coverage instructions  \* Carrier discretion  Ⓟ Bill Part B MAC  Ⓑ Bill DME MAC

⊛ **V2321**   Lenticular lens, per lens, trifocal Ⓑ Qp Qh 🦽    A

*IOM: 100-02, 15, 120; 100-04, 3, 10.4*

✳ **V2399**   Specialty trifocal (by report) Ⓑ Qp Qh    A

Bill on paper. Requires report of type of trifocal lens and optical lab invoice.

## Variable Asphericity/Sphericity Lenses

✳ **V2410**   Variable asphericity lens, single vision, full field, glass or plastic, per lens Ⓑ Qp Qh 🦽    A

✳ **V2430**   Variable asphericity lens, bifocal, full field, glass or plastic, per lens Ⓑ Qp Qh 🦽    A

✳ **V2499**   Variable sphericity lens, other type Ⓑ Qp Qh    A

Bill on paper. Requires report of other ptical lab invoice.

## Contact Lenses

If a CPT procedure code for supply of contact lens is reported, recode with specific lens type listed below (per lens).

✳ **V2500**   Contact lens, PMMA, spherical, per lens Ⓑ Qp Qh 🦽    A

Requires prior authorization for patients under age 21.

✳ **V2501**   Contact lens, PMMA, toric or prism ballast, per lens Ⓑ Qp Qh 🦽    A

Requires prior authorization for clients under age 21.

✳ **V2502**   Contact lens, PMMA, bifocal, per lens Ⓑ Qp Qh 🦽    A

Requires prior authorization for clients under age 21. Bill on paper. Requires optical lab invoice.

✳ **V2503**   Contact lens PMMA, color vision deficiency, per lens Ⓑ Qp Qh 🦽    A

Requires prior authorization for clients under age 21. Bill on paper. Requires optical lab invoice.

✳ **V2510**   Contact lens, gas permeable, spherical, per lens Ⓑ Qp Qh 🦽    A

Requires prior authorization for clients under age 21.

✳ **V2511**   Contact lens, gas permeable, toric, prism ballast, per lens Ⓑ Qp Qh 🦽    A

Requires prior authorization for clients under age 21.

✳ **V2512**   Contact lens, gas permeable, bifocal, per lens Ⓑ Qp Qh 🦽    A

Requires prior authorization for clients under age 21.

✳ **V2513**   Contact lens, gas permeable, extended wear, per lens Ⓑ Qp Qh 🦽    A

Requires prior authorization for clients under age 21.

⊛ **V2520**   Contact lens, hydrophilic, spherical, per lens Ⓑ Ⓑ Qp Qh 🦽    A

Requires prior authorization for clients under age 21.

*IOM: 100-03, 1, 80.1; 100-03, 1, 80.4*

⊛ **V2521**   Contact lens, hydrophilic, toric, or prism ballast, per lens Ⓑ Ⓑ Qp Qh 🦽    A

Requires prior authorization for clients under age 21.

*IOM: 100-03, 1, 80.1; 100-03, 1, 80.4*

⊛ **V2522**   Contact lens, hydrophilic, bifocal, per lens Ⓑ Ⓑ Qp Qh 🦽    A

Requires prior authorization for clients under age 21.

*IOM: 100-03, 1, 80.1; 100-03, 1, 80.4*

⊛ **V2523**   Contact lens, hydrophilic, extended wear, per lens Ⓑ Ⓑ Qp Qh 🦽    A

Requires prior authorization for clients under age 21.

*IOM: 100-03, 1, 80.1; 100-03, 1, 80.4*

✳ **V2530**   Contact lens, scleral, gas impermeable, per lens (for contact lens modification, *see* 92325) Ⓑ Qp Qh 🦽    A

Requires prior authorization for clients under age 21.

⊛ **V2531**   Contact lens, scleral, gas permeable, per lens (for contact lens modification, *see* 92325) Ⓑ Qp Qh 🦽    A

Requires prior authorization for clients under age 21. Bill on paper. Requires optical lab invoice.

*IOM: 100-03, 1, 80.5*

✳ **V2599**   Contact lens, other type Ⓑ Ⓑ Qp Qh A

Requires prior authorization for clients under age 21. Bill on paper. Requires report of other type of contact lens and optical invoice.

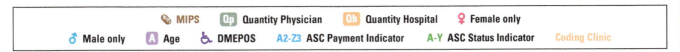

🐾 MIPS    Qp Quantity Physician    Qh Quantity Hospital    ♀ Female only

♂ Male only    Ⓐ Age    🦽 DMEPOS    A2-Z3 ASC Payment Indicator    A-Y ASC Status Indicator    Coding Clinic

## Low Vision Aids

If a CPT procedure code for supply of low vision aid is reported, recode with specific systems listed below.

**✳ V2600** Hand held low vision aids and other nonspectacle mounted aids Ⓑ Qp Qh   A

Requires prior authorization.

**✳ V2610** Single lens spectacle mounted low vision aids Ⓑ Qp Qh   A

Requires prior authorization.

**✳ V2615** Telescopic and other compound lens system, including distance vision telescopic, near vision telescopes and compound microscopic lens system Ⓑ Qp Qh   A

Requires prior authorization. Bill on paper. Requires optical lab invoice.

## Prosthetic Eye

**⚙ V2623** Prosthetic eye, plastic, custom Ⓑ Qp Qh &   A

DME regional carrier. Requires prior authorization. Bill on paper. Requires optical lab invoice.

**✳ V2624** Polishing/resurfacing of ocular prosthesis Ⓑ Qp Qh &   A

Requires prior authorization. Bill on paper. Requires optical lab invoice.

**✳ V2625** Enlargement of ocular prosthesis Ⓑ Qp Qh &   A

Requires prior authorization. Bill on paper. Requires optical lab invoice.

**✳ V2626** Reduction of ocular prosthesis Ⓑ Qp Qh &   A

Requires prior authorization. Bill on paper. Requires optical lab invoice.

**⚙ V2627** Scleral cover shell Ⓑ Qp Qh &   A

DME regional carrier

Requires prior authorization. Bill on paper. Requires optical lab invoice.

*IOM: 100-03, 4, 280.2*

**✳ V2628** Fabrication and fitting of ocular conformer Ⓑ Qp Qh &   A

Requires prior authorization. Bill on paper. Requires optical lab invoice.

**✳ V2629** Prosthetic eye, other type Ⓑ Qp Qh   A

Requires prior authorization. Bill on paper. Requires optical lab invoice.

## Intraocular Lenses

**⚙ V2630** Anterior chamber intraocular lens Ⓑ Qp Qh &   N1  N

*IOM: 100-02, 15, 120*

**⚙ V2631** Iris supported intraocular lens Ⓑ Qp Qh &   N1  N

*IOM: 100-02, 15, 120*

**⚙ V2632** Posterior chamber intraocular lens Ⓑ Qp Qh &   N1  N

*IOM: 100-02, 15, 120*

**Figure 52**  Posterior intraocular lens.

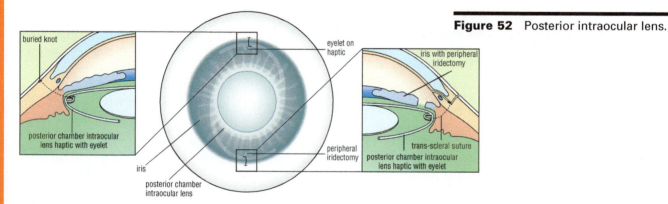

buried knot

posterior chamber intraocular lens haptic with eyelet

iris

posterior chamber intraocular lens

eyelet on haptic

peripheral iridectomy

iris with peripheral iridectomy

trans-scleral suture

posterior chamber intraocular lens haptic with eyelet

▶ New   ↻ Revised   ✔ Reinstated   ~~deleted~~ Deleted   ⊘ Not covered or valid by Medicare

⚙ Special coverage instructions   ✳ Carrier discretion   Ⓑ Bill Part B MAC   Ⓑ Bill DME MAC

## Miscellaneous Vision Services

✳ **V2700**  Balance lens, per lens ⑧ Qp Qh ♿  A

⊘ **V2702**  Deluxe lens feature ⑧ Qp Qh  E1

*IOM: 100-02, 15, 120; 100-04, 3, 10.4*

✳ **V2710**  Slab off prism, glass or plastic, per lens ⑧ Qp Qh  A

✳ **V2715**  Prism, per lens ⑧ Qp Qh ♿  A

✳ **V2718**  Press-on lens, Fresnel prism, per lens ⑧ Qp Qh ♿  A

✳ **V2730**  Special base curve, glass or plastic, per lens ⑧ Qp Qh  A

✿ **V2744**  Tint, photochromatic, per lens ⑧ Qp Qh ♿  A

Requires prior authorization.

*IOM: 100-02, 15, 120; 100-04, 3, 10.4*

✿ **V2745**  Addition to lens, tint, any color, solid, gradient or equal, excludes photochroatic, any lens material, per lens ⑧ Qp Qh ♿  A

Includes photochromatic lenses (V2744) used as sunglasses, which are prescribed in addition to regular prosthetic lenses for aphakic patient will be denied as not medically necessary.

*IOM: 100-02, 15, 120; 100-04, 3, 10.4*

✿ **V2750**  Anti-reflective coating, per lens ⑧ Qp Qh ♿  A

Requires prior authorization.

*IOM: 100-02, 15, 120; 100-04, 3, 10.4*

✿ **V2755**  U-V lens, per lens ⑧ Qp Qh ♿  A

*IOM: 100-02, 15, 120; 100-04, 3, 10.4*

✳ **V2756**  Eye glass case ⑧ Qp Qh  E1

✳ **V2760**  Scratch resistant coating, per lens ⑧ Qp Qh ♿  E1

✿ **V2761**  Mirror coating, any type, solid, gradient or equal, any lens material, per lens ⑧ Qp Qh  B

*IOM: 100-02, 15, 120; 100-04, 3, 10.4*

✿ **V2762**  Polarization, any lens material, per lens ⑧ Qp Qh ♿  E1

*IOM: 100-02, 15, 120; 100-04, 3, 10.4*

✳ **V2770**  Occluder lens, per lens ⑧ Qp Qh ♿  A

Requires prior authorization.

✳ **V2780**  Oversize lens, per lens ⑧ Qp Qh ♿  A

Requires prior authorization.

✳ **V2781**  Progressive lens, per lens ⑧ Qp Qh  B

Requires prior authorization.

✿ **V2782**  Lens, index 1.54 to 1.65 plastic or 1.60 to 1.79 glass, excludes polycarbonate, per lens ⑧ Qp Qh ♿  A

Do not bill in addition to V2784

*IOM: 100-02, 15, 120; 100-04, 3, 10.4*

✿ **V2783**  Lens, index greater than or equal to 1.66 plastic or greater than or equal to 1.80 glass, excludes polycarbonate, per lens ⑧ Qp Qh ♿  A

Do not bill in addition to V2784

*IOM: 100-02, 15, 120; 100-04, 3, 10.4*

✿ **V2784**  Lens, polycarbonate or equal, any index, per lens ⑧ Qp Qh ♿  A

Covered only for patients with functional vision in one eye-in this situation, an impact-resistant material is covered for both lenses if eyeglasses are covered. Claims with V2784 that do not meet this coverage criterion will be denied as not medically necessary.

*IOM: 100-02, 15, 120; 100-04, 3, 10.4*

✳ **V2785**  Processing, preserving and transporting corneal tissue ⑧ Qp Qh  F4 F

For ASC, bill on paper. Must attach eye bank invoice to claim.

For Hospitals, bill charges for corneal tissue to receive cost based reimbursement.

*IOM: 100- 4, 4, 200.1*

✿ **V2786**  Specialty occupational multifocal lens, per lens ⑧ Qp Qh ♿  E1

*IOM: 100-02, 15, 120; 100-04, 3, 10.4*

◠ **V2787**  Astigmatism correcting function of intraocular lens ⑧  E1

*Medicare Statute 1862(a)(7)*

⊘ **V2788**  Presbyopia correcting function of intraocular lens ⑧  E1

*Medicare Statute 1862a7*

✳ **V2790**  Amniotic membrane for surgical reconstruction, per procedure ⑧ Qp Qh  N1 N

✳ **V2797**  Vision supply, accessory and/or service component of another HCPCS vision code ⑧ Qp Qh  E1

✳ **V2799**  Vision item or service, miscellaneous ⑧  A

Bill on paper. Requires report of miscellaneous service and optical lab invoice.

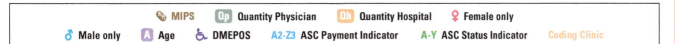

🖥 MIPS   Qp Quantity Physician   Qh Quantity Hospital   ♀ Female only
♂ Male only   Ⓐ Age   ♿ DMEPOS   A2-Z3 ASC Payment Indicator   A-Y ASC Status Indicator   Coding Clinic

## HEARING SERVICES (V5000-V5999)

These codes are for non-physician services.

### Assessments and Evaluations

⊘ **V5008**  Hearing screening Ⓑ ⓆⱣ Ⓠⱨ    E1
   *IOM: 100-02, 16, 90*

⊘ **V5010**  Assessment for hearing aid Ⓑ ⓆⱣ Ⓠⱨ    E1
   *Medicare Statute 1862a7*

⊘ **V5011**  Fitting/orientation/checking of hearing aid Ⓑ ⓆⱣ Ⓠⱨ    E1
   *Medicare Statute 1862a7*

⊘ **V5014**  Repair/modification of a hearing aid Ⓑ    E1
   *Medicare Statute 1862a7*

⊘ **V5020**  Conformity evaluation Ⓑ    E1
   *Medicare Statute 1862a7*

### Monaural Hearing Aid

⊘ **V5030**  Hearing aid, monaural, body worn, air conduction Ⓑ    E1
   *Medicare Statute 1862a7*

⊘ **V5040**  Hearing aid, monaural, body worn, bone conduction Ⓑ    E1
   *Medicare Statute 1862a7*

⊘ **V5050**  Hearing aid, monaural, in the ear Ⓑ    E1
   *Medicare Statute 1862a7*

⊘ **V5060**  Hearing aid, monaural, behind the ear Ⓑ    E1
   *Medicare Statute 1862a7*

### Miscellaneous Services and Supplies

⊘ **V5070**  Glasses, air conduction Ⓑ    E1
   *Medicare Statute 1862a7*

⊘ **V5080**  Glasses, bone conduction Ⓑ    E1
   *Medicare Statute 1862a7*

⊘ **V5090**  Dispensing fee, unspecified hearing aid Ⓑ    E1
   *Medicare Statute 1862a7*

⊘ **V5095**  Semi-implantable middle ear hearing prosthesis Ⓑ    E1
   *Medicare Statute 1862a7*

⊘ **V5100**  Hearing aid, bilateral, body worn Ⓑ    E1
   *Medicare Statute 1862a7*

⊘ **V5110**  Dispensing fee, bilateral Ⓑ    E1
   *Medicare Statute 1862a7*

### Hearing Aids

⊘ **V5120**  Binaural, body Ⓑ    E1
   *Medicare Statute 1862a7*

⊘ **V5130**  Binaural, in the ear Ⓑ    E1
   *Medicare Statute 1862a7*

⊘ **V5140**  Binaural, behind the ear Ⓑ    E1
   *Medicare Statute 1862a7*

⊘ **V5150**  Binaural, glasses Ⓑ    E1
   *Medicare Statute 1862a7*

⊘ **V5160**  Dispensing fee, binaural Ⓑ    E1
   *Medicare Statute 1862a7*

⊘ **V5171**  Hearing aid, contralateral routing device, monaural, in the ear (ITE) Ⓑ    E1
   *Medicare Statute 1862a7*

⊘ **V5172**  Hearing aid, contralateral routing device, monaural, in the canal (ITC) Ⓑ    E1
   *Medicare Statute 1862a7*

⊘ **V5181**  Hearing aid, contralateral routing device, monaural, behind the ear (BTE) Ⓑ    E1
   *Medicare Statute 1862a7*

⊘ **V5190**  Hearing aid, contralateral routing, monaural, glasses Ⓑ    E1
   *Medicare Statute 1862a7*

⊘ **V5200**  Dispensing fee, contralateral, monaural Ⓑ    E1
   *Medicare Statute 1862a7*

⊘ **V5211**  Hearing aid, contralateral routing system, binaural, ITE/ITE Ⓑ    E1
   *Medicare Statute 1862a7*

⊘ **V5212**  Hearing aid, contralateral routing system, binaural, ITE/ITC Ⓑ    E1
   *Medicare Statute 1862a7*

⊘ **V5213**  Hearing aid, contralateral routing system, binaural, ITE/BTE Ⓑ    E1
   *Medicare Statute 1862a7*

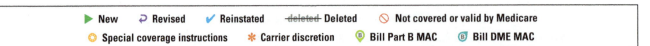

▶ New   ↻ Revised   ✔ Reinstated   ~~deleted~~ Deleted   ⊘ Not covered or valid by Medicare
⊙ Special coverage instructions   ✳ Carrier discretion   Ⓑ Bill Part B MAC   Ⓑ Bill DME MAC

⊘ **V5214** Hearing aid, contralateral routing system, binaural, ITC/ITC  E1

*Medicare Statute 1862a7*

⊘ **V5215** Hearing aid, contralateral routing system, binaural, ITC/BTE  E1

*Medicare Statute 1862a7*

⊘ **V5221** Hearing aid, contralateral routing system, binaural, BTE/BTE  E1

*Medicare Statute 1862a7*

⊘ **V5230** Hearing aid, contralateral routing system, binaural, glasses ⑧  E1

*Medicare Statute 1862a7*

⊘ **V5240** Dispensing fee, contralateral routing system, binaural ⑧  E1

*Medicare Statute 1862a7*

⊘ **V5241** Dispensing fee, monaural hearing aid, any type ⑧  E1

*Medicare Statute 1862a7*

⊘ **V5242** Hearing aid, analog, monaural, CIC (completely in the ear canal) ⑧  E1

*Medicare Statute 1862a7*

⊘ **V5243** Hearing aid, analog, monaural, ITC (in the canal) ⑧  E1

*Medicare Statute 1862a9*

⊘ **V5244** Hearing aid, digitally programmable analog, monaural, CIC ⑧  E1

*Medicare Statute 1862a7*

⊘ **V5245** Hearing aid, digitally programmable, analog, monaural, ITC ⑧  E1

*Medicare Statute 1862a7*

⊘ **V5246** Hearing aid, digitally programmable analog, monaural, ITE (in the ear) ⑧ E1

*Medicare Statute 1862a7*

⊘ **V5247** Hearing aid, digitally programmable analog, monaural, BTE (behind the ear) ⑧  E1

*Medicare Statute 1862a7*

⊘ **V5248** Hearing aid, analog, binaural, CIC ⑧ E1

*Medicare Statute 1862a7*

⊘ **V5249** Hearing aid, analog, binaural, ITC ⑧ E1

*Medicare Statute 1862a7*

⊘ **V5250** Hearing aid, digitally programmable analog, binaural, CIC ⑧  E1

*Medicare Statute 1862a7*

⊘ **V5251** Hearing aid, digitally programmable analog, binaural, ITC ⑧  E1

*Medicare Statute 1862a7*

⊘ **V5252** Hearing aid, digitally programmable, binaural, ITE ⑧  E1

*Medicare Statute 1862a7*

⊘ **V5253** Hearing aid, digitally programmable, binaural, BTE ⑧  E1

*Medicare Statute 1862a7*

⊘ **V5254** Hearing aid, digital, monaural, CIC ⑧E1

*Medicare Statute 1862a7*

⊘ **V5255** Hearing aid, digital, monaural, ITC ⑧E1

*Medicare Statute 1862a7*

⊘ **V5256** Hearing aid, digital, monaural, ITE ⑧E1

*Medicare Statute 1862a7*

⊘ **V5257** Hearing aid, digital, monaural, BTE ⑧  E1

*Medicare Statute 1862a7*

⊘ **V5258** Hearing aid, digital, binaural, CIC ⑧ E1

*Medicare Statute 1862a7*

⊘ **V5259** Hearing aid, digital, binaural, ITC ⑧ E1

*Medicare Statute 1862a7*

⊘ **V5260** Hearing aid, digital, binaural, ITE ⑧ E1

*Medicare Statute 1862a7*

⊘ **V5261** Hearing aid, digital, binaural, BTE ⑧ E1

*Medicare Statute 1862a7*

⊘ **V5262** Hearing aid, disposable, any type, monaural ⑧  E1

*Medicare Statute 1862a7*

⊘ **V5263** Hearing aid, disposable, any type, binaural ⑧  E1

*Medicare Statute 1862a7*

⊘ **V5264** Ear mold/insert, not disposable, any type ⑧  E1

*Medicare Statute 1862a7*

⊘ **V5265** Ear mold/insert, disposable, any type ⑧  E1

*Medicare Statute 1862a7*

⊘ **V5266** Battery for use in hearing device ⑧  E1

*Medicare Statute 1862a7*

⊘ **V5267** Hearing aid or assistive listening device/supplies/accessories, not otherwise specified ⑧  E1

*Medicare Statute 1862a7*

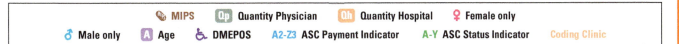

🐾 MIPS  **Qp** Quantity Physician  **Qh** Quantity Hospital  ♀ Female only
♂ Male only  **A** Age  &. DMEPOS  A2-Z3 ASC Payment Indicator  A-Y ASC Status Indicator  Coding Clinic

## Assistive Listening Devices

⊘ **V5268**   Assistive listening device, telephone
amplifier, any type Ⓑ                          E1

*Medicare Statute 1862a7*

⊘ **V5269**   Assistive listening device, alerting, any
type Ⓑ                                         E1

*Medicare Statute 1862a7*

⊘ **V5270**   Assistive listening device, television
amplifier, any type Ⓑ                          E1

*Medicare Statute 1862a7*

⊘ **V5271**   Assistive listening device, television
caption decoder Ⓑ                              E1

*Medicare Statute 1862a7*

⊘ **V5272**   Assistive listening device, TDD Ⓑ        E1

*Medicare Statute 1862a7*

⊘ **V5273**   Assistive listening device, for use with
cochlear implant Ⓑ                             E1

*Medicare Statute 1862a7*

⊘ **V5274**   Assistive listening device, not otherwise
specified Ⓑ Qp Qh                              E1

*Medicare Statute 1862a7*

⊘ **V5275**   Ear impression, each Ⓑ                   E1

*Medicare Statute 1862a7*

⊘ **V5281**   Assistive listening device, personal FM/
DM system, monaural (1 receiver,
transmitter, microphone), any
type Ⓑ Qp Qh                                   E1

*Medicare Statute 1862a7*

⊘ **V5282**   Assistive listening device, personal FM/
DM system, binaural (2 receivers,
transmitter, microphone), any
type Ⓑ Qp Qh                                   E1

*Medicare Statute 1862a7*

⊘ **V5283**   Assistive listening device, personal FM/
DM neck, loop induction
receiver Ⓑ Qp Qh                               E1

*Medicare Statute 1862a7*

⊘ **V5284**   Assistive listening device, personal FM/
DM, ear level receiver Ⓑ Qp Qh                 E1

*Medicare Statute 1862a7*

⊘ **V5285**   Assistive listening device, personal FM/
DM, direct audio input
receiver Ⓑ Qp Qh                               E1

*Medicare Statute 1862a7*

⊘ **V5286**   Assistive listening device, personal blue
tooth FM/DM receiver Ⓑ Qp Qh                   E1

*Medicare Statute 1862a7*

⊘ **V5287**   Assistive listening device, personal FM/
DM receiver, not otherwise
specified Ⓑ Qp Qh                              E1

*Medicare Statute 1862a7*

⊘ **V5288**   Assistive listening device, personal FM/
DM transmitter assistive listening
device Ⓑ Qp Qh                                 E1

*Medicare Statute 1862a7*

⊘ **V5289**   Assistive listening device, personal FM/
DM adapter/boot coupling device for
receiver, any type Ⓑ Qp Qh                     E1

*Medicare Statute 1862a7*

⊘ **V5290**   Assistive listening device, transmitter
microphone, any type Ⓑ Qp Qh                   E1

*Medicare Statute 1862a7*

## Other Supllies and Miscellaneous Services

⊘ **V5298**   Hearing aid, not otherwise
classified Ⓑ                                   E1

*Medicare Statute 1862a7*

⊛ **V5299**   Hearing service, miscellaneous Ⓑ          B

*IOM: 100-02, 16, 90*

## Repair/Modification

⊘ **V5336**   Repair/modification of augmentative
communicative system or device
(excludes adaptive hearing aid) Ⓓ              E1

*Medicare Statute 1862a7*

## Speech, Language, and Pathology Screening

These codes are for non-physician services.

⊘ **V5362**   Speech screening Ⓑ                       E1

*Medicare Statute 1862a7*

⊘ **V5363**   Language screening Ⓑ                     E1

*Medicare Statute 1862a7*

⊘ **V5364**   Dysphagia screening Ⓑ                    E1

*Medicare Statute 1862a7*

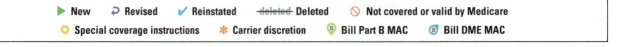

▶ New    ↻ Revised    ✔ Reinstated    ~~deleted~~ Deleted    ⊘ Not covered or valid by Medicare
⊛ Special coverage instructions    ✱ Carrier discretion    Ⓑ Bill Part B MAC    Ⓓ Bill DME MAC

# APPENDIX A

## Jurisdiction List for DMEPOS HCPCS Codes

Deleted codes are valid for dates of service on or before the date of deletion. The jurisdiction list includes codes that are not payable by Medicare. Please consult the Medicare contractor in whose jurisdiction a claim would be filed in order to determine coverage under Medicare.

**NOTE: All Local Carrier language has been changed to Part B MAC**

| HCPCS | DESCRIPTION | JURISDICTION |
|-------|-------------|--------------|
| A0021 - A0999 | Ambulance Services | Part B MAC |
| A4206 - A4209 | Medical, Surgical, and Self-Administered Injection Supplies | Part B MAC if incident to a physician's service (not separately payable). If other, DME MAC. |
| A4210 | Needle Free Injection Device | DME MAC |
| A4211 | Medical, Surgical, and Self-Administered Injection Supplies | Part B MAC if incident to a physician's service (not separately payable). If other, DME MAC. |
| A4212 | Non Coring Needle or Stylet with or without Catheter | Part B MAC |
| A4213 - A4215 | Medical, Surgical, and Self-Administered Injection Supplies | Part B MAC if incident to a physician's service (not separately payable). If other, DME MAC. |
| A4216 - A4218 | Saline | Part B MAC if incident to a physician's service (not separately payable). If other, DME MAC. |
| A4220 | Refill Kit for Implantable Pump | Part B MAC |
| A4221 - A4236 | Self-Administered Injection and Diabetic Supplies | DME MAC |
| A4244 - A4250 | Medical, Surgical, and Self-Administered Injection Supplies | Part B MAC if incident to a physician's service (not separately payable). If other, DME MAC. |
| A4252 - A4259 | Diabetic Supplies | DME MAC |
| A4261 | Cervical Cap for Contraceptive Use | Part B MAC |
| A4262 - A4263 | Lacrimal Duct Implants | Part B MAC |
| A4264 | Contraceptive Implant | Part B MAC |
| A4265 | Paraffin | Part B MAC if incident to a physician's service (not separately payable). If other, DME MAC. |
| A4266 - A4269 | Contraceptives | Part B MAC |
| A4270 | Endoscope Sheath | Part B MAC |
| A4280 | Accessory for Breast Prosthesis | DME MAC |
| A4281 - A4286 | Accessory for Breast Pump | DME MAC |
| A4290 | Sacral Nerve Stimulation Test Lead | Part B MAC |
| A4300 - A4301 | Implantable Catheter | Part B MAC |
| A4305 - A4306 | Disposable Drug Delivery System | Part B MAC if incident to a physician's service (not separately payable). If other, DME MAC. |

| HCPCS | DESCRIPTION | JURISDICTION |
|-------|-------------|--------------|
| A4310 - A4358 | Incontinence Supplies/ Urinary Supplies | If provided in the physician's office for a temporary condition, the item is incident to the physician's service & billed to the Part B MAC. If provided in the physician's office or other place of service for a permanent condition, the item is a prosthetic device & billed to the DME MAC. |
| A4360 - A4435 | Urinary Supplies | If provided in the physician's office for a temporary condition, the item is incident to the physician's service & billed to the Part B MAC. If provided in the physician's office or other place of service for a permanent condition, the item is a prosthetic device & billed to the DME MAC. |
| A4450 - A4456 | Tape; Adhesive Remover | Part B MAC if incident to a physician's service (not separately payable), or if supply for implanted prosthetic device. If other, DME MAC. |
| A4458-A4459 | Enema Bag/System | DME MAC |
| A4461-A4463 | Surgical Dressing Holders | Part B MAC if incident to a physician's service (not separately payable). If other, DME MAC. |
| A4465 - A4467 | Non-elastic Binder and Garment, Strap, Covering | DME MAC |
| A4470 | Gravlee Jet Washer | Part B MAC |
| A4480 | Vabra Aspirator | Part B MAC |
| A4481 | Tracheostomy Supply | Part B MAC if incident to a physician's service (not separately payable). If other, DME MAC. |
| A4483 | Moisture Exchanger | DME MAC |
| A4490 - A4510 | Surgical Stockings | DME MAC |
| A4520 | Diapers | DME MAC |
| A4550 | Surgical Trays | Part B MAC |
| A4553 - A4554 | Underpads | DME MAC |
| A4555 - A4558 | Electrodes; Lead Wires; Conductive Paste | Part B MAC if incident to a physician's service (not separately payable). If other, DME MAC. |
| A4559 | Coupling Gel | Part B MAC if incident to a physician's service (not separately payable). If other, DME MAC. |
| A4561 - A4563 | Pessary; Vaginal Insert | Part B MAC |

| HCPCS | DESCRIPTION | JURISDICTION |
|---|---|---|
| A4565-A4566 | Sling | Part B MAC |
| A4570 | Splint | Part B MAC |
| A4575 | Topical Hyperbaric Oxygen Chamber, Disposable | DME MAC |
| A4580 - A4590 | Casting Supplies & Material | Part B MAC |
| A4595 | TENS Supplies | Part B MAC if incident to a physician's service (not separately payable). If other, DME MAC. |
| A4600 | Sleeve for Intermittent Limb Compression Device | DME MAC |
| A4601-A4602 | Lithium Replacement Batteries | DME MAC |
| A4604 | Tubing for Positive Airway Pressure Device | DME MAC |
| A4605 | Tracheal Suction Catheter | DME MAC |
| A4606 | Oxygen Probe for Oximeter | DME MAC |
| A4608 | Transtracheal Oxygen Catheter | DME MAC |
| A4611 - A4613 | Oxygen Equipment Batteries and Supplies | DME MAC |
| A4614 | Peak Flow Rate Meter | Part B MAC if incident to a physician's service (not separately payable). If other, DME MAC. |
| A4615 - A4629 | Oxygen & Tracheostomy Supplies | Part B MAC if incident to a physician's service (not separately payable). If other, DME MAC. |
| A4630 - A4640 | DME Supplies | DME MAC |
| A4641 - A4642 | Imaging Agent; Contrast Material | Part B MAC |
| A4648 | Tissue Marker, Implanted | Part B MAC |
| A4649 | Miscellaneous Surgical Supplies | Part B MAC if incident to a physician's service (not separately payable), or if supply for implanted prosthetic device or implanted DME. If other, DME MAC. |
| A4650 | Implantable Radiation Dosimeter | Part B MAC |
| A4651 - A4932 | Supplies for ESRD | DME MAC (not separately payable) |
| A5051 - A5093 | Additional Ostomy Supplies | If provided in the physician's office for a temporary condition, the item is incident to the physician's service & billed to the Part B MAC. If provided in the physician's office or other place of service for a permanent condition, the item is a prosthetic device & billed to the DME MAC. |

| HCPCS | DESCRIPTION | JURISDICTION |
|---|---|---|
| A5102 - A5200 | Additional Incontinence and Ostomy Supplies | If provided in the physician's office for a temporary condition, the item is incident to the physician's service & billed to the Part B MAC. If provided in the physician's office or other place of service for a permanent condition, the item is a prosthetic device & billed to the DME MAC. |
| A5500 - A5514 | Therapeutic Shoes | DME MAC |
| A6000 | Non-Contact Wound Warming Cover | DME MAC |
| A6010-A6024 | Surgical Dressing | Part B MAC if incident to a physician's service (not separately payable) or if supply for implanted prosthetic device or implanted DME. If other, DME MAC. |
| A6025 | Silicone Gel Sheet | Part B MAC if incident to a physician's service (not separately payable) or if supply for implanted prosthetic device or implanted DME. If other, DME MAC. |
| A6154 - A6411 | Surgical Dressing | Part B MAC if incident to a physician's service (not separately payable) or if supply for implanted prosthetic device or implanted DME. If other, DME MAC. |
| A6412 | Eye Patch | Part B MAC if incident to a physician's service (not separately payable) or if supply for implanted prosthetic device or implanted DME. If other, DME MAC. |
| A6413 | Adhesive Bandage | Part B MAC if incident to a physician's service (not separately payable) or if supply for implanted prosthetic device or implanted DME. If other, DME MAC. |
| A6441 - A6457 | Surgical Dressing | Part B MAC if incident to a physician's service (not separately payable) or if supply for implanted prosthetic device or implanted DME. If other, DME MAC. |
| A6460 - A6461 | Surgical Dressing | Part B MAC |
| A6501 - A6512 | Surgical Dressing | Part B MAC if incident to a physician's service (not separately payable) or if supply for implanted prosthetic device or implanted DME. If other, DME MAC. |
| A6513 | Compression Burn Mask | DME MAC |
| A6530 - A6549 | Compression Gradient Stockings | DME MAC |
| A6550 | Supplies for Negative Pressure Wound Therapy Electrical Pump | DME MAC |
| A7000 - A7002 | Accessories for Suction Pumps | DME MAC |
| A7003 - A7039 | Accessories for Nebulizers, Aspirators and Ventilators | DME MAC |

| HCPCS | DESCRIPTION | JURISDICTION |
|---|---|---|
| A7040 - A7041 | Chest Drainage Supplies | Part B MAC |
| A7044 - A7047 | Respiratory Accessories | DME MAC |
| A7048 | Vacuum Drainage Supply | Part B MAC |
| A7501-A7527 | Tracheostomy Supplies | DME MAC |
| A8000-A8004 | Protective Helmets | DME MAC |
| A9150 | Non-Prescription Drugs | Part B MAC |
| A9152 - A9153 | Vitamins | Part B MAC |
| A9155 | Artificial Saliva | Part B MAC |
| A9180 | Lice Infestation Treatment | Part B MAC |
| A9270 | Noncovered Items or Services | DME MAC |
| A9272 | Disposable Wound Suction Pump | DME MAC |
| A9273 | Hot Water Bottles, Ice Caps or Collars, and Heat and/or Cold Wraps | DME MAC |
| A9274 - A9278 | Glucose Monitoring | DME MAC |
| A9279 | Monitoring Feature/ Device | DME MAC |
| A9280 | Alarm Device | DME MAC |
| A9281 | Reaching/Grabbing Device | DME MAC |
| A9282 | Wig | DME MAC |
| A9283 | Foot Off Loading Device | DME MAC |
| A9284- A9286 | Non-electric Spirometer, Inversion Devices and Hygienic Items | DME MAC |
| A9300 | Exercise Equipment | DME MAC |
| A9500 - A9700 | Supplies for Radiology Procedures | Part B MAC |
| A9900 | Miscellaneous DME Supply or Accessory | Part B MAC if used with implanted DME. If other, DME MAC. |
| A9901 | Delivery | DME MAC |
| A9999 | Miscellaneous DME Supply or Accessory | Part B MAC if used with implanted DME. If other, DME MAC. |
| B4034 - B9999 | Enteral and Parenteral Therapy | DME MAC |
| D0120 - D9999 | Dental Procedures | Part B MAC |
| E0100 - E0105 | Canes | DME MAC |
| E0110 - E0118 | Crutches | DME MAC |
| E0130 - E0159 | Walkers | DME MAC |
| E0160 - E0175 | Commodes | DME MAC |
| E0181 - E0199 | Decubitus Care Equipment | DME MAC |
| E0200 - E0239 | Heat/Cold Applications | DME MAC |
| E0240 - E0248 | Bath and Toilet Aids | DME MAC |
| E0249 | Pad for Heating Unit | DME MAC |

| HCPCS | DESCRIPTION | JURISDICTION |
|---|---|---|
| E0250 - E0304 | Hospital Beds | DME MAC |
| E0305 - E0326 | Hospital Bed Accessories | DME MAC |
| E0328 - E0329 | Pediatric Hospital Beds | DME MAC |
| E0350 - E0352 | Electronic Bowel Irrigation System | DME MAC |
| E0370 | Heel Pad | DME MAC |
| E0371 - E0373 | Decubitus Care Equipment | DME MAC |
| E0424 - E0484 | Oxygen and Related Respiratory Equipment | DME MAC |
| E0485 - E0486 | Oral Device to Reduce Airway Collapsibility | DME MAC |
| E0487 | Electric Spirometer | DME MAC |
| E0500 | IPPB Machine | DME MAC |
| E0550 - E0585 | Compressors/Nebulizers | DME MAC |
| E0600 | Suction Pump | DME MAC |
| E0601 | CPAP Device | DME MAC |
| E0602 - E0604 | Breast Pump | DME MAC |
| E0605 | Vaporizer | DME MAC |
| E0606 | Drainage Board | DME MAC |
| E0607 | Home Blood Glucose Monitor | DME MAC |
| E0610 - E0615 | Pacemaker Monitor | DME MAC |
| E0616 | Implantable Cardiac Event Recorder | Part B MAC |
| E0617 | External Defibrillator | DME MAC |
| E0618 - E0619 | Apnea Monitor | DME MAC |
| E0620 | Skin Piercing Device | DME MAC |
| E0621 - E0636 | Patient Lifts | DME MAC |
| E0637 - E0642 | Standing Devices/Lifts | DME MAC |
| E0650 - E0676 | Pneumatic Compressor and Appliances | DME MAC |
| E0691 - E0694 | Ultraviolet Light Therapy Systems | DME MAC |
| E0700 | Safety Equipment | DME MAC |
| E0705 | Transfer Board | DME MAC |
| E0710 | Restraints | DME MAC |
| E0720 - E0745 | Electrical Nerve Stimulators | DME MAC |
| E0746 | EMG Device | Part B MAC |
| E0747 - E0748 | Osteogenic Stimulators | DME MAC |
| E0749 | Implantable Osteogenic Stimulators | Part B MAC |
| E0755- E0770 | Stimulation Devices | DME MAC |
| E0776 | IV Pole | DME MAC |
| E0779 - E0780 | External Infusion Pumps | DME MAC |
| E0781 | Ambulatory Infusion Pump | DME MAC |

| HCPCS | DESCRIPTION | JURISDICTION |
|---|---|---|
| E0782 - E0783 | Infusion Pumps, Implantable | Part B MAC |
| E0784 | Infusion Pumps, Insulin | DME MAC |
| E0785 - E0786 | Implantable Infusion Pump Catheter | Part B MAC |
| E0791 | Parenteral Infusion Pump | DME MAC |
| E0830 | Ambulatory Traction Device | DME MAC |
| E0840 - E0900 | Traction Equipment | DME MAC |
| E0910 - E0930 | Trapeze/Fracture Frame | DME MAC |
| E0935 - E0936 | Passive Motion Exercise Device | DME MAC |
| E0940 | Trapeze Equipment | DME MAC |
| E0941 | Traction Equipment | DME MAC |
| E0942 - E0945 | Orthopedic Devices | DME MAC |
| E0946 - E0948 | Fracture Frame | DME MAC |
| E0950 - E1298 | Wheelchairs | DME MAC |
| E1300 - E1310 | Whirlpool Equipment | DME MAC |
| E1352 - E1392 | Additional Oxygen Related Equipment | DME MAC |
| E1399 | Miscellaneous DME | Part B MAC if implanted DME. If other, DME MAC. |
| E1405 - E1406 | Additional Oxygen Equipment | DME MAC |
| E1500 - E1699 | Artificial Kidney Machines and Accessories | DME MAC (not separately payable) |
| E1700 - E1702 | TMJ Device and Supplies | DME MAC |
| E1800 - E1841 | Dynamic Flexion Devices | DME MAC |
| E1902 | Communication Board | DME MAC |
| E2000 | Gastric Suction Pump | DME MAC |
| E2100 - E2101 | Blood Glucose Monitors with Special Features | DME MAC |
| E2120 | Pulse Generator for Tympanic Treatment of Inner Ear | DME MAC |
| E2201 - E2397 | Wheelchair Accessories | DME MAC |
| E2402 | Negative Pressure Wound Therapy Pump | DME MAC |
| E2500 - E2599 | Speech Generating Device | DME MAC |
| E2601 - E2633 | Wheelchair Cushions and Accessories | DME MAC |
| E8000 - E8002 | Gait Trainers | DME MAC |
| G0008 - G0067 | Misc. Professional Services | Part B MAC |
| G0068 - G0070 | Infusion Drug Professional Services | DME MAC |
| G0071 - G0329 | Misc. Professional Services | Part B MAC |

| HCPCS | DESCRIPTION | JURISDICTION |
|---|---|---|
| G0333 | Dispensing Fee | DME MAC |
| G0337 - G0343 | Misc. Professional Services | Part B MAC |
| G0372 | Misc. Professional Services | Part B MAC |
| G0378 - G0490 G0491-G9987 | Misc. Professional Services | Part B MAC |
| J0120 - J1094 | Injection | Part B MAC if incident to a physician's service or used in an implanted infusion pump. If other, DME MAC. |
| J1095 - J9591 | Ophthalmic Drug | Part B MAC |
| J1100 - J2786 | Injection | Part B MAC if incident to a physician's service or used in an implanted infusion pump. If other, DME MAC. |
| J2787 | Ophthalmic Drug | Part B MAC |
| J2788 - J3570 | Injection | Part B MAC if incident to a physician's service or used in an implanted infusion pump. If other, DME MAC. |
| J3590 - J9591 | Unclassified Biologicals | Part B MAC |
| J7030 - J7131 | Miscellaneous Drugs and Solutions | Part B MAC if incident to a physician's service or used in an implanted infusion pump. If other, DME MAC. |
| J7170 - J7179 | Clotting Factors | Part B MAC |
| J7180 - J7195 | Antihemophilic Factor | Part B MAC |
| J7196 - J7197 | Antithrombin III | Part B MAC |
| J7198 | Anti-inhibitor; per I.U. | Part B MAC |
| J7199 - J7211 | Other Hemophilia Clotting Factors | Part B MAC |
| J7296 - J7307 | Contraceptives | Part B MAC |
| J7308 - J7309 | Aminolevulinic Acid HCL | Part B MAC |
| J7310 | Ganciclovir, Long-Acting Implant | Part B MAC |
| J7311 - J7316 | Ophthalmic Drugs | Part B MAC |
| J7318 - J7329 | Hyaluronan | Part B MAC |
| J7330 | Autologous Cultured Chondrocytes, Implant | Part B MAC |
| J7336 | Capsaicin | Part B MAC |
| J7340 | Carbidopa/Levodopa | Part B MAC if incident to a physician's service or used in an implanted infusion pump. If other, DME MAC. |
| J7342 - J7345 | Ciprofloxacin otic & Topical Aminolevulinic Acid | Part B MAC |
| J7500 - J7599 | Immunosuppressive Drugs | Part B MAC if incident to a physician's service or used in an implanted infusion pump. If other, DME MAC. |
| J7604 - J7699 | Inhalation Solutions | Part B MAC if incident to a physician's service. If other, DME MAC. |

| HCPCS | DESCRIPTION | JURISDICTION |
|-------|-------------|--------------|
| J7799 -J7999 | NOC Drugs, Other than Inhalation Drugs | Part B MAC if incident to a physician's service or used in an implanted infusion pump. If other, DME MAC. |
| J8498 | Anti-emetic Drug | DME MAC |
| J8499 | Prescription Drug, Oral, Non Chemotherapeutic | Part B MAC if incident to a physician's service. If other, DME MAC. |
| J8501 - J8999 | Oral Anti-Cancer Drugs | DME MAC |
| J9000 - J9999 | Chemotherapy Drugs | Part B MAC if incident to a physician's service or used in an implanted infusion pump. If other, DME MAC. |
| K0001 - K0108 | Wheelchairs | DME MAC |
| K0195 | Elevating Leg Rests | DME MAC |
| K0455 | Infusion Pump used for Uninterrupted Administration of Epoprostenal | DME MAC |
| K0462 | Loaner Equipment | DME MAC |
| K0552 - K0605 | External Infusion Pump Supplies & Continuous Glucose Monitor | DME MAC |
| K0606 - K0609 | Defibrillator Accessories | DME MAC |
| K0669 | Wheelchair Cushion | DME MAC |
| K0672 | Soft Interface for Orthosis | DME MAC |
| K0730 | Inhalation Drug Delivery System | DME MAC |
| K0733 | Power Wheelchair Accessory | DME MAC |
| K0738 | Oxygen Equipment | DME MAC |
| K0739 | Repair or Nonroutine Service for DME | Part B MAC if implanted DME. If other, DME MAC. |
| K0740 | Repair or Nonroutine Service for Oxygen Equipment | DME MAC |
| K0743 - K0746 | Suction Pump and Dressings | DME MAC |
| K0800 - K0899 | Power Mobility Devices | DME MAC |
| K0900 | Custom DME, other than Wheelchair | DME MAC |
| L0112 - L4631 | Orthotics | DME MAC |
| L5000 - L5999 | Lower Limb Prosthetics | DME MAC |
| L6000 - L7499 | Upper Limb Prosthetics | DME MAC |
| L7510 - L7520 | Repair of Prosthetic Device | Part B MAC if repair of implanted prosthetic device. If other, DME MAC. |
| L7600 - L8485 | Prosthetics | DME MAC |
| L8499 | Unlisted Procedure for Miscellaneous Prosthetic Services | Part B MAC if implanted prosthetic device. If other, DME MAC. |
| L8500 - L8501 | Artificial Larynx; Tracheostomy Speaking Valve | DME MAC |

| HCPCS | DESCRIPTION | JURISDICTION |
|-------|-------------|--------------|
| L8505 | Artificial Larynx Accessory | DME MAC |
| L8507 | Voice Prosthesis, Patient Inserted | DME MAC |
| L8509 | Voice Prosthesis, Inserted by a Licensed Health Care Provider | Part B MAC for dates of service on or after 10/01/2010. DME MAC for dates of service prior to 10/01/2010 |
| L8510 | Voice Prosthesis | DME MAC |
| L8511 - L8515 | Voice Prosthesis | Part B MAC if used with tracheoesophageal voice prostheses inserted by a licensed health care provider. If other, DME MAC |
| L8701 - L8702 | Assist Device | DME MAC |
| L8600 - L8699 | Prosthetic Implants | Part B MAC |
| L9900 | Miscellaneous Orthotic or Prosthetic Component or Accessory | Part B MAC if used with implanted prosthetic device. If other, DME MAC. |
| M0075 - M1071 | Medical Services | Part B MAC |
| P2028 - P9615 | Laboratory Tests | Part B MAC |
| Q0035 | Cardio-kymography | Part B MAC |
| Q0081 | Infusion Therapy | Part B MAC |
| Q0083 - Q0085 | Chemotherapy Administration | Part B MAC |
| Q0091 | Smear Preparation | Part B MAC |
| Q0092 | Portable X-ray Setup | Part B MAC |
| Q0111 - Q0115 | Miscellaneous Lab Services | Part B MAC |
| Q0138-Q0139 | Ferumoxytol Injection | Part B MAC |
| Q0144 | Azithromycin Dihydrate | Part B MAC if incident to a physician's service. If other, DME MAC. |
| Q0161 - Q0181 | Anti-emetic | DME MAC |
| Q0477 - Q0509 | Ventricular Assist Devices | Part B MAC |
| Q0510 - Q0514 | Drug Dispensing Fees | DME MAC |
| Q0515 | Sermorelin Acetate | Part B MAC |
| Q1004 - Q1005 | New Technology IOL | Part B MAC |
| Q2004 | Irrigation Solution | Part B MAC |
| Q2009 | Fosphenytoin | Part B MAC |
| Q2017 | Teniposide | Part B MAC |
| Q2026-Q2028 | Injectable Dermal Fillers | Part B MAC |
| Q2034 - Q2039 | Influenza Vaccine | Part B MAC |
| Q2041 - Q2043 | Cellular Immunotherapy | Part B MAC |
| Q2049-Q2050 | Doxorubicin | Part B MAC if incident to a physician's service or used in an implanted infusion pump. If other, DME MAC. |
| Q2052 | IVIG Demonstration | DME MAC |
| Q3001 | Supplies for Radiology Procedures | Part B MAC |

| HCPCS | DESCRIPTION | JURISDICTION |
|---|---|---|
| Q3014 | Telehealth Originating Site Facility Fee | Part B MAC |
| Q3027 - Q3028 | Vaccines | Part B MAC |
| Q3031 | Collagen Skin Test | Part B MAC |
| Q4001 - Q4051 | Splints and Casts | Part B MAC |
| Q4074 | Inhalation Drug | Part B MAC if incident to a physician's service. If other, DME MAC. |
| Q4081 | Epoetin | Part B MAC |
| Q4082 | Drug Subject to Competitive Acquisition Program | Part B MAC |
| Q4100 - Q4204 | Skin Substitutes | Part B MAC |
| Q5001 - Q5010 | Hospice Services | Part B MAC |
| Q5101-Q5111 | Injection | Part B MAC if incident to a physician's service or used in an implanted infusion pump. If other, DME MAC. |
| Q9950 - Q9954 | Imaging Agents | Part B MAC |
| Q9955 - Q9957 | Microspheres | Part B MAC |
| Q9958 - Q9983 | Imaging Agents & Radiology Supplies | Part B MAC |
| Q9991 - Q9992 | Injection | Part B MAC if incident to a physician's service or used in an implanted infusion pump. If other, DME MAC. |
| R0070 - R0076 | Diagnostic Radiology Services | Part B MAC |
| V2020 - V2025 | Frames | DME MAC |
| V2100 - V2513 | Lenses | DME MAC |

| HCPCS | DESCRIPTION | JURISDICTION |
|---|---|---|
| V2520 - V2523 | Hydrophilic Contact Lenses | Part B MAC if incident to a physician's service. If other, DME MAC. |
| V2530 - V2531 | Contact Lenses, Scleral | DME MAC |
| V2599 | Contact Lens, Other Type | Part B MAC if incident to a physician's service. If other, DME MAC. |
| V2600 - V2615 | Low Vision Aids | DME MAC |
| V2623 - V2629 | Prosthetic Eyes | DME MAC |
| V2630 - V2632 | Intraocular Lenses | Part B MAC |
| V2700 - V2780 | Miscellaneous Vision Service | DME MAC |
| V2781 | Progressive Lens | DME MAC |
| V2782 - V2784 | Lenses | DME MAC |
| V2785 | Processing—Corneal Tissue | Part B MAC |
| V2786 | Lens | DME MAC |
| V2787 - V2788 | Intraocular Lenses | Part B MAC |
| V2790 | Amniotic Membrane | Part B MAC |
| V2797 | Vision Supply | DME MAC |
| V2799 | Miscellaneous Vision Service | Part B MAC if supply for an implanted prosthetic device. If other, DME MAC |
| V5008 - V5299 | Hearing Services | Part B MAC |
| V5336 | Repair/Modification of Augmentative Communicative System or Device | DME MAC |
| V5362 - V5364 | Speech Screening | Part B MAC |

## GENERAL CORRECT CODING POLICIES FOR NATIONAL CORRECT CODING INITIATIVE POLICY MANUAL FOR MEDICARE SERVICES

Current Procedural Terminology (CPT) codes, descriptions and other data only are copyright 2018 American Medical Association. All rights reserved.

CPT® is a registered trademark of the American Medical Association.

Applicable FARS\DFARS Restrictions Apply to Government Use.

Fee schedules, relative value units, conversion factors, prospective payment systems, and/or related components are not assigned by the AMA, are not part of CPT, and the AMA is not recommending their use. The AMA does not directly or indirectly practice medicine or dispense medical services. The AMA assumes no liability for the data contained or not contained herein.

## Chapter I

## Revision Date 1/1/2019

## GENERAL CORRECT CODING POLICIES

### A. Introduction

Healthcare providers utilize HCPCS/CPT codes to report medical services performed on patients to Medicare Carriers (A/B MACs processing practitioner service claims) and Fiscal Intermediaries (FIs). HCPCS (Healthcare Common Procedure Coding System) consists of Level I CPT (Current Procedural Terminology) codes and Level II codes. CPT codes are defined in the American Medical Association's (AMA) *CPT Manual* which is updated and published annually. HCPCS Level II codes are defined by the Centers for Medicare & Medicaid Services (CMS) and are updated throughout the year as necessary. Changes in CPT codes are approved by the AMA CPT Editorial Panel which meets three times per year.

CPT and HCPCS Level II codes define medical and surgical procedures performed on patients. Some procedure codes are very specific defining a single service [e.g., CPT code 93000 (electrocardiogram)] while other codes define procedures consisting of many services [e.g., CPT code 58263 (vaginal hysterectomy with removal of tube(s) and ovary(s) and repair of enterocele)]. Because many procedures can be performed by different approaches, different methods, or in combination with other procedures, there are often multiple HCPCS/CPT codes defining similar or related procedures.

CPT and HCPCS Level II code descriptors usually do not define all services included in a procedure. There are often services inherent in a procedure or group of procedures. For example, anesthesia services include certain preparation and monitoring services.

The CMS developed the NCCI to prevent inappropriate payment of services that should not be reported together. Prior to April 1, 2012, NCCI PTP edits were placed into either the "Column One/Column Two Correct Coding Edit Table" or the "Mutually Exclusive Edit Table." However, on April 1, 2012, the edits in the "Mutually Exclusive Edit Table" were moved to the "Column One/Column Two Correct Coding Edit Table" so that all the NCCI PTP edits are currently contained in this single table. Combining the two tables simplifies researching NCCI edits and online use of NCCI tables. Each edit table contains edits which are pairs of HCPCS/CPT codes that in general should not be reported together. Each edit has a column one and column two HCPCS/CPT code. If a provider reports the two codes of an edit pair, the column two code is denied, and the column one code is

eligible for payment. However, if it is clinically appropriate to utilize an NCCI-associated modifier, both the column one and column two codes are eligible for payment. (NCCI-associated modifiers and their appropriate use are discussed elsewhere in this chapter.)

When the NCCI was first established and during its early years, the "Column One/Column Two Correct Coding Edit Table" was termed the "Comprehensive/Component Edit Table." This latter terminology was a misnomer. Although the column two code is often a component of a more comprehensive column one code, this relationship is not true for many edits. In the latter type of edit the code pair edit simply represents two codes that should not be reported together. For example, a provider shall not report a vaginal hysterectomy code and total abdominal hysterectomy code together.

In this chapter, Sections B–Q address various issues relating to NCCI PTP edits.

Medically Unlikely Edits (MUEs) prevent payment for an inappropriate number/quantity of the same service on a single day. An MUE for a HCPCS/CPT code is the maximum number of units of service (UOS) under most circumstances reportable by the same provider for the same beneficiary on the same date of service. The ideal MUE value for a HCPCS/CPT code is one that allows the vast majority of appropriately coded claims to pass the MUE. More information concerning MUEs is discussed in Section V of this chapter.

In this Manual many policies are described utilizing the term "physician." Unless indicated differently the usage of this term does not restrict the policies to physicians only but applies to all practitioners, hospitals, providers, or suppliers eligible to bill the relevant HCPCS/CPT codes pursuant to applicable portions of the Social Security Act (SSA) of 1965, the Code of Federal Regulations (CFR), and Medicare rules. In some sections of this Manual, the term "physician" would not include some of these entities because specific rules do not apply to them. For example, Anesthesia Rules [e.g., CMS Internet-only Manual, Publication 100-04 (Medicare Claims Processing Manual), Chapter 12 (Physician/Nonphysician Practitioners), Section 50(Payment for Anesthesiology Services)] and Global Surgery Rules [e.g., CMS Internet-only Manual, Publication 100-04 (Medicare Claims Processing Manual), Chapter 12 (Physician/Nonphysician Practitioners), Section 40 (Surgeons and Global Surgery)] do not apply to hospitals.

Providers reporting services under Medicare's hospital outpatient prospective payment system (OPPS) shall report all services in accordance with appropriate Medicare Internet-only Manual (IOM) instructions.

Physicians must report services correctly. This manual discusses general coding principles in Chapter I and principles more relevant to other specific groups of HCPCS/CPT codes in the other chapters. There are certain types of improper coding that physicians must avoid.

Procedures shall be reported with the most comprehensive CPT code that describes the services performed. Physicians must not unbundle the services described by a HCPCS/CPT code. Some examples follow:

- A physician shall not report multiple HCPCS/CPT codes when a single comprehensive HCPCS/CPT code describes these services. For example if a physician performs a vaginal hysterectomy on a uterus weighing less than 250 grams with bilateral salpingo-oophorectomy, the physician shall report CPT code 58262 (Vaginal hysterectomy, for uterus 250 g or less; with removal of tube(s), and/or ovary(s)). The physician shall not report CPT code 58260 (Vaginal hysterectomy, for uterus 250 g or less;) plus CPT code 58720 (Salpingo-oophorectomy, complete or partial, unilateral or bilateral (separate procedure)).
- A physician shall not fragment a procedure into component parts. For example, if a physician performs an anal endoscopy with biopsy, the physician shall report CPT code 46606 (Anoscopy; with biopsy, single or multiple). It is improper to unbundle this procedure and report CPT code 46600(Anoscopy; diagnostic,...) plus CPT code 45100 (Biopsy of anorectal wall, anal approach...). The latter code is not intended to be utilized with an endoscopic procedure code.
- A physician shall not unbundle a bilateral procedure code into two unilateral procedure codes. For example if a physician performs bilateral mammography, the physician shall report CPT code 77066 (Diagnostic mammography . . . bilateral). The physician shall not report CPT code 77065 (Diagnostic mammography . . . unilateral) with two units of service or 77065LT plus 77065RT.
- A physician shall not unbundle services that are integral to a more comprehensive procedure. For example, surgical access is integral to a surgical procedure. A physician shall not report CPT code 49000 (Exploratory laparotomy,...) when performing an open abdominal procedure such as a total abdominal colectomy (e.g., CPT code 44150).

Physicians must avoid downcoding. If a HCPCS/CPT code exists that describes the services performed, the physician must report this code rather than report a less comprehensive code with other codes describing the services not included in the less comprehensive code. For example if a physician performs a unilateral partial mastectomy with axillary lymphadenectomy, the provider shall report CPT code 19302 (Mastectomy, partial...; with axillary lymphadenectomy). A physician shall not report CPT code 19301 (Mastectomy, partial...) plus CPT code 38745 (Axillary lymphadenectomy; complete).

Physicians must avoid upcoding. A HCPCS/CPT code may be reported only if all services described by that code have been performed. For example, if a physician performs a superficial axillary lymphadenectomy (CPT code 38740), the physician shall not report CPT code 38745 (Axillary lymphadenectomy; complete).

Physicians must report units of service correctly. Each HCPCS/CPT code has a defined unit of service for reporting purposes. A physician shall not report units of service for a HCPCS/CPT code using a criterion that differs from the code's defined unit of service. For example, some therapy codes are reported in fifteen minute increments (e.g., CPT codes 97110-97124).

Others are reported per session (e.g., CPT codes 92507, 92508). A physician shall not report a "per session" code using fifteen minute increments. CPT code 92507 or 92508 should be reported with one unit of service on a single date of service.

MUE and NCCI PTP edits are based on services provided by the same physician to the same beneficiary on the same date of service. Physicians shall not inconvenience beneficiaries nor increase risks to beneficiaries by performing services on different dates of service to avoid MUE or NCCI PTP edits.

In 2010 the *CPT Manual* modified the numbering of codes so that the sequence of codes as they appear in the *CPT Manual* does not necessarily correspond to a sequential numbering of codes. In the *National Correct Coding Initiative Policy Manual for Medicare Services,* use of a numerical range of codes reflects all codes that numerically fall within the range regardless of their sequential order in the *CPT Manual*.

This chapter addresses general coding principles, issues, and policies. Many of these principles, issues, and policies are addressed further in subsequent chapters dealing with specific groups of HCPCS/CPT codes. In this chapter examples are often utilized to clarify principles, issues, or policies. The examples do not represent the only codes to which the principles, issues, or policies apply.

## B. Coding Based on Standards of Medical/Surgical Practice

Most HCPCS/CPT code defined procedures include services that are integral to them. Some of these integral services have specific CPT codes for reporting the service when not performed as an integral part of another procedure. For example, CPT code 36000 (introduction of needle or intracatheter into a vein) is integral to all nuclear medicine procedures requiring injection of a radiopharmaceutical into a vein. CPT code 36000 is not separately reportable with these types of nuclear medicine procedures. However, CPT code 36000 may be reported alone if the only service provided is the introduction of a needle into a vein. Other integral services do not have specific CPT codes. (For example, wound irrigation is integral to the treatment of all wounds and does not have a HCPCS/CPT code.) Services integral to HCPCS/CPT code defined procedures are included in those procedures based on the standards of medical/surgical practice. It is inappropriate to separately report services that are integral to another procedure with that procedure.

Many NCCI PTP edits are based on the standards of medical/surgical practice. Services that are integral to another service are component parts of the more comprehensive service. When integral component services have their own HCPCS/CPT codes, NCCI PTP edits place the comprehensive service in column one and the component service in column two. Since a component service integral to a comprehensive service is not separately reportable, the column two code is not separately reportable with the column one code.

Some services are integral to large numbers of procedures. Other services are integral to a more limited number of procedures. Examples of services integral to a large number of procedures include:

- Cleansing, shaving and prepping of skin
- Draping and positioning of patient
- Insertion of intravenous access for medication administration

- Insertion of urinary catheter
- Sedative administration by the physician performing a procedure (see Chapter II, Anesthesia Services)
- Local, topical or regional anesthesia administered by the physician performing the procedure
- Surgical approach including identification of anatomical landmarks, incision, evaluation of the surgical field, debridement of traumatized tissue, lysis of adhesions, and isolation of structures limiting access to the surgical field such as bone, blood vessels, nerve, and muscles including stimulation for identification or monitoring
- Surgical cultures
- Wound irrigation
- Insertion and removal of drains, suction devices, and pumps into same site
- Surgical closure and dressings
- Application, management, and removal of postoperative dressings and analgesic devices (peri-incisional)
- Application of TENS unit
- Institution of Patient Controlled Anesthesia
- Preoperative, intraoperative and postoperative documentation, including photographs, drawings, dictation, or transcription as necessary to document the services provided
- Surgical supplies, except for specific situations where CMS policy permits separate payment

Although other chapters in this Manual further address issues related to the standards of medical/surgical practice for the procedures covered by that chapter, it is not possible because of space limitations to discuss all NCCI PTP edits based on the principle of the standards of medical/surgical practice. However, there are several general principles that can be applied to the edits as follows:

1. The component service is an accepted standard of care when performing the comprehensive service.
2. The component service is usually necessary to complete the comprehensive service.
3. The component service is not a separately distinguishable procedure when performed with the comprehensive service.

Specific examples of services that are not separately reportable because they are components of more comprehensive services follow:

### Medical:

1. Since interpretation of cardiac rhythm is an integral component of the interpretation of an electrocardiogram, a rhythm strip is not separately reportable.
2. Since determination of ankle/brachial indices requires both upper and lower extremity Doppler studies, an upper extremity Doppler study is not separately reportable.
3. Since a cardiac stress test includes multiple electrocardiograms, an electrocardiogram is not separately reportable.

### Surgical:

1. Since a myringotomy requires access to the tympanic membrane through the external auditory canal, removal of impacted cerumen from the external auditory canal is not separately reportable.
2. A "scout" bronchoscopy to assess the surgical field, anatomic landmarks, extent of disease, etc., is not separately reportable with an open pulmonary procedure such as a pulmonary lobectomy. By contrast, an initial diagnostic bronchoscopy is separately reportable. If the diagnostic bronchoscopy is performed at the same patient encounter as the open pulmonary procedure and does not duplicate an earlier diagnostic bronchoscopy by the same or another physician, the diagnostic bronchoscopy may be reported with modifier –58 appended to the open pulmonary procedure code to indicate a staged procedure. A cursory examination of the upper airway during a bronchoscopy with the bronchoscope shall not be reported separately as a laryngoscopy. However, separate endoscopies of anatomically distinct areas with different endoscopes may be reported separately (e.g., thoracoscopy and mediastinoscopy).
3. If an endoscopic procedure is performed at the same patient encounter as a non-endoscopic procedure to ensure no intraoperative injury occurred or verify the procedure was performed correctly, the endoscopic procedure is not separately reportable with the non-endoscopic procedure.
4. Since a colectomy requires exposure of the colon, the laparotomy and adhesiolysis to expose the colon are not separately reportable.

## C. Medical/Surgical Package

Most medical and surgical procedures include pre-procedure, intra-procedure, and post-procedure work. When multiple procedures are performed at the same patient encounter, there is often overlap of the pre-procedure and post-procedure work. Payment methodologies for surgical procedures account for the overlap of the pre-procedure and post-procedure work.

The component elements of the pre-procedure and post-procedure work for each procedure are included component services of that procedure as a standard of medical/surgical practice. Some general guidelines follow:

1. Many invasive procedures require vascular and/or airway access. The work associated with obtaining the required access is included in the pre-procedure or intra-procedure work. The work associated with returning a patient to the appropriate post-procedure state is included in the post-procedure work.

Airway access is necessary for general anesthesia and is not separately reportable. There is no CPT code for elective endotracheal intubation. CPT code 31500 describes an emergency endotracheal intubation and shall not be reported for elective endotracheal intubation. Visualization of the airway is a component part of an endotracheal intubation, and CPT codes describing procedures that visualize the airway (e.g., nasal endoscopy, laryngoscopy, bronchoscopy) shall not be reported with an endotracheal intubation. These CPT codes describe diagnostic and therapeutic endoscopies, and it is a misuse of these codes to report visualization of the airway for endotracheal intubation.

Intravenous access (e.g., CPT codes 36000, 36400, 36410) is not separately reportable when performed with many types of procedures (e.g., surgical procedures, anesthesia procedures, radiological procedures requiring intravenous contrast, nuclear medicine procedures requiring intravenous radiopharmaceutical).

After vascular access is achieved, the access must be maintained by a slow infusion (e.g., saline) or injection of heparin or saline into a "lock". Since these services are necessary for maintenance of the vascular access, they are not separately reportable with the vascular access CPT codes or procedures requiring vascular access as a standard of medical/surgical practice. CPT codes 37211-37214 (Transcatheter therapy with infusion for thrombolysis) shall not be reported for use of an anticoagulant to maintain vascular access.

The global surgical package includes the administration of fluids and drugs during the operative procedure. CPT codes 96360-96377 shall not be reported separately for that operative procedure. Under **OPPS**, the administration of fluids and drugs during or for an operative procedure are included services and are not separately reportable (e.g., CPT codes 96360-96377).

When a procedure requires more invasive vascular access services (e.g., central venous access, pulmonary artery access), the more invasive vascular service is separately reportable if it is not typical of the procedure and the work of the more invasive vascular service has not been included in the valuation of the procedure.

Insertion of a central venous access device (e.g., central venous catheter, pulmonary artery catheter) requires passage of a catheter through central venous vessels and, in the case of a pulmonary artery catheter, through the right atrium and ventricle. These services often require the use of fluoroscopic guidance. Separate reporting of **CPT** codes for right heart catheterization, selective venous catheterization, or pulmonary artery catheterization is not appropriate when reporting a CPT code for insertion of a central venous access device. Since CPT code 77001 describes fluoroscopic guidance for central venous access device procedures, CPT codes for more general fluoroscopy (e.g., 76000, 76001, 77002) shall not be reported separately. *(CPT code 76001 was deleted January 1, 2019.)*

2.  Medicare Anesthesia Rules prevent separate payment for anesthesia services by the same physician performing a surgical or medical procedure. The physician performing a surgical or medical procedure shall not report **CPT** codes 96360-96377 for the administration of anesthetic agents during the procedure. If it is medically reasonable and necessary that a separate provider (anesthesia practitioner) perform anesthesia services (e.g., monitored anesthesia care) for a surgical or medical procedure, a separate anesthesia service may be reported by the second provider.

Under **OPPS**, anesthesia for a surgical procedure is an included service and is not separately reportable. For example, a provider shall not report **CPT** codes 96360-96377 for anesthesia services.

When anesthesia services are not separately reportable, physicians and facilities shall not unbundle components of anesthesia and report them in lieu of an anesthesia code.

3.  If an endoscopic procedure is performed at the same patient encounter as a non-endoscopic procedure to ensure no intraoperative injury occurred or verify the procedure was performed correctly, the endoscopic procedure is not separately reportable with the non-endoscopic procedure.
4.  Many procedures require cardiopulmonary monitoring either by the physician performing the procedure or an anesthesia practitioner. Since these services are integral to the procedure, they are not separately reportable. Examples of these services include cardiac monitoring, pulse oximetry, and ventilation management (e.g., 93000-93010, 93040-93042, 94760, 94761, 94770).
5.  A biopsy performed at the time of another more extensive procedure (e.g., excision, destruction, removal) is separately reportable under specific circumstances.

If the biopsy is performed on a separate lesion, it is separately reportable. This situation may be reported with anatomic modifiers or modifier -59.

The biopsy is not separately reportable if *utilized for* the purpose of assessing margins of resection or verifying resectability.

If a biopsy is performed and submitted for pathologic evaluation that will be completed after the more extensive procedure is performed, the biopsy is not separately reportable with the more extensive procedure.

If a single lesion is biopsied multiple times, only one biopsy code may be reported with a single unit of service. If multiple lesions are non-endoscopically biopsied, a biopsy code may be reported for each lesion appending a modifier indicating that each biopsy was performed on a separate lesion. For endoscopic biopsies, multiple biopsies of a single or multiple lesions are reported with one unit of service of the biopsy code. If it is medically reasonable and necessary to submit multiple biopsies of the same or different lesions for separate pathologic examination, the medical record must identify the precise location and separate nature of each biopsy.

6.  Exposure and exploration of the surgical field is integral to an operative procedure and is not separately reportable. For example, an exploratory laparotomy (CPT code 49000) is not separately reportable with an intra-abdominal procedure. If exploration of the surgical field results in additional procedures other than the primary procedure, the additional procedures may generally be reported separately. However, a procedure designated by the CPT code descriptor as a "separate procedure" is not separately reportable if performed in a region anatomically related to the other procedure(s) through the same skin incision, orifice, or surgical approach.
7.  If a definitive surgical procedure requires access through diseased tissue (e.g., necrotic skin, abscess, hematoma, seroma), a separate service for this access (e.g., debridement, incision and drainage) is not separately reportable. Types of procedures to which this principle applies include, but are not limited to, -ectomy, -otomy, excision, resection, -plasty, insertion, revision, replacement, relocation, removal or closure. For example, debridement of skin and subcutaneous tissue at the site of an abdominal incision made to perform an intra-abdominal procedure is not separately reportable. (See Chapter IV, Section H (General Policy Statements), Subsection #11 for guidance on reporting debridement with open fractures and dislocations.)
8.  If removal, destruction, or other form of elimination of a lesion requires coincidental elimination of other pathology, only the primary procedure may be reported. For example, if an area of pilonidal disease contains an abscess, incision and drainage of the abscess during the procedure to excise the area of pilonidal disease is not separately reportable.
9.  An excision and removal (–ectomy) includes the incision and opening (–otomy) of the organ. A HCPCS/CPT code for an –otomy procedure shall not be reported with an –ectomy code for the same organ.
10. Multiple approaches to the same procedure are mutually exclusive of one another and shall not be reported separately.

For example, both a vaginal hysterectomy and abdominal hysterectomy should not be reported separately.

11. If a procedure utilizing one approach fails and is converted to a procedure utilizing a different approach, only the completed procedure may be reported. For example, if a laparoscopic hysterectomy is converted to an open hysterectomy, only the open hysterectomy procedure code may be reported.

12. If a laparoscopic procedure fails and is converted to an open procedure, the physician shall not report a diagnostic laparoscopy in lieu of the failed laparoscopic procedure. For example, if a laparoscopic cholecystectomy is converted to an open cholecystectomy, the physician shall not report the failed laparoscopic cholecystectomy nor a diagnostic laparoscopy.

13. If a diagnostic endoscopy is the basis for and precedes an open procedure, the diagnostic endoscopy may be reported with modifier -58 appended to the open procedure code. However, the medical record must document the medical reasonableness and necessity for the diagnostic endoscopy. A scout endoscopy to assess anatomic landmarks and extent of disease is not separately reportable with an open procedure. When an endoscopic procedure fails and is converted to another surgical procedure, only the completed surgical procedure may be reported. The endoscopic procedure is not separately reportable with the completed surgical procedure.

14. Treatment of complications of primary surgical procedures is separately reportable with some limitations. The global surgical package for an operative procedure includes all intra-operative services that are normally a usual and necessary part of the procedure. Additionally the global surgical package includes all medical and surgical services required of the surgeon during the postoperative period of the surgery to treat complications that do not require return to the operating room. Thus, treatment of a complication of a primary surgical procedure is not separately reportable (1) if it represents usual and necessary care in the operating room during the procedure or (2) if it occurs postoperatively and does not require return to the operating room. For example, control of hemorrhage is a usual and necessary component of a surgical procedure in the operating room and is not separately reportable. Control of postoperative hemorrhage is also not separately reportable unless the patient must be returned to the operating room for treatment. In the latter case, the control of hemorrhage may be separately reportable with modifier -78.

## D. Evaluation and Management (E&M) Services

Medicare Global Surgery Rules define the rules for reporting evaluation and management (E&M) services with procedures covered by these rules. This section summarizes some of the rules.

All procedures on the Medicare Physician Fee Schedule are assigned a Global period of 000, 010, 090, XXX, YYY, ZZZ, or MMM. The global concept does not apply to XXX procedures. The global period for YYY procedures is defined by the Carrier (A/B MAC processing practitioner service claims). All procedures with a global period of ZZZ are related to another procedure, and the applicable global period for the ZZZ code is determined by the related procedure. Procedures with a global period of MMM are maternity procedures.

Since NCCI PTP edits are applied to same day services by the same provider to the same beneficiary, certain Global Surgery Rules are applicable to NCCI. An E&M service is separately reportable on the same date of service as a procedure with a global period of 000, 010, or 090 under limited circumstances.

If a procedure has a global period of 090 days, it is defined as a major surgical procedure. If an E&M is performed on the same date of service as a major surgical procedure for the purpose of deciding whether to perform this surgical procedure, the E&M service is separately reportable with modifier -57. Other preoperative E&M services on the same date of service as a major surgical procedure are included in the global payment for the procedure and are not separately reportable. NCCI does not contain edits based on this rule because Medicare Carriers (A/B MACs processing practitioner service claims) have separate edits.

If a procedure has a global period of 000 or 010 days, it is defined as a minor surgical procedure. In general E&M services on the same date of service as the minor surgical procedure are included in the payment for the procedure. The decision to perform a minor surgical procedure is included in the payment for the minor surgical procedure and shall not be reported separately as an E&M service. However, a significant and separately identifiable E&M service unrelated to the decision to perform the minor surgical procedure is separately reportable with modifier -25. The E&M service and minor surgical procedure do not require different diagnoses. If a minor surgical procedure is performed on a new patient, the same rules for reporting E&M services apply. The fact that the patient is "new" to the provider is not sufficient alone to justify reporting an E&M service on the same date of service as a minor surgical procedure. NCCI contains many, but not all, possible edits based on these principles.

Example: If a physician determines that a new patient with head trauma requires sutures, confirms the allergy and immunization status, obtains informed consent, and performs the repair, an E&M service is not separately reportable. However, if the physician also performs a medically reasonable and necessary full neurological examination, an E&M service may be separately reportable.

For major and minor surgical procedures, postoperative E&M services related to recovery from the surgical procedure during the postoperative period are included in the global surgical package as are E&M services related to complications of the surgery. Postoperative visits unrelated to the diagnosis for which the surgical procedure was performed unless related to a complication of surgery may be reported separately on the same day as a surgical procedure with modifier 24 ("Unrelated Evaluation and Management Service by the Same Physician or Other Qualified Health Care Professional During a Postoperative Period").

Procedures with a global surgery indicator of "XXX" are not covered by these rules. Many of these "XXX" procedures are performed by physicians and have inherent pre-procedure, intra-procedure, and post-procedure work usually performed each time the procedure is completed. This work shall not be reported as a separate E&M code. Other "XXX" procedures are not usually performed by a physician and have no physician work relative value units associated with them. A physician shall not report a separate E&M code with these procedures for the supervision of others performing the procedure or for the interpretation of the procedure. With most "XXX" procedures, the physician may, however, perform a significant and separately identifiable E&M service on the same date of service which may be reported by appending modifier -25 to the E&M code. This E&M service may be related to the same diagnosis necessitating performance of the "XXX" procedure but cannot include any work inherent in the "XXX" procedure, supervision of others performing the "XXX" procedure, or time for interpreting the result of the "XXX" procedure. Appending modifier -25 to a significant, separately identifiable E&M service when performed on the same date of service as an "XXX" procedure is correct coding.

# E. Modifiers and Modifier Indicators

1. The AMA *CPT Manual* and CMS define modifiers that may be appended to HCPCS/CPT codes to provide additional information about the services rendered. Modifiers consist of two alphanumeric characters.

Modifiers may be appended to HCPCS/CPT codes only if the clinical circumstances justify the use of the modifier. A modifier shall not be appended to a HCPCS/CPT code solely to bypass an NCCI PTP edit if the clinical circumstances do not justify its use. If the Medicare program imposes restrictions on the use of a modifier, the modifier may only be used to bypass an NCCI PTP edit if the Medicare restrictions are fulfilled.

Modifiers that may be used under appropriate clinical circumstances to bypass an NCCI edit include:

Anatomic modifiers: E1-E4, FA, F1-F9, TA, T1-T9, LT, RT, LC, LD, RC, LM, RI

Global surgery modifiers: -24, -25, -57, -58, -78, -79

Other modifiers: -27,-59, -91, XE, XS, XP, XU

Modifiers 76 ("repeat procedure or service by same physician") and 77 ("repeat procedure by another physician") are not NCCI-associated modifiers. Use of either of these modifiers does not bypass an NCCI PTP edit.

Each NCCI PTP edit has an assigned modifier indicator. A modifier indicator of "0" indicates that NCCI-associated modifiers cannot be used to bypass the edit. A modifier indicator of "1" indicates that NCCI-associated modifiers may be used to bypass an edit under appropriate circumstances. A modifier indicator of "9" indicates that the edit has been deleted, and the modifier indicator is not relevant.

It is very important that NCCI-associated modifiers only be used when appropriate. In general these circumstances relate to separate patient encounters, separate anatomic sites or separate specimens. (See subsequent discussion of modifiers in this section.) Most edits involving paired organs or structures (e.g., eyes, ears, extremities, lungs, kidneys) have NCCI PTP modifier indicators of "1" because the two codes of the code pair edit may be reported if performed on the contralateral organs or structures. Most of these code pairs should not be reported with NCCI-associated modifiers when performed on the ipsilateral organ or structure unless there is a specific coding rationale to bypass the edit. The existence of the NCCI PTP edit indicates that the two codes generally cannot be reported together unless the two corresponding procedures are performed at two separate patient encounters or two separate anatomic locations. However, if the two corresponding procedures are performed at the same patient encounter and

in contiguous structures, NCCI-associated modifiers generally should not be utilized.

The appropriate use of most of these modifiers is straightforward. However, further explanation is provided about modifiers -25, -58, and -59. Although modifier -22 is not a modifier that bypasses an NCCI PTP edit, its use is occasionally relevant to an NCCI PTP edit and is discussed below.

a) **Modifier -22:** Modifier -22 is defined by the *CPT Manual* as "Increased Procedural Services." This modifier shall not be reported unless the service(s) performed is(are) substantially more extensive than the usual service(s) included in the procedure described by the HCPCS/CPT code reported.

Occasionally a provider may perform two procedures that should not be reported together based on an NCCI PTP edit. If the edit allows use of NCCI-associated modifiers to bypass it and the clinical circumstances justify use of one of these modifiers, both services may be reported with the NCCI-associated modifier. However, if the NCCI PTP edit does not allow use of NCCI-associated modifiers to bypass it and the procedure qualifies as an unusual procedural service, the physician may report the column one HCPCS/CPT code of the NCCI PTP edit with modifier -22. The Carrier (A/B MAC processing practitioner service claims) may then evaluate the unusual procedural service to determine whether additional payment is justified.

For example, CMS limits payment for CPT code 69990 (microsurgical techniques, requiring use of operating microscope . . .) to procedures listed in the Internet-only Manual (IOM) (*Claims Processing Manual*, Publication 100-04, 12-§20.4.5). If a physician reports CPT code 69990 with two other CPT codes and one of the codes is not on this list, an NCCI PTP edit with the code not on the list will prevent payment for CPT code 69990. Claims processing systems do not determine which procedure is linked with CPT code 69990. In situations such as this, the physician may submit his claim to the local carrier (A/B MAC processing practitioner service claims) for readjudication appending modifier 22 to the CPT code. Although the carrier (A/B MAC processing practitioner service claims) cannot override an NCCI PTP edit that does not allow use of NCCI-associated modifiers, the carrier (A/B MAC processing practitioner service claims) has discretion to adjust payment to include use of the operating microscope based on modifier 22.

b) **Modifier -25:** The *CPT Manual* defines modifier -25 as a "significant, separately identifiable evaluation and management service by the same physician or other qualified health care professional on the same day of the procedure or other service." Modifier -25 may be appended to an evaluation and management (E&M) CPT code to indicate that the E&M service is significant and separately identifiable from other services reported on the same date of service. The E&M service may be related to the same or different diagnosis as the other procedure(s).

Modifier -25 may be appended to E&M services reported with minor surgical procedures (global period of 000 or 010 days) or procedures not covered by global surgery rules (global indicator of XXX). Since minor surgical procedures and XXX procedures include pre-procedure, intra-procedure, and post-procedure work inherent in the procedure, the provider shall not report an E&M service for this work. Furthermore, Medicare Global Surgery rules prevent the reporting of a separate E&M service for the work associated with the decision to perform a minor surgical procedure whether the patient is a new or established patient.

c) **Modifier -58:** Modifier -58 is defined by the *CPT Manual* as a "staged or related procedure or service by the same physician or other qualified health care professional during the postoperative period." It may be used to indicate that a procedure was followed by a second procedure during the post-operative period of the first procedure. This situation may occur because the second procedure was planned prospectively, was more extensive than the first procedure, or was therapy after a diagnostic surgical service. Use of modifier -58 will bypass NCCI PTP edits that allow use of NCCI-associated modifiers.

If a diagnostic endoscopic procedure results in the decision to perform an open procedure, both procedures may be reported with modifier -58 appended to the HCPCS/CPT code for the open procedure. However, if the endoscopic procedure preceding an open procedure is a "scout" procedure to assess anatomic landmarks and/or extent of disease, it is not separately reportable.

Diagnostic endoscopy is never separately reportable with another endoscopic procedure of the same organ(s) when performed at the same patient encounter. Similarly, diagnostic laparoscopy is never separately reportable with a surgical laparoscopic procedure of the same body cavity when performed at the same patient encounter.

If a planned laparoscopic procedure fails and is converted to an open procedure, only the open procedure may be reported. The failed laparoscopic procedure is not separately reportable. The NCCI contains many, but not all, edits bundling laparoscopic procedures into open procedures. Since the number of possible code combinations bundling a laparoscopic procedure into an open procedure is much greater than the number of such edits in NCCI, the principle stated in this paragraph is applicable regardless of whether the selected code pair combination is included in the NCCI tables. A provider shall not select laparoscopic and open HCPCS/CPT codes to report because the combination is not included in the NCCI tables.

d) Modifier -59: Modifier -59 is an important NCCI-associated modifier that is often used incorrectly. For the NCCI its primary purpose is to indicate that two or more procedures are performed at different anatomic sites or different patient encounters. One function of NCCI PTP edits is to prevent payment for codes that report overlapping services except in those instances where the services are "separate and distinct." Modifier 59 shall only be used if no other modifier more appropriately describes the relationships of the two or more procedure codes. The *CPT Manual* defines modifier -59 as follows:

**Modifier -59: Distinct Procedural Service:** Under certain circumstances, it may be necessary to indicate that a procedure or service was distinct or independent from other non E/M services performed on the same day. Modifier -59 is used to identify procedures/services other than E/M services that are not normally reported together, but are appropriate under the circumstances. Documentation must support a different session, different procedure or surgery, different site or organ system, separate incision/excision, separate lesion, or separate injury (or area of injury in extensive injuries) not ordinarily encountered or performed on the same day by the same individual. However, when another already established modifier is appropriate, it should be used rather than modifier -59. Only if no more descriptive modifier is available, and the use of modifier -59 best explains the circumstances, should modifier -59 be used. Note: Modifier 59 should not be

appended to an E/M service. To report a separate and distinct E/M service with a non-E/M service performed on the same date, see modifier 25.

NCCI PTP edits define when two procedure HCPCS/CPT codes may not be reported together except under special circumstances. If an edit allows use of NCCI-associated modifiers, the two procedure codes may be reported together when the two procedures are performed at different anatomic sites or different patient encounters. Carrier (A/B MAC processing practitioner service claims) processing systems utilize NCCI-associated modifiers to allow payment of both codes of an edit. Modifier -59 and other NCCI-associated modifiers shall **NOT** be used to bypass an NCCI PTP edit unless the proper criteria for use of the modifier are met. Documentation in the medical record must satisfy the criteria required by any NCCI-associated modifier used.

Some examples of the appropriate use of modifier -59 are contained in the individual chapter policies.

One of the common misuses of modifier -59 is related to the portion of the definition of modifier -59 allowing its use to describe "different procedure or surgery." The code descriptors of the two codes of a code pair edit usually represent different procedures or surgeries. The edit indicates that the two procedures/surgeries cannot be reported together if performed at the same anatomic site and same patient encounter. The provider cannot use modifier -59 for such an edit based on the two codes being different procedures/surgeries. However, if the two procedures/surgeries are performed at separate anatomic sites or at separate patient encounters on the same date of service, modifier -59 may be appended to indicate that they are different procedures/surgeries on that date of service.

There are several exceptions to this general principle about misuse of modifier -59 that apply to some code pair edits for procedures performed at the same patient encounter.

(1) When a diagnostic procedure precedes a surgical or non-surgical therapeutic procedure and is the basis on which the decision to perform the surgical or non-surgical therapeutic procedure is made, that diagnostic procedure may be considered to be a separate and distinct procedure as long as (a) it occurs before the therapeutic procedure and is not interspersed with services that are required for the therapeutic intervention; (b) it clearly provides the information needed to decide whether to proceed with the therapeutic procedure; and (c) it does not constitute a service that would have otherwise been required during the therapeutic intervention. If the diagnostic procedure is an inherent component of the surgical or non-surgical therapeutic procedure, it shall not be reported separately.

(2) When a diagnostic procedure follows a surgical procedure or non-surgical therapeutic procedure, that diagnostic procedure may be considered to be a separate and distinct procedure as long as (a) it occurs after the completion of the therapeutic procedure and is not interspersed with or otherwise commingled with services that are only required for the therapeutic intervention, and (b) it does not constitute a service that would have otherwise been required during the therapeutic intervention. If the post-procedure diagnostic procedure is an inherent component or otherwise included (or not separately payable) post-procedure service of the surgical procedure or non-surgical therapeutic procedure, it shall not be reported separately.

(3) There is an appropriate use for modifier 59 that is applicable only to codes for which the unit of service is a mea-

sure of time (e.g., per 15 minutes, per hour). If two separate and distinct timed services are provided in separate and distinct time blocks, modifier 59 may be used to identify the services. The separate and distinct time blocks for the two services may be sequential to one another or split. When the two services are split, the time block for one service may be followed by a time block for the second service followed by another time block for the first service. All Medicare rules for reporting timed services are applicable. For example, the total time is calculated for all related timed services performed. The number of reportable units of service is based on the total time, and these units of service are allocated between the HCPCS/CPT codes for the individual services performed. The physician is not permitted to perform multiple services, each for the minimal reportable time, and report each of these as separate units of service. (e.g., A physician or therapist performs eight minutes of neuromuscular reeducation (CPT code 97112) and eight minutes of therapeutic exercises (CPT code 97110). Since the physician or therapist performed 16 minutes of related timed services, only one unit of service may be reported for one, not each, of these codes.)

Use of modifier -59 to indicate different procedures/surgeries does not require a different diagnosis for each HCPCS/CPT coded procedure/surgery. Additionally, different diagnoses are not adequate criteria for use of modifier -59. The HCPCS/CPT codes remain bundled unless the procedures/surgeries are performed at different anatomic sites or separate patient encounters.

From an NCCI perspective, the definition of different anatomic sites includes different organs, different anatomic regions, or different lesions in the same organ. It does not include treatment of contiguous structures of the same organ. For example, treatment of the nail, nail bed, and adjacent soft tissue constitutes treatment of a single anatomic site. Treatment of posterior segment structures in the ipsilateral eye constitutes treatment of a single anatomic site. Arthroscopic treatment of a shoulder injury in adjoining areas of the ipsilateral shoulder constitutes treatment of a single anatomic site.

If the same procedure is performed at different anatomic sites, it does not necessarily imply that a HCPCS/CPT code may be reported with more than one unit of service (UOS) for the procedure. Determining whether additional UOS may be reported depends in part upon the HCPCS/CPT code descriptor including the definition of the code's unit of service, when present.

Example #1: The column one/column two code edit with column one CPT code 38221 (Diagnostic bone marrow biopsy) and column two CPT code 38220 (Diagnostic bone marrow, aspiration) includes two distinct procedures when performed at separate anatomic sites (e.g., contralateral iliac bones) or separate patient encounters. In these circumstances, it would be acceptable to use modifier -59. However, if both 38221 and 38220 are performed on the same iliac bone at the same patient encounter which is the usual practice, modifier -59 shall NOT be used. Although CMS does not allow separate payment for CPT code 38220 with CPT code 38221 when bone marrow aspiration and biopsy are performed on the same iliac bone at a single patient encounter, a physician may report CPT code 38222 Diagnostic bone marrow; biopsy(ies) and aspiration(s).

Example #2: The procedure to procedure edit with column one CPT code 11055 (paring or cutting of benign hyperkeratotic lesion ...) and column two CPT code 11720 (debridement of nail(s) by any method; 1 to 5) may be bypassed with modifier 59 only if the paring/cutting of a benign hyperkeratotic lesion is performed on a different digit (e.g., toe) than one that has nail debridement. Modifier 59 shall not be used to bypass the edit if the two procedures are performed on the same digit.

e) Modifiers XE, XS, XP, XU: These modifiers were effective January 1, 2015. These modifiers were developed to provide greater reporting specificity in situations where modifier 59 was previously reported and may be utilized in lieu of modifier 59 whenever possible. (Modifier 59 should only be utilized if no other more specific modifier is appropriate.) Although NCCI will eventually require use of these modifiers rather than modifier 59 with certain edits, physicians may begin using them for claims with dates of service on or after January 1, 2015. The modifiers are defined as follows:

XE – "Separate encounter, A service that is distinct because it occurred during a separate encounter" This modifier shall only be used to describe separate encounters on the same date of service.

XS – "Separate Structure, A service that is distinct because it was performed on a separate organ/structure"

XP – "Separate Practitioner, A service that is distinct because it was performed by a different practitioner"

XU – "Unusual Non-Overlapping Service, The use of a service that is distinct because it does not overlap usual components of the main service"

## F. Standard Preparation/Monitoring Services for Anesthesia

With few exceptions anesthesia HCPCS/CPT codes do not specify the mode of anesthesia for a particular procedure. Regardless of the mode of anesthesia, preparation and monitoring services are not separately reportable with anesthesia service HCPCS/CPT codes when performed in association with the anesthesia service. However, if the provider of the anesthesia service performs one or more of these services prior to and unrelated to the anticipated anesthesia service or after the patient is released from the anesthesia practitioner's postoperative care, the service may be separately reportable with modifier -59.

## G. Anesthesia Service Included in the Surgical Procedure

Under the CMS Anesthesia Rules, with limited exceptions, Medicare does not allow separate payment for anesthesia services performed by the physician who also furnishes the medical or surgical service. In this case, payment for the anesthesia service is included in the payment for the medical or surgical procedure. For example, separate payment is not allowed for the physician's performance of local, regional, or most other anesthesia including nerve blocks if the physician also performs the medical or surgical procedure. However, Medicare allows separate reporting for moderate conscious sedation services (CPT codes 99151-99153) when provided by same physician performing a medical or surgical procedure except for those procedures listed in Appendix G of the *CPT Manual*.

CPT codes describing anesthesia services (00100-01999) or services that are bundled into anesthesia shall not be reported in addition to the surgical or medical procedure requiring the anesthesia services if performed by the same physician. Examples of improperly reported services that are bundled into the anesthesia service when anesthesia is provided by the physician performing the medical or surgical procedure include introduction of needle or intracatheter into a vein (CPT code 36000), venipuncture (CPT code 36410), intravenous infusion/injection (CPT codes 96360-96368, 96374-96377) or cardiac assessment (e.g., CPT codes 93000-93010, 93040-93042). However, if these services are not related to the delivery of an anesthetic agent, or are not an inherent component of the procedure or global service, they may be reported separately.

The physician performing a surgical or medical procedure shall not report an epidural/subarachnoid injection (CPT codes 62320-62327) or nerve block (CPT codes 64400-64530) for anesthesia for that procedure.

## H. HCPCS/CPT Procedure Code Definition

The HCPCS/CPT code descriptors of two codes are often the basis of an NCCI PTP edit. If two HCPCS/CPT codes describe redundant services, they shall not be reported separately. Several general principles follow:

1. A family of CPT codes may include a CPT code followed by one or more indented CPT codes. The first CPT code descriptor includes a semicolon. The portion of the descriptor of the first code in the family preceding the semicolon is a common part of the descriptor for each subsequent code of the family. For example,

   CPT code 70120   Radiologic examination, mastoids; less than 3 views per side
   CPT code 70130   Complete, minimum of 3 views per side

   The portion of the descriptor preceding the semicolon ("Radiologic examination, mastoids") is common to both CPT codes 70120 and 70130. The difference between the two codes is the portion of the descriptors following the semicolon. Often as in this case, two codes from a family may not be reported separately. A physician cannot report CPT codes 70120 and 70130 for a procedure performed on ipsilateral mastoids at the same patient encounter. It is important to recognize, however, that there are numerous circumstances when it may be appropriate to report more than one code from a family of codes. For example, CPT codes 70120 and 70130 may be reported separately if the two procedures are performed on contralateral mastoids or at two separate patient encounters on the same date of service.

2. If a HCPCS/CPT code is reported, it includes all components of the procedure defined by the descriptor. For example, CPT code 58291 includes a vaginal hysterectomy with "removal of tube(s) and/or ovary(s)." A physician cannot report a salpingo-oophorectomy (CPT code 58720) separately with CPT code 58291.

3. CPT code descriptors often define correct coding relationships where two codes may not be reported separately with one another at the same anatomic site and/or same patient encounter. A few examples follow:
   a) A "partial" procedure is not separately reportable with a "complete" procedure.
   b) A "partial" procedure is not separately reportable with a "total" procedure.
   c) A "unilateral" procedure is not separately reportable with a "bilateral" procedure.
   d) A "single" procedure is not separately reportable with a "multiple" procedure.
   e) A "with" procedure is not separately reportable with a "without" procedure.
   f) An "initial" procedure is not separately reportable with a "subsequent" procedure.

## I. *CPT Manual* and CMS Coding Manual Instructions

CMS often publishes coding instructions in its rules, manuals, and notices. Physicians must utilize these instructions when reporting services rendered to Medicare patients.

The *CPT Manual* also includes coding instructions which may be found in the "Introduction", individual chapters, and appendices. In individual chapters the instructions may appear at the beginning of a chapter, at the beginning of a subsection of the chapter, or after specific CPT codes. Physicians should follow *CPT Manual* instructions unless CMS has provided different coding or reporting instructions.

The American Medical Association publishes *CPT Assistant* which contains coding guidelines. CMS does not review nor approve the information in this publication. In the development of NCCI PTP edits, CMS occasionally disagrees with the information in this publication. If a physician utilizes information from *CPT Assistant* to report services rendered to Medicare patients, it is possible that Medicare Carriers (A/B MACs processing practitioner service claims) and Fiscal Intermediaries may utilize different criteria to process claims.

## J. CPT "Separate Procedure" Definition

If a CPT code descriptor includes the term "separate procedure", the CPT code may not be reported separately with a related procedure. CMS interprets this designation to prohibit the separate reporting of a "separate procedure" when performed with another procedure in an anatomically related region often through the same skin incision, orifice, or surgical approach.

A CPT code with the "separate procedure" designation may be reported with another procedure if it is performed at a separate patient encounter on the same date of service or at the same patient encounter in an anatomically unrelated area often through a separate skin incision, orifice, or surgical approach. Modifier -59 or a more specific modifier (e.g., anatomic modifier) may be appended to the "separate procedure" CPT code to indicate that it qualifies as a separately reportable service.

## K. Family of Codes

The *CPT Manual* often contains a group of codes that describe related procedures that may be performed in various combinations. Some codes describe limited component services, and other codes describe various combinations of component services. Physicians must utilize several principles in selecting the correct code to report:

1. A HCPCS/CPT code may be reported if and only if all services described by the code are performed.

2. The HCPCS/CPT code describing the services performed shall be reported. A physician shall not report multiple codes corresponding to component services if a single comprehensive code describes the services performed. There are limited exceptions to this rule which are specifically identified in this Manual.

3. HCPCS/CPT code(s) corresponding to component service(s) of other more comprehensive HCPCS/CPT code(s) shall not be reported separately with the more comprehensive HCPCS/CPT code(s) that include the component service(s).

4. If the HCPCS/CPT codes do not correctly describe the procedure(s) performed, the physician shall report a "not otherwise specified" CPT code rather than a HCPCS/CPT code that most closely describes the procedure(s) performed.

## L. More Extensive Procedure

The *CPT Manual* often describes groups of similar codes differing in the complexity of the service. Unless services are performed at separate patient encounters or at separate anatomic sites, the less complex service is included in the more complex service and is not separately reportable. Several examples of this principle follow:

1. If two procedures only differ in that one is described as a "simple" procedure and the other as a "complex" procedure, the "simple" procedure is included in the "complex" procedure and is not separately reportable unless the two procedures are performed at separate patient encounters or at separate anatomic sites.

2. If two procedures only differ in that one is described as a "simple" procedure and the other as a "complicated" procedure, the "simple" procedure is included in the "complicated" procedure and is not separately reportable unless the two procedures are performed at separate patient encounters or at separate anatomic sites.

3. If two procedures only differ in that one is described as a "limited" procedure and the other as a "complete" procedure, the "limited" procedure is included in the "complete" procedure and is not separately reportable unless the two procedures are performed at separate patient encounters or at separate anatomic sites.

4. If two procedures only differ in that one is described as an "intermediate" procedure and the other as a "comprehensive" procedure, the "intermediate" procedure is included in the "comprehensive" procedure and is not separately reportable unless the two procedures are performed at separate patient encounters or at separate anatomic sites.

5. If two procedures only differ in that one is described as a "superficial" procedure and the other as a "deep" procedure, the "superficial" procedure is included in the "deep" procedure and is not separately reportable unless the two procedures are performed at separate patient encounters or at separate anatomic sites.

6. If two procedures only differ in that one is described as an "incomplete" procedure and the other as a "complete" procedure, the "incomplete" procedure is included in the "complete" procedure and is not separately reportable unless the two procedures are performed at separate patient encounters or at separate anatomic sites.

7. If two procedures only differ in that one is described as an "external" procedure and the other as an "internal" procedure, the "external" procedure is included in the "internal" procedure and is not separately reportable unless the two

procedures are performed at separate patient encounters or at separate anatomic sites.

## M. Sequential Procedure

Some surgical procedures may be performed by different surgical approaches. If an initial surgical approach to a procedure fails and a second surgical approach is utilized at the same patient encounter, only the HCPCS/CPT code corresponding to the second surgical approach may be reported. If there are different HCPCS/CPT codes for the two different surgical approaches, the two procedures are considered "sequential", and only the HCPCS/CPT code corresponding to the second surgical approach may be reported. For example, a physician may begin a cholecystectomy procedure utilizing a laparoscopic approach and have to convert the procedure to an open abdominal approach. Only the CPT code for the open cholecystectomy may be reported. The CPT code for the failed laparoscopic cholecystectomy is not separately reportable.

## N. Laboratory Panel

The *CPT Manual* defines organ and disease specific panels of laboratory tests. If a laboratory performs all tests included in one of these panels, the laboratory *shall* report the CPT code for the panel. If the laboratory repeats one of these component tests as a medically reasonable and necessary service on the same date of service, the CPT code corresponding to the repeat laboratory test may be reported with modifier -91 appended *(See Chapter X, Section C [Oran or Disease Oriented Panels]).*

## O. Misuse of Column Two Code with Column One Code (Misuse of Code Edit Rationale)

CMS manuals and instructions often describe groups of HCPCS/CPT codes that should not be reported together for the Medicare program. Edits based on these instructions are often included as misuse of column two code with column one code.

A HCPCS/CPT code descriptor does not include exhaustive information about the code. Physicians who are not familiar with a HCPCS/CPT code may incorrectly report the code in a context different than intended. The NCCI has identified HCPCS/CPT codes that are incorrectly reported with other HCPCS/CPT codes as a result of the misuse of the column two code with the column one code. If these edits allow use of NCCI-associated modifiers (modifier indicator of "1"), there are limited circumstances when the column two code may be reported on the same date of service as the column one code. Two examples follow:

1. Three or more HCPCS/CPT codes may be reported on the same date of service. Although the column two code is misused if reported as a service associated with the column one code, the column two code may be appropriately reported with a third HCPCS/CPT code reported on the same date of service. For example, CMS limits separate payment for use of the operating microscope for microsurgical techniques (CPT code 69990) to a group of procedures listed in the online *Claims Processing Manual* (Chapter 12, Section

20.4.5 (Allowable Adjustments)). The NCCI has edits with column one codes of surgical procedures not listed in this section of the manual and column two CPT code of 69990. Some of these edits allow use of NCCI-associated modifiers because the two services listed in the edit may be performed at the same patient encounter as a third procedure for which CPT code 69990 is separately reportable.

2. There may be limited circumstances when the column two code is separately reportable with the column one code. For example, the NCCI has an edit with column one CPT code of 80061 (lipid profile) and column two CPT code of 83721 (LDL cholesterol by direct measurement). If the triglyceride level is less than 400 mg/dl, the LDL is a calculated value utilizing the results from the lipid profile for the calculation, and CPT code 83721 is not separately reportable. However, if the triglyceride level is greater than 400 mg/dl, the LDL may be measured directly and may be separately reportable with CPT code 83721 utilizing an NCCI-associated modifier to bypass the edit.

Misuse of code as an edit rationale may be applied to procedure to procedure edits where the column two code is not separately reportable with the column one code based on the nature of the column one coded procedure. This edit rationale may also be applied to code pairs where use of the column two code with the column one code is deemed to be a coding error.

## P. Mutually Exclusive Procedures

Many procedure codes cannot be reported together because they are mutually exclusive of each other. Mutually exclusive procedures cannot reasonably be performed at the same anatomic site or same patient encounter. An example of a mutually exclusive situation is the repair of an organ that can be performed by two different methods. Only one method can be chosen to repair the organ. A second example is a service that can be reported as an "initial" service or a "subsequent" service. With the exception of drug administration services, the initial service and subsequent service cannot be reported at the same patient encounter.

## Q. Gender-Specific Procedures (formerly Designation of Sex)

The descriptor of some HCPCS/CPT codes includes a gender-specific restriction on the use of the code. HCPCS/CPT codes specific for one gender should not be reported with HCPCS/CPT codes for the opposite gender. For example, CPT code 53210 describes a total urethrectomy including cystostomy in a female, and CPT code 53215 describes the same procedure in a male. Since the patient cannot have both the male and female procedures performed, the two CPT codes cannot be reported together.

## R. Add-on Codes

Some codes in the *CPT Manual* are identified as "add-on" codes which describe a service that can only be reported in addition to a primary procedure. *CPT Manual* instructions specify the primary procedure code(s) for most add-on codes. For other add-on codes, the primary procedure code(s) is(are) not specified. When the *CPT Manual* identifies specific primary codes, the add-on code shall not be reported as a supplemental service for other HCPCS/CPT codes not listed as a primary code.

Add-on codes permit the reporting of significant supplemental services commonly performed in addition to the primary procedure. By contrast, incidental services that are necessary to accomplish the primary procedure (e.g., lysis of adhesions in the course of an open cholecystectomy) are not separately reportable with an add-on code. Similarly, complications inherent in an invasive procedure occurring during the procedure are not separately reportable. For example, control of bleeding during an invasive procedure is considered part of the procedure and is not separately reportable.

In general, NCCI procedure to procedure edits do not include edits with most add-on codes because edits related to the primary procedure(s) are adequate to prevent inappropriate payment for an add-on coded procedure. (I.e., if an edit prevents payment of the primary procedure code, the add-on code shall not be paid.) However, NCCI does include edits for some add-on codes when coding edits related to the primary procedures must be supplemented. Examples include edits with add-on HCPCS/CPT codes 69990 (microsurgical techniques requiring use of operating microscope) and 95940/95941/G0453 (intraoperative neurophysiology testing).

HCPCS/CPT codes that are not designated as add-on codes shall not be misused as an add-on code to report a supplemental service. A HCPCS/CPT code may be reported if and only if all services described by the CPT code are performed. A HCPCS/CPT code shall not be reported with another service because a portion of the service described by the HCPCS/CPT code was performed with the other procedure. For example: If an ejection fraction is estimated from an echocardiogram study, it would be inappropriate to additionally report CPT code 78472 (cardiac blood pool imaging with ejection fraction) with the echocardiography (CPT code 93307). Although the procedure described by CPT code 78472 includes an ejection fraction, it is measured by gated equilibrium with a radionuclide which is not utilized in echocardiography.

## S. Excluded Service

The NCCI does not address issues related to HCPCS/CPT codes describing services that are excluded from Medicare coverage or are not otherwise recognized for payment under the Medicare program.

## T. Unlisted Procedure Codes

The *CPT Manual* includes codes to identify services or procedures not described by other HCPCS/CPT codes. These unlisted procedure codes are generally identified as XXX99 or XXXX9 codes and are located at the end of each section or subsection of the manual. If a physician provides a service that is not accurately described by other HCPCS/CPT codes, the service shall be reported utilizing an unlisted procedure code. A physician shall not report a CPT code for a specific procedure if it does not accurately describe the service performed. It is inappropriate to report the best fit HCPCS/CPT code unless it accurately describes the service performed, and all components of the HCPCS/CPT code were performed. Since unlisted procedure codes may be reported for a very diverse group of services, the NCCI generally does not include edits with these codes.

## U. Modified, Deleted, and Added Code Pairs/Edits

**Information moved to Introduction chapter, Section (Purpose), Page Intro-5 of this Manual.**

## V. Medically Unlikely Edits (MUEs)

To lower the Medicare Fee-For-Service Paid Claims Error Rate, CMS has established units of service edits referred to as Medically Unlikely Edit(s) (MUEs).

An MUE for a HCPCS/CPT code is the maximum number of units of service (UOS) under most circumstances allowable by the same provider for the same beneficiary on the same date of service. The ideal MUE value for a HCPCS/CPT code is the unit of service that allows the vast majority of appropriately coded claims to pass the MUE.

All practitioner claims submitted to Carriers (A/B MACs processing practitioner service claims), outpatient facility services claims (Type of Bill 13X, 14X, 85X) submitted to Fiscal Intermediaries (A/B MACs processing facility claims), and supplier claims submitted to Durable Medical Equipment (DME) MACs are tested against MUEs.

Prior to April 1, 2013, each line of a claim was adjudicated separately against the MUE value for the HCPCS/CPT code reported on that claim line. If the units of service on that claim line exceeded the MUE value, the entire claim line was denied.

In the April 1, 2013 version of MUEs, CMS began introducing date of service (DOS) MUEs. Over time CMS will convert many, but not all, MUEs to DOS MUEs. Since April 1, 2013, MUEs are adjudicated either as claim line edits or DOS edits. If the MUE is adjudicated as a claim line edit, the units of service (UOS) on each claim line are compared to the MUE value for the HCPCS/CPT code on that claim line. If the UOS exceed the MUE value, all UOS on that claim line are denied. If the MUE is adjudicated as a DOS MUE, all UOS on each claim line for the same date of service for the same HCPCS/CPT code are summed, and the sum is compared to the MUE value. If the summed UOS exceed the MUE value, all UOS for the HCPCS/CPT code for that date of service are denied. Denials due to claim line MUEs or DOS MUEs may be appealed to the local claims processing contractor. DOS MUEs are utilized for HCPCS/CPT codes where it would be extremely unlikely that more UOS than the MUE value would ever be performed on the same date of service for the same patient.

The MUE files on the CMS NCCI website display an "MUE Adjudication Indicator" (MAI) for each HCPCS/CPT code. An MAI of "1" indicates that the edit is a claim line MUE. An MAI of "2" or "3" indicates that the edit is a DOS MUE.

If a HCPCS/CPT code has an MUE that is adjudicated as a claim line edit, appropriate use of CPT modifiers (e.g., -59, -76, -77, -91, anatomic) may be used to the same HCPCS/CPT code on separate lines of a claim. Each line of the claim with that HCPCS/CPT code will be separately adjudicated against the MUE value for that HCPCS/CPT code. Claims processing contractors have rules limiting use of these modifiers with some HCPCS/CPT codes.

MUEs for HCPCS codes with an MAI of "2" are absolute date of service edits. These are "per day edits based on policy".

HCPCS codes with an MAI of "2" have been rigorously reviewed and vetted within CMS and obtain this MAI designation because UOS on the same date of service (DOS) in excess of the MUE value would be considered impossible because it was contrary to statute, regulation or subregulatory guidance. This subregulatory guidance includes clear correct coding policy that is binding on both providers and CMS claims processing contractors. Limitations created by anatomical or coding limitations are incorporated in correct coding policy, both in the HIPAA mandated coding descriptors and CMS approved coding guidance as well as specific guidance in CMS and NCCI manuals. For example, it would be contrary to correct coding policy to report more than one unit of service for CPT 94002 "ventilation assist and management . . . initial day" because such usage could not accurately describe two initial days of management occurring on the same date of service as would be required by the code descriptor. As a result, claims processing contractors are instructed that an MAI of "2" denotes a claims processing restriction for which override during processing, reopening, or redetermination would be contrary to CMS policy.

MUEs for HCPCS codes with an MAI of "3" are "per day edits based on clinical benchmarks". MUEs assigned an MAI of "3" are based on criteria (e.g., nature of service, prescribing information) combined with data such that it would be possible but medically highly unlikely that higher values would represent correctly reported medically necessary services. If contractors have evidence (e.g., medical review) that UOS in excess of the MUE value were actually provided, were correctly coded and were medically necessary, the contractor may bypass the MUE for a HCPCS code with an MAI of "3" during claim processing, reopening or redetermination, or in response to effectuation instructions from a reconsideration or higher level appeal.

Both the MAI and MUE value for each HCPCS/CPT code are based on one or more of the following criteria:

(1) Anatomic considerations may limit units of service based on anatomic structures. For example,
   a) The MUE value for an appendectomy is "1" since there is only one appendix.
   b) The MUE for a knee brace is "2" because there are two knees and Medicare policy does not cover back-up equipment.
   c) The MUE value for a lumbar spine procedure reported per lumbar vertebra or per lumbar interspace cannot exceed "5" since there are only five lumbar vertebrae or interspaces.
   d) The MUE value for a procedure reported per lung lobe cannot exceed "5" since there are only five lung lobes (three in right lung and two in left Lung).

(2) CPT code descriptors/CPT coding instructions in the *CPT Manual* may limit units of service. For example,
   a) A procedure described as the "initial 30 minutes" would have an MUE value of 1 because of the use of the term "initial". A different code may be reported for additional time.
   b) If a code descriptor uses the plural form of the procedure, it must not be reported with multiple units of service. For example, if the code descriptor states "biopsies", the code is reported with "1" unit of service regardless of the number of biopsies performed.
   c) The MUE value for a procedure with "per day", "per week", or "per month" in its code descriptor is "1" because MUEs are based on number of services per day of service.

d) The MUE value of a code for a procedure described as "unilateral" is "1" if there is a different code for the procedure described as "bilateral".

e) The code descriptors of a family of codes may define different levels of service, each having an MUE of "1". For example, CPT codes 78102-78104 describe bone marrow imaging. CPT code 78102 is reported for imaging a "limited area". CPT code 78103 is reported for imaging "multiple areas". CPT code 78104 is reported for imaging the "whole body".

f) The MUE value for CPT code 86021 (Antibody identification; leukocyte antibodies) is "1" because the code descriptor is plural including testing for any and all leukocyte antibodies. On a single date of service only one specimen from a patient would be tested for leukocyte antibodies.

(3) Edits based on established CMS policies may limit units of service (UOS). For example,

a) The MUE value for a surgical or diagnostic procedure may be based on the bilateral surgery indicator on the Medicare Physician Fee Schedule Database(MPFSDB)

   i. If the bilateral surgery indicator is "0", a bilateral procedure must be reported with "1" UOS. There is no additional payment for the code if reported as a unilateral or bilateral procedure because of anatomy or physiology. Alternatively, the code descriptor may specifically state that the procedure is a unilateral procedure, and there is a separate code for a bilateral procedure.

   ii. If the bilateral surgery indicator is "1", a bilateral surgical procedure must be reported with "1" UOS and modifier 50 (bilateral modifier). A bilateral diagnostic procedure may be reported with "2" UOS on one claim line, "1" UOS and modifier 50 on one claim line, or "1" UOS with modifier RT on one claim line plus "1" UOS and modifier LT on a second claim line.

   iii. If the bilateral surgery indicator is "2", a bilateral procedure must be reported with "1" UOS. The procedure is priced as a bilateral procedure because (1) the code descriptor defines the procedure as bilateral; (2) the code descriptor states that the procedure is performed unilaterally or bilaterally; or (3) the procedure is usually performed as a bilateral procedure.

   iv. If the bilateral surgery indicator is "3", a bilateral surgical procedure must be reported with "1" UOS and modifier 50 (bilateral modifier). A bilateral diagnostic procedure may be reported with "2" UOS on one claim line, "1" UOS and modifier 50 on one claim line, or 1 UOS with modifier RT on one claim line plus "1" UOS and modifier LT on a second claim line.

b) The MUE value for a code may be "1" where the code descriptor does not specify a UOS and CMS considers the default UOS to be "per day".

c) The MUE value for a code may be "0" because the code is listed as invalid, not covered, bundled, not separately payable, statutorily excluded, not reasonable and necessary, etc. based on

   i. The Medicare Physician Fee Schedule Database

   ii. Outpatient Prospective Payment System Addendum B

   iii. Alpha-Numeric HCPCS Code File

   iv. DMEPOS Jurisdiction List

   v. Medicare Internet-Only Manual

(4) The nature of an analyte may limit units of service and is in general determined by one of three considerations:

a) The nature of the specimen may limit the units of service. For example, CPT code 81575 describes a creatinine clearance test and has an MUE of "1" because the test requires a 24 hour urine collection.

b) The physiology, pathophysiology, or clinical application of the analyte is such that a maximum unit of service for a single date of service can be determined. For example, the MUE for CPT code 82747 (RBC folic acid) is "1" because the test result would not be expected to change during a single day, and thus it is not necessary to perform the test more than once on a single date of service.

(5) The nature of a procedure/service may limit units of service and is in general determined by the amount of time required to perform a procedure/service (e.g., overnight sleep studies) or clinical application of a procedure/service (e.g., motion analysis tests).

a) The MUE for many surgical or medical procedures is "1" because the procedure is rarely, if ever, performed more than one time per day (e.g., colonoscopy, motion analysis tests).

b) The MUE value for a procedure is "1" because of the amount of time required to perform the procedure (e.g., overnight sleep study).

(6) The nature of equipment may limit units of service and is in general determined by the number of items of equipment that would be utilized (e.g., cochlear implant or wheelchair). For example, the MUE value for a wheelchair code is "1" because only one wheelchair is used at one time and Medicare policy does not cover back-up equipment.

(7) Although clinical judgment considerations and determinations are based on input from numerous physicians and certified coders are sometimes initially utilized to establish some MUE values, these values are subsequently validated or changed based on submitted and/or paid claims data.

(8) Prescribing information is based on FDA labeling as well as off-label information published in CMS approved drug compendia. See below for additional information about how prescribing information is utilized in determining MUE values.

(9) Submitted and paid claims data (100%) from a six month period is utilized to ascertain the distribution pattern of UOS typically reported for a given HCPCS/CPT code.

(10) Published policies of the Durable Medical Equipment (DME) Medicare Administrative Contractors (MACs) may limit units of service for some durable medical equipment, prosthetics, orthotics, and supplies (DMEPOS). For example,

a) The MUE values for many ostomy and urological supply codes, nebulizer codes, and CPAP accessory codes are typically based on a three month supply of items.

b) The MUE values for surgical dressings, parenteral and enteral nutrition, immunosuppressive drugs, and oral anti-cancer drugs are typically based on a one month supply.

c) The MUE values take into account the requirement for reporting certain codes with date spans.

d) The MUE value of a code may be 0 if the item is non-covered, not medically necessary, or not separately payable.

e) The MUE value of a code may be 0 if the code is invalid for claim submission to the DME MAC.

UOS denied based on an MUE may be appealed. Because a denial of services due to an MUE is a coding denial, not a medical necessity denial, the presence of an Advanced Beneficiary Notice of Noncoverage (ABN) shall not shift liability to the beneficiary for UOS denied based on an MUE. If during reopening or redetermination medical records are provided with respect to an MUE denial for an edit with an MAI of "3", contractors will review the records to determine if the provider actually furnished units in excess of the MUE, if the codes were used correctly, and whether the services were medically reasonable and necessary. If the units were actually provided but one of the other conditions is not met, a change in denial reason may be warranted (for example, a change from the MUE denial based on incorrect coding to a determination that the item/service is not reasonable and necessary under section 1862(a)(1)). This may also be true for certain edits with an MAI of "1". CMS interprets the notice delivery requirements under §1879 of the Social Security Act (the Act) as applying to situations in which a provider expects the initial claim determination to be a reasonable and necessary denial. Consistent with NCCI guidance, denials resulting from MUEs are not based on any of the statutory provisions that give liability protection to beneficiaries under section 1879 of the Social Security Act. Thus, ABN issuance based on an MUE is NOT appropriate. A provider/ supplier may not issue an ABN in connection with services denied due to an MUE and cannot bill the beneficiary for units of service denied based on an MUE.

HCPCS J code and drug related C and Q code MUEs are based on prescribing information and 100% claims data for a six month period of time. Utilizing the prescribing information the highest total daily dose for each drug was determined. This dose and its corresponding units of service were evaluated against paid and submitted claims data. Some of the guiding principles utilized in developing these edits are as follows:

(1) If the prescribing information defined a maximum daily dose, this value was used to determine the MUE value. For some drugs there is an absolute maximum daily dose. For others there is a maximum "recommended" or "usual" dose. In the latter of the two cases, the daily dose calculation was evaluated against claims data.

(2) If the maximum daily dose calculation is based on actual body weight, a dose based on a weight range of 110-150 kg was evaluated against the claims data. If the maximum daily dose calculation is based on ideal body weight, a dose based on a weight range of 90-110 kg was evaluated against claims data. If the maximum daily dose calculation is based on body surface area (BSA), a dose based on a BSA range of 2.4-3.0 square meters was evaluated against claims data.

(3) For "as needed" (PRN) drugs and drugs where maximum daily dose is based on patient response, prescribing information and claims data were utilized to establish MUE values.

(4) Published off label usage of a drug was considered for the maximum daily dose calculation.

(5) The MUE values for some drug codes are set to 0. The rationale for such values include but are not limited to: discontinued manufacture of drug, non-FDA approved compounded drug, practitioner MUE values for oral antineoplastic, oral anti-emetic, and oral immune suppressive drugs which should be billed to the DME MACs, and outpatient hospital MUE values for inhalation drugs which should be billed to the DME MACs, and Practitioner/ASC MUE values for HCPCS C codes describing medications that would not be related to a procedure performed in an ASC.

Non-drug related HCPCS/CPT codes may be assigned an MUE of 0 for a variety of reasons including, but not limited to: outpatient hospital MUE value for surgical procedure only performed as an inpatient procedure, noncovered service, bundled service, or packaged service.

The MUE files on the CMS NCCI website display an "Edit Rationale" for each HCPCS/CPT code. Although an MUE may be based on several rationales, only one is displayed on the website. One of the listed rationales is "Data." This rationale indicates that 100% claims data from a six month period of time was the major factor in determining the MUE value. If a physician appeals an MUE denial for a HCPCS/CPT code where the MUE is based on "Data," the reviewer will usually confirm that (1) the correct code is reported; (2) the correct UOS is utilized; (3) the number of reported UOS were performed; and (4) all UOS were medically reasonable and necessary.

The first MUEs were implemented January 1, 2007. Additional MUEs are added on a quarterly basis on the same schedule as NCCI updates. Prior to implementation proposed MUEs are sent to numerous national healthcare organizations for a sixty day review and comment period.

Many surgical procedures may be performed bilaterally. Instructions in the CMS *Internet-only Manual* (Publication 100-04 *Medicare Claims Processing Manual*, Chapter 12 (Physicians/Nonphysician Practitioners), Section 40.7.B. and Chapter 4 (Part B Hospital (Including Inpatient Hospital Part B and OPPS)), Section 20.6.2 require that bilateral surgical procedures be reported using modifier 50 with one unit of service *unless the code descriptor defines the procedure as "bilateral". If the code descriptor defines the procedure as a "bilateral" procedure, it shall be reported with one unit of service without modifier 50*. If a bilateral surgical procedure is performed at different sites bilaterally, one unit of service may be reported for each site. That is, the HCPCS/CPT code may be reported with modifier 50 and one unit of service for each site at which it was performed bilaterally.

Some A/B MACs allow providers to report repetitive services performed over a range of dates on a single line of a claim with multiple units of service. If a provider reports services in this fashion, the provider should report the "from date" and "to date" on the claim line. Contractors are instructed to divide the units of service reported on the claim line by the number of days in the date span and round to the nearest whole number. This number is compared to the MUE value for the code on the claim line.

Suppliers billing services to the DME MACs typically report some HCPCS codes for supply items for a period exceeding a single day. The DME MACs have billing rules for these codes. For some codes the DME MACs require that the "from date" and "to date" be reported. The MUEs for these codes are based on the maximum number of units of service that may be reported for a single date of service. For other codes the DME MACs permit multiple days' supply items to be reported on a single claim line where the "from date" and "to date" are the same. The DME MACs have rules allowing supply items for a maximum number of days to be reported at one time for each of these types of codes. The MUE values for these codes are based on the maximum number of days that may be reported at one time. As with all MUEs, the MUE value does not represent a utilization guideline. Suppliers shall not assume that they may report units of service up to the MUE value on each date of service. Suppliers may only report supply items that are medically reasonable and necessary.

Most MUE values are set so that a provider or supplier would only very occasionally have a claim line denied. If a provider encounters a code with frequent denials due to the MUE, or frequent use of a CPT modifier to bypass the MUE, the provider or supplier should consider the following: (1) Is the HCPCS/CPT code being used correctly? (2) Is the unit of service being counted correctly? (3) Are all reported services medically reasonable and necessary? and (4) Why does the provider's or supplier's practice differ from national patterns? A provider or supplier may choose to discuss these questions with the local Medicare contractor or a national healthcare organization whose members frequently perform the procedure.

Most MUE values are published on the CMS MUE webpage https://www.cms.gov/Medicare/Coding/NationalCorrectCod InitEd/MUE.html. However, some MUE values are not published and are confidential. These values shall not be published in oral or written form by any party that acquires one or more of them.

MUEs are not utilization edits. Although the MUE value for some codes may represent the commonly reported units of service (e.g., MUE of "1" for appendectomy), the usual units of service for many HCPCS/CPT codes is less than the MUE value. Claims reporting units of service less than the MUE value may be subject to review by claims processing contractors, Program Safeguard Contractors (PSCs), Zoned Program Integrity Contractors (ZPICs), Recovery Audit Contractors (RACs), and Department of Justice (DOJ).

Since MUEs are coding edits rather than medical necessity edits, claims processing contractors may have units of service edits that are more restrictive than MUEs. In such cases, the more restrictive claims processing contractor edit would be applied to the claim. Similarly, if the MUE is more restrictive than a claims processing contractor edit, the more restrictive MUE would apply.

A provider, supplier, healthcare organization, or other interested party may request reconsideration of an MUE value for a HCPCS/CPT code *by CMS by writing the NCCI/MUE contractor.* Written request*s* proposing an alternative MUE with rationale may be sent to *the entity and address identified on the CMS NCCI website (http://www.cms.gov/Medicare/Coding/NationalCorrectCodInitED/index.html).*

## W. Add-on Code Edit Tables

Add-on codes are discussed in Chapter I, Section R (Add-on Codes). CMS publishes a list of add-on codes and their primary codes annually prior to January 1. The list is updated quarterly based on the AMA's "CPT Errata" documents or implementation of new HCPCS/CPT add-on codes. CMS identifies add-on codes and their primary codes based on CPT Manual instructions, CMS interpretation of HCPCS/CPT codes, and CMS coding instructions.

The NCCI program includes three Add-on Code Edit Tables, one table for each of three "Types" of add-on codes. Each table lists the add-on code with its primary codes. An add-on code, with one exception, is eligible for payment if and only if one of its primary codes is also eligible for payment.

The "Type I Add-on Code Edit Table" lists add-on codes for which the CPT Manual or HCPCS tables define all acceptable primary codes. Claims processing contractors should not allow other primary codes with Type I add-on codes. CPT code 99292 (Critical care, evaluation and management of the critically ill or critically injured patient; each additional 30 minutes (List separately in addition to code for primary service)) is included as a Type I add-on code since its only primary code is CPT code 99291 (Critical care, evaluation and management of the critically ill or critically injured patient; first 30-74 minutes). For Medicare purposes, CPT code 99292 may be eligible for payment to a physician without CPT code 99291 if another physician of the same specialty and physician group reports and is paid for CPT code 99291.

The "Type II Add-on Code Edit Table" lists add-on codes for which the CPT Manual and HCPCS tables do not define any primary codes. Claims processing contractors should develop their own lists of acceptable primary codes.

The "Type III Add-on Code Edit Table" lists add-on codes for which the CPT Manual or HCPCS tables define some, but not all, acceptable primary codes. Claims processing contractors should allow the listed primary codes for these add-on codes but may develop their own lists of additional acceptable primary codes.

Although the add-on code and primary code are normally reported for the same date of service, there are unusual circumstances where the two services may be reported for different dates of service (e.g., CPT codes 99291 and 99292).

The first Add-On Code edit tables were implemented April 1, 2013. For subsequent years, new Add-On Code edit tables will be published to be effective for January 1 of the new year based on changes in the new year's CPT Manual. CMS also issues quarterly updates to the Add-On Code edit tables if required due to publication of new HCPCS/CPT codes or changes in add-on codes or their primary codes. The changes in the quarterly update files (April 1, July 1, or October 1) are retroactive to the implementation date of that year's annual Add-On Code edit files unless the files specify a different effective date for a change. Since the first Add-On Code edit files were implemented on April 1, 2013, changes in the July 1 and October 1 quarterly updates for 2013 were retroactive to April 1, 2013 unless the files specified a different effective date for a change.

# FIGURE CREDITS

1. From Little J et al: *Dental management of the medically compromised patient,* ed 9, St. Louis, 2017, Mosby. *(Courtesy Medtronic, Minneapolis)*
2. From Franklin I, Dawson P, Rodway A: *Essentials of Clinical Surgery,* ed 2, 2012, Saunders.
3. Modified from Grosfeld J et al: *Pediatric surgery,* ed 7, Philadelphia, 2012, Mosby.
4. Modified from Hsu J, Michael J, Fisk J: *AAOS atlas of orthoses and assistive devices,* ed 4, Philadelphia, 2008, Mosby.
5. From Wold G: *Basic Geriatric Nursing,* ed 5, St. Louis, 2011, Mosby.
6. Modified from Roberts J, Hedges J: *Clinical procedures in emergency medicine,* ed 6, St. Louis, 2013, Saunders.
7. From Auerbach P: *Wilderness medicine,* ed 7, Philadelphia, 2016, Mosby. *(Courtesy Black Diamond Equipment, Ltd.)*
8. *(Original to book).*
9. Modified from Abeloff M et al: *Clinical oncology,* ed 5, Philadelphia, 2013, Churchill Livingstone.
10. *(Original to book).*
11. Modified from Duthie E, Katz P, Malone M: *Practice of geriatrics,* ed 4, Philadelphia, 2007, Saunders.
12. Modified from Roberts J, Hedges J: *Clinical procedures in emergency medicine,* ed 6, St. Louis, 2013, Saunders.
13. From Young A, Proctor D: *Kinn's the medical assistant,* ed 13, St. Louis, 2016, Saunders.
14. From Bonewit-West K: *Clinical procedures for medical assistants,* ed 9, Philadelphia, 2015, WB Saunders.
15. From Roberts J, Hedges J: *Clinical procedures in emergency medicine,* ed 6, St. Louis, 2013, Saunders.
16. From Yeo: *Shackelford's surgery of the alimentary tract,* ed 7, Philadelphia, 2012, Saunders.
17. Redrawn from Bragg D, Rubin P, Hricak H: *Oncologic imaging,* ed 2, 2002, Saunders.
18. From Roberts J, Hedges J: *Clinical procedures in emergency medicine,* ed 6, St. Louis, 2013, Saunders. *(Courtesy Atrium Medical Corp., Hudson, NH 03051)*
19. **A** From Auerbach P: *Wilderness medicine,* ed 7, Philadelphia, 2016, Mosby. **B** Modified from Hsu J, Michael J, Fisk J: *AAOS atlas of orthoses and assistive devices,* ed 4, Philadelphia, 2008, Mosby.
20. Modified from Lusardi M, Nielsen C: *Orthotics and prosthetics in rehabilitation,* ed 3, St. Louis, 2013, Butterworth-Heinemann.
21. Modified from Lusardi M, Nielsen C: *Orthotics and prosthetics in rehabilitation,* ed 3, St. Louis, 2013, Butterworth-Heinemann.
22. Modified from Lusardi M, Nielsen C: *Orthotics and prosthetics in rehabilitation,* ed 3, St. Louis, 2013, Butterworth-Heinemann.
23. From Buck C: *The Next Step, Advanced Medical Coding 2019/2020 edition,* St. Louis, 2017, Saunders.
24. From Jardins T: *Clinical Manifestations and Assessment of Respiratory Disease,* ed 7, St. Louis, 2015, Elsevier.
25. From Hsu J, Michael J, Fisk J: *AAOS atlas of orthoses and assistive devices,* ed 4, Philadelphia, 2008, Mosby.
26. Modified from Hsu J, Michael J, Fisk J: *AAOS atlas of orthoses and assistive devices,* ed 4, Philadelphia, 2008, Mosby.
27. Modified from Hsu J, Michael J, Fisk J: *AAOS atlas of orthoses and assistive devices,* ed 4, Philadelphia, 2008, Mosby.
28. From Didomenico, Lawrence A., and Nik Gatalyak. "End-Stage Ankle Arthritis." *Clinics in Podiatric Medicine and Surgery* 29.3 (2012): 391-412.
29. Cameron, Michelle H., and Linda G. Monroe. *Physical Rehabilitation for the Physical Therapist Assistant,* ed 1, St. Louis, 2011, Saunders.
30. From Rowe, Dale E., and Avinash L. Jadhav. "Care of the Adolescent with Spina Bifida." *Pediatric Clinics of North America* 55.6 (2008): 1359-374.
31. Modified from Lusardi M, Nielsen C: *Orthotics and prosthetics in rehabilitation,* ed 3, St. Louis, 2013, Butterworth-Heinemann.
32. From Hsu J, Michael J, Fisk J: *AAOS atlas of orthoses and assistive devices,* ed 4, Philadelphia, 2008, Mosby.
33. *(Original to book.)*
34. From Hochberg, Marc C. *Rheumatology,* ed 5, Philadelphia, 2011, Mosby.
35. Modified from Hsu J, Michael J, Fisk J: *AAOS atlas of orthoses and assistive devices,* ed 4, Philadelphia, 2008, Mosby.
36. From Coughlin, Michael J., Roger A. Mann, and Charles L. Saltzman. *Surgery of the Foot and Ankle,* ed 9, Philadelphia, 2013, Mosby.
37. From Canale S: *Campbell's operative orthopaedics,* ed 12, St. Louis, 2012, Mosby.
38. From Sorrentino, Sheila A., and Bernie Gorek. *Mosby's Textbook for Long-term Care Nursing Assistants,* ed 7, St. Louis, 2014, Mosby.
39. From Pedretti, Lorraine Williams, Heidi McHugh. Pendleton, and Winifred Schultz-Krohn. *Pedretti's Occupational Therapy: Practice Skills for Physical Dysfunction,* ed 7, St. Louis, 2013, Elsevier.
40. From Skirven, Terri M. *Rehabilitation of the Hand and Upper Extremity,* ed 6, Philadelphia, 2010, Mosby.
41. From Lusardi M, Nielsen C: *Orthotics and prosthetics in rehabilitation,* ed 3, St. Louis, 2013, Butterworth-Heinemann. *(Courtesy Michael Curtain)*
42. Schickendantz, Mark S. "Diagnosis and Treatment of Elbow Disorders in the Overhead Athlete." *Hand Clinics* 18.1 (2002): 65-75.
43. Modified from Bland K, Copeland E: *The breast: comprehensive management of benign and malignant disorders,* ed 4, St. Louis, 2009, Saunders.
44. From Shah, Jatin P., Snehal G. Patel, Bhuvanesh Singh, and Jatin P. Shah. *Jatin Shah's Head and Neck Surgery and Oncology,* ed 4, Philadelphia, 2012, Mosby, 2012. From Subburaj, K., C. Nair, S. Rajesh, S.m. Meshram, and B. Ravi. "Rapid Development of Auricular Prosthesis Using CAD and Rapid Prototyping Technologies." *International Journal of Oral and Maxillofacial Surgery* 36.10 (2007): 938-43.
45. From Weinzweig J: *Plastic surgery secrets,* ed 2, Philadelphia, 2010, Hanley & Belfus, p 543.
46. Modified from Mann D: *Heart failure: a companion to Braunwald's heart disease,* ed 3, Philadelphia, 2015, Saunders.
47. Modified from Roberts J, Hedges J: *Clinical procedures in emergency medicine,* ed 6, Philadelphia, 2013, Saunders.
48. From Yanoff M, Duker J: *Ophthalmology,* ed 4, St. Louis, 2014, Mosby.
49. From Feldman M, Friedman L, Brandt L: *Sleisenger and Fordtran's gastrointestinal and liver disease,* ed 10, Philadelphia, 2015, Saunders.
50. From Katz V et al: *Comprehensive gynecology,* ed 7, Philadelphia, 2016, Mosby.
51. From Young A, Proctor D: *Kinn's the medical assistant,* ed 13, St. Louis, 2016, Saunders.
52. From Yanoff M, Duker J: *Ophthalmology,* ed 4, St. Louis, 2014, Mosby.